Epigenetics and Human Health

Epigenetics and Human Health

Edited by Augustus Drew

**hayle
medical**

New York

Hayle Medical,
750 Third Avenue, 9th Floor,
New York, NY 10017, USA

Visit us on the World Wide Web at:
www.haylemedical.com

ISBN: 978-1-63241-652-0

Cataloging-in-Publication Data

Epigenetics and human health / edited by Augustus Drew.
  p. cm.
Includes bibliographical references and index.
ISBN 978-1-63241-652-0
1. Epigenetics. 2. Medical genetics. 3. Human genetics. 4. Health. I. Drew, Augustus.
RB155 .E65 2019
616.042--dc23

Table of Contents

Preface

Epigenetics refers to the study of heritable phenotype changes which occur independently of alterations in the primary DNA sequence. Epigenetic processes play a crucial role in human development before birth. These processes are crucial to fetal development. In this stage, a single cell differentiates into a variety of different cell types, which later form cohesive tissues, organs and organ systems. The study of food nutrients and their effects on human health through epigenetic modifications is known as nutriepigenomics. If metabolic disturbances occur during the time of human development, then epigenetic alterations may lead to permanent changes in the tissues and organ structures resulting in diseases. This book elucidates the concepts and innovative models around prospective developments with respect to epigenetics and human health. It studies, analyzes and upholds the pillars of epigenetics and human health and its utmost significance in modern times. The extensive content of this book provides the readers with a thorough understanding of the subject.

This book unites the global concepts and researches in an organized manner for a comprehensive understanding of the subject. It is a ripe text for all researchers, students, scientists or anyone else who is interested in acquiring a better knowledge of this dynamic field.

I extend my sincere thanks to the contributors for such eloquent research chapters. Finally, I thank my family for being a source of support and help.

Editor

1

GLI2 promoter hypermethylation in saliva of children with a respiratory allergy

Sabine A. S. Langie[1,2]* [iD], Matthieu Moisse[3], Katarzyna Szarc vel Szic[1,4], Ellen Van Der Plas[1,7], Gudrun Koppen[1], Sofie De Prins[1], Tijs Louwies[1], Vera Nelen[5], Guy Van Camp[6], Diether Lambrechts[3], Greet Schoeters[1,7,8], Wim Vanden Berghe[4] and Patrick De Boever[1,2]

Abstract

Background: The prevalence of respiratory allergy in children is increasing. Epigenetic DNA methylation changes are plausible underlying molecular mechanisms.

Results: Saliva samples collected in substudies of two longitudinal birth cohorts in Belgium (FLEHS1 & FLEHS2) were used to discover and confirm DNA methylation signatures that can differentiate individuals with respiratory allergy from healthy subjects. Genome-wide analysis with Illumina Methylation 450K BeadChips revealed 23 differentially methylated gene regions (DMRs) in saliva from 11y old allergic children (N=26) vs. controls (N=20) in FLEHS1. A subset of 7 DMRs was selected for confirmation by iPLEX MassArray analysis. First, iPLEX analysis was performed in the same 46 FLEHS1 samples for analytical confirmation of the findings obtained during the discovery phase. iPLEX results correlated significantly with the 450K array data (P <0.0001) and confirmed 4 out of the 7 DMRs. Aiming for additional biological confirmation, the 7 DMRs were analyzed using iPLEX in a substudy of an independent birth cohort (FLEHS2; N=19 cases vs. 20 controls, aged 5 years). One DMR in the *GLI2* promoter region showed a consistent statistically significant hypermethylation in individuals with respiratory allergy across the two birth cohorts and technologies. In addition to its involvement in TGF-β signaling and T-helper differentiation, *GLI2* has a regulating role in lung development.

Conclusion: *GLI2* is considered an interesting candidate DNA methylation marker for respiratory allergy.

Keywords: DNA methylation, Saliva, Respiratory allergy, Illumina Methylation 450K BeadChip, GLI2

Background

Respiratory allergies are increasing in frequency and severity and are the most common allergies in Europe and worldwide. The European Federation of Allergy and Airways Diseases Patients' Associations (EFA) reported in 2011 that respiratory allergies affected around 20–30% of the European population [1]. More specifically, about 113 million European citizens suffered from allergic rhinitis and 68 million from allergic asthma in 2011. Zooming in on children as a vulnerable group, the International Study of Asthma and Allergies in Childhood (ISAAC) reported in 2009 that 10 to 20% of adolescents aged 13 and 14 in Europe were suffering from allergic rhinitis [2]. Genetic predisposition is an important risk factor for developing respiratory allergies, but the rise in prevalence happened within a too short time period to be explained by genetic changes. Epigenetic modulations, such as altered DNA methylation patterns in gene regulatory sequences, due to environmental exposures are a plausible mechanisms underlying the development and progression of respiratory allergies. Changes in the DNA methylation profile are expected to express themselves in altered gene and protein expression. Such changes contribute to the biological embedding of respiratory allergy during critical developmental phases. In this context, Bégin and Nadeau noted that DNA methylation changes in several loci are associated with the allergy phenotype and environmental exposures [3].

---

* Correspondence: sabine.langie@vito.be
[1]VITO- Sustainable Health, Boeretang 200, 2400 Mol, Belgium
[2]Centre for Environmental Sciences, Hasselt University, Diepenbeek, Belgium
Full list of author information is available at the end of the article

There is an increased interest in the discovery of DNA methylation markers that can differentiate individuals with a respiratory allergy from healthy subjects [4–20]. A number of studies focus on birth cohorts and describe the identification/confirmation of DNA methylation markers, either via an epigenome-wide or gene-targeted approach, in peripheral blood of children with respiratory disorders like wheezing or (allergic) asthma [10–17]. Blood-based DNA methylation analyses involved mostly the follow-up of school-age children, while we are aware of only three reports that describe DNA methylation markers in relation to allergic asthma and wheezing in peripheral blood from pre-school children around 4 years of age [14, 15, 17]. More recently, it has been shown that saliva can be used as biofluid to perform gene-targeted DNA methylation studies [19, 21] as well as genome-wide DNA methylation analysis [22–24]. In children, especially at pre-school age, analysis of saliva may be advantageous over a blood analysis, which is invasive and kept to a minimum for study compliance and ethical reasons. We demonstrated the feasibility of assessing DNA methylation patterns in saliva using genome-wide methylation analysis and observed that patterns were consistent with those in blood; the methylation status of about 96% of the cg-sites was comparable between peripheral blood mononuclear cells (PBMC) and saliva [25]. In addition, we identified differential methylated gene regions (DMRs) in a case-control study with adults having a respiratory allergy [25].

In the current study, we aimed at discovery and confirmation of DMRs in saliva of children with respiratory allergy when comparing them to healthy control subjects.

Methods
Study design and sample collection
The Flemish Environment and Health Studies (FLEHS) were established for following internal exposure of the general Flemish population in Belgium to environmental chemicals and the associated health effects [26, 27]. The FLEHS1 birth cohort enrolled 1196 mother–child pairs between September 2002 and February 2004 via 25 maternities across Flanders, covering 20% of Flanders' area and 65 different municipalities. Details of the study and recruitment protocol have been previously reported [28]. During follow-up of the cohort at 10 years of age (*n* = 595), information on the allergy status of the children based on the ISAAC questionnaire [29] was collected. A subgroup (*n* = 99) of those followed-up at age 10 years agreed to donate saliva and blood samples and filled out an additional questionnaire at the age of 11 years. Unstimulated collection of saliva samples (2 mL) was performed using Oragene DNA OG-500 self-collection kits (DNA Genotek, Ottawa, Canada). The saliva samples were kept at room temperature until DNA extraction. Blood samples (10 mL) were collected in EDTA tubes (BD Vacutainer®, BD, Plymouth, UK) and kept less than 2 h at room temperature until further processing. Plasma was collected after centrifugation at 800×*g* for 5 min and stored at – 20 ° C for further clinical characterization.

In the second campaign, FLEHS2, 255 newborn-mother couples were recruited across the five provinces of Flanders between August 2008 and July 2009 via 10 randomly selected maternities. The study protocol has been described elsewhere [30]. The participation criteria where similar to those for FLEHS1, with the exception that mothers should have resided in Flanders for 10 years in order to be included. Health data and lifestyle information were obtained via questionnaires, including the allergy status based on the ISAAC survey. In a follow-up at 5 years of age, 78 children provided saliva samples and completed a short ISAAC-based survey mainly focused on allergy symptoms. At the age of 7 years, the participants completed a more extensive questionnaire capturing health and lifestyle data, with the main aim to confirm their allergy phenotype.

Determining IgE sensitization status and defining cases
For FLEHS1, plasma samples of the 11-year-old children were analyzed using an ImmunoCAP Phadiatop test (Thermo Fisher; performed by the medical lab AML, Antwerp) to determine specific IgE sensitization status for a mix of airborne allergens: birch, cat, dog, house dust mites (*Dermatophagoides pteronyssinus*), and grass pollen. A cutoff value 0.35 kUA/L was used to define an IgE-positive status [31]. Note that children occasionally express respiratory allergy symptoms due to food allergies. To rule these out, blood samples were analyzed for a food allergen mix (ImmunoCAP Fx5mix; egg, cow milk, fish, wheat, peanut, and soy allergens; available from Thermo Fisher and performed by the medical lab AML, Antwerp).

Twenty-six children participating in the current substudy of the FLEHS1 birth cohort were considered to have a respiratory allergy if they reported (either self-reported or doctor's diagnosed) at least one respiratory allergy symptom (occurrence of asthma, hay fever, other types of rhinitis, wheezing, or runny nose, in the past year and ever; as questioned in accordance with the ISAAC questionnaire [29]) and Phadiatop IgE ≥ 0.35 kU/L. Twenty control subjects were assigned that did not report any (doctor's diagnosed) allergy symptoms, and Phadiatop and FX5 IgE < 0.35 kU/L.

Due to the unavailability of blood samples to measure IgE levels in the FLEHS2 cohort, cases and controls were identified as (1) cases = doctor's diagnosed and/or self-reported respiratory allergy symptoms (*n* = 19) and (2) controls = no self-reported and/or diagnosed allergies plus ≤ 1 reported incidence of family history for allergy

($n = 20$). Both the questionnaires completed at age 5 and age 7 were consulted to define cases and were checked for misreporting.

Since the Flemish birth cohorts were designed as environmental health surveys, and less as a clinical study into allergy, all respiratory allergy subtypes (e.g., allergic asthma, rhinitis, hay fever, house dust mite) were combined into one group of respiratory allergy cases to increase the sample size and power of the study.

DNA extraction and bisulfite treatment

Genomic DNA was extracted from saliva using the Oragene PrepIT kit (DNA Genotek, Ottawa, Canada) according to the manufacturer's instructions. About 500 ng of gDNA was bisulfite converted using the EZ DNA methylation kit (Zymo Research, Cambridge Bioscience, Cambridge, UK) according to the manufacturer's instructions. Bisulfite conversion and quality control was performed as previously described [25].

Infinium HumanMethylation450 BeadChip Array and data processing

Genome-wide DNA methylation profiles were generated with Infinium HumanMethylation450 BeadChip Array (Illumina, San Diego, CA, USA) according to the standard Infinium HD Assay Methylation Protocol Guide (Part #15019519, Illumina). The BeadChip images were captured using the Illumina iScan. The raw array data were uploaded to the Gene Expression Omnibus (GEO) database and have accession number GSE110128.

Raw data analysis, QC, normalization, cell-count estimation, and methylation β value conversions were performed using the R-packages minfi [32] and IMA [33]. In brief, the raw Red/Green channel data from the 450K-Illumina methylation array were read by the "read.450k.exp" function, converted to methylation values by "preprocessRaw" and subsequently normalized using "preprocessSWAN," an implementation of the Subset-quantile Within Array Normalization (SWAN) normalization procedure [34]. Principal component analysis and unsupervised clustering were used to check for sample outliers. All samples passed quality controls and were loaded into the R-package IMA for further processing/filtering. Samples having > 75% of CpG sites with a detection p value > 1e–05 were removed (all samples passed this filter). Cg-probes with a detection p value greater than 0.01 in all samples and cg-probes on the X and Y chromosomes were removed.

The normalized β values of the 450K BeadChip data were converted to M values ($M = \log2(\beta/(1 - \beta))$) for statistical analysis [35] and differential methylation between samples (respiratory allergy cases vs. healthy controls) was estimated with linear models using R-package Limma [36]. Gender, batch effect, and differences in cell composition were included as covariates. Resulting p values were corrected for multiple testing using the Benjamini-Hochberg procedure (p_{adj}). Results in tables and figures are presented as median β values ± standard deviation.

To estimate the proportion of various salivary cell types, the statistical deconvolution method described by Houseman et al. and implemented in "minfi" as the "estimateCellCountsMset" function was used [37]. Reference methylomes from leukocyte subtypes were obtained from the study of Reinius et al. [38]. Buccal epithelial cell reference methylomes were obtained from the GEO dataset GSE48472 [39].

iPLEX MassArray analysis

Differentially methylated CpG sites in the identified DMRs were further confirmed using iPLEX MassArray analysis by Agena Bioscience (Hamburg, Germany) according to the manufacturer's protocol (iPLEX® Pro Application Guide, SQNM-USG-CUS-030 Rev 3.0; CO-12-274, 2012). Briefly, the iPLEX technique targets individual CpG sites and allows simultaneous analysis of multiple CpGs in a single-well reaction. PCR- and extension primers (probes) were automatically developed with SEQUENOM's MassARRAY Designer Software for each CpG that had to be investigated, and were run as 7 multiplexes and 1 singleplex. One microliter of the bisulfite-treated DNA (5–10 ng/µL) was added to 100 nM of a primer mix (500 nM each primer) in a 5-µL reaction. Amplification was carried out as follows: 95 °C for 2 min, then 45 cycles of 95 °C for 30 s, 56 °C for 30 s, and 72 °C for 60 s, followed by 72 °C for 5 min. After PCR, the unincorporated dNTPs are neutralized with SAP treatment. Resulting primer extension products were Resin treated to remove access salt and were analyzed with MALDI-TOF MS as each primer and its extension products have a unique molecular mass. The peak heights are indicative for the methylation status. The spectra were acquired using the MassARRAY® Analyzer instrument, and raw data were processed with TyperAnalyzer software according to the MassARRAY® Analyzer User's Guide.

Statistical analysis

DMRs were identified with comb-p analysis [40], using the list of uncorrected p values for all CpG sites as calculated from the differential methylation analysis together with their chromosomal location. This statistical procedure combines adjacent p values, performs false discovery adjustment, and finds regions of enrichment. For these regions, it assigns a combined Stouffer-Liptak p value based on the uncorrected p values and finally corrects for multiple testing using the Sidak correction, yielding adjusted p values (p_{adj}). The generated output is a list of regions that are differently methylated, and an aggregated, adjusted p value is assigned to each region [40]. A region with an adjusted p value < 0.05 was deemed differently methylated.

Two different methods were applied to correct for differences in cell proportions in the FLEHS1 study. In a first step, we applied the full reference-based deconvolution method, according to Houseman et al. (as described above), and corrected our methylation data for the following cell proportions: granulocytes, CD4+ T cells, CD8+ T cells, B cells, monocytes, NK cells, and buccal cells. In parallel, normalized β values were corrected for the buccal and granulocyte cell fractions only (using GEO GSE35069 and GSE48472 as granulocyte and buccal reference methylomes). The estimated granulocyte and buccal cell fractions were also used to correct the FLEHS1 iPLEX data. For the FLEHS2 study, no Illumina data were available and cell counts could not be estimated. As such, for comparison of the iPLEX data between FLEHS1 and FLEHS2, non-corrected data were analyzed with SPSS statistics. Figure 1 gives an overview of the performed data analysis and various cell correction methods.

Using SPSS statistics, correlations between methylation in saliva samples detected by 450K BeadChip or iPLEX MassArray were analyzed via the Spearman correlation coefficient (ρ). The iPLEX MassArray data were analyzed by General Linear Models, Univariate Analysis of Variance to identify statistical differences in methylation levels of the DMR between respiratory allergy cases and healthy controls. The methylation level of a DMR was calculated as the mean methylation of the CpGs in that region. The models for the analyses on the FLEHS1 data were corrected for buccal and granulocyte cell count, gender, and batch in which samples were analyzed (since there was a gap of a year between the analysis of the 2 batches). The FLEHS2 samples were analyzed as one batch, and the models using these data were only corrected for gender. A p value below 0.05 was considered statistically significant. A DMR region was considered "confirmed" when the region reached statistical significance and a delta beta difference in the same direction as the original finding.

Functional analysis

Biological interpretation and identification of interactions between molecules using network analysis via Ingenuity Pathway Analysis (IPA) was performed (http://www.ingenuity.com/). The freely available "ChromHMM from ENCODE/Broad" tool [41–43], as part of the

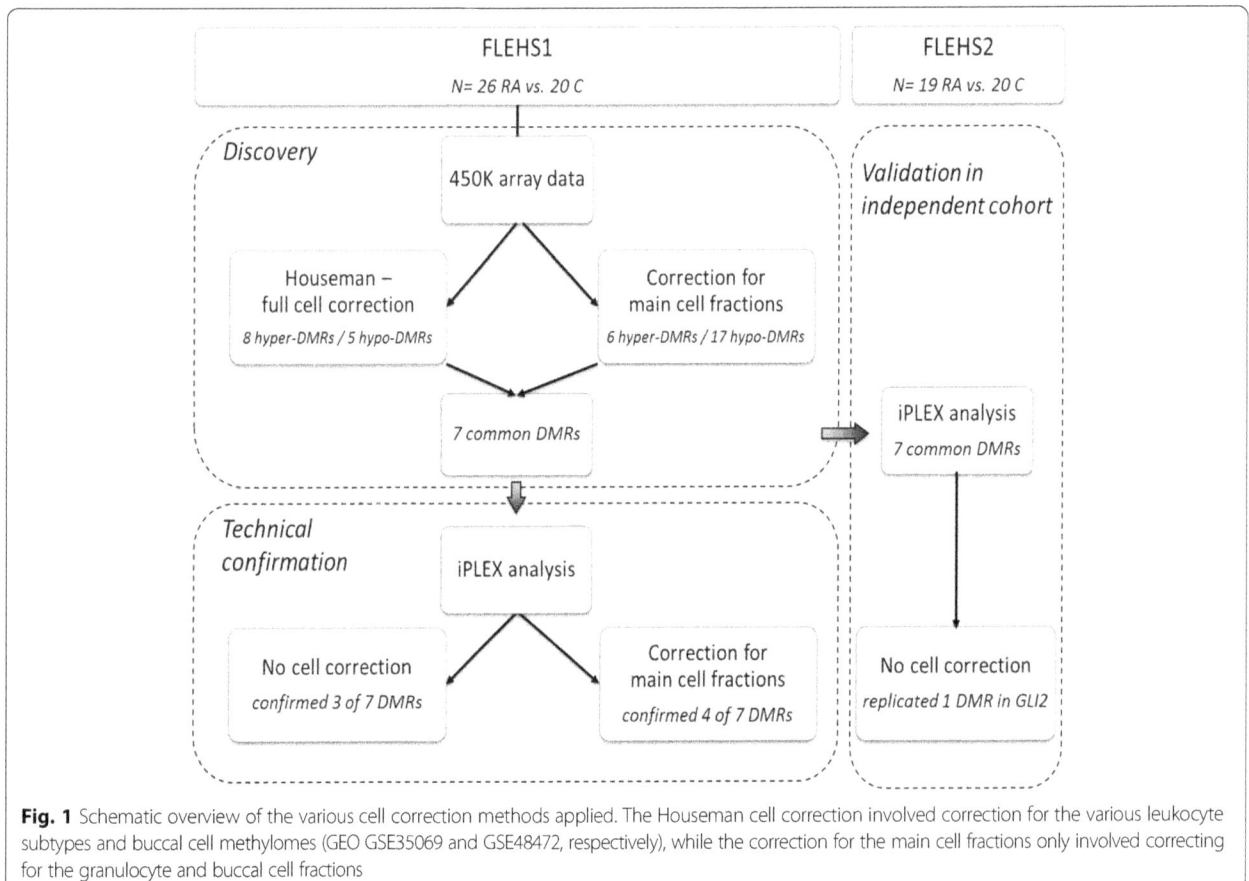

Fig. 1 Schematic overview of the various cell correction methods applied. The Houseman cell correction involved correction for the various leukocyte subtypes and buccal cell methylomes (GEO GSE35069 and GSE48472, respectively), while the correction for the main cell fractions only involved correcting for the granulocyte and buccal cell fractions

UCSC hg19 browser, was used to visualize the chromatin state segmentation of the *GLI2* DMR. ChromeHMM uses a multivariate Hidden Markov Model (HMM) and integrates multiple chromatin datasets such as ChIP-Seq data of various histone modifications to discover de novo the major re-occurring combinatorial and spatial patterns of marks. Estimation of gene expression values was computed based on the number of reads which map per kb of exon model per million mapped reads (RPKM) for each gene, for each tissue or sample, as generated by the Genotype-Tissue Expression (GTEx) project (derived from Ensembl genes hg18, UCSC genome browser) [44, 45].

Results

Characteristics of the study population

In the FLEHS1 sub-cohort, the children with respiratory allergy (17 boys and 9 girls) mainly reported rhinitis (defined as runny nose without suffering from a cold; $N = 23$), among which 14 reported also to suffer from hay fever and 8 had asthma ($N = 8$; 4 in combination with hay fever). Two children reported only hay fever without the signs of asthma or rhinitis/runny nose (so total $N = 16$ for hay fever). The median ($\pm$SE) Phadiatop IgE level detected for the allergy cases was 29.5 ± 7.0 kU/L and a mean FX5 IgE level of 0.14 ± 3.9 kU/L. Preventive medication (i.e., inhalation of (cortico)steroids, sometimes in combination or oral ingestion of a leukotriene receptor antagonist or antihistamines) was taken daily by 5 of the cases, while 11 children only used medication ($\beta2$ adrenergic receptor agonist and/or corticosteroid inhaler/nasal spray, sometimes in combination with oral intake of antihistamines, or homeopathic treatment) when experiencing an upsurge. The healthy control group consisted of 8 boys and 12 girls; median ($\pm$SE) Phadiatop and Fx5 IgE levels were 0.00 ± 0.04 and 0.00 ± 0.02, respectively.

Among the 5-year-old children with a respiratory allergy in the FLEHS2 sub-cohort, there were 8 boys and 11 girls, and for 12 of the children, it was reported that one or both of their parent suffered from 1 or more respiratory allergies. By the age of 7, there were 2 cases of asthma (1 in combination with hay fever), 12 reported symptoms of rhinitis, and 4 had a wheezing phenotype. In addition, 5 children suffered from house dust mite allergy, including 3 out of the 12 children who reported rhinitis/runny nose and the asthma case who also reported hay fever. Preventive medication (oral intake of antihistamines) was taken daily by 2 of the cases, while 2 other only used medication (oral intake of antihistamines combined with a steroid inhaler or nasal spray) when having an upsurge. The control group consisted of 11 boys and 9 girls, among which 9 children reported to have one case of respiratory allergy in their family.

Discovery of DMRs in FLEHS1 birth cohort

Following quality filtering and normalization of the Illumina 450K data, 470,562 cg-probes (96.9%) from the original 485,512 probes were kept for downstream data analyses. Comb-p analysis revealed 13 DMRs (Fig. 2) between respiratory allergy cases and controls when correcting for differences in cell composition. The parallel analysis, involving correction of the data only for the main salivary cell fractions (i.e., buccal cells and granulocytes), revealed 23 DMRs in respiratory allergy cases compared to control subjects. The 7 DMRs in common between the 2 data analysis strategies were selected for further confirmation. Four of these DMRs were hypermethylated, and 3 DMRs were hypomethylated in children with a respiratory allergy compared controls (Fig. 2, Table 1).

Confirmation of 450K methylation data by iPLEX MassArray

Analysis using iPLEX MassArray showed significant positive correlations with the Illumina 450K array data for the 7 DMRs ($p < 0.0001$; $\rho = 0.89$–0.95, except for *APOBEC1* ($\rho = 0.55$), *GRAMD1B* ($\rho = 0.80$), and *MED24* ($\rho = 0.64$)). The same polarity of the direction of the methylation changes was observed for all the studied DMRs (Table 1). However, when comparing respiratory allergy cases with control subjects, we were only able to confirm 3 of the 7 DMRs, those located in the genes *GLI2*, *GRAMD1B*, and *HTRA3*. In parallel, a cell correction analysis was performed, correcting the iPLEX data for the granulocyte and buccal cell proportions as identified from the 450K array data. These data analysis resulted in a confirmation of 4 of the 7 DMRs, located in *GLI2*, *GRAMD1B*, *HTRA3*, and *MED24* (Table 1).

Verification of DMRs in the independent birth cohort FLEHS2

The DMRs that were identified in FLEHS1 samples were further investigated using iPLEX MassArray in saliva samples obtained from children taking part in the FLEHS2 cohort. Two significant DMRs in the *GLI2* and *GRAMD1B* genes from respiratory allergy cases versus control subjects were confirmed in FLEHS 2 (Table 2). The DMR in *GLI2* was confirmed with a 7% hypermethylation in children with a respiratory allergy compared to control subjects, whereas *GRAMD1B* showed the opposite methylation change (2% hypomethylation in cases compared to controls) when compared to the results obtained for the FLEHS1 cohort (1.6% hypermethylation in cases compared to controls).

Transcriptional activity and biological interpretation of the *GLI2* DMR

The hypermethylated DMR identified by the comb-p software in the *GLI2* gene is a combination of 3 hypermethylated cg-sites: cg00637745, cg13872898, and

a

Corrected for estimated cell counts (Houseman et al.)

Corrected for granulocyte and buccal cell proportions

COL20A1
LOC105375650
FRG2
IL1A
LEP
SDHAP3

ALOX12
APOBEC1
GLI2
GRAMD1B
HTRA3
MED24
OPCML

ACDB4
ANKDD1B   C19orf35
DNAAF5
GADL1 LINC00336
LY86
MEIS1
MEIS2
MORC2-AS1
NOC2LP2
OR56A3
PIWIL2
PTPRN2
RASA3
TM9SF2

b

Cell correction method	Gene	Chromosome	DMR start	end	n_probes	p_{adj}
	ALOX12	chr17	6898737	6899888	15	0.0001
	APOBEC1	chr12	7780735	7781431	6	0.0042
	GLI2	chr2	121497333	121498521	3	<0.0001
Overlap	**GRAMD1B**	chr11	123430574	123431162	5	0.0023
	HTRA3	chr4	8291936	8292328	4	0.0091
	MED24	chr17	38183169	38183790	6	0.0055
	OPCML	chr11	132662454	132662963	4	0.0006
	COL20A1	chr20	61953800	61954258	4	0.0009
Reference based	**FRG2**	chr4	190938632	190939230	4	0.0018
correction	IL1A	chr2	113544231	113544348	3	0.0136
according to	**LEP**	chr7	127880931	127881440	7	<0.0001
Houseman et al.	**LOC105375650**	chr8	96085269	96085994	5	<0.0001
	SDHAP3	chr5	1594281	1595048	11	0.0004
	ACBD4	chr17	43221219	43221807	5	0.0211
	ANKDD1B	chr5	74907591	74908170	5	0.0107
	C19orf35	chr19	2281918	2282568	7	0.0060
	DNAAF5	chr7	807595	808081	5	0.0029
	GADL1	chr3	30936069	30936531	9	0.0076
	LINC00336	chr6	33560952	33561449	9	0.0238
Corrected for	PIWIL2	chr8	22132562	22133076	12	0.0003
granulocyte and	LY86	chr6	6588692	6589075	5	0.0139
buccal cell	MEIS1	chr2	66672336	66672841	4	0.0007
proportions	MEIS2	chr15	37388126	37389585	3	0.0029
	MORC2-AS1	chr22	31317763	31318444	3	0.0448
	NOC2LP2	chr2	132202003	132202537	7	0.0001
	OR56A3	chr11	5959657	5960213	6	0.0176
	PTPRN2	chr7	158045979	158046358	6	0.0018
	RASA3	chr13	114881440	114881968	4	0.0074
	TM9SF2	chr13	100217961	100219013	6	<0.0001

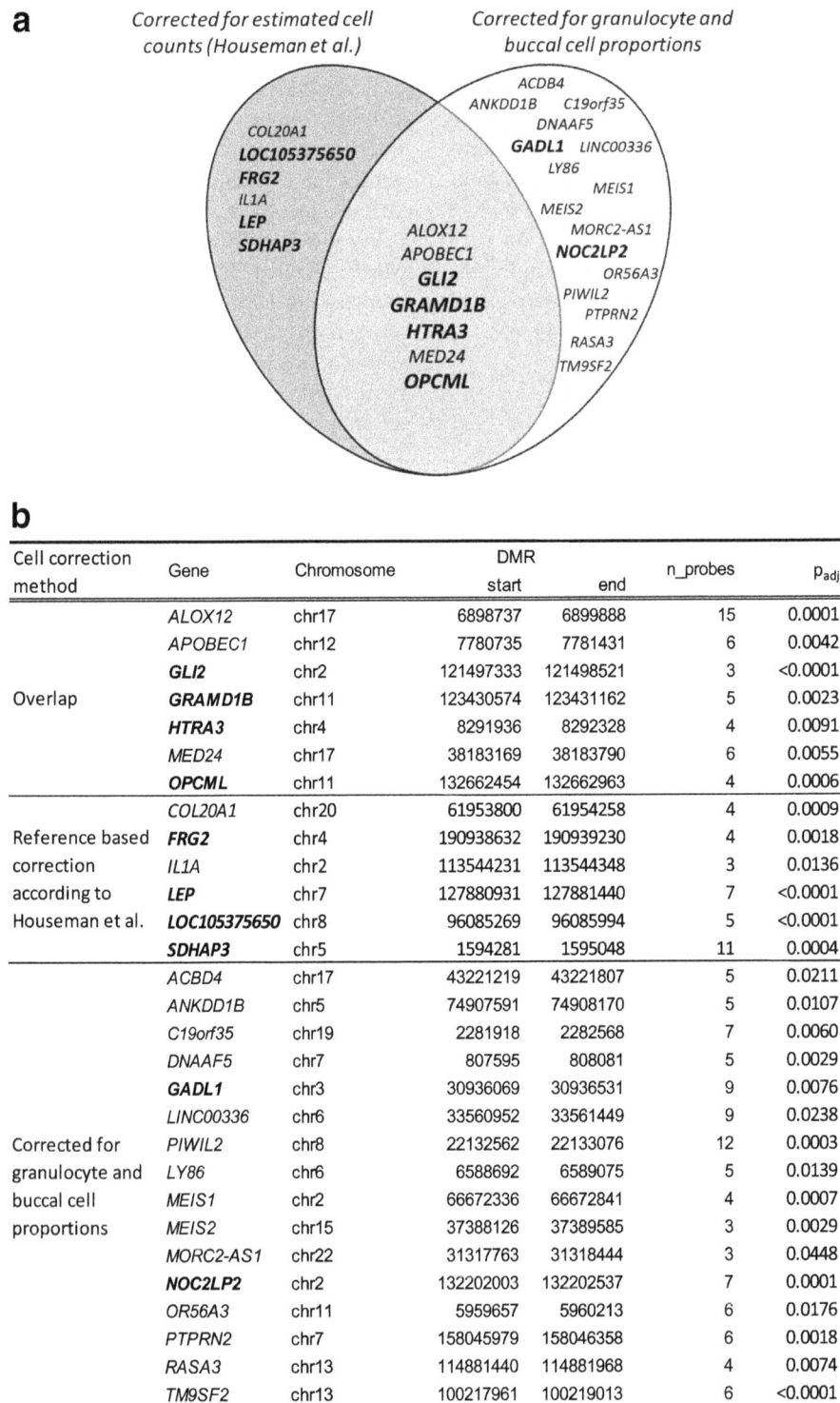

Fig. 2 Overview of identified DMRs in FLEHS1 birth cohort. **a** Seven gene regions showed an overlap between the DMRs identified via cell correction according to Houseman et al. and those after correction for the granulocyte and buccal cell proportions. Hyper-methylated gene regions are shown in bold; all other DMRs were hypo-methylated in respiratory allergy cases compared to controls. **b** The location of the DMRs in the genome and the number of significantly different methylation probes were analyzed (corresponding to CpG-sites) in these gene regions

Table 1 iPLEX MassArray confirmation of the 7 DMRs identified with 450K array in FLEHS1 saliva samples

Gene	450K array data				iPLEX MassArray data				
	Allergy Beta ± SD	Control Beta ± SD	Delta beta	p_{adj}[a]	Allergy Beta ± SD	Control Beta ± SD	Delta beta	p[b]	p[c]
ALOX12	0.35 ± 0.10	0.39 ± 0.07	− 0.044	0.0001	0.24 ± 0.08	0.26 ± 0.05	− 0.021	0.109	0.102
APOBEC1	0.84 ± 0.09	0.86 ± 0.07	− 0.022	0.0042	0.76 ± 0.23	0.83 ± 0.20	− 0.068	0.109	0.102
GLI2	0.74 ± 0.10	0.73 ± 0.07	0.009	< 0.0001	0.63 ± 0.12	0.61 ± 0.09	0.020	0.034*	0.035*
GRAMD1B	0.16 ± 0.04	0.15 ± 0.03	0.010	0.0023	0.10 ± 0.03	0.08 ± 0.03	0.016	0.002*	0.002*
HTRA3	0.66 ± 0.07	0.65 ± 0.05	0.013	0.0091	0.56 ± 0.07	0.53 ± 0.06	0.030	0.036*	0.011*
MED24	0.53 ± 0.02	0.54 ± 0.02	− 0.011	0.0055	0.40 ± 0.04	0.40 ± 0.03	− 0.001	0.328	0.036*
OPCML	0.66 ± 0.07	0.65 ± 0.09	0.003	0.0006	0.50 ± 0.08	0.48 ± 0.12	0.021	0.125	0.140

[a]Corrected for estimated cell counts (according to Houseman et al.), batch, and gender and adjusted for multiple testing
[b]Corrected for batch and gender
[c]Corrected for estimated buccal and granulocyte cell fractions, batch, and gender
Genes given in bold are significantly differentially methylated (*p <0.05)

cg17870997. This DMR is located in an intragenic CpG shore, 707 bp upstream from CpG-island 56. According to the UCSC genome browser h19 (based on data from the Bernstein Lab at the Broad Institute—part of the ENCODE consortium), the region is enriched for H3K4Me1 and H3K27Ac histone marks (Additional file 1: Figure S1), which are associated with enhancers or enhanced transcription, respectively [46]. Indeed, based on the Chromatin State Segmentation database from ENCODE/Broad Institute ([42, 43]; available through the UCSC genome browser h19), several enhancers and promoters are located within the DMR in *GLI2*. More specifically, using available data from H1-hESC embryonic stem cells, cg00637745 and cg13872898 seem to be located at the start of or within a weak promoter, while cg17870997 is located at the beginning of an active promoter. When considering data from the normal human lung fibroblast cell lines (NHLF), cg00637745 and cg13872898 were indicated to be located in a weakly transcribed region and cg17870997 in a weak enhancer

Table 2 iPLEX MassArray verification of the seven identified DMRs in the independent birth cohort FLEHS2

Gene	FLEHS2 iPLEX MassArray data			
	Allergy Beta ± SD	Control Beta ± SD	Delta beta	p[a]
ALOX12	0.24 ± 0.05	0.26 ± 0.06	− 0.016	0.443
APOBEC1	0.79 ± 0.17	0.82 ± 0.16	− 0.036	0.348
GLI2	0.72 ± 0.08	0.65 ± 0.10	0.071	0.017*
GRAMD1B	0.08 ± 0.03	0.10 ± 0.03	− 0.020	0.035*
HTRA3	0.59 ± 0.08	0.55 ± 0.06	0.041	0.057
MED24	0.37 ± 0.04	0.39 ± 0.04	− 0.016	0.207
OPCML	0.47 ± 0.08	0.50 ± 0.10	− 0.030	0.317

[a]Corrected for gender
Genes given in bold are significantly differentially methylated (*p <0.05)

region. Data on the GM12878 lymphoblastoid EBV-immortalized cell line suggest that the DMR is a polycomb-repressed region. RNA-Seq data generated by the GTEx project revealed *GLI2* gene expression to be significantly expressed in lung (1.394 RPKM) and salivary gland (0.902 RPKM) tissues and repressed in blood cells (Additional file 2: Figure S2).

The IPA tool was used to grow a network for GLI2, visualizing interactions with up- or downstream molecules. The network was simplified by keeping only the nearest neighbors of GLI2 (Fig. 3a) and overlaying the network with biological functions (Fig. 3b). According to the IPA Knowledge Base, the network included sonic hedgehog (SHH) signaling molecules (incl. GLI proteins) and key inflammatory molecules such as IL4, IL6, IL10, and IL13, as well as IL6 receptor and several chemokine receptors (CCR). Six molecules were linked to integrin-linked kinase (ILK) signaling, 10 molecules play a role in the Th1/Th2 activation pathway, and several transcription regulators (NFκB, RELA, GLI3) are involved in protein kinase A signaling. Interestingly, all molecules could be linked to 2 main functions: respiratory system development (incl. GLI family proteins, SHH, TGFB1, and cyclins) or lung inflammation (incl. cytokines and chemokine receptors).

Discussion

This study identified hypermethylation in a CpG shore of the *GLI2* gene promoter, which discriminates school-age children with a respiratory allergy from healthy control children using saliva samples. The observations were made in a discovery case-control study (FLEHS1) and confirmed in an independent case-control study (FLEHS2). The discovery was initially performed with Illumina 450K arrays and confirmed with gene-specific iPLEX MassArray technology.

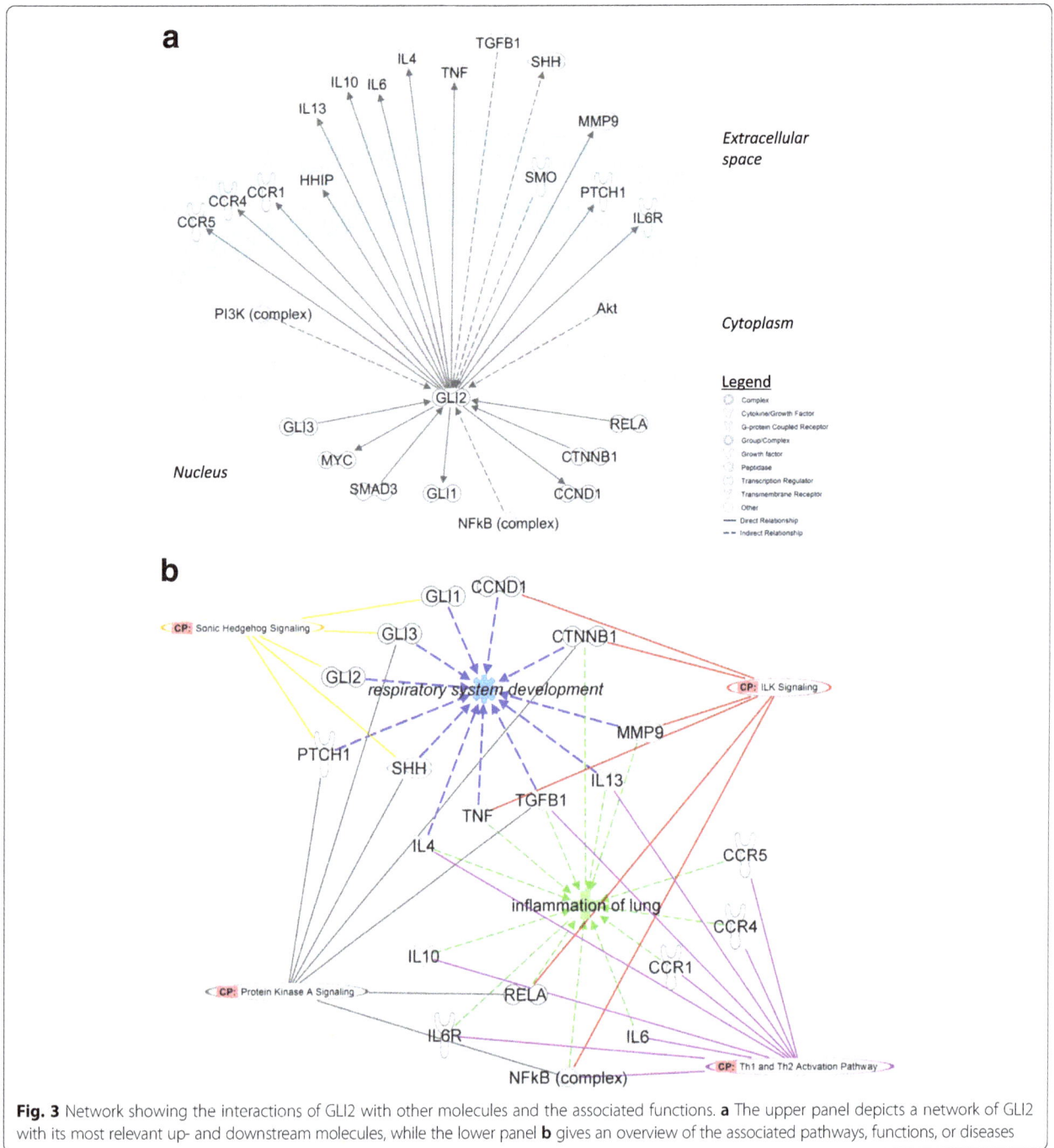

Fig. 3 Network showing the interactions of GLI2 with other molecules and the associated functions. **a** The upper panel depicts a network of GLI2 with its most relevant up- and downstream molecules, while the lower panel **b** gives an overview of the associated pathways, functions, or diseases

GLI2 DNA methylation differences in respiratory allergy

GLI2, together with GLI1 and GLI3, belongs to the GLI family of zinc-finger DNA-binding proteins [47, 48]. More specifically, it belongs to the type 2 zinc-finger protein subclass of the GLI family and is therefore characterized as transcription factor which bind DNA through zinc finger motifs. GLI2 is a key mediator of the SHH signaling pathway in vertebrates ([47–49]; Fig. 3). The SHH signaling pathway has an essential role in embryonic development and is critical for maintenance of

tissue polarity [48]. Indeed, aberrant DNA methylation in the *GLI2* gene and other HH pathway members has been studied in relation to developmental disorders (including pre-eclampsia and Down syndrome) [50–54] and cancer [55–57]. Several GWAS studies indicate a role of HH pathway molecules in the etiology of asthma [58, 59], and the recent study by Murk and DeWan [60] reported a possible interaction between *GLI2* and the major asthma susceptibility gene *ADAM33*. However, as far as we know, there are no reports in the literature on differential methylation in *GLI2* in relation to respiratory allergy.

In the current study, we identified a DMR in the *GLI2* gene that distinguishes children with a respiratory allergy from healthy controls. According to UCSC genome browser and ENCODE data, this DMR is located in a CpG shore encompassing several enhancers and promoters (Additional file 1: Figure S1), suggesting that this region is involved in the active transcription of *GLI2*. Irizarry et al. previously observed strong inverse relationships between differentially methylated CpG shores and transcription of associated genes (incl. hypermethylation leading to reduced expression of the studied tissue-specific differentially methylated gene regions), supporting a functional role for CpG shores [61, 62]. In their study, this association was especially confirmed for shores located within 2 kb of an annotated transcriptional start site, but the possibility of additional regulatory functions for shores located in intragenic regions (as is the case for our identified *GLI2* DMR) was left open. In addition, according to the recently revised *GLI2* exon/intron structure nomenclature by Sadam et al. [63], our *GLI2* DMR under investigation appears to be located at an alternative transcription start sites (TSS) in exon III. These findings underscore the importance of the studied gene region in the regulation of *GLI2*.

Aiding in the discovery of the *GLI2* DMR in the current study was the use of alternative cell correction methods to reduce false positive hits and to account for possible differences in cell composition between the reference data generated using adults opposed to the children's profiles studied in the current study. Correcting peripheral blood DNA methylation array data for differences in cell composition is generally performed according to the reference-based deconvolution method described by Houseman et al. [37]. For saliva, the most practical approach was to use blood plus buccal reference datasets [22, 25] to perform cell correction. Note that the Houseman correction does not discriminate between the various granulocyte subtypes, which might be important in future allergy studies because the proportion of eosinophils can change in individuals with allergy.

We previously identified with a reference-free deconvolution method [64] two underlying cell types in saliva that correlated significantly with the buccal and granulocyte cell fractions that were estimated to be the main cell type constituents in saliva according to the reference-based method [65]. A complementary approach was therefore to correct methylation array data for the buccal and granulocyte cell fractions only, in parallel to the full referenced-based deconvolution method. This enabled us to look at DMRs in common between both approaches and discovering true positive and biologically significant DNA

methylation markers. The information on the cell fractions was also used to adjust the gene-targeted iPLEX methylation data. This is considered as strength of our study because it is not a common practice to correct gene-targeted methylation data for differences in cell proportions, mainly because data on cell counts (e.g., assed via flow cytometry) are usually not available or cannot be estimated in gene-targeted methylation studies.

A limitation of our study is that all respiratory allergy subtypes (e.g., allergic asthma, rhinitis, hay fever) were combined into one group of respiratory allergy cases. The reason is being that the Flemish birth cohorts were mainly designed as an environmental health survey. These studies were developed in context of general health monitoring and were not geared towards molecular studies into respiratory allergy. Hence, the number of cases with full clinical characterization is limited. Nevertheless, we used information from the ISAAC questionnaire and Phadiatop IgE levels to divide the cases further into specific respiratory allergy subtypes. Although the numbers per group were quite low to perform robust statistical analysis, we observed that hypermethylation of the *GLI2* DMR was mainly associated with rhinitis in the FLEHS1 cohort (Additional file 3: Table S1) and with house dust mite allergy in the FLEHS2 cohort (Additional file 3: Table S2). However, considering the small sample sizes in our study, the complex spectrum of respiratory allergy phenotypes, and other factors possibly modulating DNA methylation (e.g., medication use), we warn for extrapolation of our findings.

In general, gene hypermethylation is assumed to lead to decreased gene and protein expression. However, concerning the complexity of HH signaling with its feedback loops and the bi-functional nature of GLI2, it is hard to give a straightforward interpretation of the biological/phenotypic consequences of the *GLI2* DMR hypermethylation. GLI proteins bind DNA at consensus GLI-family binding sites and directly modulate to the expression of HH target genes, some of which are involved in HH pathway feedback (e.g., *GLI1*, *PTCH1*) [48]. In addition, as determined by posttranscriptional and post-translational processing, GLI2 as well as GLI3 contains an amino-terminal repressor (R) and a carboxyterminal activator (A) domain. Thus, the ratio of GLIA relative to GLIR in the cell regulates the GLI-dependent transcription of target genes. GLI1 lacks the repressor domain and acts thus as an activator. GLI2A can act as a repressor and activator of transcription, whereas GLI3 has primarily a repressor function [66]. According to Sadam et al. [63], our *GLI2* DMR is located near a TSS and, considering the various possible splice variants, the identified DMR should be involved in the transcription of both GLI2A and GLI2R. So regardless the complexity of GLI2-dependent transcription, in the sections below, we describe the plausible pathways via which *GLI2* hypermethylation could increase the risk of respiratory allergies.

The role of GLI2 in T-helper cell differentiation
HH signaling mediated by the HH-responsive transcription factor GLI2 has multiple roles in T-lymphocyte development and differentiation. In recent research, Furmanski et al. [47] demonstrated in Gli2Δ mice (carrying a truncated form of Gli2 that acts as a permanent transcriptional activator of Hh target genes) that (1) GLI2A promotes Th2 differentiation (via IL4 and GATA3) in T cells, (2) *Il4* is a novel target gene of Gli2-dependent Hh signaling, and (3) an allergic disease pathology was observed in house dust mite-treated Gli2A mice—showing increased eosinophil recruitment indicating enhanced inflammation, in parallel to a higher proportion of CD4$^+$ T cells in the lung producing IL4 and IL-13, and goblet cell hyperplasia. In addition, the same group recently showed that GLI activity is induced in multiple leukocytes in a murine model of asthma and that expression of GLI2R decreases the recruitment of CD4+ Th2 cells to the allergic lung [67]. However, they reported that the allergic disease pathology was not significantly different from the WT. Still, both GLI2A and GLI2R might be closely involved in immune system development and Th2-mediated diseases. In addition, Kugler et al. indicated that it is ultimately the balance between GLI2A and GLI3R accumulation and the resulting target gene transcription in the nucleus that influences the pathway output [68].

Alternatively, GLI-dependent transcription can also be triggered by non-HH ligands, such as transforming growth factor β (TGF-β) [69]. Interestingly, associations between GLI2 and TGF-β1 were observed in our IPA network analysis (Fig. 3). In addition, knockdown of *GLI2* in human CD4+ CD25 regulatory T cells showed that GLI2 is also necessary for TGF-β1 transcription. In its activated state, GLI2 can bind on six assumed GLI binding sites in human TGF-β promotors. Thus, GLI2 can enhance TGF-β1 transcription in naïve CD4+ T cells [70]. TGF-β is produced by several immune-related cell types including CD4+ CD25 regulatory T cells, macrophages, and fibroblasts [70, 71]. TGF-β has been reported to play a key role in asthma because it mediates leukocyte chemotaxis to the lungs and thus genesis and maintenance of an inflammatory response. Furthermore, it was suggested that high TGF-β levels in the airways correlate with asthma severity, with eosinophils representing about 70–80% of all cells expressing TGF-1 in these patients' airways (reviewed by [71]). In an alternative hypothesis, *GLI2* hypermethylation could lead to reduced expression of TGF-β1, resulting in enhanced immune Th-cell differentiation and pro-inflammatory cytokine production. However, TGF-β1 has also been

reported to have anti-inflammatory and immunosuppressive properties, as reflected by the inhibition of immune cell differentiation (Th1 and Th2 cells and B cells) and cytokine production (IFN-γ and IL-2) [71]. Moreover, TGF-β has been described as a key molecule in the repair of the airway epithelium in allergic diseases such as asthma and allergic rhinitis [71]. In addition, enhanced expression of GLI2 also modulates TCR repertoire selection and results in lower CD4+/CD8+ ratio [49]. Based on the anti-inflammatory role of TGF-β1, another hypothesis might be that *GLI2* hypermethylation could lead to reduced expression of TGF-β1, resulting in enhanced immune Th-cell differentiation and pro-inflammatory cytokine production.

Extensive research has been done to elucidate the role of regulators of the Th differentiation (transcription factors, cytokines, and other immune derived cell molecules), but little is known about the contribution of non-immune factors, such as HH pathway-associated genes like *GLI2*. A recent report demonstrates that hedgehog pathways and TGF-β signaling both converge to GLI2 [72]. The crosstalk of these signaling pathways and their role in respiratory allergic diseases requires further investigation.

The role of GLI2 in lung development
GLI2 is natively expressed in the lung mesenchyme (mucus connective tissue) near the epithelial border, and it is important for proper epithelial mesenchymal signaling during early long development [73]. Estimation of gene expression (derived from Ensembl genes hg18, UCSC genome browser) showed reasonable expression of *GLI2* in the lung and salivary gland (Additional file 2: Figure S2), but no or negligible expression in blood cells. It is important to notice that the function of GLI2 can be dependent of the type of tissue in which it is expressed, but GLI2 is important for lung development [73] and altered expression might thus have an influence on the risk to develop respiratory allergies when *GLI2* methylation status is altered.

GLI2 is also suggested to be the primary GLI transcription factor transducing SHH-regulated lung growth. SHH is crucial in branching morphogenesis and formation of mature airways through branching events of bronchi and mesenchyme proliferation [68]. It is clear that in embryonic lung development, expression of SHH and its signaling molecules are highly regulated and SHH exerts its effect on different cellular components [68]. Rutter et al. [73] describe that *gli2*-null lungs show defective airway branching, left pulmonary isomerism, and severe lung hypoplasia. In combination with loss in cellular proliferation, this leads to a lung that is not able to support life at birth. Although there is a reduction in wet lung weight in *gli3*-null mouse, both *gli1*- and *gli3*-null mice still develop functional lungs. The analysis of different *gli*-null mice led to the suggestion that GLI2 primarily acts as a transcriptional activator of the lung [73]. It was also discussed that *Shh*-null mice have single lobed hypoplastic lungs, with decreased epithelium, mesenchyme, and malformations of the trachea. In addition, Rutter et al. showed that the levels of cyclins D1, D2, and E1 are linked to *GLI2* expression in the developing lung, suggesting that it may be involved in the regulation of cell cycle components. An overexpression of GLI2 resulted in an increase of these cyclins, leading to cellular proliferation and to an increase in wet lung weight [73]. Thus, when assuming a direct association between methylation and gene expression, one can speculate that suppression of *GLI2* is in association with a decreased expression of cyclins. As such, it can be postulated that *GLI2* hypermethylation is involved in the suppression of the cell cycle, with a possible negative effect on lung development and an increased chance of developing respiratory allergy.

Conclusions

We found hypermethylation in the *GLI2* gene in saliva from school-age children with a respiratory allergy when compared to saliva from healthy control subjects. The interpretation of the biological effects of the observed *GLI2* hypermethylation is not straightforward because the gene is under different levels of control. Posttranscriptional modifications to GLI2A and GLI2R and feedback loops in the HH signaling pathway complicate the usually assumed one-to-one relation between hypermethylation and decreased gene/protein expression. We suggest that *GLI2* hypermethylation can trigger inflammatory pathways dependent on IL4 and TGF-β1 signaling. In addition, *GLI2* is one of the main downstream effectors of the SHH pathway, which plays a role in branching of the bronchi and immune system regulation.

Overall, this study warrants further investigation into the mechanism linking *GLI2* to respiratory allergic disease in order to highlight the importance of differential methylation of *GLI2* in respiratory allergy and to define its potential for early identification of individuals at risk for respiratory allergy development.

Abbreviations

ALOX12: Arachidonate 12-lipoxygenase; APOBEC1: Apolipoprotein B mRNA editing enzyme, catalytic polypeptide 1; CCR: Chemokine receptors; CD: Cluster of differentiation; DMRs: Differentially methylated gene regions; EFA: European Federation of Allergy and Airways Diseases Patients' Associations; FLEHS: Flemish Environment and Health Studies; GATA3: GATA-binding protein 3; GLI: GLI family of zinc-finger DNA-binding proteins; GRAMD1B: GRAM domain containing 1B; H3K27Ac: Acetylated histone H3 at lysine 27; H3K4Me1: Monomethylated histone H3 at lysine 4; HH: Hedgehog; HTRA3: High-temperature requirement factor A3; IFN-γ: Interferon gamma; IgE: Immunoglobulin E; IL: Interleukin; IPA: Ingenuity Pathway Analysis; ISAAC: International Study of Asthma and Allergies in Childhood; MED24: Mediator complex subunit 24; NFκB: Nuclear factor kappa-light-chain-enhancer of activated B cells; NHLF: Normal Human Lung Fibroblasts; OPCML: Opioid-binding protein/cell adhesion molecule-like; PBMC: Peripheral blood mononuclear cells; RELA: Nuclear factor NF-kappa-B p65 subunit; RPKM: Reads per kb of exon model per million mapped reads; SHH: Sonic hedgehog; TGF-β: Transforming growth factor-β; Th: T-helper cell

Acknowledgements

We thank our study volunteers for participating in this study. The FLEHS studies were commissioned, financed, and steered by the Flemish Government (Department of Economy, Science and Innovations, Agency for Care and Health and Department of Environment), and relevant FLEHS data has been made available by the FLEHS Supervisory Board. The support of the Provincial Institute of Hygiene for field work is acknowledged. A special thanks goes to Anne Schepers, at the Laboratory of Cancer Research and Clinical Oncology, Center for Medical Genetics, University of Antwerp, for the excellent work with the Infinium HumanMethylation450 BeadChip Arrays. Last but not least, we are thankful for the technical support given by Karen Hollanders, Stijn Van Uytsel, and Sophie Breemans.

Funding

SL was the beneficiary of a post-doctoral grant from the AXA Research Fund and the Cefic-LRI Innovative Science Award 2013 and has currently a post-doctoral fellowship (12L5216N) provided by The Research Foundation-Flanders (FWO) and the Flemish Institute of Technological Research (VITO). The methylation work was funded by the Cefic-LRI Innovative Science Award 2013. PDB is recipient of a Bill & Melinda Gates Foundation Grand Challenges Exploration Grant (OPP119403) in the field of saliva biomarker discovery.

Authors' contributions

SL, GK, GS, and PDB conceived and designed the experiments. SL, SDP, TL, and VN facilitated the field work. SL, EVP, and KSVS performed the experiments. MM, SL, and PDB analyzed the data. SL, GVC, WVB, DL, and PDB contributed the reagents/materials/analysis tools. SL, MM, WVD, and PDB wrote the paper. SL, MM, WVD, and PDB evaluated and interpreted the results. All authors evaluated and approved the manuscript.

Competing interests

In relation to this work, VITO applied for the patent "RESPIRATORY ALLERGY - Allergim 1," which was published on 8/12/2016 (WO 2016/193151 A1).

Author details

[1]VITO- Sustainable Health, Boeretang 200, 2400 Mol, Belgium. [2]Centre for Environmental Sciences, Hasselt University, Diepenbeek, Belgium. [3]Laboratory for Translational Genetics, Center for Cancer Biology, VIB and KU Leuven, Campus Gasthuisberg, Leuven, Belgium. [4]Proteinchemistry, Proteomics & Epigenetic Signaling (PPES), Department of Biomedical Sciences, University of Antwerp, Wilrijk, Belgium. [5]Environment and Health unit, Provincial Institute of Hygiene, Antwerp, Belgium. [6]Center for Medical Genetics, University of Antwerp and Antwerp University hospital, Antwerp, Belgium. [7]Department of Biomedical Sciences, University of Antwerp, Wilrijk, Belgium. [8]Department of Environmental Medicine, Institute of Public Health, University of Southern Denmark, Odense, Denmark.

References

1. European Federation of Allergy and Airways Diseases Patients Associations (EFA). EFA book on respiratory allergies—raise awareness, relieve the burden, 2011.
2. Ait-Khaled N, Pearce N, Anderson HR, Ellwood P, Montefort S, Shah J. Global map of the prevalence of symptoms of rhinoconjunctivitis in children: the International Study of Asthma and Allergies in Childhood (ISAAC) phase three. Allergy. 2009;64(1):123–48.
3. Bégin P, Nadeau KC. Epigenetic regulation of asthma and allergic disease. Allergy Asthma Clin Immunol. 2014;10(1):27.
4. Li JY, Zhang Y, Lin XP, Ruan Y, Wang Y, Wang CS, et al. Association between DNA hypomethylation at IL13 gene and allergic rhinitis in house dust mite-sensitized subjects. Clin Exp Allergy. 2016;46(2):298–307.
5. Calzada D, Aguerri M, Baos S, Lahoz C, Cardaba B. Epigenetic regulation analyses of FOXP3 in olive pollen allergy. J Investig Allergol Clin Immunol. 2015;25(3):222–4.
6. Pascual M, Suzuki M, Isidoro-Garcia M, Padron J, Turner T, Lorente F, et al. Epigenetic changes in B lymphocytes associated with house dust mite allergic asthma. Epigenetics. 2011;6(9):1131–7.
7. Perera F, Tang WY, Herbstman J, Tang D, Levin L, Miller R, et al. Relation of DNA methylation of 5′-CpG island of ACSL3 to transplacental exposure to airborne polycyclic aromatic hydrocarbons and childhood asthma. PLoS One. 2009;4(2):e4488.
8. DeVries A, Wlasiuk G, Miller SJ, Bosco A, Stern DA, Lohman IC, et al. Epigenome-wide analysis links SMAD3 methylation at birth to asthma in children of asthmatic mothers. J Allergy Clin Immunol. 2017;140(2):534-542. doi: https://doi.org/10.1016/j.jaci.2016.10.041.
9. North ML, Ellis AK. The role of epigenetics in the developmental origins of allergic disease. Ann Allergy Asthma Immunol. 2011;106(5):355–61. quiz 62
10. Yang IV, Pedersen BS, Liu A, O'Connor GT, Teach SJ, Kattan M, et al. DNA methylation and childhood asthma in the inner city. J Allergy Clin Immunol. 2015;136(1):69–80.
11. Mukherjee N, Lockett GA, Merid SK, Melen E, Pershagen G, Holloway JW, et al. DNA methylation and genetic polymorphisms of the Leptin gene interact to influence lung function outcomes and asthma at 18 years of age. International Journal of Molecular Epidemiology and Genetics. 2016; 7(1):1–17.
12. Acevedo N, Reinius LE, Greco D, Gref A, Orsmark-Pietras C, Persson H, et al. Risk of childhood asthma is associated with CpG-site polymorphisms, regional DNA methylation and mRNA levels at the GSDMB/ORMDL3 locus. Hum Mol Genet. 2015;24(3):875–90.
13. Guthikonda K, Zhang H, Nolan VG, Soto-Ramirez N, Ziyab AH, Ewart S, et al. Oral contraceptives modify the effect of GATA3 polymorphisms on the risk of asthma at the age of 18 years via DNA methylation. Clin Epigenetics. 2014;6(1):17.
14. Lluis A, Depner M, Gaugler B, Saas P, Casaca VI, Raedler D, et al. Increased regulatory T-cell numbers are associated with farm milk exposure and lower atopic sensitization and asthma in childhood. J Allergy Clin Immunol. 2014; 133(2):551–9.
15. Michel S, Busato F, Genuneit J, Pekkanen J, Dalphin JC, Riedler J, et al. Farm exposure and time trends in early childhood may influence DNA methylation in genes related to asthma and allergy. Allergy. 2013;68(3):355–64.
16. Reinius LE, Gref A, Sääf A, Acevedo N, Joerink M, Kupczyk M, et al. DNA methylation in the neuropeptide S receptor 1 (NPSR1) promoter in relation to asthma and environmental factors. PLoS One. 2013;8(1):e53877.
17. Morales E, Bustamante M, Vilahur N, Escaramis G, Montfort M, de Cid R, et al. DNA hypomethylation at ALOX12 is associated with persistent wheezing in childhood. Am J Respir Crit Care Med. 2012;185(9):937–43.
18. Wang CM, Chang CB, Chan MW, Wen ZH, Wu SF. Dust mite allergen-specific immunotherapy increases IL4 DNA methylation and induces Der p-specific T cell tolerance in children with allergic asthma. Cell Mol Immunol. 2017. doi: https://doi.org/10.1038/cmi.2017.26.
19. Gaffin JM, Raby BA, Petty CR, Hoffman EB, Baccarelli AA, Gold DR, et al. β-2 adrenergic receptor gene methylation is associated with decreased asthma severity in Inner-City School Children. Clin Exp Allergy. 2014;44(5):681–9.
20. Chen W, Boutaoui N, Brehm JM, Han YY, Schmitz C, Cressley A, et al. ADCYAP1R1 and asthma in Puerto Rican children. Am J Respir Crit Care Med. 2013;187(6):584–8.
21. Brunst KJ, Leung YK, Ryan PH, Khurana Hershey GK, Levin L, Ji H, et al. Forkhead box protein 3 (FOXP3) hypermethylation is associated with diesel exhaust exposure and risk for childhood asthma. J Allergy Clin Immunol. 2013;131(2):592–4.
22. Smith AK, Kilaru V, Klengel T, Mercer KB, Bradley B, Conneely KN, et al. DNA extracted from saliva for methylation studies of psychiatric traits: evidence tissue specificity and relatedness to brain. Am J Med Genet B Neuropsychiatr Genet. 2015;168B(1):36–44.
23. Thompson TM, Sharfi D, Lee M, Yrigollen CM, Naumova OY, Grigorenko EL. Comparison of whole-genome DNA methylation patterns in whole blood, saliva, and lymphoblastoid cell lines. Behav Genet. 2013;43(2):168–76.
24. Wu HC, Wang Q, Chung WK, Andrulis IL, Daly MB, John EM, et al. Correlation of DNA methylation levels in blood and saliva DNA in young girls of the LEGACY Girls study. Epigenetics. 2014;9(7):929–33.
25. Langie SA, Szarc Vel Szic K, Declerck K, Traen S, Koppen G, Van Camp G, et al. Whole-genome saliva and blood DNA methylation profiling in individuals with a respiratory allergy. PLoS One. 2016;11(3):e0151109.
26. Flemish Center of Expertise on Environment and Health. Secondary Flemish Center of Expertise on Environment and Health. http://www.milieu-en-gezondheid.be/en/home.
27. Schoeters G, Den Hond E, Colles A, Loots I, Morrens B, Keune H, et al. Concept of the Flemish human biomonitoring programme. Int J Hyg Environ Health. 2012;215(2):102–8.
28. Koppen G, Den Hond E, Nelen V, Van De Mieroop E, Bruckers L, Bilau M, et al. Organochlorine and heavy metals in newborns: results from the Flemish environment and health survey (FLEHS 2002-2006). Environ Int. 2009;35(7):1015–22.
29. Asher MI, Keil U, Anderson HR, Beasley R, Crane J, Martinez F, et al. International Study of Asthma and Allergies in Childhood (ISAAC): rationale and methods. Eur Respir J. 1995;8(3):483–91.
30. Remy S, Govarts E, Bruckers L, Paulussen M, Wens B, Hond ED, et al. Expression of the sFLT1 gene in cord blood cells is associated to maternal arsenic exposure and decreased birth weight. PLoS One. 2014;9(3):e92677.
31. Paganelli R, Ansotegui IJ, Sastre J, Lange CE, Roovers MH, de Groot H, et al. Specific IgE antibodies in the diagnosis of atopic disease. Clinical evaluation of a new in vitro test system, UniCAP, in six European allergy clinics. Allergy. 1998;53(8):763–8.
32. Aryee MJ, Jaffe AE, Corrada-Bravo H, Ladd-Acosta C, Feinberg AP, Hansen KD, et al. Minfi: a flexible and comprehensive Bioconductor package for the analysis of Infinium DNA methylation microarrays. Bioinformatics (Oxford, England). 2014;30(10):1363–9.
33. Wang D, Yan L, Hu Q, Sucheston LE, Higgins MJ, Ambrosone CB, et al. IMA: an R package for high-throughput analysis of Illumina's 450K Infinium methylation data. Bioinformatics (Oxford, England). 2012;28(5):729–30.
34. Maksimovic J, Gordon L, Oshlack A. SWAN: subset-quantile within array normalization for Illumina Infinium HumanMethylation450 BeadChips. Genome Biol. 2012;13(6):R44.
35. Du P, Zhang X, Huang CC, Jafari N, Kibbe WA, Hou L, et al. Comparison of beta-value and M-value methods for quantifying methylation levels by microarray analysis. BMC Bioinformatics. 2010;11:587.
36. Smyth GK. Linear models and empirical Bayes methods for assessing differential expression in microarray experiments. Stat Appl Genet Mol Biol. 2004;3:Article3.
37. Houseman EA, Accomando WP, Koestler DC, Christensen BC, Marsit CJ, Nelson HH, et al. DNA methylation arrays as surrogate measures of cell mixture distribution. BMC Bioinformatics. 2012;13:86.
38. Reinius LE, Acevedo N, Joerink M, Pershagen G, Dahlen SE, Greco D, et al. Differential DNA methylation in purified human blood cells: implications for cell lineage and studies on disease susceptibility. PLoS One. 2012;7(7):e41361.
39. Slieker RC, Bos SD, Goeman JJ, Bovee JV, Talens RP, van der Breggen R, et al. Identification and systematic annotation of tissue-specific differentially methylated regions using the Illumina 450k array. Epigenetics Chromatin. 2013;6(1):26.
40. Pedersen BS, Schwartz DA, Yang IV, Kechris KJ. Comb-p: software for combining, analyzing, grouping and correcting spatially correlated P-values. Bioinformatics (Oxford, England). 2012;28(22):2986–8.
41. Ernst J, Kellis M. ChromHMM: automating chromatin-state discovery and characterization. Nat Methods. 2012;9(3):215–6.
42. Ernst J, Kellis M. Discovery and characterization of chromatin states for systematic annotation of the human genome. Nat Biotechnol. 2010;28(8):817–25.
43. Ernst J, Kheradpour P, Mikkelsen TS, Shoresh N, Ward LD, Epstein CB, et al. Mapping and analysis of chromatin state dynamics in nine human cell types. Nature. 2011;473(7345):43–9.

44. GTEx Consortium. The Genotype-Tissue Expression (GTEx) project. Nat Genet. 2013;45(6):580-5. doi:https://doi.org/10.1038/ng.2653.

45. Mele M, Ferreira PG, Reverter F, DeLuca DS, Monlong J, Sammeth M, et al. Human genomics. The human transcriptome across tissues and individuals. Science (New York, NY). 2015;348(6235):660-5.

46. Shlyueva D, Stampfel G, Stark A. Transcriptional enhancers: from properties to genome-wide predictions. Nat Rev Genet. 2014;15(4):272–86.

47. Furmanski AL, Saldana JI, Ono M, Sahni H, Paschalidis N, D'Acquisto F, et al. Tissue-derived hedgehog proteins modulate Th differentiation and disease. J Immunol (Baltimore, Md : 1950). 2013;190(6):2641–9.

48. Rimkus TK, Carpenter RL, Qasem S, Chan M, Lo HW. Targeting the sonic hedgehog signaling pathway: review of smoothened and GLI inhibitors. Cancers (Basel). 2016;8(2). doi: https://doi.org/10.3390/cancers8020022.

49. Rowbotham NJ, Hager-Theodorides AL, Furmanski AL, Crompton T. A novel role for hedgehog in T-cell receptor signaling: implications for development and immunity. Cell Cycle (Georgetown, Tex). 2007;6(17):2138–42.

50. Cofer ZC, Cui S, EauClaire SF, Kim C, Tobias JW, Hakonarson H, et al. Methylation microarray studies highlight PDGFA expression as a factor in biliary atresia. PLoS One. 2016;11(3):e0151521.

51. Kolarova J, Tangen I, Bens S, Gillessen-Kaesbach G, Gutwein J, Kautza M, et al. Array-based DNA methylation analysis in individuals with developmental delay/intellectual disability and normal molecular karyotype. European Journal of Medical Genetics. 2015;58(8):419–25.

52. Yuen RK, Penaherrera MS, von Dadelszen P, DE MF, Robinson WP. DNA methylation profiling of human placentas reveals promoter hypomethylation of multiple genes in early-onset preeclampsia. Eur J Hum Genet. 2010;18(9):1006–12.

53. Mendioroz M, Do C, Jiang X, Liu C, Darbary HK, Lang CF, et al. Trans effects of chromosome aneuploidies on DNA methylation patterns in human Down syndrome and mouse models. Genome Biol. 2015;16:263.

54. Lu XL, Wang L, Chang SY, Shangguan SF, Wang Z, Wu LH, et al. Sonic hedgehog signaling affected by promoter hypermethylation induces aberrant Gli2 expression in spina bifida. Mol Neurobiol. 2016;53(8):5413–24.

55. Hovestadt V, Jones DT, Picelli S, Wang W, Kool M, Northcott PA, et al. Decoding the regulatory landscape of medulloblastoma using DNA methylation sequencing. Nature. 2014;510(7506):537–41.

56. Frigola J, Song J, Stirzaker C, Hinshelwood RA, Peinado MA, Clark SJ. Epigenetic remodeling in colorectal cancer results in coordinate gene suppression across an entire chromosome band. Nat Genet. 2006;38(5):540–9.

57. Stefanska B, Kurzava L, Lubecka K, Beetch M, Flower K, Flanagan JM. Epigenetic regulation of WNT and hedgehog oncogenic signaling in breast cancer cells in response to dietary polyphenols. FASEB J. 2017;31(1 Supplement):646.63.

58. Li X, Howard TD, Moore WC, Ampleford EJ, Li H, Busse WW, et al. Importance of hedgehog interacting protein and other lung function genes in asthma. J Allergy Clin Immunol. 2011;127(6):1457–65.

59. Xu M, Tantisira KG, Wu A, Litonjua AA, J-h C, Himes BE, et al. Genome wide association study to predict severe asthma exacerbations in children using random forests classifiers. BMC Medical Genetics. 2011;12:90.

60. Murk W, DeWan AT. Genome-wide search identifies a gene-gene interaction between 20p13 and 2q14 in asthma. BMC Genet. 2016;17(1):102. https://doi.org/10.1186/s12863-016-0370-3.

61. Irizarry RA, Ladd-Acosta C, Wen B, Wu Z, Montano C, Onyango P, et al. The human colon cancer methylome shows similar hypo- and hypermethylation at conserved tissue-specific CpG island shores. Nat Genet. 2009;41(2):178–86.

62. Stirzaker C, Taberlay PC, Statham AL, Clark SJ. Mining cancer methylomes: prospects and challenges. Trends Genet. 2014;30(2):75–84.

63. Sadam H, Liivas U, Kazantseva A, Pruunsild P, Kazantseva J, Timmusk T, et al. GLI2 cell-specific activity is controlled at the level of transcription and RNA processing: consequences to cancer metastasis. Biochim Biophys Acta (BBA) - Mol Basis Dis. 2016;1862(1):46–55.

64. Houseman EA, Kile ML, Christiani DC, Ince TA, Kelsey KT, Marsit CJ. Reference-free deconvolution of DNA methylation data and mediation by cell composition effects. BMC Bioinformatics. 2016;17:259.

65. Langie SA, Moisse M, Declerck K, Koppen G, Godderis L, Vanden Berghe W, et al. Salivary DNA methylation profiling: aspects to consider for biomarker identification. Basic Clin Pharmacol Toxicol. 2017;121(3):93-101. doi: https://doi.org/10.1111/bcpt.12721.

66. Sasaki H, Nishizaki Y, Hui C, Nakafuku M, Kondoh H. Regulation of Gli2 and Gli3 activities by an amino-terminal repression domain: implication of Gli2 and Gli3 as primary mediators of Shh signaling. Development. 1999;126(17):3915–24.

67. Standing ASI, Yánez DC, Ross R, Crompton T, Furmanski AL. Frontline science: Shh production and Gli signaling is activated in vivo in lung, enhancing the Th2 response during a murine model of allergic asthma. J Leukoc Biol. 2017;102(4):965–76.

68. Kugler MC, Joyner AL, Loomis CA, Munger JS. Sonic hedgehog signaling in the lung. From development to disease. Am J Respir Cell Mol Biol. 2015;52(1):1–13.

69. Zhang J, Tian X-J, Xing J. Signal transduction pathways of EMT induced by TGF-β, SHH, and WNT and their crosstalks. Journal of Clinical Medicine. 2016;5(4):41.

70. Furler RL, Uittenbogaart CH. GLI2 regulates TGF-beta1 in human CD4+ T cells: implications in cancer and HIV pathogenesis. PLoS One. 2012;7(7):e40874.

71. Tirado-Rodriguez B, Ortega E, Segura-Medina P, Huerta-Yepez S. TGF-β: an important mediator of allergic disease and a molecule with dual activity in cancer development. J Immunol Res. 2014;2014:15.

72. Liang R, Šumová B, Cordazzo C, Mallano T, Zhang Y, Wohlfahrt T, et al. The transcription factor GLI2 as a downstream mediator of transforming growth factor-β-induced fibroblast activation in SSc. Ann Rheum Dis. 2017;76(4):756–64.

73. Rutter M, Wang J, Huang Z, Kuliszewski M, Post M. Gli2 influences proliferation in the developing lung through regulation of cyclin expression. Am J Respir Cell Mol Biol. 2010;42(5):615–25.

2

TET1 exerts its anti-tumor functions via demethylating DACT2 and SFRP2 to antagonize Wnt/β-catenin signaling pathway in nasopharyngeal carcinoma cells

Jiangxia Fan[†], Yan Zhang[†], Junhao Mu, Xiaoqian He, Bianfei Shao, Dishu Zhou, Weiyan Peng, Jun Tang, Yu Jiang, Guosheng Ren and Tingxiu Xiang[*]

Abstract

Background: TET1 is a tumor suppressor gene (TSG) that codes for ten-eleven translocation methyl cytosine dioxygenase1 (TET1) catalyzing the conversion of 5-methylcytosine to 5-hydroxy methyl cytosine as a first step of TSG demethylation. Its hypermethylation has been associated with cancer pathogenesis. However, whether TET1 plays any role in nasopharyngeal carcinoma (NPC) remains unclear. This study investigated the expression and methylation of TET1 in NPC and confirmed its role and mechanism as a TSG.

Results: TET1 expression was downregulated in NPC tissues compared with nasal septum deviation tissues. Demethylation of TET1 in HONE1 and HNE1 cells restored its expression with downregulated methylation, implying that TET1 was silenced by promoter hypermethylation. Ectopic expression of TET1 suppressed the growth of NPC cells, induced apoptosis, arrested cell division in G0/G1 phase, and inhibited cell migration and invasion, confirming TET1 TSG activity. TET1 decreased the expression of nuclear β-catenin and downstream target genes. Furthermore, TET1 could cause Wnt antagonists (DACT2, SFRP2) promoter demethylation and restore its expression in NPC cells.

Conclusions: Collectively, we conclude that TET1 exerts its anti-tumor functions in NPC cells by suppressing Wnt/β-catenin signaling via demethylation of Wnt antagonists (DACT2 and SFRP2).

Keywords: *TET1*, Tumor suppressor, Nasopharyngeal carcinoma, Wnt pathway, Demethylation

Background

The worldwide incidence and mortality of nasopharyngeal carcinoma (NPC) is very low, but it is high in southern China [1, 2]. Radiation therapy is currently the primary treatment in the earlier stage, and combined with chemo-radiotherapy in the late stage, but distant metastasis and recurrence are frequent [3, 4]. As NPC is regulated by genetic and epigenetic factors [5, 6], biomarkers would help to improve treatment and outcomes. In NPC, many tumor suppressor genes (TSGs), such as *PCDH20* [7], *WIF1* [7, 8], *RASSF1* [9], *ADAMTS18* [10], *PTPRG* [11], *CDH4* [12], *CDH11* [13], *SOX11* [14], and *DACT2* [15],

are silenced by hyper-methylation. Some are associated with Wnt/β-catenin pathway activation [7, 8, 13, 15, 16].

The ten-eleven translocation (TET) proteins, TET1, TET2, and TET3 are highly active DNA cytosine oxygenases that maintain TSGs in an unmethylated state by conversion of 5-methyl cytosine (5mC) to 5-hydroxymethyl cytosine (5hmC) or by competition with DNA methyltransferases resulting in passive demethylation [17, 18]. Its C-terminal region is the catalytic domain, and the N-terminal region has a conserved CXXC domain [19], which identifies cytosine. TET1 contains three nuclear localization signals, indicating potential activity in the nucleus [20]. The *TET1* gene is located at chromosome 10q21.3, and it was first described in a patient with acute myeloid leukemia associated with a chromosome translocation [21, 22]. *TET1* is active as a TSG in breast

* Correspondence: larissaxiang@163.com
[†]Jiangxia Fan and Yan Zhang contributed equally to this work.
Chongqing Key Laboratory of Molecular Oncology and Epigenetics, the First Affiliated Hospital of Chongqing Medical University, Chongqing, China

[23], colon [24], gastric [25], prostate [26], hepatocellular [27], and renal carcinoma [28]. Its hyper-methylation has been associated with cancer pathogenesis. Li et al. showed that TET1, TET2, and TET3 are highly expressed in normal tissues, but only TET1 is downregulated in nasopharyngeal carcinoma cells [29]. Therefore, this study investigated the expression and methylation of TET1 in NPC and confirmed its role as a TSG. TET1 catalyzed several TSG demethylations to renew their expression, and suppressed Wnt/β-catenin pathway. Thus, *TET1* and its candidate target genes all are potential NPC biomarkers.

Methods

Tumor cell lines and tumor samples

The HNE1 and HONE1 nasopharyngeal carcinoma cell lines were obtained from Prof. Qian Tao, the Chinese University of Hong Kong, Hong Kong, China. The cells were maintained in RPMI 1640 (Gibco BRL, MD, USA) supplemented with 10% fetal bovine serum (FBS; PAA Laboratories, Linz, Austria), 100 U/ml penicillin (Gibco-BRL), and 100 μg/ml streptomycin (Gibco-BRL) at 37 °C in humidified air with 5% CO_2. Normal nasal tissues were obtained from the patients of nasal septum deviation (NSD); surgical margin tissues and nasopharyngeal carcinoma tissues were obtained from surgical patients treated at the Otolaryngology Surgery Department of the First Affiliated Hospital of Chongqing Medical University.

DNA and RNA extraction

Genomic DNA was extracted from cell lines and NPC tissues using a QIA amp DNA Mini Kit following the manufacturer's instructions (Qiagen, Hilden, Germany). Total RNA was extracted from cell lines and NPC tissues using TRIzol reagent (Invitrogen, Carlsbad, CA, USA). Total DNA and RNA were quantified by gel electrophoresis. Samples were stored at – 80 °C until used.

5-aza-2′-deoxycytidine (*Aza*) and (trichostatin A) *TSA* treatments

Aza and TSA treatments were performed as described previously [30, 31]. HNE1 and HONE1 cells were treated with final concentration 10 μmol/l Aza (Sigma-Aldrich, Steinheim, Germany) for 3 days with or without 100 nmol/l TSA (Sigma-Aldrich) for another 24 h.

Semi-quantitative RT-PCR and quantitative real-time PCR (qRT-PCR)

Semi-quantitative RT-PCR was performed with a 10 μl reaction mixture containing 2 μl cDNA using Go-taq (Promega, Madison, WI, USA). β-actin was amplified as the control and 32 cycles for TET1 and target genes. The primer sequences are listed in Table 1. qPCR of TET1 in NPC tissues and cell lines were normalized against β-actin. qRT-PCR was using SYBR® Green PCR Master Mix (Thermo Fisher Scientific, Hong Kong, China) in the HT7500 system (Applied Biosystems).

Bisulfite genomic sequencing and methylation-specific PCR

Bisulfite modification of DNA and methylation-specific PCR (MSP) were performed as previously described [32, 33]. Bisulfite-treated DNA was amplified with primers specific for methylated or non-methylated TET1. For bisulfite genomic sequencing (BGS), bisulfite-treated DNA was amplified using the primers shown in Table 1. The PCR products were cloned into eight to ten randomly chosen colonies using pCR4-Topo vector (Invitrogen Corporation, Carlsbad, CA) and then sequenced.

Construction of plasmids and stable cell lines

The TET1 plasmid contains the catalytic domain (CD) including the Cys-rich and DSBH regions. Both pcDNA3.1-Flag-HA-TET1-CD-His (pcDNA3.1-TET1-CD) plasmid with the CD regions (enzymatically active) and pcDNA3.1-Flag-HA-TET1-CD-mut-His (pcDNA3.1-TET1-CD-mut) plasmid with two amino acid substitutions in CD regions (enzymatically inactive) were gifts from Prof. Qian Tao (Chinese University of Hong Kong, Hong Kong, China) [29]. pN3myc-TET1-CD (pcDNA3.1-myc-TET1) was constructed by EcoRI and XbaI enzyme digestion pcDNA3.1-Flag-HA-TET1-CD-His and subcloned into pcNDA3.1-N3myc plasmids, which was validated by RT-PCR and sequencing. And pTopflash and pFopflash were used in our previous work [34].

pcDNA3.1 vector and pcDNA3.1-TET1-CD, pcDNA3.1-TET1-CD-mut were transfected into cells using Lipofectamine2000 (Invitrogen Corporation, Carlsbad, CA, USA) according to the manufacturer's protocol. Stable cells were confirmed by RT-PCR and Western blot.

Dot-blot analysis

Genomic DNA was purified, sonicated, denatured in $2 \times$ DNA denaturing buffer, and incubated at 95 °C for 10 min before spotting onto polyvinylidene difluoride (PVDF; Bio-Rad, Hercules, CA, USA) membranes. Equal amounts of DNA were allowed to spotting onto the membranes, which were then dried at room temperature. After UV cross-linking at 1200 J/m^2 and 2 h at 60 °C in incubator, membranes were blocked with 5% low-fat milk for 1 h at room temperature and incubated with primary antibodies against 5-hmC (1:5000; #39769; active motif), 5mC (1:1000; #28692;Cell Signaling Technology) overnight at 4 °C with gentle agitation. Membranes were incubated with secondary antibodies and read to detect DNA using

Table 1 List of primers used in this study

PCR	Primer	Sequence (5'-3')	Product size (bp)	PCR Cycles	Annealing temperature (°C)
RT-PCR	TET1F	AGGACCAAGTGTTGCTGCTGT	219	32	55
	TET1R	ATCACAGCAGTTGGACAGTGG			
	β-actinF	TCCTGTGGCATCCACGAAACT	315	23	55
	β-actinR	GAAGCATTTGCGGTGGACGAT			
qRT-PCR	DKK1F	CTGCATGCGTCACGCTATGT	161		60
	DKK1R	AGGTGGTTCTTCTGGAATAC			
	DKK2F	ACCCGCTGCAATAATGGAATC	99		60
	DKK2R	ATGGTTGCGATCTCTATGCCG			
	Snail1F	GAGGCGGTGGCAGACTAG	159		60
	Snail1R	GACACATCGGTCAGACCAG			
	DKK3F	CACCCTCAATGAGATGTTCC	161		60
	DKK3R	TGGTCTCATTGTGATAGCTG			
	DACT1F	CTGGAGGAGAAGTTCTTGGA	161		60
	DACT1R	TCCAGGTGCTCTTCAGATGT			
	DACT2F	AGCCGTGGGGCACATTCTG	173		60
	DACT2R	CCAGGTCCTGCCGATACTTG			
	SFRP1F	ACGAGTTGAAATCTGAGGCCATC	197		60
	SFRP1R	ACAGTCAGCCCCATTCTTCAG			
	SFRP2F	ATCCTGGAGACCAAGAGCAAGAC	142		60
	SFRP2R	TGACCAGATAGGGCGCGTTGATG			
	WNT5BF	AAATGCCACGGCGTCTCG	163		60
	WNT5BR	GGGTGAAGCGGCTGTTGA			
	WNT3F	ACGAGAACTCCCCCAACTTT	170		60
	WNT3R	GATGCAGTGGCATTTTTCCT			
	WNT5AF1	CGGTGTACAACCTGGCTGATG	101		60
	WNT5AR1	CACCTTGCGGAAGTCTGCC			
	WNT7AF	CTGGAACTGCTCTGCACTGGGA	129		60
	WNT7AR	GTACAGGCAGCTGTGATGGCGT			
	WNT7BF	TTTGGCGTCCTCTACGTGAAG	145		60
	WNT7BR	CCCCGATCACAATGATGGCA			
	EcadF	TACACTGCCCAGGAGCCAGA	103		60
	EcadR	TGGCACCAGTGTCCGGATTA			
	NcadF	CGAATGGATGAAAGACCCATCC	174		60
	NcadR	GGAGCCACTGCCTTCATAGTCAA			
	β-actinF1	GTCTTCCCCTCCATCGTG	113		60
	β-actinR1	AGGGTGAGGATGCCTCTCTT			
MSP	TET1m4	GTCGGTAGGCGTTTTTCGC	173	40	60
	TET1m8	CCCAACTCACCGCTAACCG			
	TET1u4	GAGTTGGTAGGTGTTTTTTGT	175	40	58
	TET1u8	CCCAACTCACCACTAACCA			
	DKK1m1	ATTTTGTAGTCGAATCGGTAC	127	40	60
	DKK1m2	CCGAATAACTCCCGCTACG			
	DKK1u1	TGATTTTGTAGTTGAATTGGTAT	131	40	58
	DKK1u2	ACCCAAATAACTCCCACTACA			

Table 1 List of primers used in this study *(Continued)*

PCR	Primer	Sequence (5'-3')	Product size (bp)	PCR Cycles	Annealing temperature (°C)
	DKK2m1	AGAGTTAAATCGTCGAGATTTC	146	40	60
	DKK2m2	CTAAAAACAATCAAATACGAAACG			
	DKK2u1	GGAGAGTTAAATTGTTGAGATTTT	149	40	58
	DKK2u2	ACTAAAAACAATCAAATACAAAACA			
	DKK3m3	TTTCGGGTATCGGCGTTGTC	148	40	60
	DKK3m4	ACTAAACCGAATTACGCTACG			
	DKK3u3	GTTTTTTTGGGTATTGGTGTTGTT	135	40	58
	DKK3u4	CAACTAAACCAAATTACACTACA			
	DACT1m3	CGGGATAGTAGTAGTCGGC	118	40	60
	DACT1m4	CGCTAAAACTACGACCGCG			
	DACT1u3	GTTGGGATAGTAGTAGTTGGT	123	40	58
	DACT1u4	AAACACTAAAACTACAACCACA			
	DACT2m3	CGTGTAGATTTCGTTTTTCGC	200	40	60
	DACT2m4	CCGAAAATCCGCCCGACG			
	DACT2u3	TGTGTGTAGATTTTGTTTTTTGT	203	40	58
	DACT2u4	CCCCAAAAATCCACCCAACA			
	SFRP1m1	TGTAGTTTTCGGAGTTAGTGTCGCGC	126	40	60
	SFRP1m2	CCTACGATCGAAAACGACGCGAACG			
	SFRP1u1	GTTTTGTAGTTTTTGGAGTTAGTGTTGTGT	137	40	58
	SFRP1u2	CTCAACCTACAATCAAAAACAACACAAACA			
	SFRP2m1	GGAGTTTTTCGGAGTTGCGC	128	40	60
	SFRP2m2	CTCTTCGCTAAATACGACTCG			
	SFRP2u1	GTTGGAGTTTTTTGGAGTTGTGT	133	40	58
	SFRP2u2	CTCTCTTCACTAAATACAACTCA			
BGS	TET1BGS1	TTGTTTTTTTATTGTGGATTTTTG	384	40	60
	TET1BGS2	AACCCACCCCTAAAACAAC			
Chip-PCR	DACT2F	CGTGCAGACCCCGCCCTC	113		60
	DACT2R	GATCCCGAGCTGTGTCGCG			
	SFRP2F	TGTCCCGCTTCTCCGCG	98		60
	SFRP2R	GAGTTCGAGCTTGTCCCG			
	Wnt5AF	CTCTCCGTGGAACAGTTGC	136		60
	Wnt5AR	GCAGAGCTGGGATGCGC			

enhanced chemiluminescence (ECL, Amersham Pharmacia Biotech, Piscataway, NJ, USA) at last.

Colony formation assay

Cells were stably transfected with pcDNA3.1, pcDNA3.1-TET1-CD, or pcDNA3.1-TET1-CD-mut plasmids and plated at 400 or 800 cells/well in six-well plates for HNE1 and HONE1, respectively. Following selection for 10 days with G418, colonies (≥ 50 cells/ colony) were stained with gentian violet (ICM Pharma, Singapore) and counted. All experiments were performed three times.

Cell proliferation assay

Stably transfected HNE1 and HONE1 cells were collected, counted, and plated in 96-well plates. Proliferation was assayed after 24, 48, and 72 h by the MTS Reagent (Promega, Madison, WI, USA) (absorbance 490 nm). All experiments were performed three times.

Wound healing and transwell assays

Stably transfected TET1-CD and vector plasmid-transfected HNE1 and HONE1 cells were cultured in six-well plates until confluent. The monolayers were scratched, washed with PBS, and cultured in 0% FBS-RPMI 1640.

Cells were photographed at 0, 12, and 24 h at ×100 magnification by light microscopy (Leica DMI4000B, Milton Keynes, Bucks, UK). All experiments were performed three times.

Cell migration and invasion were evaluated in 8-μm pore size Transwell chambers (Corning Life Sciences, Corning, NY, USA). The Transwell membranes were pre-coated with Matrigel (BD Biosciences) for the invasion assay. Cells stably expressing empty-vector or TET1-CD were washed twice in PBS and serum-free medium and plated into Transwell chamber inserts in 24-well plates after counting. The lower chambers contained 700 μL culture medium with 20% FBS. After incubation in FBS-free RPMI 1640 for 24 h, the cells that had migrated into the lower chamber were fixed in 4% paraformaldehyde for 30 min and stained with 0.1% crystal violet for 30 min. The nonmigrating cells in the upper chamber were removed, and the stained cells in three randomly selected fields were photographed by ×100 magnification and counted. All experiments were performed three times.

Flow cytometry analysis and apoptosis assay

For cell cycle analysis, HNE1 and HONE1 cells were seeded in six-well plates and transfected with 4 μg of TET1-CD or empty-vector control plasmids using lipofectamine 2000 (Invitrogen Corporation, Carlsbad, CA, USA) following the manufacturer's protocol. After 48 h, cells were harvested, washed, fixed in ice-cold 70% ethanol overnight at 4 °C, and treated with 100 μL of 50 mg/L propidium iodide (PI; BD Pharmingen, San Jose, CA, USA) for 30 min at 4 °C in the dark. Data were analyzed with CELL Quest software (BD Biosciences, San Jose, CA, USA). Annexin V-fluorescein isothiocyanate (FITC; BD Pharmingen) and PI double staining were used for apoptosis analysis. Briefly, the transfected cells were washed with PBS, stained with AnnexinV-FITC and PI for 5 min, and visualized immediately by flow cytometry analysis. The percentage of apoptotic cells was then calculated. All experiments were performed three times.

Western blot assay

Transfected cells were washed with ice-cold PBS and lysed using protein extraction reagent (Thermo Scientific, Rockford, IL, USA) containing phenylmethylsulfonyl fluoride and a protease inhibitor cocktail (Sigma-Aldrich, St Louis, MO). The lysate was centrifuged at 4 °C for 10 min at 10,000g, the liquid supernatant was collected, and 40 μg protein lysate aliquots were separated by sodium dodecyl sulfate-polyacrylamide gel electrophoresis (SDS-PAGE) and transferred to PVDF membranes (Bio-Rad, Hercules, CA, USA). The membranes were blocked with 5% low-fat milk for 1 h and subsequently incubated with primary antibodies (dilution 1:1000) overnight at 4 °C followed by incubation with an anti-mouse IgG or anti-rabbit IgG secondary antibody. The primary antibodies were Myc-tag (#2276; Cell Signaling Technology), active β-catenin (#19807s; Cell Signaling Technology), total β-catenin (#9562; Cell Signaling Technology), c-Myc (#13987s; Cell Signaling Technology), and cyclin D1 (#1677-1; Epitomics); β-actin (ARG62346; arigo) was used as a control. Proteins were visualized using an enhanced chemiluminescence (ECL) kit (Amersham Pharmacia Biotech, Piscataway, NJ, USA).

Immunofluorescence staining

Cells were incubated on coverslips in 24-well plates and transfected with TET1-CD. After 48 h, cells were fixed in paraformaldehyde and processed for double-label immunofluorescence by incubating with HA-tag (#3724; Cell Signaling Technology), Myc-tag (#2276; Cell Signaling Technology), total β-catenin (#2677; Cell Signaling Technology), or active β-catenin (#19807s; Cell Signaling Technology) primary antibodies at 4 °C overnight and fluorochrome-labeled secondary antibodies against mouse or rabbit IgG in the dark condition. Cells were then stained with 4′, 6-diamidino-2-phenylindole (DAPI) and subsequently visualized by a confocal laser scanning microscope and photographed.

Dual-luciferase reporter assay

Cells stably transfected with vector control and TET1-CD were plated into 24-well plates and transiently transfected with TOP/FOP-flash and Renilla luciferase reporter plasmids. The vector was the control and Renilla luciferase reporter phRL-TK was the internal control. After 48 h, cells were lysed in lysis buffer for 15 min at room temperature with shaking. Lysates were centrifuged, the supernatant was extracted, and luciferase activity was detected using a dual-luciferase reporter assay kit (Promega).

Immunohistochemistry assay

Hematoxylin and eosin (H&E) staining is used to identify normal septum deviation and cancerous tissue morphology. Immunohistochemistry (IHC) was performed using an UltraSensitive SP Kit (Maixin-Bio, Fujian, China) following the manufacturer's instructions. Normal septum deviation and NPC tissues were formalin-fixed and paraffin-embedded. Sections were deparaffinized, and following antigen retrieval by heating in a microwave in pH 6.0 sodium citrate solution, sections were incubated with TET1 (1:150; GTX124207; Gene Tex) and 5-hmC (1:150; #39769; active motif) primary antibodies at 4 °C overnight. Following incubation with secondary antibodies, and DAB and hematoxylin staining, cells were evaluated using Image-Pro Plus, version 6.0 (IPP6.0, Silver Spring, MD, USA).

The universal German semi-quantitative scoring system [35] was used to assess TET1 protein expression by the intensity of nuclei staining and number of stained cells. Briefly, each sample selected three to five random fields of vision at × 400 magnification, through the score of staining intensity(0 = no; 1 = weak; 2 = moderate; 3 = intense) was multiplied by the score of the range of stained cells (0 = 0%; 1 = 1~24%; 2 = 25~49%; 3 = 50~74%; 4 = 75~100%) to give the score of one field of vision, and then taking the average (range from 0 to 12). The scores for immunostaining were scored by two individuals who did not know the sample information. Student's t test was used for statistical analysis.

Methylated DNA immunoprecipitation (MeDIP) and Hydroxymethylated DNA immunoprecipitation (hMeDIP)

Two micrograms of sonicated DNA was denatured at 95 °C for 10 min, immediately cooled on ice for 10 min, and diluted in 500 μl of IP buffer (10 mM Na-Phosphate pH 7.0 140 mM NaCl 0.05% Triton X-100), 50 μl as input. Then, add 10 μl of anti-5mC (#28692; Cell Signaling Technology) or anti-5hmC (#39769; active motif; Cell Signaling Technology), IgG (#2729, Cell Signaling Technology) as control. After 2 h incubation at 4 °C with overhead shaking, 30 μl of 50% protein A/G-Sepharose magnetic beads were added and incubated for another 2 h. Put the tube on the magnetic beam for 5 min and discard supernatant. After five washes with IP buffer, DNA was eluted with Proteinase K for 2 h, then purified using the QIAQuick PCR Purification Kit (Qiagen) according to the manufacturer's instructions. DNA was analyzed by quantitative real-time PCR by using a SYBR GreenER kit (Invitrogen). Primers sequences are provided in Table 1. Fold enrichment was calculated as follows: %Input = 10% × 2^($CT^{input}-CT^{sample}$).

Statistical analysis

Continuous variables were reported as the mean value ± standard deviation (SD) compared by Student's t test. Categorical values were compared by the chi-square test or Fisher's exact test. Differences accepted for significance was $p < 0.05$. All data analyses were carried out

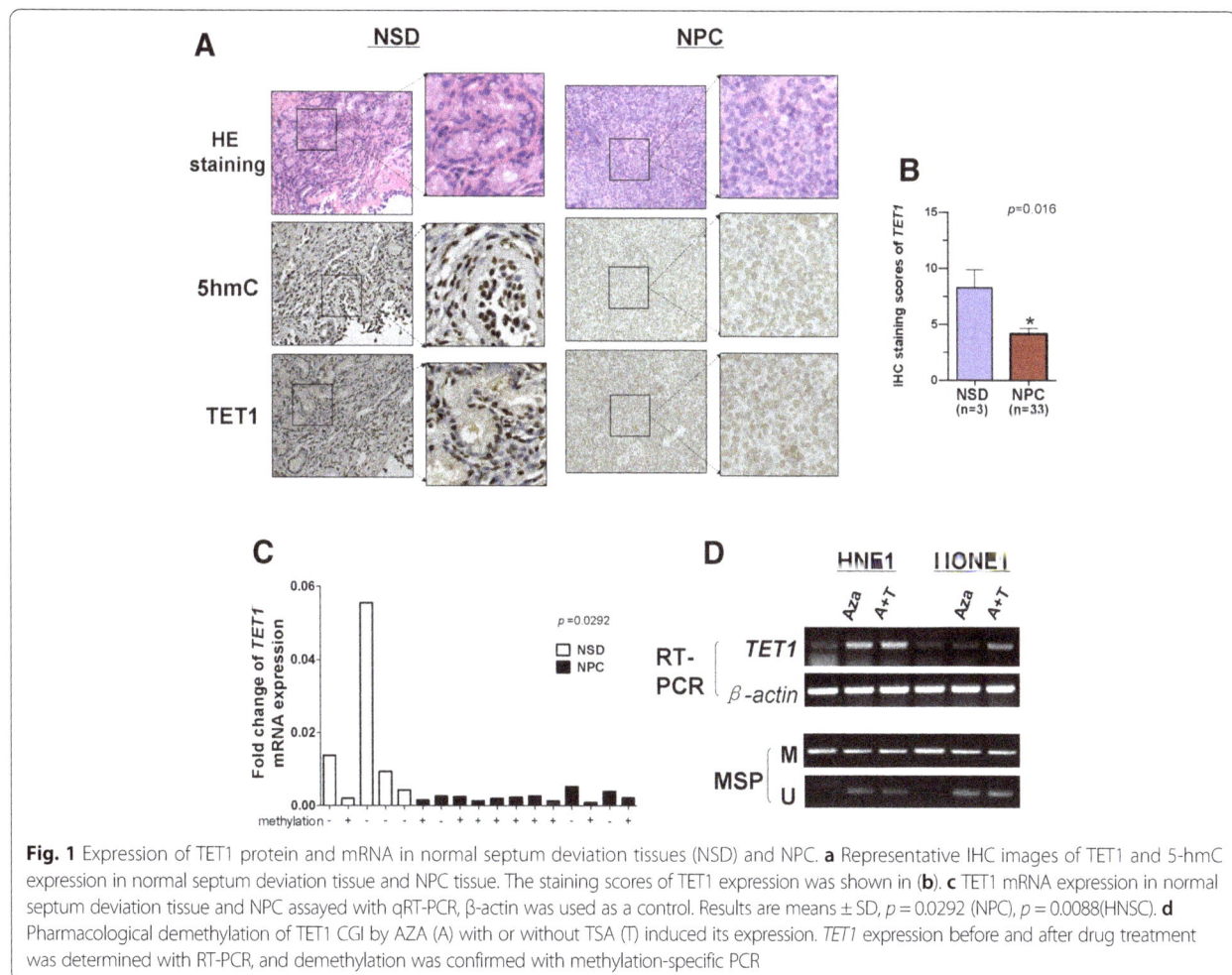

Fig. 1 Expression of TET1 protein and mRNA in normal septum deviation tissues (NSD) and NPC. a Representative IHC images of TET1 and 5-hmC expression in normal septum deviation tissue and NPC tissue. The staining scores of TET1 expression was shown in (b). c TET1 mRNA expression in normal septum deviation tissue and NPC assayed with qRT-PCR, β-actin was used as a control. Results are means ± SD, $p = 0.0292$ (NPC), $p = 0.0088$(HNSC). d Pharmacological demethylation of TET1 CGI by AZA (A) with or without TSA (T) induced its expression. *TET1* expression before and after drug treatment was determined with RT-PCR, and demethylation was confirmed with methylation-specific PCR

with the statistical analysis software package SPSS22.0 (SPSS Inc., Chicago, IL, USA). All biostatistics calculations were performed using Prism (Graphpad Software, Inc., La Jolla, California).

Results

TET1 expression is downregulated in NPC cell lines

Our previous studies found that TET1, 2, and 3 are expressed in human adult and fetal tissues and that only TET1 was downregulated in NPC cell lines [29]. H&E staining showed normal epithelial and cancer cell morphology and IHC staining showed that both TET1 and 5hmC expression were higher in 3 normal septum deviation than in 33 NPC tissues (Fig. 1a, b). Unfortunately, there was no correlation between TET1 expression and clinical and pathological features (Table 2). qRT-PCR was used to assay *TET1* mRNA expression and revealed that it was higher in normal nasal tissues than NPC ($p = 0.0292$), and most samples with low TET1 expression show considerably high methylation in CpG island of TET1 promoter (Fig. 1c). When methylated or silenced HNE1 and HONE1 nasopharyngeal cells were treated with the demethylation reagent 5-aza-2'-deoxycytidine (Aza) with or without trichostatin A (TSA) histone deacetylase, PCR confirmed that *TET1* expression was restored with a significant decrease of *TET1* promoter methylation (Fig. 1d). The results indicate that CpG methylation of *TET1* promoter mediated its silencing in NPC cells.

TET1 promoter is frequently methylated in NPC tissues

The CpG islands of TET1 and primer design for MSP have been shown in previous study [29]. Methylation-specific PCR was used to assay 55 NPCs and 9 surgical margin tissue samples. Hyper-methylation of the *TET1* promoter was observed in 45/55 (81.8%) NPCs and 4/9 (44.4%) in surgical margin tissues, indicating that methylation of the TET1 promoter was a common event in NPC (Fig. 2a). BGS analysis further confirmed the MSP data (Fig. 2b).

Ectopic expression of TET1 suppresses NPC cell growth mediated by its catalytic domain

As TET1 was downregulated in NPC and expressed in normal septum deviation, the tumor repressive of TET1 overexpression on the growth of NPC cells was evaluated. RT-PCR and Western blotting confirmed the expression of TET1 mRNA and protein in stably transfected HNE1 and HONE1 cells, which had few intrinsic TET1 expressions (Fig. 3a, b). MTS and colony formation assays revealed that TET1 significantly suppressed cell viability at 24, 48, and 72 h (*$p < 0.05$, **$p < 0.01$, and ***$p < 0.001$, respectively) and decreased colony formation by 45–55% compared with cells transfected with empty vectors, but no difference between empty vector group and TET1-CD-mut group, i.e., with inactive catalytic domains (Fig. 3c, d). The results indicated that re-expression of TET1 with an active catalytic domain suppressed the growth of NPC cell lines.

Table 2 Association between TET1 expression and clinical characteristics in NPC tissues

Characteristics	Number ($n = 33$)	TET1 expression				p value
		None	Low	Moderate	High	
Age (years)						
≧ 48	16	2	9	4	1	0.778
< 48	17	1	8	6	2	
Gender						
Female	9	0	4	4	1	0.548
Male	24	3	13	6	2	
WHO histological type						
I (keratinizing)	5	0	2	3	0	0.401
II/III (non-keratinizing)	28	3	15	7	3	
Clinical stages						
I	6	1	4	1	0	0.255
II	13	1	8	4	0	
III	12	1	5	3	3	
IV	2	0	0	2	0	
Lymph node metastasis						
positive	21	1	9	8	3	0.179
negative	12	2	8	2	0	

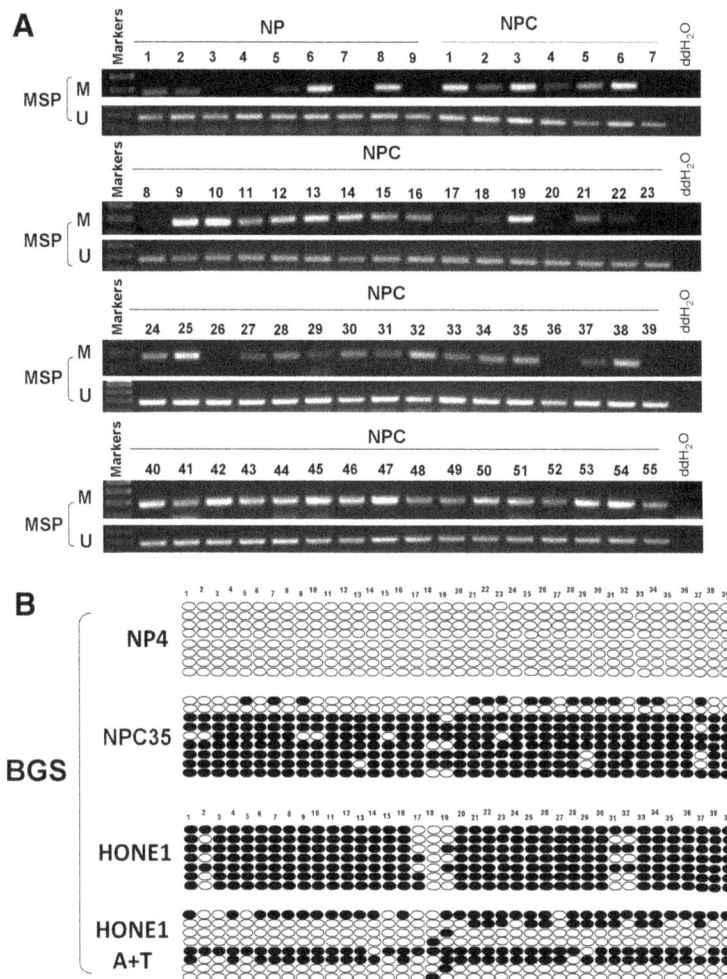

Fig. 2 The methylation status of *TET1* in NSD, surgical margin tissues, nasopharyngeal carcinoma (NPC) tissues, and nasopharyngeal carcinoma cells lines. **a** Promoter methylation of *TET1* in surgical margin tissues and nasopharyngeal carcinoma tissues as measured by MSP. M: methylated; U: unmethylated. **b** Bisulfite genomic sequencing confirmed the methylation status of *TET1* CpG sites in NSD, NPC tissues, and HONE1 cells with or without A+T treatment

TET1 induces NPC cell cycle arrest in G0-G1 phase and apoptosis

Flow cytometry was used to determine whether TET1 affected the cell cycle and apoptosis of NPC cells. TET1-transfection resulted in a 20 and 9% increase of the numbers of HNE1 and HONE1 cells in the G0/G1 phase ($p < 0.001$) compared with controls, respectively (Fig. 4a). Transfection also increased the number of apoptotic cells (Fig. 4b). These results demonstrated that TET1 inhibited the proliferation of NPC cells by inducing cell cycle arrest and promoted apoptosis.

TET1 suppresses NPC cells migration and invasion via regulating epithelial-mesenchymal transition

Transwell chamber motility showed that motility was significantly suppressed in HNE1 and HONE1 cells expressing TET1 (Fig. 5a, b). Similar results were observed in wound healing assays (all $p < 0.001$) (Fig. 5c, d). Matrigel invasiveness assays demonstrated that ectopic TFT1 expression significantly inhibited HNE1 and HONE1 cell invasion in culture medium containing 20% FBS (Fig. 6a, b). These results indicated that TET1-expression inhibited migration and invasion of NPC cells. The epithelial to mesenchymal transition (EMT) plays an important role in cancer progression and metastasis. To verify whether TET1 suppresses cell migration caused by inhibiting EMT, the expression of epithelial and mesenchymal markers was investigated. qRT-PCR showed the increase of E-cadherin and occludin and the decrease of N-cadherin, vimentin, and snail1 in TET1-expressed HNE1 and HONE1 cells (Fig. 6c). And immunofluorescence staining proved the same results in HONE1 cells (Fig. 6d). These results suggested that TET1 inhibits EMT in NPC cells.

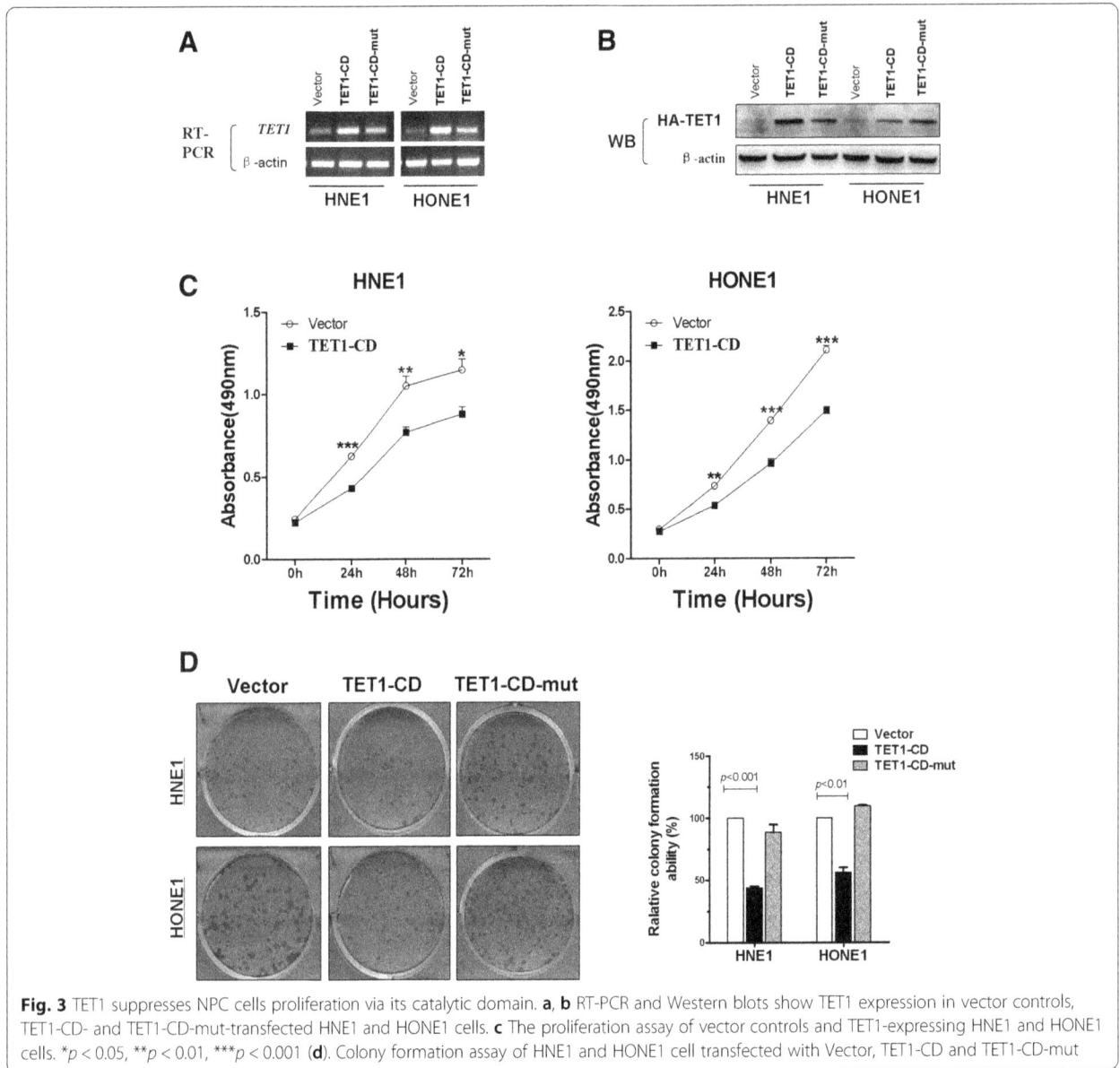

Fig. 3 TET1 suppresses NPC cells proliferation via its catalytic domain. **a, b** RT-PCR and Western blots show TET1 expression in vector controls, TET1-CD- and TET1-CD-mut-transfected HNE1 and HONE1 cells. **c** The proliferation assay of vector controls and TET1-expressing HNE1 and HONE1 cells. *$p < 0.05$, **$p < 0.01$, ***$p < 0.001$ (**d**). Colony formation assay of HNE1 and HONE1 cell transfected with Vector, TET1-CD and TET1-CD-mut

TET1 inhibits the Wnt/β-catenin signaling pathway

Aberrant activation of the Wnt/β-catenin signaling pathway was involved in NPC carcinogenesis. The evidence indicated that methylation of genes promoting negative Wnt regulators contributes to aberrant silencing and activation of Wnt/β-catenin signaling in human cancers. Western blotting, TOP/FOP-Flash, and immunofluorescence were used to investigate the effect of TET1 on Wnt/β-catenin signaling in NPC cells. The expression of β-catenin and some downstream target genes of Wnt/β-catenin were confirmed in NPC cells. Active β-catenin, c-Myc, and cyclinD1 were downregulated, with no significant change in total β-catenin in NPC cells overexpressed TET1 (Fig. 7a). TOP-flash assays found that TET1 overexpression had a significant inhibitory effect on β-catenin/TCF activity compared with FOP-flash controls (Fig. 7b). Immunofluorescence confirmed that nuclear expression of active β-catenin was decreased by TET1 overexpression, and total β-catenin has no significant change (Fig. 7c, d). Collectively, the data demonstrated that TET1 inhibited the Wnt/β-catenin signaling pathway in NPC cells.

TET1 renews expression of Wnt antagonists by demethylation of their promoter

To determine how TET1 influenced Wnt/β-catenin signaling, the expression of Wnt pathway antagonists, including DACT (DACT1,2,3), SFRP (SFRP1,2,3), DKK

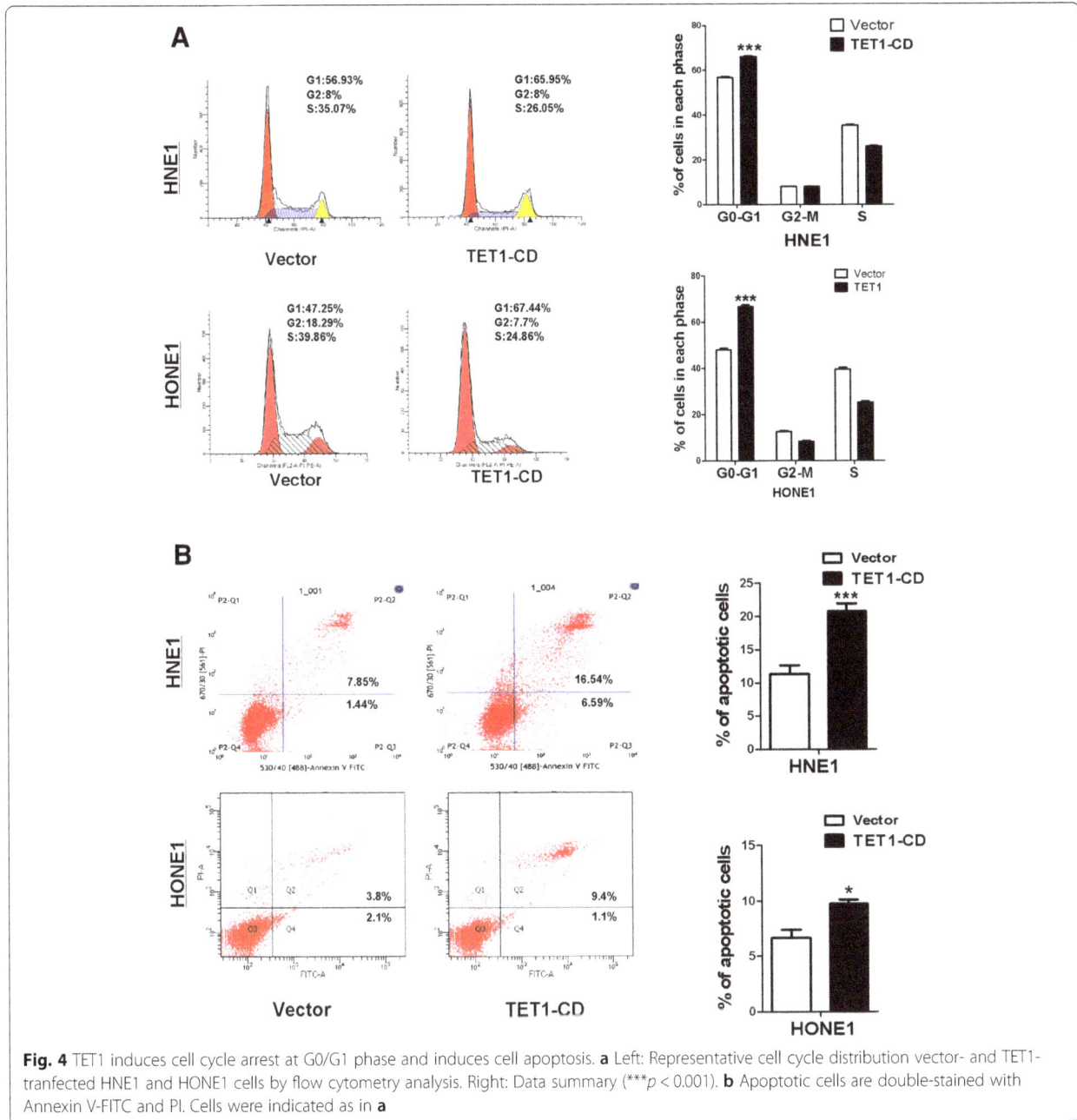

Fig. 4 TET1 induces cell cycle arrest at G0/G1 phase and induces cell apoptosis. **a** Left: Representative cell cycle distribution vector- and TET1-tranfected HNE1 and HONE1 cells by flow cytometry analysis. Right: Data summary (***$p < 0.001$). **b** Apoptotic cells are double-stained with Annexin V-FITC and PI. Cells were indicated as in **a**

(DKK1-3) family genes, and WNT proteins (include WNT1,3,3A,4, WAN5A, WNT5B, WNT7A, WNT7B) in HNSN (head and neck squamous cell normal tissues) and HNSC (head and neck squamous cell carcinoma) was analyzed. DACT (1,2,3), WNT5A, and WNT7B were significantly positive correlation with TET1($p < 0.05$), and WNT4 and WNT7A were negative correlation with TET1 in the TCGA Head and Neck Squamous cell Carcinoma database ($p < 0.05$, Additional file 1: Figure S1). We further found that *DACT2* and *WNT5B* had the low-expression and

hypermethylation in HNSC compared with HNSN (Additional file 2: Figure S2), data from TCGA (http://methhc.mbc.nctu.edu.tw/php/index.php). Based on above information, DACT (1,2,3), WNT5A, WNT5B, and WNT7B were most likely to be affected by TET1 in NPC.

Dot-blot assays were used to characterize 5hmC and 5mC expression in NPC cell lines that over-expressed TET1. TET1 re-expression in transfected TET1-silenced cells resulted in increased levels of 5hmC and decreased levels of 5mC compared with empty-vector transfected cells (Fig. 8a). To determine how TET1 influenced Wnt/

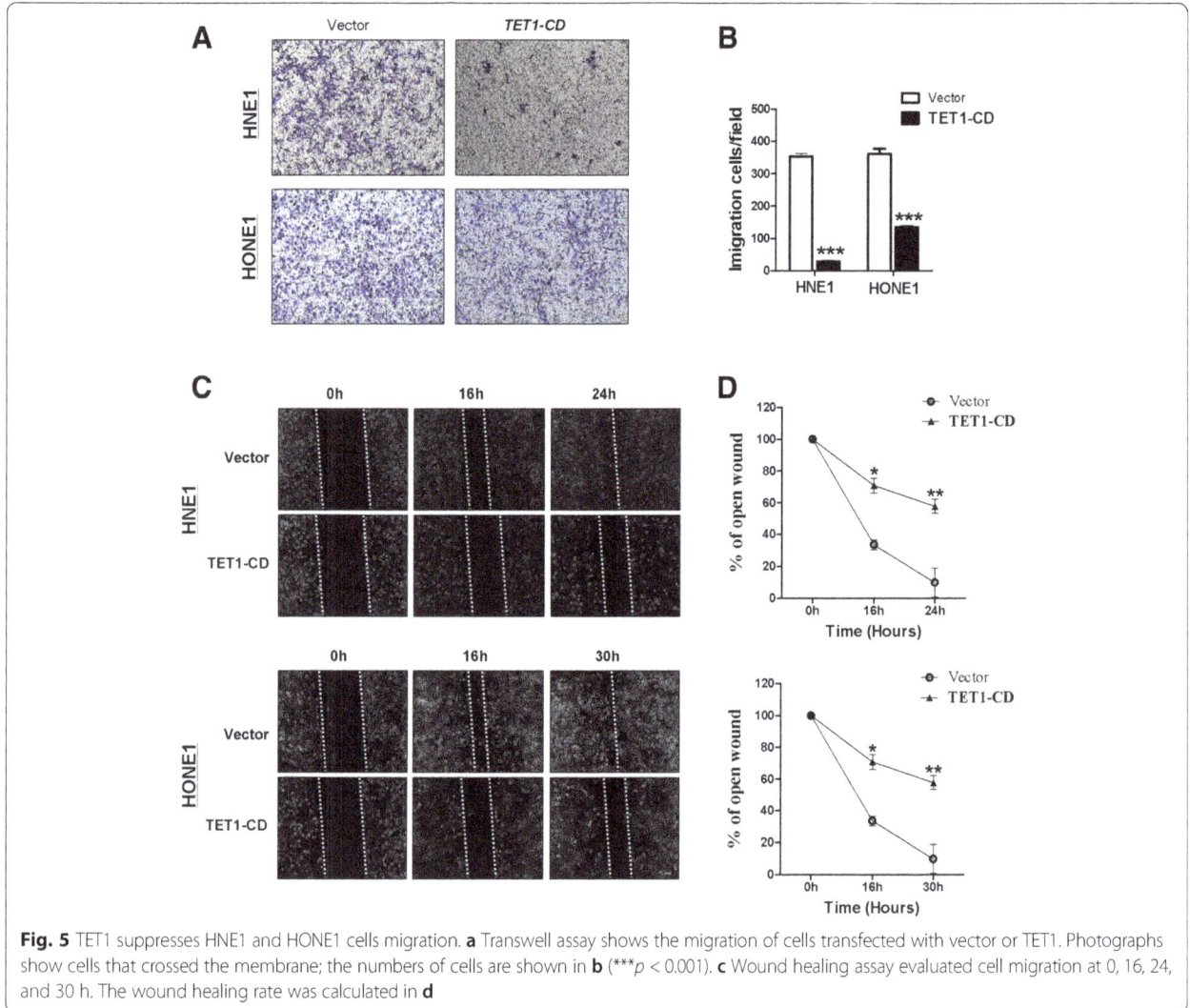

Fig. 5 TET1 suppresses HNE1 and HONE1 cells migration. **a** Transwell assay shows the migration of cells transfected with vector or TET1. Photographs show cells that crossed the membrane; the numbers of cells are shown in **b** (***$p < 0.001$). **c** Wound healing assay evaluated cell migration at 0, 16, 24, and 30 h. The wound healing rate was calculated in **d**

β-catenin signaling, the expression of Wnt pathway antagonists, including DACT family genes (*DACT1, 2, 3*), DKK (*DKK1, 2, 3*) family genes, and SFRP family genes (*SFRP1* and *SFRP2*), in TET1-transfected and vector-transfected cells was assayed by qRT-PCR and revealed an increase of *DACT2, SFRP1,* and *SFRP2* mRNA expression in TET1-transfected cells compared with vector controls (Fig. 8b). In addition to Wnt pathway antagonists, we also found that the *Wnt5A* and *Wnt5B* were upregulated in TET1-transfected NPC cells (Fig. 8b). Furthermore, we found that Wnt5B, SFRP1, and SFRP2 were hypermethylated in nasopharyngeal carcinoma tissues (Additional file 3: Figure S3), and the hypermethylation of DKKs and DACTs in nasopharyngeal carcinoma tissues was also confirmed [15, 36]. In the meantime, the reduced methylation status of DACT2, Wnt5A, and SFRP2 promoter was detected in TET1-CD-expressing tumor cells, with increased unmethylated sites at the promoter CpG regions (Fig. 8c), suggesting that TET1

really acts as a demethylase to renew expression of multiple TSGs in tumor cells. MeDIP and hMeDIP experiments were used to further confirm the demethylation of TET1; the results showed that TET1 can cause an increase of 5-hmC and reduction of 5mC in promoters of Wnt5A, SFRP2, and DACT2 in HNE1 cells (Fig. 8d). These studies suggested that TET1 can cause demethylation of Wnt5A, SFRP2, and DACT2 in nasopharyngeal carcinoma cells and restore their expression.

Discussion and conclusion

TET1 has been described as a TSG, inhibiting proliferation in renal, colorectal, and gastric cancer [24, 25, 28], and migration and invasion in the lung, breast, and prostate cancer [26, 37, 38]. This study found that TET1 was expressed in normal septum deviation and downregulated in NPC tissues as well as NPC cells, and it was methylated in most NPC tissues and cells. This implies that *TET1* was silenced by hyper-methylation in NPC.

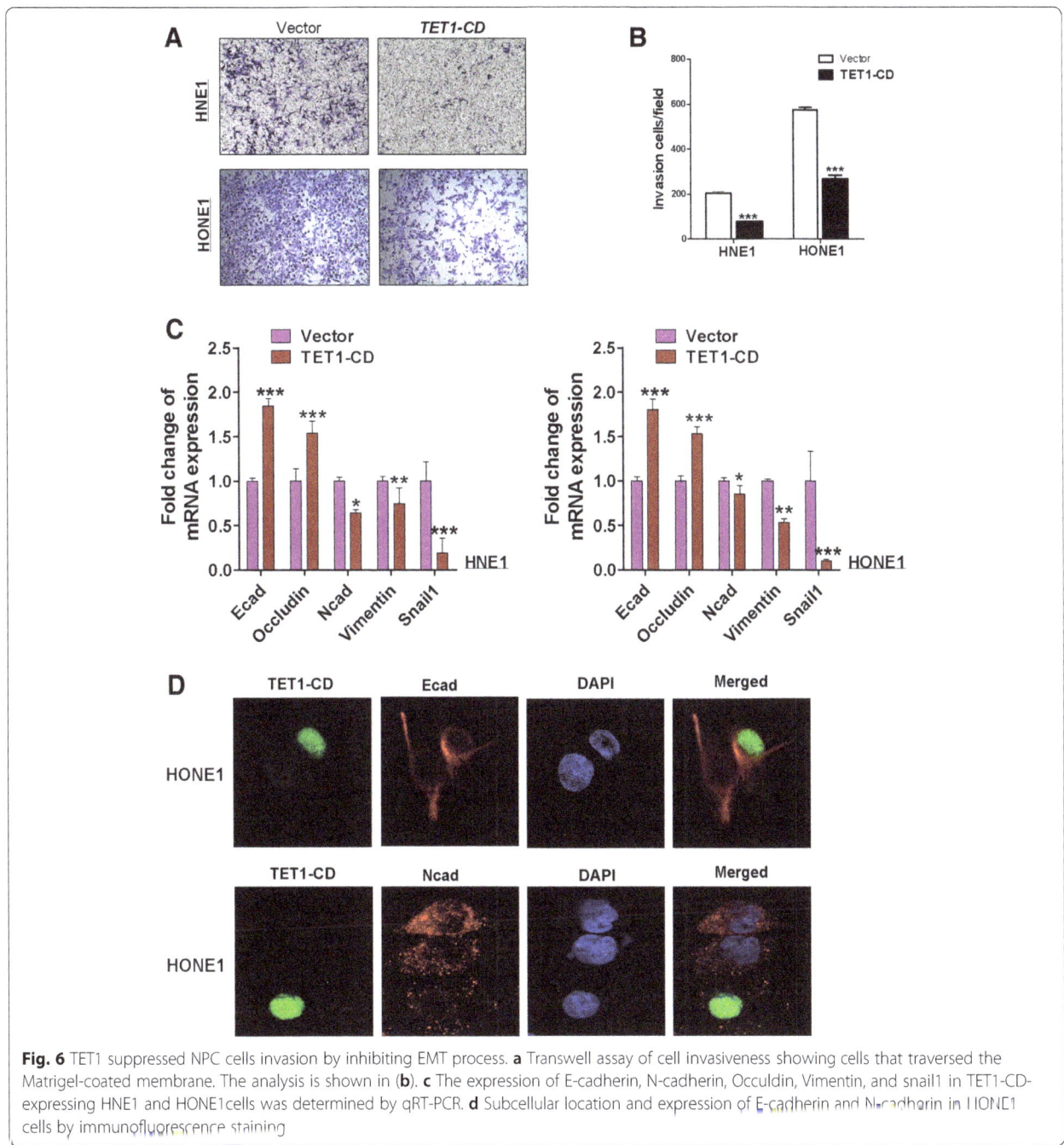

Fig. 6 TET1 suppressed NPC cells invasion by inhibiting EMT process. **a** Transwell assay of cell invasiveness showing cells that traversed the Matrigel-coated membrane. The analysis is shown in (**b**). **c** The expression of E-cadherin, N-cadherin, Occuldin, Vimentin, and snail1 in TET1-CD-expressing HNE1 and HONE1 cells was determined by qRT-PCR. **d** Subcellular location and expression of E-cadherin and N-cadherin in HONE1 cells by immunofluorescence staining

Demethylation by Aza with TSA can restore TET1 expression, but HONE1 treated only by Aza did not restore TET1 expression, indicating other mechanism involving TET1 expression. In present study, TET1 suppressed NPC cell proliferation, motility, and invasiveness. It also induced G0/G1 phase arrest and apoptosis. The results were consisted with other cancers. So, our data indicate that TET1 acts as a TSG activity in NPC.

Many TSGs act by inhibiting Wnt/β-catenin signaling, a pathway known to be sensitive to TSG methylation in NPC [15, 16, 39–41], and TET1 was previously shown

regulating the Wnt/β-catenin pathway in colorectal cancer [24]. We found that TET1 inhibits the expression of β-catenin and its target genes, cyclinD1 and c-Myc. TET1 also prevented β-catenin interaction with T-cell factor/lymphoid enhancer factor (TCF/LEF) transcription factors, which are end point mediators of Wnt signaling. These data demonstrated that TET1 suppressed NPC cell growth by regulating the Wnt/β-catenin signaling pathway.

To determine how TET1 regulated the Wnt/β-catenin signaling pathway, the expression of downstream target

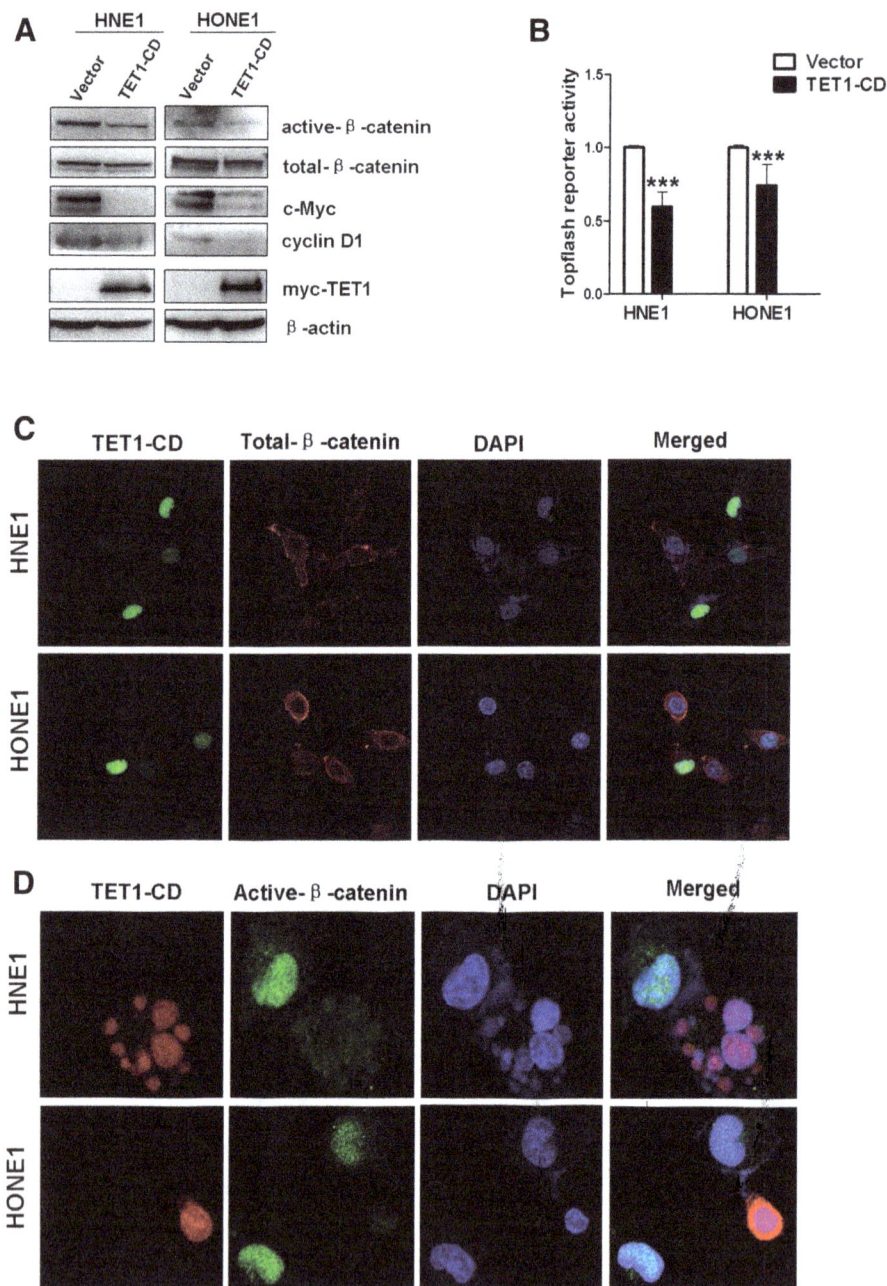

Fig. 7 TET1 inhibits Wnt/β-catenin signaling pathway in NPC. **a** Western blots of β-catenin and the downstream Wnt/β-catenin gene. **b** Top/Fop dual-luciferase reporter assay in HNE1 and HONE1 cells. Fop-flash was the control. **c, d** Subcellular location and expression of total β-catenin and active β-catenin by immunofluorescence staining

genes was assayed. It was previously demonstrated that TET1 could demethylate the PTEN gene, which codes for phosphatase and tensin homolog protein, to inhibit tumor growth in gastric cancer [42]. TET1 suppression of matrix metalloproteins in breast cancer inhibits tumor cell invasion through maintaining expression of *TIMP*2 and *TIMP3* [37]. Epigenetic disruption of Wnt/β-catenin signaling is crucial to several tumorigeneses, especially by promoter methylation of WNT antagonists [43–45].

Methylation of *SFRPs*, *DACT2*, *DKK2*, and *DKK3* was frequently detected in NPC [15]. Recent works suggest that *TET1* upregulates DKKs, which are Wnt pathway inhibitors that suppress CRC and ovarian cancer cell proliferation [24, 46]. Given the crucial role of TET1 in epigenetic modification of WNT antagonists, we thus aimed to thoroughly analyze the expression of Wnt pathway negative regulators in TET1-transfected cells. Our data clearly demonstrated that enforced expression

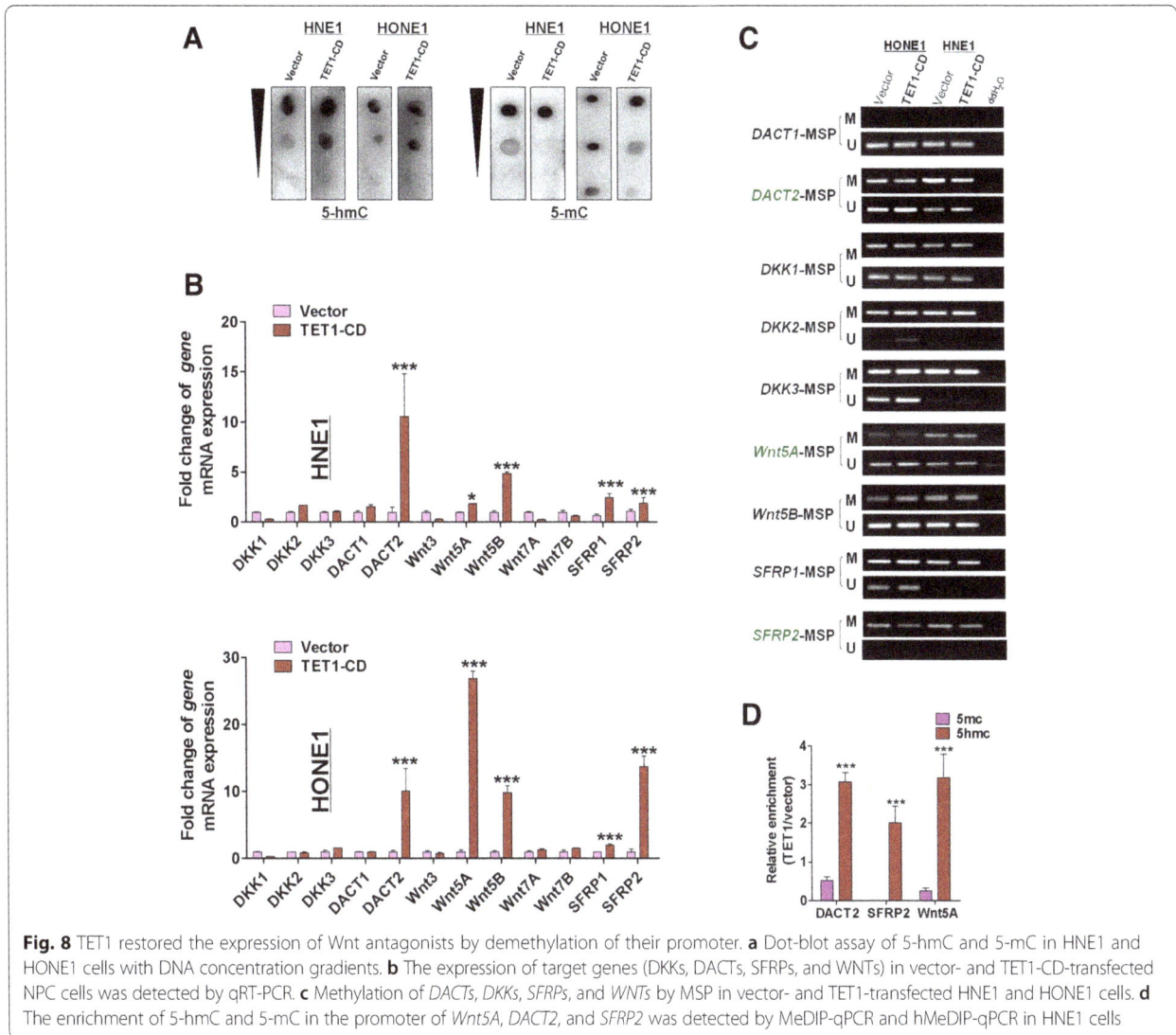

Fig. 8 TET1 restored the expression of Wnt antagonists by demethylation of their promoter. **a** Dot-blot assay of 5-hmC and 5-mC in HNE1 and HONE1 cells with DNA concentration gradients. **b** The expression of target genes (DKKs, DACTs, SFRPs, and WNTs) in vector- and TET1-CD-transfected NPC cells was detected by qRT-PCR. **c** Methylation of *DACTs*, *DKKs*, *SFRPs*, and *WNTs* by MSP in vector- and TET1-transfected HNE1 and HONE1 cells. **d** The enrichment of 5-hmC and 5-mC in the promoter of *Wnt5A*, *DACT2*, and *SFRP2* was detected by MeDIP-qPCR and hMeDIP-qPCR in HNE1 cells

of TET1 indeed significantly restore the expression of *DACT2*, *SFRP1*, and *SFRP2*, but no obvious influence to *DKKs* family, *DACT1* and *DACT3*. In addition, TET1 also increased the expression of *Wnt5A* and *Wnt5B*. And we have shown that *Wnt5B*, *SFRP1*, *SFRP2*, and *DACT2* are hypermethylated in nasopharyngeal carcinoma tissues [36]. But further analysis showed that the methylation status and 5-mC levels of *DACT2*, *SFRP2*, and *Wnt5A* promoter were decreased, accompanying with 5-hmC increased after TET1 upregulation, whereas there were no obvious changes in the promoters of *Wnt5B* and *SFRP1*, suggesting that other mechanisms are involved in *Wnt5B* and *SFRP1* upregulation in TET1 transfected cell line. Li et al. have confirmed that SFRP2 function as TSG in NPC [15]. We also demonstrated that DACT2 act as a TSG in NPC [36].

The Wnt pathway includes canonical Wnt/β-catenin and non-canonical Wnt signaling, which have different roles in cancer progression [15]. The Wnts family includes 19 members. Wnt1, Wnt3, Wnt3A, Wnt7A, Wnt7B, and Wnt8 participate in β-catenin-dependent signaling; Wnt4, Wnt5A, and Wnt11 participate in β-catenin-independent signaling. The canonical Wnt protein Wnt3A promotes the secretion of β-catenin and cancer development. The noncanonical Wnt protein, Wnt5A, inhibits Wnt3A promotion of β-catenin secretion. So far, there are conflicting reports as to whether WNT5A acts as a tumor promotion genes or a tumor suppressor in cancers. Most of the evidence shows that WNT5A overexpression promotes the proliferation, invasion, and metastasis of cells in different types of cancers by promoting the epithelial-mesenchymal transition (EMT) and stem cell-like phenotypes [47–50]. However, contradictory reports showed that increased Wnt5A expression inhibited cell proliferation and motility, and negative Wnt5A expression contributes to the tumor lymph node metastasis and poor prognosis [51–54]. Recently, it was shown that the contradictory roles of Wnt5A are due to existence of various Wnt5A isoforms [55]. Further studies will be needed to identify functions of Wnt5A in NPC.

Added up, we provided the first evidence indicating that TET1 was a TSG in NPC cells and suppressed NPC proliferation, migration, and invasiveness progression via restoring Wnt pathway antagonist expression to antagonize activity of Wnt pathway. Furthermore, this study provides important insights into the regulation of TET1 for Wnt pathway.

Abbreviations

5-hmC: 5-Hydroxymethyl cytosine; 5-mC: 5-Methyl cytosine; AnnexinV-FITC: Annexin V-fluorescein isothiocyanate; Aza: 5-Aza-2-deoxycytidine; BGS: Bisulfite genomic sequencing; DAPI: 4, 6-Diamidino- 2- phenylindole; EMT: Epithelial-to-mesenchymal transition; MSP: Methylation-specific PCR; NPC: Nasopharyngeal carcinoma; NSD: Normal nasal tissues; PVDF: Polyvinylidene difluoride; qRT-PCR: Quantitative real-time PCR; RT-PCR: Semi-quantitative RT-PCR; SDS-PAGE: Sodium dodecyl sulfate polyacrylamide gel electrophoresis; TCF/LEF: T Cell factor/lymphoid enhancer factor; TET: Ten-eleven translocation; TET1: Ten-eleven translocation methyl cytosine dioxygenase1; TSA: Trichostatin A

Acknowledgements
The authors thank Prof. Qian Tao (the Chinese University of Hong Kong, Hong Kong, China) for generously providing cell lines, primers, and plasmids. This study was supported by National Natural Science Foundation of China (#81572769,81372238) and Natural Science Foundation of Chongqing (2016ZDXM006).

Authors' contributions
JF and TX contributed to the conception and design of the research. JF and YZ performed the majority of the experiments in this study. JM, XH, BS, DZ, WP, and JT performed the experiments and analyzed the data. YJ collected the samples. JF wrote the manuscript. GR reviewed the article. TX reviewed data and the final version of the article. All authors reviewed and approved the final manuscript.

Competing interests
The authors declare that they have no competing interests.

References
1. Chan AT, Gregoire V, Lefebvre JL, Licitra L, Hui EP, Leung SF, Felip E, Group E-E-EGW. Nasopharyngeal cancer: EHNS-ESMO-ESTRO Clinical Practice Guidelines for diagnosis, treatment and follow-up. Ann Onco. 2012;23(Suppl 7):vii83–5.
2. Tao Q, Chan AT. Nasopharyngeal carcinoma: molecular pathogenesis and therapeutic developments. Expert Rev Mol Med. 2007;9:1–24.
3. Wei WI, Kwong DL. Current management strategy of nasopharyngeal carcinoma. Clin Exp Otorhinolaryngol. 2010;3:1–12.
4. Lee AW, Ma BB, Ng WT, Chan AT. Management of nasopharyngeal carcinoma: current practice and future perspective. J Clin Oncol. 2015;33:3356–64.
5. Dai W, Zheng H, Cheung AK, Lung ML. Genetic and epigenetic landscape of nasopharyngeal carcinoma. Chin Clin Oncol. 2016;5:16.
6. Li LL, Shu XS, Wang ZH, Cao Y, Tao Q. Epigenetic disruption of cell signaling in nasopharyngeal carcinoma. Chin J Cancer. 2011;30:231–9.
7. Chen T, Long B, Ren G, Xiang T, Li L, Wang Z, He Y, Zeng Q, Hong S, Hu G. Protocadherin20 acts as a tumor suppressor gene: epigenetic inactivation in nasopharyngeal carcinoma. J Cell Biochem. 2015;116:1766–75.
8. Fendri A, Khabir A, Hadri-Guiga B, Sellami-Boudawara T, Daoud J, Frikha M, Ghorbel A, Gargouri A, Mokdad-Gargouri R. Epigenetic alteration of the Wnt inhibitory factor-1 promoter is common and occurs in advanced stage of Tunisian nasopharyngeal carcinoma. Cancer Investig. 2010;28:896–903.
9. Chow LS, Lo KW, Kwong J, To KF, Tsang KS, Lam CW, Dammann R, Huang DP. RASSF1A is a target tumor suppressor from 3p21.3 in nasopharyngeal carcinoma. Int J Cancer. 2004;109:839–47.
10. Jin H, Wang X, Ying J, Wong AH, Li H, Lee KY, Srivastava G, Chan AT, Yeo W, Ma BB, et al. Epigenetic identification of ADAMTS18 as a novel 16q23.1 tumor suppressor frequently silenced in esophageal, nasopharyngeal and multiple other carcinomas. Oncogene. 2007;26:7490–8.
11. Cheung AK, Lung HL, Hung SC, Law EW, Cheng Y, Yau WL, Bangarusamy DK, Miller LD, Liu ET, Shao JY, et al. Functional analysis of a cell cycle-associated, tumor-suppressive gene, protein tyrosine phosphatase receptor type G, in nasopharyngeal carcinoma. Cancer Res. 2008;68:8137–45.
12. Du C, Huang T, Sun D, Mo Y, Feng H, Zhou X, Xiao X, Yu N, Hou B, Huang G, et al. CDH4 as a novel putative tumor suppressor gene epigenetically silenced by promoter hypermethylation in nasopharyngeal carcinoma. Cancer Lett. 2011;309:54–61.
13. Li L, Ying J, Li H, Zhang Y, Shu X, Fan Y, Tan J, Cao Y, Tsao SW, Srivastava G, et al. The human cadherin 11 is a pro-apoptotic tumor suppressor modulating cell stemness through Wnt/beta-catenin signaling and silenced in common carcinomas. Oncogene. 2012;31:3901–12.
14. Zhang S, Li S, Gao JL. Promoter methylation status of the tumor suppressor gene SOX11 is associated with cell growth and invasion in nasopharyngeal carcinoma. Cancer Cell Int. 2013;13:109.
15. Li L, Zhang Y, Fan Y, Sun K, Su X, Du Z, Tsao SW, Loh TK, Sun H, Chan AT, et al. Characterization of the nasopharyngeal carcinoma methylome identifies aberrant disruption of key signaling pathways and methylated tumor suppressor genes. Epigenomics. 2015;7:155–73.
16. Chan SL, Cui Y, van Hasselt A, Li H, Srivastava G, Jin H, Ng KM, Wang Y, Lee KY, Tsao GS, et al. The tumor suppressor Wnt inhibitory factor 1 is frequently methylated in nasopharyngeal and esophageal carcinomas. Lab Investig. 2007;87:644–50.
17. Ito S, D'Alessio AC, Taranova OV, Hong K, Sowers LC, Zhang Y. Role of Tet proteins in 5mC to 5hmC conversion, ES-cell self-renewal and inner cell mass specification. Nature. 2010;466:1129–33.
18. Tahiliani M, Koh KP, Shen Y, Pastor WA, Bandukwala H, Brudno Y, Agarwal S, Iyer LM, Liu DR, Aravind L, Rao A. Conversion of 5-methylcytosine to 5-hydroxymethylcytosine in mammalian DNA by MLL partner TET1. Science. 2009;324:930–5.
19. Frauer C, Rottach A, Meilinger D, Bultmann S, Fellinger K, Hasenoder S, Wang M, Qin W, Soding J, Spada F, Leonhardt H. Different binding properties and function of CXXC zinc finger domains in Dnmt1 and Tet1. PLoS One. 2011;6:e16627.
20. Mohr F, Dohner K, Buske C, Rawat VP. TET genes: new players in DNA demethylation and important determinants for stemness. Exp Hematol. 2011;39:272–81.
21. Ittel A, Jeandidier E, Helias C, Perrusson N, Humbrecht C, Lioure B, Mazurier I, Mayeur-Rousse C, Lavaux A, Thiebault S, et al. First description of the t(10;11) (q22;q23)/MLL-TET1 translocation in a T-cell lymphoblastic lymphoma, with subsequent lineage switch to acute myelomonocytic myeloid leukemia. Haematologica. 2013;98:e166–8.
22. Lorsbach RB, Moore J, Mathew S, Raimondi SC, Mukatira ST, Downing JR. TET1, a member of a novel protein family, is fused to MLL in acute myeloid leukemia containing the t(10;11) (q22;q23). Leukemia. 2003;17:637–41.
23. Sang Y, Cheng C, Tang XF, Zhang MF, Lv XB. Hypermethylation of TET1 promoter is a new diagnosic marker for breast cancer metastasis. Asian Pac J Cancer Prev. 2015;16:1197–200.
24. Neri F, Dettori D, Incarnato D, Krepelova A, Rapelli S, Maldotti M, Parlato C, Paliogiannis P, Oliviero S. TET1 is a tumour suppressor that inhibits colon cancer growth by derepressing inhibitors of the WNT pathway. Oncogene. 2015;34:4168–76.

25. Fu HL, Ma Y, Lu LG, Hou P, Li BJ, Jin WL, Cui DX. TET1 exerts its tumor suppressor function by interacting with p53-EZH2 pathway in gastric cancer. J Biomed Nanotechnol. 2014;10:1217–30.

26. Hsu CH, Peng KL, Kang ML, Chen YR, Yang YC, Tsai CH, Chu CS, Jeng YM, Chen YT, Lin FM, et al. TET1 suppresses cancer invasion by activating the tissue inhibitors of metalloproteinases. Cell Rep. 2012;2:568–79.

27. Lin LL, Wang W, Hu Z, Wang LW, Chang J, Qian H. Negative feedback of miR-29 family TET1 involves in hepatocellular cancer. Med Oncol. 2014;31:291.

28. Fan M, He X, Xu X. Restored expression levels of TET1 decrease the proliferation and migration of renal carcinoma cells. Mol Med Rep. 2015;12:4837–42.

29. Li L, Li C, Mao H, Du Z, Chan WY, Murray P, Luo B, Chan AT, Mok TS, Chan FK, et al. Epigenetic inactivation of the CpG demethylase TET1 as a DNA methylation feedback loop in human cancers. Sci Rep. 2016;6:26591.

30. Xiang T, Li L, Fan Y, Jiang Y, Ying Y, Putti TC, Tao Q, Ren G. PLCD1 is a functional tumor suppressor inducing G(2)/M arrest and frequently methylated in breast cancer. Cancer Biol Ther. 2010;10:520–7.

31. Li L, Xu J, Qiu G, Ying J, Du Z, Xiang T, Wong KY, Srivastava G, Zhu XF, Mok TS, et al. Epigenomic characterization of a p53-regulated 3p22.2 tumor suppressor that inhibits STAT3 phosphorylation via protein docking and is frequently methylated in esophageal and other carcinomas. Theranostics. 2018;8:61–77.

32. Tao Q, Huang H, Geiman TM, Lim CY, Fu L, Qiu GH, Robertson KD. Defective de novo methylation of viral and cellular DNA sequences in ICF syndrome cells. Hum Mol Genet. 2002;11:2091–102.

33. Tao Q, Swinnen LJ, Yang J, Srivastava G, Robertson KD, Ambinder RF. Methylation status of the Epstein-Barr virus major latent promoter C in iatrogenic B cell lymphoproliferative disease. Application of PCR-based analysis. Am J Pathol. 1999;155:619–25.

34. Li L, Ying J, Tong X, Zhong L, Su X, Xiang T, Shu X, Rong R, Xiong L, Li H, et al. Epigenetic identification of receptor tyrosine kinase-like orphan receptor 2 as a functional tumor suppressor inhibiting beta-catenin and AKT signaling but frequently methylated in common carcinomas. Cell Mol Life Sci. 2014;71:2179–92.

35. Pan X, Zhou T, Tai YH, Wang C, Zhao J, Cao Y, Chen Y, Zhang PJ, Yu M, Zhen C, et al. Elevated expression of CUEDC2 protein confers endocrine resistance in breast cancer. Nat Med. 2011;17:708–14.

36. Zhang Y, Fan J, Fan Y, Li L, He X, Xiang Q, Mu J, Zhou D, Sun X, Yang Y, et al. The new 6q27 tumor suppressor DACT2, frequently silenced by CpG methylation, sensitizes nasopharyngeal cancer cells to paclitaxel and 5-FU toxicity via β-catenin/Cdc25c signaling and G2/M arrest. Clin Epigenetics. 2018;10:26.

37. Lu HG, Zhan W, Yan L, Qin RY, Yan YP, Yang ZJ, Liu GC, Li GQ, Wang HF, Li XL, et al. TET1 partially mediates HDAC inhibitor-induced suppression of breast cancer invasion. Mol Med Rep. 2014;10:2595–600.

38. Yokoyama S, Higashi M, Tsutsumida H, Wakimoto J, Hamada T, Wiest E, Matsuo K, Kitazono I, Goto Y, Guo X, et al. TET1-mediated DNA hypomethylation regulates the expression of MUC4 in lung cancer. Genes Cancer. 2017;8:517–27.

39. Ren XY, Zhou GQ, Jiang W, Sun Y, Xu YF, Li YQ, Tang XR, Wen X, He QM, Yang XJ, et al. Low SFRP1 expression correlates with poor prognosis and promotes cell invasion by activating the Wnt/beta-catenin signaling pathway in NPC. Cancer Prev Res (Phila). 2015;8:968–77.

40. Wong AM, Kong KL, Chen L, Liu M, Zhu C, Tsang JW, Guan XY. Characterization of CACNA2D3 as a putative tumor suppressor gene in the development and progression of nasopharyngeal carcinoma. Int J Cancer. 2013;133:2284–95.

41. Chen Z, Tang C, Zhu Y, Xie M, He D, Pan Q, Zhang P, Hua D, Wang T, Jin L, et al. TrpC5 regulates differentiation through the Ca2+/Wnt5a signalling pathway in colorectal cancer. Clin Sci (Lond). 2017;131:227–37.

42. Pei YF, Tao R, Li JF, Su LP, Yu BQ, Wu XY, Yan M, Gu QL, Zhu ZG, Liu BY. TET1 inhibits gastric cancer growth and metastasis by PTEN demethylation and re-expression. Oncotarget. 2016;7:31322–35.

43. Voorham QJ, Janssen J, Tijssen M, Snellenberg S, Mongera S, van Grieken NC, Grabsch H, Kliment M, Rembacken BJ, Mulder CJ, et al. Promoter methylation of Wnt-antagonists in polypoid and nonpolypoid colorectal adenomas. BMC Cancer. 2013;13:603.

44. Rawson JB, Manno M, Mrkonjic M, Daftary D, Dicks E, Buchanan DD, Younghusband HB, Parfrey PS, Young JP, Pollett A, et al. Promoter methylation of Wnt antagonists DKK1 and SFRP1 is associated with opposing tumor subtypes in two large populations of colorectal cancer patients. Carcinogenesis. 2011;32:741–7.

45. Ying Y, Tao Q. Epigenetic disruption of the WNT/beta-catenin signaling pathway in human cancers. Epigenetics. 2009;4:307–12.

46. Duan H, Yan Z, Chen W, Wu Y, Han J, Guo H, Qiao J. TET1 inhibits EMT of ovarian cancer cells through activating Wnt/beta-catenin signaling inhibitors DKK1 and SFRP2. Gynecol Oncol. 2017;147:408–17.

47. Asem MS, Buechler S, Wates RB, Miller DL, Stack MS. Wnt5a signaling in cancer. Cancers (Basel). 2016;8:79.

48. Yap LF, Ahmad M, Zabidi MM, Chu TL, Chai SJ, Lee HM, Lim PV, Wei W, Dawson C, Teo SH, Khoo AS. Oncogenic effects of WNT5A in Epstein-Barr virus-associated nasopharyngeal carcinoma. Int J Oncol. 2014;44:1774–80.

49. Zhu N, Qin L, Luo Z, Guo Q, Yang L, Liao D. Challenging role of Wnt5a and its signaling pathway in cancer metastasis (Review). Exp Ther Med. 2014;8:3–8.

50. Qin L, Yin YT, Zheng FJ, Peng LX, Yang CF, Bao YN, Liang YY, Li XJ, Xiang YQ, Sun R, et al. WNT5A promotes stemness characteristics in nasopharyngeal carcinoma cells leading to metastasis and tumorigenesis. Oncotarget. 2015;6:10239–52.

51. Zhong Z, Shan M, Wang J, Liu T, Shi Q, Pang D. Decreased Wnt5a expression is a poor prognostic factor in triple-negative breast cancer. Med Sci Monit. 2016;22:1–7.

52. Mehdawi LM, Prasad CP, Ehrnstrom R, Andersson T, Sjolander A. Non-canonical WNT5A signaling up-regulates the expression of the tumor suppressor 15-PGDH and induces differentiation of colon cancer cells. Mol Oncol. 2016;10:1415–29.

53. Zhang Y, Du J, Zheng J, Liu J, Xu R, Shen T, Zhu Y, Chang J, Wang H, Zhang Z, et al. EGF-reduced Wnt5a transcription induces epithelial-mesenchymal transition via Arf6-ERK signaling in gastric cancer cells. Oncotarget. 2015;6:7244–61.

54. Thiele S, Gobel A, Rachner TD, Fuessel S, Froehner M, Muders MH, Baretton GB, Bernhardt R, Jakob F, Gluer CC, et al. WNT5A has anti-prostate cancer effects in vitro and reduces tumor growth in the skeleton in vivo. J Bone Miner Res. 2015;30:471–80.

55. Huang TC, Lee PT, Wu MH, Huang CC, Ko CY, Lee YC, Lin DY, Cheng YW, Lee KH. Distinct roles and differential expression levels of Wnt5a mRNA isoforms in colorectal cancer cells. PLoS One. 2017;12:e0181034.

3

Promoter methylation of the *MGAT3* and *BACH2* genes correlates with the composition of the immunoglobulin G glycome in inflammatory bowel disease

Marija Klasić[1†], Dora Markulin[1†], Aleksandar Vojta[1], Ivana Samaržija[1], Ivan Biruš[1], Paula Dobrinić[1], Nicholas T. Ventham[2], Irena Trbojević-Akmačić[3], Mirna Šimurina[3], Jerko Štambuk[3], Genadij Razdorov[3], Nicholas A. Kennedy[2,5], Jack Satsangi[2,10], Ana M. Dias[6], Salome Pinho[6], Vito Annese[7], Anna Latiano[8], Renata D'Inca[9], IBD consortium, Gordan Lauc[3,4] and Vlatka Zoldoš[1*]

Abstract

Background: Many genome- and epigenome-wide association studies (GWAS and EWAS) and studies of promoter methylation of candidate genes for inflammatory bowel disease (IBD) have demonstrated significant associations between genetic and epigenetic changes and IBD. Independent GWA studies have identified genetic variants in the *BACH2, IL6ST, LAMB1, IKZF1,* and *MGAT3* loci to be associated with both IBD and immunoglobulin G (IgG) glycosylation.

Methods: Using bisulfite pyrosequencing, we analyzed CpG methylation in promoter regions of these five genes from peripheral blood of several hundred IBD patients and healthy controls (HCs) from two independent cohorts, respectively.

Results: We found significant differences in the methylation levels in the *MGAT3* and *BACH2* genes between both Crohn's disease and ulcerative colitis when compared to HC. The same pattern of methylation changes was identified for both genes in CD19[+] B cells isolated from the whole blood of a subset of the IBD patients. A correlation analysis was performed between the *MGAT3* and *BACH2* promoter methylation and individual IgG glycans, measured in the same individuals of the two large cohorts. *MGAT3* promoter methylation correlated significantly with galactosylation, sialylation, and bisecting GlcNAc on IgG of the same patients, suggesting that activity of the GnT-III enzyme, encoded by this gene, might be altered in IBD. The correlations between the *BACH2* promoter methylation and IgG glycans were less obvious, since *BACH2* is not a glycosyltransferase and therefore may affect IgG glycosylation only indirectly.

Conclusions: Our results suggest that epigenetic deregulation of key glycosylation genes might lead to an increase in pro-inflammatory properties of IgG in IBD through a decrease in galactosylation and sialylation and an increase of bisecting GlcNAc on digalactosylated glycan structures. Finally, we showed that CpG methylation in the promoter of the *MGAT3* gene is altered in CD3[+] T cells isolated from inflamed mucosa of patients with ulcerative colitis from a third smaller cohort, for which biopsies were available, suggesting a functional role of this glyco-gene in IBD pathogenesis.

* Correspondence: vzoldos@biol.pmf.hr
†Marija Klasić and Dora Markulin contributed equally to this work.
[1]Department of Biology, Division of Molecular Biology, Faculty of Science, University of Zagreb, Horvatovac 102a, 10000 Zagreb, Croatia
Full list of author information is available at the end of the article

Background

Inflammatory bowel disease (IBD) is a chronic intestinal inflammatory condition classified in two major forms— Crohn's disease (CD) and ulcerative colitis (UC)—which exhibit etiologically and clinically distinct features. Nowadays, IBD affects 2.5–3 million people in Europe and causes considerable morbidity [1]. Despite numerous clinical, genetic, and other experimental studies, our understanding of IBD development and progression remains incomplete.

It is generally accepted that IBD represents an aberrant immune response to gut microbiota in genetically susceptible individuals [2]. Genome-wide association studies (GWAS) have identified over 200 genetic susceptibility loci, the majority of which were associated with both forms of IBD in genome-wide meta-analysis [3–7]. However, common genetic variants account only for 8.2 and 13.1% heritability of UC and CD, respectively [7]. Interaction of an individual's gut microbiome, immune system, genetic background, and environmental factors, such as smoking, diet, drugs, and physical activity [2, 8–10], makes IBD a complex etiopathogenic entity. The challenge is therefore to identify additional factors involved in the development and progression of this disease, especially given its rapidly increasing incidence. It is probable that epigenetics play a key role in the interactions between environmental, microbial, and genetic factors that participate in IBD development and progression. These include DNA methylation and histone modifications, as well as some other epigenetic mechanisms [11–13]; for a review, see [14, 15].

DNA methylation remains the most studied epigenetic modification, readily assayed in a large number of individuals/samples. Hypermethylation of gene promoters is generally associated with gene silencing, while promoter hypomethylation is associated with gene activation [16]. Environmentally changed DNA methylation pattern may contribute to the development of many complex diseases by mediating the interplay between external and internal factors and the gene expression [17–21]. There are also data to suggest that the aforementioned environmental modifiers of IBD can also affect DNA methylation [17–19, 22]. Epigenetic component of IBD has been addressed in many studies, mostly by whole genome methylation analysis performed on peripheral blood mononuclear cells (PBMCs) or mucosal tissue, revealing regions differentially methylated between the disease and healthy state, as well as between CD and UC [11–13, 23–26].

The majority of eukaryotic proteins are modified by addition of complex oligosaccharides (glycans) through the process of glycosylation. Therefore, glycans are an integral part of nearly all membrane and secreted proteins, including components of the immune system [27]. Aberrant protein glycosylation is implicated in virtually every human complex disease, including inflammation [28–31]. Previous studies have suggested that N-glycosylation of secreted and membrane proteins might be regulated epigenetically and that aberrant glycosylation profiles in disease can arise through aberrant epigenetics [32–38]. A comprehensive review about the role of protein glycosylation in IBD has been given recently [39]. N-glycosylation of serum-circulating proteins (such as the acute phase proteins; immunoglobulin G, IgG; and immunoglobulin A, IgA) or whole plasma N-glycome (i.e., N-glycans present on all plasma proteins) has been the focus of IBD biomarker discovery [36, 40–43]. In addition, our partners from IBD consortium and others established that altered glycosylation of IgG, which is a key effector of the humoral immune system, has a role in balancing inflammation at the systemic level [42–46].

GWA studies indicated associations of IBD with several loci involved in protein glycosylation [47, 48]. More recently, the first GWAS of IgG glycosylation identified 16 loci specifically associated with changes in IgG glycosylation [49]. Interestingly, five of these loci showed pleiotropy with IBD: *MGAT3*, a glyco-gene encoding for a glycosyltransferase, GnT-III; *LAMB1*, a member of transmembrane glycoprotein family of extracellular matrix; the *IL6ST*, a signal transducer shared by many cytokines; *IKZF1*; and *BACH2*, transcription factors involved in B cell differentiation, activation, and maturation. Only the *MGAT3* is a classical glyco-gene with a known function in IgG glycosylation, while the exact functional roles for other four GWAS hits in IgG glycosylation or IBD remain unknown.

In this study, we investigated promoter methylation differences in these five genes, associated with both IBD and IgG glycosylation, in peripheral whole blood of several hundred IBD patients from two independent cohorts. We also correlated promoter methylation data with IgG glycosylation data analyzed previously for the same IBD patients by our partners from the IDD consortium [43, 46, 50]. Peripheral blood was used for DNA methylation analysis and serum or plasma was used for glycan analysis, since one of our goals was the search for potential IBD biomarkers. As peripheral whole blood is a heterogeneous cell mixture with specific methylation pattern for each of the cell types [51], we also analyzed promoter methylation of our candidate genes in CD19+ B cells and CD3+ T cells isolated from peripheral blood mononuclear cells (PBMCs). B cells were of our particular interest since these cells produce IgG on their membrane and are precursors of plasma cells which secrete IgG. We have further explored if aberrant promoter methylation recorded in peripheral whole blood of IBD patients can be a proxy for epigenetic events occurring in the inflamed mucosa. To address this question, we analyzed DNA methylation from PBMCs, CD3$^+$ T cells isolated from PBMCs, and CD3$^+$ T cells isolated from inflamed colonic mucosa of UC patients from the third smaller cohort, for which biopsies were available.

Methods

Patient selection and ethics

Patients were recruited prospectively from Edinburgh, UK, and Florence, Italy, as a part of the IBD-BIOM project. The recruitment of patients from Edinburgh has been described elsewhere [13, 43]. Briefly, we recruited IBD patients prospectively as close as possible to the date of diagnosis from gastroenterology outpatient and endoscopy appointments between 2012 and 2015. We recruited symptomatic controls from gastroenterology clinics during the same period. In these individuals, we had excluded IBD and other organic bowel pathology following biochemical and/or endoscopic investigations. We recruited a further healthy volunteer cohort with no gastrointestinal symptoms. IBD patients were stratified by disease type (ulcerative colitis, UC, and Crohn's disease, CD). Detailed genetic, phenotypic, and other data regarding IBD cases are given in Additional file 1: Tables S1 and S2. Florence cohort was collected through the network of the Italian Group for IBD (IG-IBD) since the beginning of 2001 and first described in 2005 [1] following an internal validation of phenotyping. Subsequently, longitudinal update has been performed on a yearly basis.

Ethical approvals were obtained from Tayside Committee on Medical Ethics B, and all patients and controls provided written, informed consent (LREC 06/S1101/16, LREC 2000/4/192).

Florence recruitment details

IBD patients were prospectively recruited as close as possible to the date of diagnosis from gastroenterology outpatient and endoscopy appointments between years 2012 and 2015 in different tertiary referral centers in San Giovanni Rotondo, Rome, Rozzano (Milan), Padua, and Florence, Italy. Symptomatic controls were recruited in the same centers (gastroenterology clinics) during the same period. In these individuals, IBD and other organic bowel pathology were excluded by biochemical and/or endoscopic investigations. IBD patients were stratified by disease type (ulcerative colitis, UC, and Crohn's disease, CD). Samples were obtained with the same methodology (see further) and centrally collected at San Giovanni Rotondo, Italy.

Sample collection

We collected whole blood at the time of patient recruitment into 9-ml serum Z-clot activator tubes (Greiner),

allowed them to clot at 4 °C for 60 min, and then centrifuged at 2500×g for 15 min. The serum was aliquoted off and stored at – 80 °C until further analysis.

A subset of patients and controls recruited in Edinburgh (Additional file 1: Table S3) underwent immunomagnetic cell separation to obtain CD19$^+$ B cells. The methods have previously been detailed elsewhere [13]. Venepuncture using 9-ml K3 EDTA vacuette (Greiner) tubes was performed to obtain between of 18 and 36 ml of EDTA-buffered blood. An initial Ficoll (Ficoll-Paque, GE Healthcare, Bucks, UK) density gradient centrifugation was performed to obtain peripheral blood mononuclear cells. Cells labelled with antibody-coated microbeads (human CD8$^+$ and CD19$^+$ microbeads, 20 µl per 1×10^7 cells) were immunomagnetic separated using the auto-MACs Pro cell separator (Miltenyi, Germany). CD19$^+$ separations were performed following an initial CD8$^+$ depletion step. Nucleic acids were extracted using AllPrep (Qiagen, Hilden, Germany) according to the manufacturer's guidance and stored at – 80 °C.

Colonic biopsies from controls and UC patients with inactive and active form of disease were mechanically dissociated to prepare single-cell suspensions using Hanks' balanced salt solution modified medium, without calcium chloride and magnesium sulfate (HBSS) (Sigma), with penicillin/streptomycin and gentamicin. PBMCs were obtained by density gradient centrifugation using Lymphoprep. CD3$^+$ T cells (from biopsies and blood) were magnetically sorted by using the EasySep™ Human T Cell Enrichment Kit (STEMCELL) following the manufacturer's instructions. Following cell isolation, DNA extraction was performed using the Invisorb Spin Tissue Mini Kit (Stratec Molecular) following the manufacturer's instructions.

DNA methylation analysis

We analyzed promoter methylation of the candidate genes in the DNA from whole blood, as well as from the separated CD19$^+$ B cells. In addition, for the *MGAT3*, which is a glycosyltransferase with direct and known function in IgG glycosylation [52], we analyzed promoter methylation—in DNA from PBMCs, CD3$^+$ T cells isolated from PBMCs, and CD3$^+$ T cells isolated from the colonic mucosa of healthy controls and UC patients (classified according to active and inactive form of the disease) of the third independent smaller subcohort collected by the Gastroenterology Department of Centro Hospitalar do Porto-Hospital de Santo António, Portugal (Additional file 1: Table S4). All specimens were subjected to histological examination and classification. All participants gave informed consent about all clinical procedures, and research protocols were approved by the ethics committee of CHP/HSA, Portugal (233/12(179-DEFI/177-CES).

For DNA methylation analysis, 500 ng of DNA from whole blood was bisulfite converted using EZ-96 DNA Methylation Gold kit (Zymo Research, Freiburg, Germany), and 100 ng of DNA from CD19$^+$ B cells, PBMCs, and T cells was converted using EZ DNA Methylation Gold kit (Zymo Research, Freiburg, Germany) according to the manufacturer's protocol. Two to six pyrosequencing assays were developed for promoter regions of each of the five candidate genes (BACH2, MGAT3, IL6ST, IKZF1, and LAMB1). The selection of analyzed CpG sites was random for assays 2–5 of the MGAT3 gene. CpG sites within the MGAT3 assay 1 were selected based on the GEO (Gene Expression Omnibus) database where methylation data were obtained using Illumina HumanMethylation450 Bead-Chip v1.1 technology. For the BACH2 gene, assays were selected based on location of differentially methylated CpGs in different cell lines tested by ENCODE project, using Illumina HumanMethylation450 BeadChip v1.1 technology (a newer version, the Infinium MethylationE-PIC 850K was not available at the time). We used traditional bisulfite-based protocols which cannot discriminate between 5-methylcytosine (5-mC) and 5-hydroxymethylcytosine (5-hmC) as oxidative bisulfite (oxBS-450K) method can [53]. However, recent studies have shown that global DNA hydroxymethylation is very low in blood cells [54, 55]. Furthermore, hydroxymethylation is significantly depleted from promotors and CpG islands, while enriched in the gene bodies [53, 56].

Based on the estimated statistical power, we did initial screening on 60 patients for each pyrosequencing assay, after which we excluded those genes (pyrosequencing assays) that did not show any statistically significant differences between IBD patients and healthy controls. Pyrosequencing assays for LAMB1, IL6ST, and IKZF1 are shown in Additional file 2: Figure S1. We continued to analyze promoter methylation only in the BACH2 and MGAT3 genes. Specific regions were amplified using PyroMark PCR kit (Qiagen, Hilden, Germany). The cycling conditions for the BACH2 gene were as follows: initial polymerase activation step for 15 min at 95 °C followed by 50 cycles of 30 s denaturation at 95 °C, primer annealing for 30 s at primer-specific temperatures (Additional file 1: Table S5), and 30 s at 72 °C, with final extension at 72 °C for 10 min. The cycling protocol used for amplification of the MGAT3 gene fragments was described previously [35], with the annealing temperature adjusted to 55 °C for the fragment 1 performed on DNA from CD19$^+$ B cells. For quantitative measurement of DNA methylation level at specific CpG sites, PCR-amplified bisulfite-converted DNA was sequenced using the PyroMark Q24 Advanced pyrosequencing system (Qiagen) according to the manufacturer's recommendations. Sequences of PCR and pyrosequencing primers for the BACH2 and the MGAT3 genes are listed in Additional file 1: Table S5. EpiTect PCR Control DNA Set (methylated and unmethylated bisulfite-converted human DNA, Qiagen) was used as a control for PCR and pyrosequencing reactions.

Statistical analysis

The nonparametric Mann-Whitney U test was used to compare the methylation status of CpG sites encompassed by the pyrosequencing assays in the MGAT3 and BACH2 genes between the two independent groups: HC compared to each of CD or UC. Significance threshold was set at $p < 0.05$ with additional Bonferroni correction for multiple testing. Given that age was our primary concern as a potential confounder, we visualized the age in the three groups (CD, UC, and HC) for the samples included in each analysis as violin plots (Additional file 3: Figure S2) and assured there was no significant difference between the age groups ($p > 0.05$) using the Mann-Whitney U test. This was done to assure the validity and strengthen the rationale for the selection of statistical methods.

For the data of the MGAT3 promoter methylation from PBMCs, CD3$^+$ T cells isolated from blood, and CD3$^+$ T cells isolated from inflamed colonic mucosa (the Porto cohort), the Mann-Whitney U test was applied with Bonferroni correction accounting for 15 CpG sites.

Glycan analysis

Glycans present on IgG were analyzed from serum of over 1000 IBD (UC and CD) patients and healthy controls in the Edinburgh cohort using ultra performance liquid chromatography (UPLC) [43, 50]. In the Florence cohort, plasma samples of 3500 IBD patients and healthy controls was used for analysis of IgG glycopeptides by liquid chromatography coupled to mass spectrometry (LC-MS) [46]. The data for IgG glycosylation analysis were used in this work for correlation analysis with promoter methylation data of MGAT3 and BACH2 genes, with matching samples from the very same patients and healthy controls.

Isolation of IgG from blood plasma

IgG has been isolated from blood plasma by affinity chromatography using CIM Protein G 96-well plate (BIA Separations, Ajdovščina, Slovenia) and vacuum manifold (Pall Corporation, Port Washington, NY, USA) as previously described [57, 58]. In short, plasma samples (50–90 μl) were diluted with 1 × PBS, pH 7.4 in the ratio 1:7. All samples were filtered through 0.45 and 0.2-μm AcroPrep GHP filter plates (Pall Corporation) using vacuum manifold and immediately applied to pre-conditioned Protein G plate. After washing of the

Protein G plate, IgG was eluted with 0.1 mol L^{-1} formic acid and immediately neutralized with ammonium bicarbonate to pH 7.0. Protein G plate was regenerated and stored at 4 °C.

IgG glycosylation analysis using ultra-performance liquid chromatography

N-glycans from isolated IgG in the Edinburgh cohort were released with PNGase F after drying 300 μl of each IgG elution fraction, labeled with 2-aminobenzamide and excess of regents removed by clean-up using hydrophilic interaction liquid chromatography solid phase extraction (HILIC-SPE). Fluorescently labeled and purified N-glycans were separated by HILIC-UPLC using Acquity UPLC instrument (Waters, Milford, MA, USA) as previously described [43]. Samples were separated into 24 peaks [57], and the amount of N-glycans in each chromatographic peak was expressed as a percentage of total integrated area (% area).

IgG glycosylation analysis using liquid chromatography coupled to mass spectrometry

In the Florence cohort, Fc-specific IgG glycopeptides were analyzed after IgG purification, overnight trypsin digestion at 37 °C, and reverse-phase purification on Chromabond C18 beads using vacuum manifold as described [46, 59]. Samples were analyzed using nanoliquid chromatography coupled to mass spectrometry (nanoLC-MS), on a nanoACQUITY UPLC system (Waters, Milford Massachusetts, USA) coupled to quadrupole-TOF-MS (Compact; Bruker Daltonics, Bremen, Germany) equipped with a sheath-flow ESI sprayer (capillary electrophoresis ESI-MS sprayer; Agilent Technologies, Santa Clara, USA) as previously described [46]. The nanoACQUITY UPLC system and the Bruker Compact Q-TOF-MS were operated under HyStar software version 3.2.

Data was processed as described previously [46, 60]. This resulted in the extraction of 16 IgG1, 16 IgG2/3, and 11 IgG4 glycoforms. The tryptic Fc-glycopeptides for IgG2 and IgG3 subclasses have identical peptide moieties in the Caucasian population and are therefore not distinguishable with this methodology. Annotation of the spectra was done based on accurate mass according to the relevant literature [40, 57].

Correlation analysis

Methylation data for the *BACH2* (assay 2) and the *MGAT3* (assays 1 and 2) genes (obtained for the two large cohorts) were filtered according to the peak quality by rejecting peaks marked as "failed" by the pyrosequencing software. Average methylation across all assayed CpG sites was calculated for each pyrosequencing assay in each cohort. Methylation results for individual patients were matched with their corresponding glycan profiles. Sizes of datasets and patient classes obtained after including complete records (i.e., both methylation data and glycan profiles present) are shown in Additional file 1: Table S6. Individual glycan structures were represented as relative abundances and batch-corrected. Percentage of structures with bisecting N-acetylglucosamine was calculated for each cohort as a derived trait at this point. Glycan structures identified by each method were translated to Oxford notation, and only the 13 structures present in both the Edinburgh and Florence datasets were considered for correlation. We used IgG1 data from the Florence cohort, as this isoform was the most abundant. Three additional derived traits were calculated: ratios of FA2B to FA2, FA2BG1 to FA2G1, and FA2BG2 to FA2G2.

Pearson correlation between CpG methylation data and 17 glycan features (13 structures and 4 derived traits) was calculated. Significance threshold was set at $p < 0.05$ with additional Bonferroni correction for 17-fold multiple testing.

Methylation of assayed CpG sites in promoters of the *BACH2* and *MGAT3* genes was correlated with measured glycan structures. Pearson correlation coefficient along with the associated p value was calculated between average CpG methylation (for all genes/assays) and each measured IgG glycan structure. Calculation was done on pairwise complete observations. Only correlations with the p value below 0.01 were considered further. Next, correlation coefficients for all CpG assays were calculated, which was used to rank glycan structures according to regulation by the assayed region. Glycan structures with the strongest correlation (either positive or negative) to CpG methylation were then used to explain regulatory effects. All calculations and data visualizations were done in R language and environment for statistical computing (R Foundation for Statistical Computing, Vienna, Austria). Visualization of correlations was done using the R package "corrplot."

Results
Promoter methylation of the candidate genes in whole blood and B cells of IBD patients

In order to assess the level of methylation in CpG islands of the five candidate genes (*BACH2*, *MGAT3*, *IKZF1*, *LAMB1*, and *IL6ST*), associated with both IBD and IgG glycosylation by GWAS, we developed several pyrosequencing assays for each of the genes (Fig. 1 and Additional file 2: Figure S1). We performed initial screening of the pyrosequencing assays on 60 patients. Overall cytosine methylation levels were very low for *LAMB1* (average value per group < 8%), for *IL6ST* (< 3.5%), and for *IKZF1* (< 4%) in the assayed portion of their promoters; therefore, we

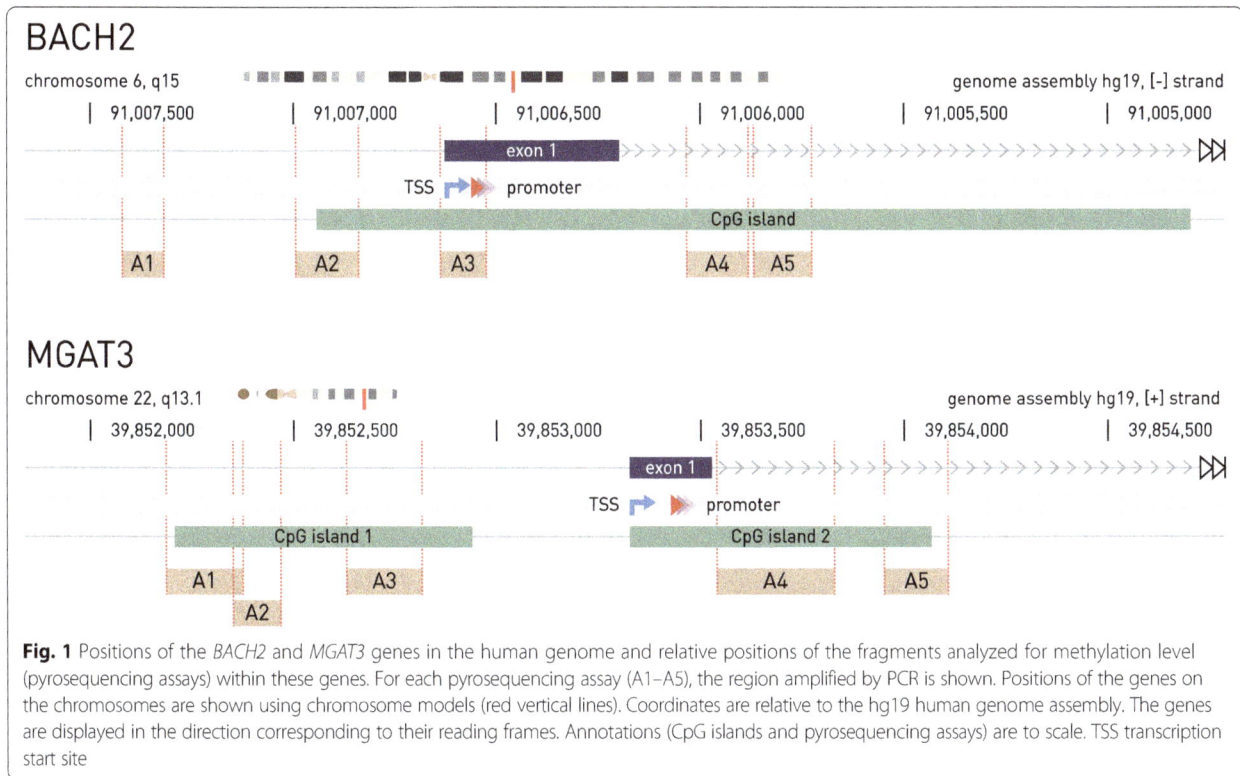

Fig. 1 Positions of the *BACH2* and *MGAT3* genes in the human genome and relative positions of the fragments analyzed for methylation level (pyrosequencing assays) within these genes. For each pyrosequencing assay (A1–A5), the region amplified by PCR is shown. Positions of the genes on the chromosomes are shown using chromosome models (red vertical lines). Coordinates are relative to the hg19 human genome assembly. The genes are displayed in the direction corresponding to their reading frames. Annotations (CpG islands and pyrosequencing assays) are to scale. TSS transcription start site

could not identify differential methylation. We then excluded these genes from further analysis.

MGAT3 and *BACH2* promoter methylation was analyzed in several hundred IBD patients and healthy controls from two independent cohorts (Additional file 1: Tables S1 and S2). In these genes, we analyzed methylation level at 47 CpGs covered by five pyrosequencing assays in the *BACH2* gene: 21 CpG sites were in the promoter region, 1 CpG site was in first exon, and 25 CpG sites were located in the first intron of the gene. A total of 32 CpG sites, covered by five pyrosequencing assays, was analyzed for *MGAT3*: 18 CpG sites were located in the promoter region and 14 CpG sites in the first intron (Fig. 1). Most of those CpG sites were located within CpG islands of the both genes. We found differential CpG methylation between IBD patients and HC within the assay A2, located at 213–368 bp upstream (relative to the gene orientation) of the TSS in the *BACH2* promoter and within the assays A1 and A2, located in the CpG island 1 of the *MGAT3* gene. The same pattern of differential methylation at these CpG sites was observed in whole blood of patients and HC from two large independent cohorts (Fig. 2). CpG methylation level was generally low (up to 20%) in the assayed portion of the *BACH2* promoter; however, significant differences between HC and CD methylation level were recorded at CpG sites 4, 5, 6, and 8 (Fig. 2a). For the assayed portion of the *MGAT3* promoter, general

methylation level was high, with all CpG sites showing a reproducibly significant difference between HC and both CD and UC. CpG sites 2, 13, and 15 showed significant differences only for CD but not for UC. Direction of change was different for the two genes—differentially methylated CpG sites within the *BACH2* promoter were hypomethylated, while those for the *MGAT3* gene were hypermethylated in disease compared to healthy individuals.

These results were confirmed on CD19+ B cells isolated from peripheral whole blood of the independent, smaller patient sample from the Edinburgh cohort (67 samples). The CpG sites 1–5 and 12–13 in the *MGAT3* promoter were differentially methylated between CD and HC. Only CpG site 5 within the assay A2 of the *BACH2* gene showed change in the methylation level between HC and CD in CD19+ B cells (Fig. 2b). There were no differences in the methylation level of the same CpG sites within assayed fragments of the *BACH2* and *MGAT3* genes between UC and HC.

It is worth noting that the same pattern of CpG methylation differences was observed in PBMCs of the IBD patients and HC from both large independent cohorts, and most of the CpG sites within the assayed portion of the *MGAT3* promoter were also differentially methylated in CD19+ B cells from the subset of IBD patients from the Edinburgh cohort (Fig. 2a, b).

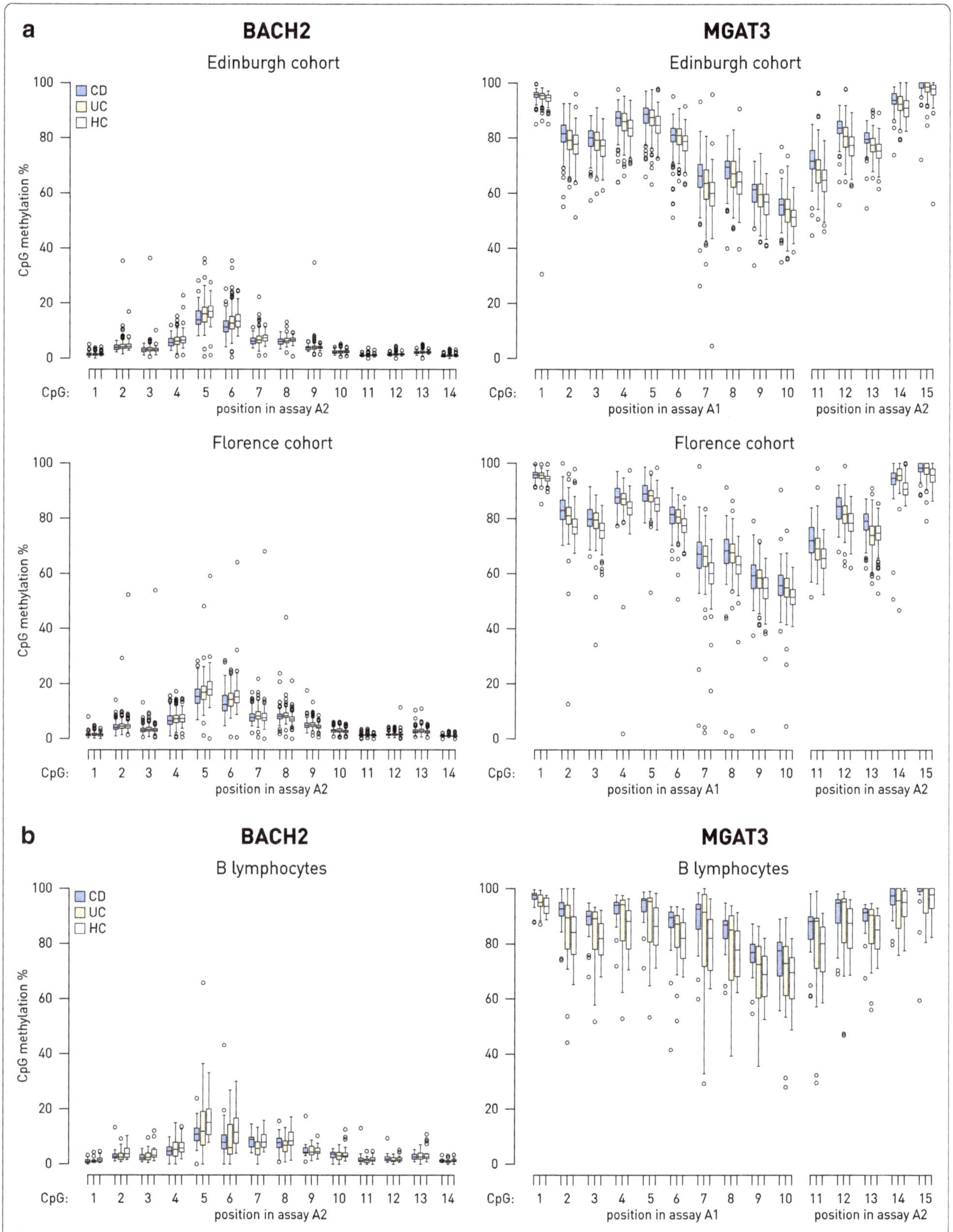

Fig. 2 (See legend on next page.)

Fig. 2 Box plot of CpG methylation in peripheral whole blood for the *BACH2* and *MGAT3* genes in the Edinburgh and Florence cohorts and in B cells from a subset of patients from Edinburgh cohort. Groups were compared using the Mann-Whitney *U* test with significance threshold of $p = 0.05$, corrected for multiple testing using the Bonferroni method. **a** Methylation levels were generally low in the assayed portion of the *BACH2* gene promoter, with significant differences between HC and CD methylation at CpG sites 4, 5, 6, and 8 (replicated in both cohorts). For the *MGAT3* gene, general methylation level was high, with all CpG sites showing a reproducibly significant difference between HC and both CD and UC, except for CpG sites 2, 13, and 15 for which reproducible significant differences were found only between HC and CD. **b** In B cells, isolated from PBMCs of a subset of the patients from the Edinburg cohort, differential methylation was found at the CpG position 5 of the *BACH2* gene (assay 2) between HC and CD, while for the *MGAT3* gene, differentially methylated were CpG sites 1–5, 12, and 13 between HC and CD. CD Crohn's disease, UC ulcerative colitis, HC healthy controls

Promoter methylation of the *MGAT3* gene in CD3⁺ T cells from PBMCs and inflamed colonic mucosa of UC patients

We included in our investigation biopsy samples of UC patients from an independent cohort from the Gastro-enterology Department of Centro Hospitalar do Porto-Hospital de Santo António, Portugal. Given the technical challenges in obtaining DNA and RNA from a small number of purified cells from inflamed colonic mucosa, a subset of patients with active and inactive phase of UC was selected for methylation analysis from three sources: (1) PBMCs, (2) CD3⁺ T cells isolated from PBMCs, and (3) CD3⁺ T cells isolated from colonic mucosa (see also Additional file 1: Table S4).

Inter-individual variation of *MGAT3* methylation level measured from PBMCs and from CD3⁺ T cells isolated from PBMCs was quite large—it varied from 47 to 94% and from 26 to 90%, respectively. Therefore, we could not find any difference in CpG methylation level between UC patients and HC in assayed fragments of the *MGAT3* promoter, neither in PBMCs nor in CD3⁺ T cells isolated from PBMCs. However, we recorded a total of 7 (out of 15) differentially methylated CpG sites in CD3⁺ T cells isolated from colonic mucosa of UC patients with active disease compared with HC (Fig. 3). Overall, the methylation level of CpGs within assayed fragments of the *MGAT3* promoter was high in CD3⁺ T cells from healthy colonic mucosa (between 77 and 98%). When compared to inflamed mucosa of UC patients with active phase of the disease, the same CpG sites were hypomethylated, with the highest difference at the CpG position 10 (13.24%; $p = 5.08 \times 10^{-5}$; Fig. 3). In inactive UC, no significant differences could be found after Bonferroni correction for multiple testing.

It is worth noting that the methylation pattern in CD3⁺ T cells isolated from inflamed colonic mucosa differed from the methylation patterns in PBMCs and for CD3⁺ T cells isolated from PBMCs. The latter two were very similar and had much lower methylation levels than that measured for CD3⁺ T cells from inflamed colonic mucosa (Fig. 3). Also, *MGAT3* methylation level was increased in UC compared with HC when measured from PBMCs or CD3⁺ T cells isolated from PBMCs (hypermethylation), while it was decreased (hypomethylation) when measured from CD3⁺ T cells isolated from inflamed colonic mucosa in comparison with healthy mucosa.

Correlation between the *MGAT3* and *BACH2* promoter methylation and IgG glycosylation

There were statistically significant correlations that replicated across assays and cohorts between the *MGAT3* promoter methylation and glycan structures FA2, FA2G2, FA2BG2, and FA2G2S1, as well as the derived trait of the ratio of FA2B to FA2 (Fig. 4a). All correlations except with FA2 were negative. No reproducible significant correlations could be found between *BACH2* promoter methylation and the glycan structures (Fig. 4a).

In order to infer a mechanistic pathway of the observed correlations, we mapped them to the glycan biosynthesis pathways (Fig. 4b). The ratio of bisecting glycans to FA2 was taken as an indicator of *MGAT3* (GnT-III) activity. This interpretation allowed us to infer lower GnT-III enzymatic activity when the promoter of the *MGAT3* gene was methylated. Increase in *MGAT3* promoter methylation correlated with a decrease in certain galactosylated and sialylated structures (Fig. 4b). In addition to the decreased levels of bisecting GlcNAc on non-galactosylated glycans (B/FA2), the most significant effect of the *MGAT3* promoter methylation on IgG glycome composition was a decrease of IgG galactosylation.

Discussion

Results from this study strongly indicate that the *MGAT3* and *BACH2* genes play an important role in IBD pathogenesis and suggest a possible disease pathway mediated by the pro-inflammatory properties of IgG antibodies acquired by alterations in Fc glycosylation. Our recent study, performed on a large cohort of over 1000 IBD patients, reported a significant difference in IgG glycome composition in both UC and CD compared to healthy controls [43, 46]. We found a decrease in quantity of galacosylated glycans in both CD and UC, as well as a decrease in sialylated glycans and an increase of bisecting GlcNAc on digalactosylated glycan structures on IgG in CD. Indeed, alternative *N*-glycosylation of an IgG molecule influences its function—pro-inflammatory and anti-inflammatory activity depends on the

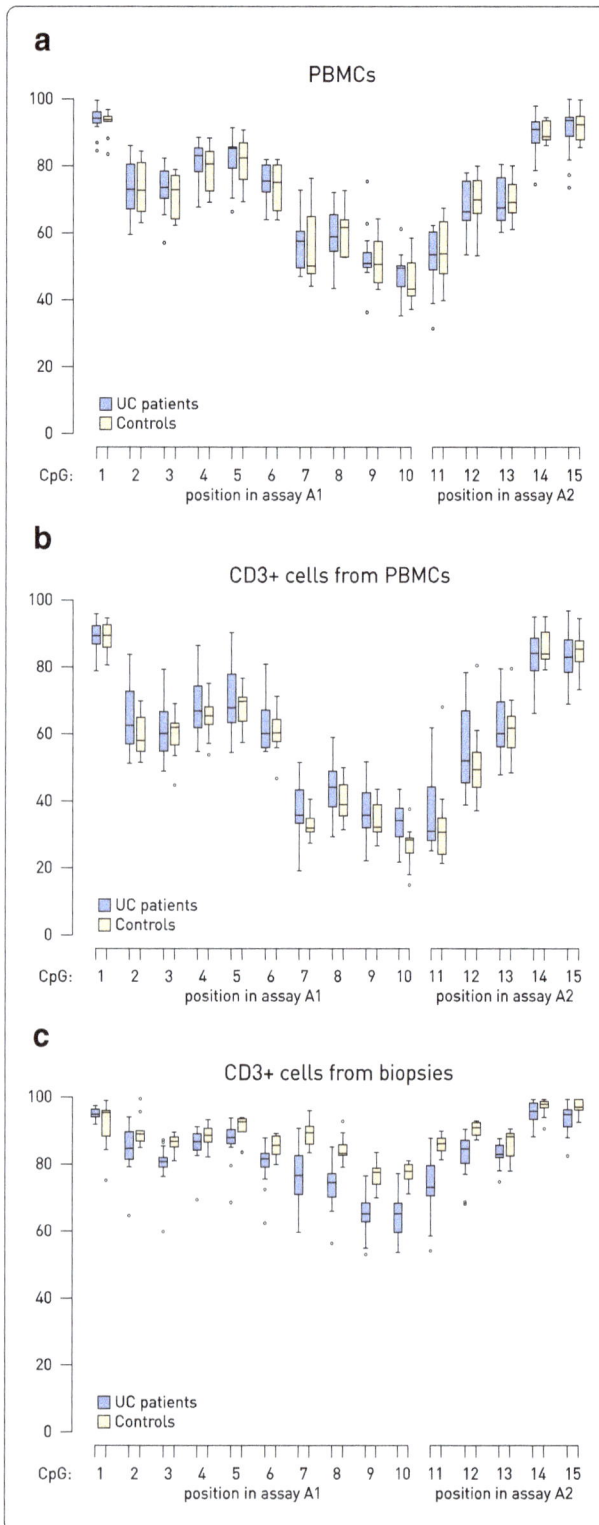

a PBMCs

b CD3+ cells from PBMCs

c CD3+ cells from biopsies

Fig. 3 Box plot of CpG methylation level in the *MGAT3* gene promoter (assays A1 and A2) analyzed from PBMCs (**a**), CD3+ T cells isolated from PBMCs (**b**), and CD3+ T cells isolated from inflamed colonic mucosa (**c**) from the independent cohort of Porto. Changes between UC patients with active disease and HC were statistically significant only in CD3+ T cells isolated from inflamed colonic mucosa at CpG positions 3 and 7–12 (*p* < 0.05 after Bonferroni correction for 15 hypotheses). PBMC peripheral blood mononuclear cells, UC ulcerative colitis, HC healthy controls

glycans added on the Cy2 domain of its Fc region [29]. These glycans are of a biantennary complex type with or without bisecting GlcNAc, core fucose, galactose, and sialic acid residues [61]. Recently, this was confirmed in a large multi-centric study of IgG glycome in IBD [46]. Therefore, glycan changes observed on IgG in peripheral blood of UC and CD patients are obviously associated with increased inflammatory potential of IgG, suggesting functional relevance of IgG glycosylation for IBD.

Here, we propose a possible mechanism underlying the aberrant IgG glycosylation pattern observed in IBD [43, 46]. Out of five candidate genes analyzed in this work, the *MGAT3*, a glycosyltransferase which participates in synthesis of IgG glycans, and the *BACH2*, a transcription factor and a master regulator of a network of genes relevant for B cell integrity [62, 63], showed differential methylation in peripheral blood of both CD and UC patients when compared to healthy individuals. Even though we identified changes in methylation level for both UC and CD compared to HC, the differences were more pronounced for CD. This is concordant with other studies that explored either whole genome methylation or promoter methylation of candidate genes in IBD [11]. The extent of the change in IgG glycome composition was also consistently higher in CD than UC compared to HC [43, 46].

The protein encoded by the *MGAT3* gene (*N*-acetyl-glucosaminyltransferase III, GnT-III) is responsible for significant functional alteration of glycans on the Fc region of an IgG antibody. The GnT-III adds *N*-acetylglucosamine (GlcNAc) on β1,4-linked mannose in the three-mannose core of *N*-glycans, producing bisecting GlcNAc structures. In the same CD patients, who showed changed *MGAT3* promoter methylation level in peripheral blood cells, a significant increase in the percentage of bisecting GlcNAc on glycans of circulating IgG antibodies was recorded, too. The association of the *MGAT3* with both IgG *N*-glycosylation [49] and Crohn's disease [4, 5] suggests that *N*-glycans with bisecting GlcNAc could be involved in CD pathogenesis through functional effect on IgG antibody.

Correlations between *BACH2* and *MGAT3* promoter methylation and glycan structures have given further insight into the changes of IgG glycosylation pattern mediated by those two genes (Fig. 4b). The *MGAT3*

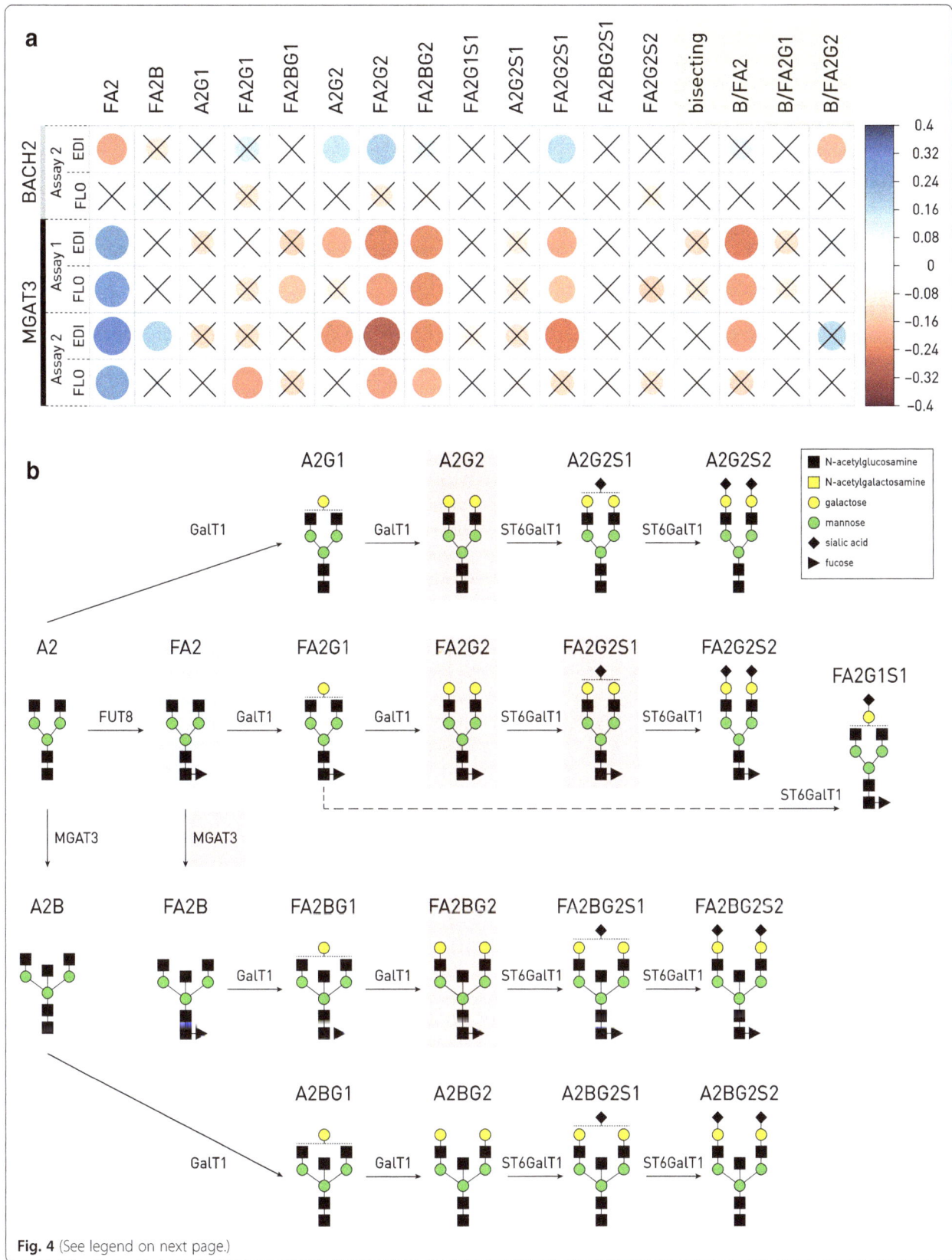

Fig. 4 (See legend on next page.)

(See figure on previous page.)

Fig. 4 Correlations between CpG methylation in the *BACH2* and *MGAT3* gene promoters and glycan structures measured from the same individuals of the Edinburgh and Florence cohorts, mapped to the glycan biosynthesis pathways. **a** Correlation coefficients between average CpG methylation in the assayed gene promoter fragments and glycan structure percentages are shown as blue (positive) or red (negative correlation) circles with their size and shade proportional to the correlation coefficient. Correlations without statistical significance (*p* > 0.05 after Bonferroni correction for multiple testing) are crossed. Columns represent 13 individual glycan structures and four derived traits (beige box). EDI Edinburgh cohort, FLO Florence cohort, Bisecting, percentage of all structures with bisecting *N*-acetylglucosamine, B/FA2 ratio of FA2B to FA2 structures, B/FA2G1 ratio of FA2BG1 to FA2G1 structures, B/FA2G2 ratio of FA2BG2 to FA2G2 structures. **b** Glycan biosynthesis pathways with the glycan structures, labels, and the enzymes mapped to correlation results for the *MGAT3* gene. Light blue rectangles indicate positive, while light red rectangles indicate negative correlation between the glycan structures or traits and CpG methylation levels. Only correlations replicated across assays and/or cohorts are shown. The red rectangle around the MGAT3 enzyme reflects the negative correlation between CpG methylation and the derived trait B/FA2, which effectively measures enzyme activity at this step. MGAT3 *N*-acetilglucosaminyltransferase III (GnT-III), FUT8 fucosyltransferase 8, GalT1 galactosyltranserase 1, ST6GalT1 Beta-galactoside alpha-2,6-sialyltransferase 1

promoter methylation probably led to decreased GnT-III enzymatic activity, as revealed by negative correlation between methylation and total bisecting glycans to FA2 ratio. Namely, GnT-III adds a bisecting GlcNAc to FA2. A further proof is the positive correlation between the *MGAT3* promoter methylation and FA2, since it is not surprising that substrate accumulates when enzyme activity is decreased. More complex effects were observed on galactosylation and sialylation. The negative correlation between *MGAT3* methylation and galactosylation of both, glycans with (FA2BG2) and without bisecting GlcNAc (FA2G2), suggests that the effect of increased galactosylation is not caused only by steric effects of bisecting GlcNAc, but also through some indirect effects of *MGAT3* expression on galactosyltransferase activity. It seems as though galactosylation and sialylation are co-regulated with the addition of a bisecting GlcNAc catalyzed by GnT-III. Furthermore, Dekkers and co-workers recently reported that transfection of cells with *MGAT3* causes an increase of IgG galactosylation [64].

Much weaker correlation was observed between *BACH2* methylation and IgG glycosylation. This was expected since *BACH2* is not a glycosyltransferase and thus is not directly involved in glycan biosynthetic pathways. However, weak positive correlations with A2G2, FA2G2, and FA2G2S1 structures, which involve galactosylation and sialylation, were observed, as well as weak negative correlation with fucosylated bianntenary structure FA2. This is interesting because GWA studies associated *BACH2* with IgG galactosylation [49] as well as with various immune and inflammatory diseases including IBD [4, 5, 65–67] in which IgG acquires pro-inflammatory properties through decrease in galactosylation, sialylation, and fucosylation [43, 46]. Since *BACH2* is orchestrating a gene regulatory network in B cells [62], we believe that some glyco-genes are also regulated by this transcription factor. Indeed, our in silico analysis identified several glyco-genes, mostly galactosyltransferases (including *B4GALT1* and *B4GALT2*), to possess putative AP-1 and NFE2 binding sites for *BACH2* transcription factor [63], suggesting that these galactosyltransferases could be controlled by BACH2

(Additional file 1: Tables S7 and S8). Our present efforts are focused on functional studies with hope to reveal a more complete view of the *BACH2* role in IgG glycosylation.

Since DNA methylation pattern is tissue-specific, our goal was to ascertain if CpG methylation from blood could be a proxy for CpG methylation of the same candidate gene in the tissue where the inflammation is taking place. In fact, IBD is an immune-mediated disorder in which T cells are actively implicated in development of gut-mucosa inflammation [68]. Previous evidence has suggested that *N*-glycosylation of intestinal T cells is associated with UC pathogenesis and disease severity [50, 69]. Therefore, we analyzed *MGAT3* promoter methylation in CD3$^+$ T cells isolated from PBMCs and from intestinal mucosa of UC patients with active and inactive form of the disease and compared with *MGAT3* promoter methylation from PBMCs of the same patients from the Porto cohort. We found 7 out of 15 differentially methylated CpG sites in CD3$^+$ T cells isolated from colonic mucosa of UC patients with active form of the disease compared to CD3$^+$ T cells from mucosa of healthy individuals. On the other hand, there were no differences in *MGAT3* promoter methylation between patients with either active or inactive form of UC and healthy controls neither in PBMCs nor in CD3$^+$ T cells isolated from PBMCs. This could be due to high dispersion in the methylation level when measured from PBMCs (47–94%) and CD3$^+$ T cells isolated from PBMCs (26–90%), probably due to small sample size and dispersion in age. Namely, cell composition changes across age in whole blood, and it can explain dispersion of CpG methylation level observed in our sample [70]. Considering much smaller dispersion in values of methylation level (65–97%) measured from CD3$^+$ T cells from *lamina propria*, the differences could be used as a signature for inflammation.

Conclusions

Taken together, our results suggest that the aberrant methylation observed in the *MGAT3* gene in CD3$^+$ T cells from intestinal mucosa of UC patients, B cells from peripheral blood, and the whole peripheral blood in UC and CD patients is a possible mechanism underlying inflammation due to a change in the immune system—either through the change of glycans on Fc region of IgGs or by modulating the glycosylation profile of glycoproteins on intestinal T cells. Others [24] have shown that some of their candidate genes changed promoter methylation level in whole biopsies, while some of the genes showed changes only in some cell types of the heterogeneous cell population from the epithelial and non-epithelial cells, pointing out the importance of cell separation from mucosal biopsies. Interestingly, one of the genes that showed differential methylation in the non-epithelial fraction, representing immune and stromal cells, was *FUT7*, the fucosyltransferase involved in sialyl Lewis X synthesis, a ligand in selectin-mediated adhesion of leukocytes to activated endothelium. Furthermore, Dias and collaborators proposed a molecular mechanism in IBD involving another glyco-gene, the *MGAT5* (GnT-V), responsible for branching of *N*-glycans. They showed decreased expression of branched *N*-glycans on T cell receptor (TCR) of *lamina propria* associated with disease severity in patients with active UC [50]. Dysregulation of *N*-glycan branching on TCR contributes to a decreased threshold of T cell activation leading to a hyper-immune response which is a feature of UC patients. Taken together, our results and those of others suggest an important role of aberrant protein glycosylation (partly through epigenetic mechanisms) in IBD through dysregulation of the immune system. Also, in IBD diagnosis and treatment, it is important to find a non-invasive, specific, and clinically useful biomarkers in order to identify high-risk patients. Using *MGAT3* hypermethylation together with the glycan traits as markers from peripheral blood of IBD patients seems promising in the disease identification.

Abbreviations
CD: Crohn's disease; EWAS: Epigenome-wide association study; GlcNAc: *N*-acetylglucosamine; GWAS: Genome-wide association study; HC: Healthy control; IBD: Inflammatory bowel disease; IgG: Immunoglobulin G; LC-MS: Liquid chromatography coupled to mass spectrometry; PBMCs: Peripheral blood mononuclear cells; UC: Ulcerative colitis

Acknowledgements
The authors would like to thank Stephanie Scott for her organizational and administrical contribution. The study has been funded by the EU FP7 grant European Commission IBD-BIOM (contract # 305479), EU FP7 Regional Potential Grant INTEGRA-Life (contract # 315997), European Structural and Investment Funds grant for the Croatian National Centre of Research Excellence in Personalized Healthcare (contract # KK.01.1.1.01.0010), and Croatian Science Foundation grant EpiGlycoIgG (contract # 3361). Financial support from Portugal (PI: SSP): FEDER—Fundo Europeu de Desenvolvimento Regional funds through the COMPETE 2020—Operacional Programme for Competitiveness and Internationalisation (POCI), Portugal 2020, and by

Portuguese funds through FCT—Fundação para a Ciência e a Tecnologia/Ministério da Ciência, Tecnologia e Inovação in the framework of the project (POCI-01/0145-FEDER-016601; PTDC/DTP-PIC/0560/2014) was received. SSP also acknowledges the European Crohn's and Colitis Organization (ECCO) and the "Broad Medical Research program at Crohn's and Colitis Foundation of America-CCFA" for funding. SSP acknowledges the Portuguese Group of Study on IBD (GEDII) for funding. A.M.D. [PD/BD/105982/2014] also acknowledges FCT for funding.

IBD-BIOM consortium: Daniel Kolarich (Department of Biomolecular Systems, Max Planck Institute of Colloids and Interfaces, Potsdam, Germany), Manfred Wuhrer (Center for Proteomics and Metabolomics, Leiden University Medical Center, Leiden, The Netherlands; Division of BioAnalytical Chemistry, VU University Amsterdam, Amsterdam, the Netherlands), Dermot P. B. McGovern (F. Widjaja Family Foundation Inflammatory Bowel and Immunobiology Research Institute, Cedars-Sinai Medical Center, Los Angeles), Iain K. Pemberton (IP Research Consulting SAS, Paris, France), Daniel IR Spencer (Ludger Ltd., Culham Science Centre, Oxford, UK, Daryl L. Fernandes (Ludger Ltd., Culham Science Centre, Oxford, UK), Rahul Kalla, Kate O'Leary, Alex T Adams, Hazel Drummond, Elaine Nimmo, Ray Boyapati, David C Wilson (Centre for Genetics and Molecular Medicine, University of Edinburgh, Edinburgh, UK), Ray Doran (Ludger Ltd., Culham Science Centre, Oxford, UK), Igor Rudan (all, Centre for Population Health Sciences, University of Edinburgh, Edinburgh, UK), Paolo Lionetti (Paediatric Gastroenterology Unit, AOU Meyer, Viale Pieraccini, Florence, Italy), Natalia Manetti (Department of Medical and Surgical Sciences, Division of Gastroenterology, University Hospital Careggi, Florence, Italy), Fabrizio Bossa (Department of Medical Sciences, Division of Gastroenterology, IRCCS-CSS Hospital, Viale Cappuccini, Rotondo, Italy), Paola Cantoro, Anna Kohn (Division of Gastroenterology, S. Camillo Hospital, Rome, Italy), Giancarlo Sturniolo (Gastrointestinal Unit, University of Padua, Padua, Italy), Silvio Danese (IBD Unit, Humanitas Research Institute, Rozzano, Milan, Italy), Mariek Pierik (Maastricht University Medical Centre (MUMC), Maastricht, the Netherlands), and David C. Wilson (Centre for Genetics and Molecular Medicine, University of Edinburgh, Edinburgh, UK).

Funding
This independent research was generously supported by the following grants: EU FP7 research grant IBD-BIOM (contract # 305479) to JS, VA, GL, and VZ; EU FP7 Regional Potential Grant INTEGRA-Life (contract # 315997) to GL and VZ; European Structural and Investment Funds grant for the Croatian National Centre of Research Excellence in Personalized Healthcare (contract # KK.01.1.1.01.0010) to GL and VZ; Croatian Science Foundation grant EpiGlycoIgG (contract # 3361) to VZ; FEDER COMPETE 2020 POCI, Portugal 2020, and Portuguese funds through FCT (contracts # POCI-01/0145-FEDER-016601 and PTDC/DTP-PIC/0560/2014) to SP; and FTC (contract # PD/BD/105982/2014) to AMD.

Authors' contributions
Study design was conceived by VZ, AV, GL, and SP. Sample provision was provided by JS, NTV, NAK, ERN, VA, RD'I, and SP. Blood and biopsy processing was conducted by AMD and AL. DNA methylation analyses were carried out by MK, DM, PD, IS, and IB. Glycan analysis was carried out by IT, JŠ, MŠ, and GR. Statistical and correlation analyses were carried out by AV, MK, and DM. Drafting of the manuscript was carried out by VZ, AV, MK, DM, and IT-A. All authors were involved in critical review, editing, revision, and approval of the final manuscript.

Author details
[1]Department of Biology, Division of Molecular Biology, Faculty of Science, University of Zagreb, Horvatovac 102a, 10000 Zagreb, Croatia. [2]Gastrointestinal Unit, Centre for Genomics and Molecular Medicine, University of Edinburgh, Edinburgh EH4 6XU, UK. [3]Genos Glycoscience Research Laboratory, Borongajska cesta 83h, 10000 Zagreb, Croatia. [4]Faculty of Pharmacy and Biochemistry, University of Zagreb, Zagreb, Croatia. [5]IBD Pharmacogenetics, University of Exeter, Exeter, UK. [6]Institute of Molecular Pathology and Immunology of the University of Porto (IPATIMUP), Porto,

Portugal. [7]Department of Medical and Surgical Sciences, Division of Gastroenterology, University Hospital Careggi, Florence, Italy. [8]Department of Medical Sciences, Division of Gastroenterology, IRCCS-CSS Hospital, Viale Cappuccini, Rotondo, Italy. [9]Gastrointestinal Unit, University of Padua, Padua, Italy. [10]Translational Gastroenterology Unit, Nuffield Department of Medicine, University of Oxford, Oxford, UK.

References

1. Burisch J, Pedersen N, Čuković-Čavka S, Brinar M, Kaimakliotis I, Duricova D, Shonová O, Vind I, Avnstrøm S, Thorsgaard N, et al. East–West gradient in the incidence of inflammatory bowel disease in Europe: the ECCO-EpiCom inception cohort. Gut. 2013;63:588–97.

2. Xavier RJ, Podolsky DK. Unravelling the pathogenesis of inflammatory bowel disease. Nature. 2007;448:427–34.

3. Anderson CA, Boucher G, Lees CW, Franke A, D'Amato M, Taylor KD, Lee JC, Goyette P, Imielinski M, Latiano A, et al. Meta-analysis identifies 29 additional ulcerative colitis risk loci, increasing the number of confirmed associations to 47. Nat Genet. 2011;43:246–52.

4. Franke A, Balschun T, Sina C, Ellinghaus D, Häsler R, Mayr G, Albrecht M, Wittig M, Buchert E, Nikolaus S, et al. Genome-wide association study for ulcerative colitis identifies risk loci at 7q22 and 22q13 (IL17REL). Nat Genet. 2010;42:292–4.

5. Franke A, McGovern DP, Barrett JC, Wang K, Radford-Smith GL, Ahmad T, Lees CW, Balschun T, Lee J, Roberts R, et al. Genome-wide meta-analysis increases to 71 the number of confirmed Crohn's disease susceptibility loci. Nat Genet. 2010;42:1118–25.

6. Jostins L, Ripke S, Weersma RK, Duerr RH, McGovern DP, Hui KY, Lee JC, Schumm LP, Sharma Y, Anderson CA, et al. Host-microbe interactions have shaped the genetic architecture of inflammatory bowel disease. Nature. 2012;491:119–24.

7. Liu JZ, van Sommeren S, Huang H, Ng SC, Alberts R, Takahashi A, Ripke S, Lee JC, Jostins L, Shah T, et al. Association analyses identify 38 susceptibility loci for inflammatory bowel disease and highlight shared genetic risk across populations. Nat Genet. 2015;47:979–86.

8. Bonaz BL, Bernstein CN. Brain-gut interactions in inflammatory bowel disease. Gastroenterology. 2013;144:36–49.

9. Pituch-Zdanowska A, Banaszkiewicz A, Albrecht P. The role of dietary fibre in inflammatory bowel disease. Gastroenterol Rev. 2015;3:135–41.

10. Rubin DT, Hanauer SB. Smoking and inflammatory bowel disease. Eur J Gastroenterol Hepatol. 2000;12:855–62.

11. McDermott E, Ryan EJ, Tosetto M, Gibson D, Burrage J, Keegan D, Byrne K, Crowe E, Sexton G, Malone K, et al. DNA methylation profiling in inflammatory bowel disease provides new insights into disease pathogenesis. J Crohn's Colitis. 2015;10:77–86.

12. Nimmo ER, Prendergast JG, Aldhous MC, Kennedy NA, Henderson P, Drummond HE, Ramsahoye BH, Wilson DC, Semple CA, Satsangi J. Genome-wide methylation profiling in Crohn's disease identifies altered epigenetic regulation of key host defense mechanisms including the Th17 pathway. Inflamm Bowel Dis. 2012;18:889–99.

13. Ventham NT, Kennedy NA, Adams AT, Kalla R, Heath S, O'Leary KR, Drummond H, consortium IB, consortium IC, Wilson DC, et al: Integrative epigenome-wide analysis demonstrates that DNA methylation may mediate genetic risk in inflammatory bowel disease. Nat Commun 2016, 7:13507.

14. Low D. DNA methylation in inflammatory bowel disease and beyond. World J Gastroenterol. 2013;19:5238.

15. Ventham NT, Kennedy NA, Nimmo ER, Satsangi J. Beyond gene discovery in inflammatory bowel disease: the emerging role of epigenetics. Gastroenterology. 2013;145:293–308.

16. Jones PA. Functions of DNA methylation: islands, start sites, gene bodies and beyond. Nat Rev Genet. 2012;13:484–92.

17. Ambatipudi S, Cuenin C, Hernandez-Vargas H, Ghantous A, Le Calvez-Kelm F, Kaaks R, Barrdahl M, Boeing H, Aleksandrova K, Trichopoulou A, et al. Tobacco smoking-associated genome-wide DNA methylation changes in the EPIC study. Epigenomics. 2016;8:599–618.

18. Barrès R, Yan J, Egan B, Treebak Jonas T, Rasmussen M, Fritz T, Caidahl K, Krook A, O'Gorman Donal J, Zierath Juleen R. Acute exercise remodels promoter methylation in human skeletal muscle. Cell Metab. 2012;15:405–11.

19. Olszak T, An D, Zeissig S, Vera MP, Richter J, Franke A, Glickman JN, Siebert R, Baron RM, Kasper DL, Blumberg RS. Microbial exposure during early life has persistent effects on natural killer T cell function. Science. 2012;336:489–93.

20. Symonds ME, Sebert SP, Budge H. The impact of diet during early life and its contribution to later disease: critical checkpoints in development and their long-term consequences for metabolic health. Proc Nutr Soc. 2009;68:416.

21. Vaissiere T, Hung RJ, Zaridze D, Moukeria A, Cuenin C, Fasolo V, Ferro G, Paliwal A, Hainaut P, Brennan P, et al. Quantitative analysis of DNA methylation profiles in lung cancer identifies aberrant DNA methylation of specific genes and its association with gender and cancer risk factors. Cancer Res. 2009;69:243–52.

22. Milagro FI, Mansego ML, De Miguel C, Martinez JA. Dietary factors, epigenetic modifications and obesity outcomes: progresses and perspectives. Mol Asp Med. 2013;34:782–812.

23. Adams AT, Kennedy NA, Hansen R, Ventham NT, O'Leary KR, Drummond HE, Noble CL, El-Omar E, Russell RK, Wilson DC, et al. Two-stage genome-wide methylation profiling in childhood-onset Crohn's disease implicates epigenetic alterations at the VMP1/MIR21 and HLA loci. Inflamm Bowel Dis. 2014;20:1784–93.

24. Cooke J, Zhang H, Greger L, Silva A-L, Massey D, Dawson C, Metz A, Ibrahim A, Parkes M. Mucosal genome-wide methylation changes in inflammatory bowel disease. Inflamm Bowel Dis. 2012;18:2128–37.

25. Harris RA, Nagy-Szakal D, Mir SAV, Frank E, Szigeti R, Kaplan JL, Bronsky J, Opekun A, Ferry GD, Winter H, Kellermayer R. DNA methylation-associated colonic mucosal immune and defense responses in treatment-naïve pediatric ulcerative colitis. Epigenetics. 2014;9:1131–7.

26. Karatzas PS, Gazouli M, Safioleas M, Mantzaris GJ. DNA methylation changes in inflammatory bowel disease. Ann Gastroenterol. 2014;27:125–32.

27. Hart GW, Copeland RJ. Glycomics hits the big time. Cell. 2010;143:672–6.

28. Böhm S, Kao D, Nimmerjahn F. Sweet and sour: the role of glycosylation for the anti-inflammatory activity of immunoglobulin G. In: Fc Receptors. Basel: Springer International Publishing; 2014. p. 393–417. 393–417.

29. Kaneko Y. Anti-inflammatory activity of immunoglobulin G resulting from Fc sialylation. Science. 2006;313:670–3.

30. National Research Council (U.S.). Committee on Assessing the Importance and Impact of Glycomics and Glycosciences., National Research Council (U.S.). Board on Chemical Sciences and Technology., National Research Council (U.S.). Board on Life Sciences.: Transforming glycoscience: a roadmap for the future. Washington, D.C.: National Academies Press; 2012.

31. Stowell SR, Ju T, Cummings RD. Protein glycosylation in cancer. Annu Rev Pathol: Mech Dis. 2015;10:473–510.

32. Horvat T, Deželjin M, Redžić I, Barišić D, Herak Bosnar M, Lauc G, Zoldoš V. Reversibility of membrane N-Glycome of HeLa cells upon treatment with epigenetic inhibitors. PLoS One. 2013;8:e54672.

33. Horvat T, Mužinić A, Barišić D, Bosnar MH, Zoldoš V. Epigenetic modulation of the HeLa cell membrane N-glycome. Biochim Biophys Acta Gen Subj. 2012;1820:1412–9.

34. Horvat T, Zoldoš V, Lauc G. Evolutional and clinical implications of the epigenetic regulation of protein glycosylation. Clin Epigenetics. 2011;2:425–32.

35. Klasić M, Krištić J, Korać P, Horvat T, Markulin D, Vojta A, Reiding KR, Wuhrer M, Lauc G, Zoldoš V. DNA hypomethylation upregulates expression of the MGAT3 gene in HepG2 cells and leads to changes in N-glycosylation of secreted glycoproteins. Sci Rep. 2016;6:24363.

36. Saldova R, Dempsey E, Pérez-Garay M, Mariño K, Watson JA, Blanco-Fernández A, Struwe WB, Harvey DJ, Madden SF, Peracaula R, et al. 5-AZA-2′-deoxycytidine induced demethylation influences N-glycosylation of secreted glycoproteins in ovarian cancer. Epigenetics. 2011;6:1362–72.

37. Vojta A, Samaržija I, Bočkor L, Zoldoš V. Glyco-genes change expression in cancer through aberrant methylation. Biochim Biophys Acta Gen Subj. 2016; 1860:1776–85.

38. Zoldoš V, Horvat T, Novokmet M, Cuenin C, Mužinić A, Pučić M, Huffman JE, Gornik O, Polašek O, Campbell H, et al. Epigenetic silencing of HNF1A associates with changes in the composition of the human plasma N-glycome. Epigenetics. 2012;7:164–72.

39. Theodoratou E, Campbell H, Ventham NT, Kolarich D, Pučić-Baković M, Zoldoš V, Fernandes D, Pemberton IK, Rudan I, Kennedy NA, et al. The role of glycosylation in IBD. Nat Rev Gastroenterol Hepatol. 2014;11(10):588–600.

40. Arnold JN, Wormald MR, Sim RB, Rudd PM, Dwek RA. The impact of glycosylation on the biological function and structure of human immunoglobulins. Annu Rev Immunol. 2007;25:21–50.

41. Miyahara K, Nouso K, Saito S, Hiraoka A, Harada K, Takahashi S, Morimoto Y, Kobayashi S, Ikeda F, Miyake Y, et al. Serum glycan markers for evaluation of disease activity and prediction of clinical course in patients with ulcerative colitis. PLoS One. 2013;8:e74861.

42. Shinzaki S, Iijima H, Nakagawa T, Egawa S, Nakajima S, Ishii S, Irie T, Kakiuchi Y, Nishida T, Yasumaru M, et al. IgG oligosaccharide alterations are a novel diagnostic marker for disease activity and the clinical course of inflammatory bowel disease. Am J Gastroenterol. 2008;103:1173–81.

43. Trbojevic Akmacic I, Ventham NT, Theodoratou E, Vuckovic F, Kennedy NA, Kristic J, Nimmo ER, Kalla R, Drummond H, Stambuk J, et al. Inflammatory bowel disease associates with proinflammatory potential of the immunoglobulin G glycome. Inflamm Bowel Dis. 2015;21:1237–47.

44. Plomp R, Ruhaak LR, Uh HW, Reiding KR, Selman M, Houwing-Duistermaat JJ, Slagboom PE, Beekman M, Wuhrer M. Subclass-specific IgG glycosylation is associated with markers of inflammation and metabolic health. Sci Rep. 2017;7:12325.

45. Schwab I, Nimmerjahn F. Intravenous immunoglobulin therapy: how does IgG modulate the immune system? Nat Rev Immunol. 2013;13:176–89.

46. Simurina M, de Haan N, Vuckovic F, Kennedy NA, Stambuk J, Falck D, Trbojevic-Akmacic I, Clerc F, Razdorov G, Khon A, et al: Glycosylation of immunoglobulin G associates with clinical features of inflammatory bowel diseases. Gastroenterology. 2018;154(5):1320–1333.e10.

47. Barrett JC, Lee JC, Lees CW, Prescott NJ, Anderson CA, Phillips A, Wesley E, Parnell K, Zhang H, Drummond H, et al. Genome-wide association study of ulcerative colitis identifies three new susceptibility loci, including the HNF4A region. Nat Genet. 2009;41:1330–4.

48. McGovern DPB, Jones MR, Taylor KD, Marciante K, Yan X, Dubinsky M, Ippoliti A, Vasiliauskas E, Berel D, Derkowski C, et al. Fucosyltransferase 2 (FUT2) non-secretor status is associated with Crohn's disease. Hum Mol Genet. 2010;19:3468–76.

49. Lauc G, Huffman JE, Pucic M, Zgaga L, Adamczyk B, Muzinic A, Novokmet M, Polasek O, Gornik O, Kristic J, et al. Loci associated with N-glycosylation of human immunoglobulin G show pleiotropy with autoimmune diseases and haematological cancers. PLoS Genet. 2013;9:e1003225.

50. Dias AM, Dourado J, Lago P, Cabral J, Marcos-Pinto R, Salgueiro P, Almeida CR, Carvalho S, Fonseca S, Lima M, et al. Dysregulation of T cell receptor N-glycosylation: a molecular mechanism involved in ulcerative colitis. Hum Mol Genet. 2014;23:2416–27.

51. Reinius LE, Acevedo N, Joerink M, Pershagen G, Dahlen SE, Greco D, Soderhall C, Scheynius A, Kere J. Differential DNA methylation in purified human blood cells: implications for cell lineage and studies on disease susceptibility. PLoS One. 2012;7:e41361.

52. Krištić J, Zoldoš V, Lauc G. Complex genetics of protein N-glycosylation. In: Endo T, Seeberger PH, Hart GW, Wong C-H, Taniguchi N, editors. Glycoscience: biology and medicine. Tokyo: Springer Japan; 2014. p. 1–7.

53. Stewart SK, Morris TJ, Guilhamon P, Bulstrode H, Bachman M, Balasubramanian S, Beck S. oxBS-450K: a method for analysing hydroxymethylation using 450K BeadChips. Methods. 2015;72:9–15.

54. Kroeze LI, Aslanyan MG, van Rooij A, Koorenhof-Scheele TN, Massop M, Carell T, Boezeman JB, Marie JP, Halkes CJ, de Witte T, et al. Characterization of acute myeloid leukemia based on levels of global hydroxymethylation. Blood. 2014;124:1110–8.

55. Sanchez-Guerra M, Zheng Y, Osorio-Yanez C, Zhong J, Chervona Y, Wang S, Chang D, McCracken JP, Diaz A, Bertazzi PA, et al. Effects of particulate matter exposure on blood 5-hydroxymethylation: results from the Beijing truck driver air pollution study. Epigenetics. 2015;10:633–42.

56. Yu M, Hon GC, Szulwach KE, Song CX, Zhang L, Kim A, Li X, Dai Q, Shen Y, Park B, et al. Base-resolution analysis of 5-hydroxymethylcytosine in the mammalian genome. Cell. 2012;149:1368–80.

57. Pucic M, Knezevic A, Vidic J, Adamczyk B, Novokmet M, Polasek O, Gornik O, Supraha-Goreta S, Wormald MR, Redzic I, et al. High throughput isolation and glycosylation analysis of IgG-variability and heritability of the IgG glycome in three isolated human populations. Mol Cell Proteomics. 2011; M111(010090):10.

58. Trbojevic-Akmacic I, Ugrina I, Lauc G. Comparative analysis and validation of different steps in glycomics studies. Methods Enzymol. 2017;586:37–55.

59. Selman MH, Derks RJ, Bondt A, Palmblad M, Schoenmaker B, Koeleman CA, van de Geijn FE, Dolhain RJ, Deelder AM, Wuhrer M. Fc specific IgG glycosylation profiling by robust nano-reverse phase HPLC-MS using a sheath-flow ESI sprayer interface. J Proteome. 2012;75:1318–29.

60. Jansen BC, Falck D, de Haan N, Hipgrave Ederveen AL, Razdorov G, Lauc G, Wuhrer M. LaCyTools: a targeted liquid chromatography-mass spectrometry data processing package for relative quantitation of glycopeptides. J Proteome Res. 2016;15:2198–210.

61. Fujii S, Nishiura T, Nishikawa A, Miura R, Taniguchi N. Structural heterogeneity of sugar chains in immunoglobulin G. Conformation of immunoglobulin G molecule and substrate specificities of glycosyltransferases. J Biol Chem. 1990;265:6009–18.

62. Igarashi K, Ochiai K, Itoh-Nakadai A, Muto A. Orchestration of plasma cell differentiation by Bach2 and its gene regulatory network. Immunol Rev. 2014;261:116–25.

63. Kuwahara M, Suzuki J, Tofukuji S, Yamada T, Kanoh M, Matsumoto A, Maruyama S, Kometani K, Kurosaki T, Ohara O, et al. The Menin–Bach2 axis is critical for regulating CD4 T-cell senescence and cytokine homeostasis. Nat Commun. 2014;5:3555.

64. Dekkers G, Plomp R, Koeleman CA, Visser R, von Horsten HH, Sandig V, Rispens T, Wuhrer M, Vidarsson G. Multi-level glyco-engineering techniques to generate IgG with defined Fc-glycans. Sci Rep. 2016;6:36964.

65. Chu X, Pan C-M, Zhao S-X, Liang J, Gao G-Q, Zhang X-M, Yuan G-Y, Li C-G, Xue L-Q, Shen M, et al. A genome-wide association study identifies two new risk loci for Graves' disease. Nat Genet. 2011;43:897–901.

66. Dubois PCA, Trynka G, Franke L, Hunt KA, Romanos J, Curtotti A, Zhernakova A, Heap GAR, Ádány R, Aromaa A, et al. Multiple common variants for celiac disease influencing immune gene expression. Nat Genet. 2010;42:295–302.

67. Sawcer S, Hellenthal G, Pirinen M, Spencer CC, Patsopoulos NA, Moutsianas L, Dilthey A, Su Z, Freeman C, Hunt SE, et al. Genetic risk and a primary role for cell-mediated immune mechanisms in multiple sclerosis. Nature. 2011; 476:214–9.

68. Macdonald TT, Monteleone G. Immunity, inflammation, and allergy in the gut. Science. 2005;307:1920–5.

69. Vossenkamper A, Hundsrucker C, Page K, van Maurik A, Sanders TJ, Stagg AJ, Das L, MacDonald TT. A CD3-specific antibody reduces cytokine production and alters phosphoprotein profiles in intestinal tissues from patients with inflammatory bowel disease. Gastroenterology. 2014;147:172–83.

70. Jaffe AE, Irizarry RA. Accounting for cellular heterogeneity is critical in epigenome-wide association studies. Genome Biol. 2014;15:R31.

4

Long non-coding RNAs: implications in targeted diagnoses, prognosis, and improved therapeutic strategies in human non- and triple-negative breast cancer

Rubén Rodríguez Bautista[1,2], Alette Ortega Gómez[1*] (iD), Alfredo Hidalgo Miranda[3], Alejandro Zentella Dehesa[4], Cynthia Villarreal-Garza[5], Federico Ávila-Moreno[6,7] and Oscar Arrieta[1]

Abstract

Triple-negative breast cancer (TNBC) has been clinically difficult to manage because of tumor aggressiveness, cellular and histological heterogeneity, and molecular mechanisms' complexity. All this in turn leads us to evaluate that tumor biological behavior is not yet fully understood. Additionally, the heterogeneity of tumor cells represents a great biomedicine challenge in terms of the complex molecular—genetical-transcriptional and epigenetical—mechanisms, which have not been fully elucidated on human solid tumors.

Recently, human breast cancer, but specifically TNBC is under basic and clinical-oncology research in the discovery of new molecular biomarkers and/or therapeutic targets to improve treatment responses, as well as for seeking algorithms for patient stratification, seeking a positive impact in clinical-oncology outcomes and life quality on breast cancer patients. In this sense, important knowledge is emerging regarding several cancer molecular aberrations, including higher genetic mutational rates, LOH, CNV, chromosomal, and epigenetic alterations, as well as transcriptome aberrations in terms of the total gene-coding ribonucleic acids (RNAs), known as mRNAs, as well as non-coding RNA (ncRNA) sequences. In this regard, novel investigation fields have included microRNAs (miRNAs), as well as long ncRNAs (lncRNAs), which have been importantly related and are likely involved in the induction, promotion, progression, and/or clinical therapeutic response trackers of TNBC. Based on this, in general terms according with the five functional archetype classification, the lncRNAs may be involved in the regulation of several molecular mechanisms which include genetic expression, epigenetic, transcriptional, and/or post-transcriptional mechanisms, which are nowadays not totally understood.

Here, we have reviewed the main dis-regulated and functionally non- and well-characterized lncRNAs and their likely involvement, from a molecular enrichment and mechanistic point of view, as tumor biomarkers for breast cancer and its specific histological subtype, TNBC. In reference to the abovementioned, it has been described that some lncRNA expression profiles correspond or are associated with the TNBC histological subtype, potentially granting their use for TNBC malignant progression, diagnosis, tumor clinical stage, and likely therapy. Based on this, lncRNAs have been proposed as potential biomarkers which might represent potential predictive tools in the differentiated breast carcinomas versus TNBC malignant disease. Finally, elucidation of the specific or multi-functional archetypal of lncRNAs in breast cancer and TNBC could be fundamental, as these molecular intermediary-regulator "lncRNAs" are widely involved in the

(Continued on next page)

* Correspondence: ortega.alette@gmail.com
[1]Thoracic Oncology Unit and Laboratory of Personalized Medicine, Instituto Nacional de Cancerología (INCan), San Fernando #22, Section XVI, Tlalpan, 14080 Mexico City, Mexico
Full list of author information is available at the end of the article

(Continued from previous page)

genome expression, epigenome regulation, and transcriptional and post-transcriptional tumor biology, which in turn will probably represent a new prospect in clinical and/or therapeutic molecular targets for the oncological management of breast carcinomas in general and also for TNBC patients.

Keywords: Breast cancer, Triple negative, Biomarkers, lncRNA

Background

The most recent worldwide cancer statistics estimated a total of 2.4 million new cases and 533,000 deaths due to breast cancer (BC) in 2015, thus making it the fifth leading cause of cancer years of life lost between 2005 and 2015 for both sexes. For women specifically, one in 14 will develop BC between birth and 79 years of age, becoming the leading cause of cancer death for women worldwide [1]. In 2017, 252,710 new breast malignant clinical cases and 40,610 BC deaths were expected to occur in the USA [2].

In addition to the known histopathological classification (tumor cell differentiation status) and TNM (tumor size, lymph node involvement, and metastasis) stage, BC has also been classified on the basis of protein and genetic expression status [3]. In this regard, Perou et al. have defined at least five genetically distinct subtypes with different molecular significance on inter-tumor subtypes [4], but also by intra-tumor heterogeneity in BC subtypes [5]. Based on the above, intra-tumor heterogeneity has been proposed as having striking morphological, genetic, and behavioral variability explained in part by the cancer stem cells population presence, clonal evolution, and malignancy capacity [6, 7]. Additionally in BC, other molecular-genetic alterations exist based on well-known non-coding RNAs (ncRNAs), including micro-ncRNAs (microRNAs) and long-ncRNAs (lncRNAs), both of which have been identified and histopathologically associated to BCs, as triple-negative BC (TNBC) [8, 9], but particularly some lncRNAs, in others as LOC339535 also named LINK-A, have functionally been associated to TNBC malignancy with poorer prognosis and progression-free survival in TNBC patients [10], as well as for HOTAIR, which has been involved in promoting or increasing malignancy in TNBC patients, compared with non-TNBC patients, probably representing a new target therapy in TNBC [11].

TNBC as a heterogeneous group of breast tumors has been characterized by the lack of expression of hormone receptors, namely estrogen receptor alpha (ER-α) and progesterone receptor (PR), with a low expression of receptor tyrosine kinase ErbB2 (also known as HER2/neu). In TNBC, additional molecular-genetic features have been identified including BRCA1/2 mutation frequency (11.2–20.0%) [12–15], which may be higher in approximately 20–40%, according to the ethnic origin [16], furthermore including additional molecular deficiencies, in others as some frequent somatic mutations on TP53 (62%) and PIK3CA (10%) [12, 13].

In addition to the mutation status, TNBC tumors also display alterations on the genetic copy number variations, genetic expression levels, and patterns, which have been associated with basal-like tumors including a high proportion of the basal histological BC subgroup (70–80%) [17]. Besides TNBCs exhibiting poor survival rates due to their highly aggressive and metastatic capacities, they are associated with higher recurrence behavior in local and distant lymph nodes and have higher proliferative rates [18–20], probably explained in part by the genetic-molecular aberrations.

Approximately, on average, 12 to 24% of women diagnosed with BC correspond to the TNBC subtype. TNBC represents a subgroup of particular interest, since it generally affects young women and tends to have a poor response to standard chemotherapy [21–23].

In TNBC, the US Food and Drug Administration (FDA) and the European Medicines Agency (EMA) have not yet approved a specific targeted agent for clinical treatment in the adjuvant, neoadjuvant, or metastatic settings. Currently, radiotherapy and a combination of chemotherapeutic agents like anthracyclines, alkylating agents, taxanes, or platinum salts are used for treating TNBC patients [24]. Thus, efficient targeted therapeutic regimens are urgently needed in TNBC for clinical management, since currently these patients have low rates of disease-free survival (DFS), overall survival (OS), and 5-year survival, in addition to a low survival 12–18 months after distant recurrence [25, 26].

TNBC tumors have been characterized by high levels of genetic instability, with a median of 1.7 (range 0.16–5.23) mutations/Mb [27, 28], and feature complex patterns of copy number gains and losses throughout the genome [29]. Epigenetically TNBCs are characterized by extensive hypomethylation, which leads to increased genome-wide instability [30]. Recently, Mathe et al. have shown that the changes in the epigenome, based on DNA methylation levels, are associated with tumor progression in TNBC [31–33].

Recent reports have shown that lncRNAs are involved in almost all human biological processes including transcriptional regulation or interference, telomere maintenance, epigenetic mechanisms modulation, imprinting, post-transcriptional and translational control, structural organization, cellular differentiation, embryo development, and pathological dysfunctions as well as non-malignant diseases, using redundant DNA, RNA, and/or protein-binding mechanisms, according to particular cases [34–36]. As it occurs for other malignant diseases, lncRNAs have been involved in the tumorigenic promotion and progression processes leading to BC development and prognosis [37].

Liu et al. proposed a TNBC classification based on mRNA coding genes and lncRNA expression profiles. This new classification could offer a more robust data matrix to establish a molecular stratification bioinformatics-algorithm that clarifies knowledge of molecular subtypes and establishes subtype-specific targets [38]. Additionally, genome-wide association studies on cancer have revealed that more than 80% of cancer-associated single-nucleotide polymorphisms occur in non-coding genetic regions. This suggests that a significant fraction of the genetic etiology of BC could be related to lncRNA expression profile and functionality [39]. Also, research involving genetic sequence control (promoters vs. enhancers) is necessary, in order to explain why, how, and where lncRNAs are expressed in human homeostasis as well as during a pathologic process [40].

In recent years, therapeutic strategies for TNBC have recorded a high number of failures in the development of chemical agents, due to the fact that recently it has been proposed to include molecular wide studies to identify additional potential biomarkers, as well as genetic-epigenetic targets, probably involved. In this regard, epigenetic targeted pathways have widely been proposed as pharmacological strategies, among these histone deacetylase inhibitors (HDACis) alone and/or in combination strategies have promising activity in TNBC-targeted treatments. Therefore, future research should be focusing on the personalized approach, which will benefit more from each kind of epigenetic agents, including panobinostat, vorinostat, and entinostat [41]. In addition, by identifying reliable treatment biomarkers, such as lncRNAs, which are implicated in epigenetic mechanisms through the recruitment of the chromatin modification complexes, in other proteins based on the polycomb repressor complex-2 (PRC2) and/or LSD1/CoREST (REST co-repressor) REST complexes, involved in the histone repressor (H3K27me3) versus activation (H3K4me2/3) code, as it has been previously described for the lncRNA HOTAIR, suggesting a scaffold functionality archetype [42], as lncRNAs have functionally been classified by five archetypes (described in Fig. 1).

In brief, the present review summarizes the current knowledge regarding lncRNA expression patterns and probable functional association with their role in BC biology and as expressed molecular biomarkers, potentially involved as therapeutic targets. In this regard, we aim to generate a systematic and deep understanding of tumor biology of TNBC, so clinicians will, in the near future, be able to offer tailored treatments in accord to the lncRNA stratification and/or specific lncRNA expression patterns in potentially different patient subgroups in BC and TNBC.

Targeted therapy efficacy in the TNBC treatment: probable lncRNAs involved

Due to the lack of knowledge on molecular targets, chemotherapy is the only available systemic treatment for TNBC and therefore adjuvant chemotherapy is recommended for TNBC operable tumors with stages I–III [43, 44]. However, systemic therapy before surgery, neoadjuvant chemotherapy (NAC), is the most appropriate approach for patients with locally advanced BC with the objectives to improve surgical options (resectability and breast conservation techniques), determine in vivo tumor sensitivity to treatment, and improve long-term survival outcomes with the pathological complete response (pCR) as an informative biomarker of those parameters [45–48]. Even with what is deemed as a poor overall survival, it is evident that subsets of TNBC patients respond better to standard care using chemotherapy combinations, and when pCR after NAC is achieved; excellent long-term survival is expected [49]. Nevertheless, a substantial proportion (30–40%) of patients with early-stage TNBC develop metastatic disease [50].

In this sense, the triple-negative paradox on TNBC patients is mainly driven by a subgroup of cells on the bulk tumor with residual disease after NAC [50]. For this reason, the search for new biomarkers would allow the prediction of a group of TNBC patients who would better respond to standard chemotherapy, thus eliminating the need to administer unnecessary, highly toxic, and costly chemotherapy treatments in patients who might benefit from more personalized treatments.

Researchers have proposed new targeted therapies based on results from clinical trials in an attempt to improve the outcome of TNBC patients. Retrospective analyses and previous trials have shown striking pCR rates in patients with high *BRCA1* mutation rates (between 72 and 90%) with a single neoadjuvant treatment using DNA crosslinking platinum salts (e.g., cisplatinum) [51, 52]. For example, TNBC patients with positive *BRCA* mutations treated with carboplatin have better response rates compared to those treated with docetaxel monotherapy [53]. Other studies have evaluated poly (ADP-Ribose) polymerase (PARP) inhibitors either alone or in combination with cytotoxic treatment. However, response to these schemes is limited to patients with BRCA-mutated BC [54, 55].

Likewise, hyper-activation of the PI3K/AKT signaling pathway is associated to oncogenic alterations in TNBC,

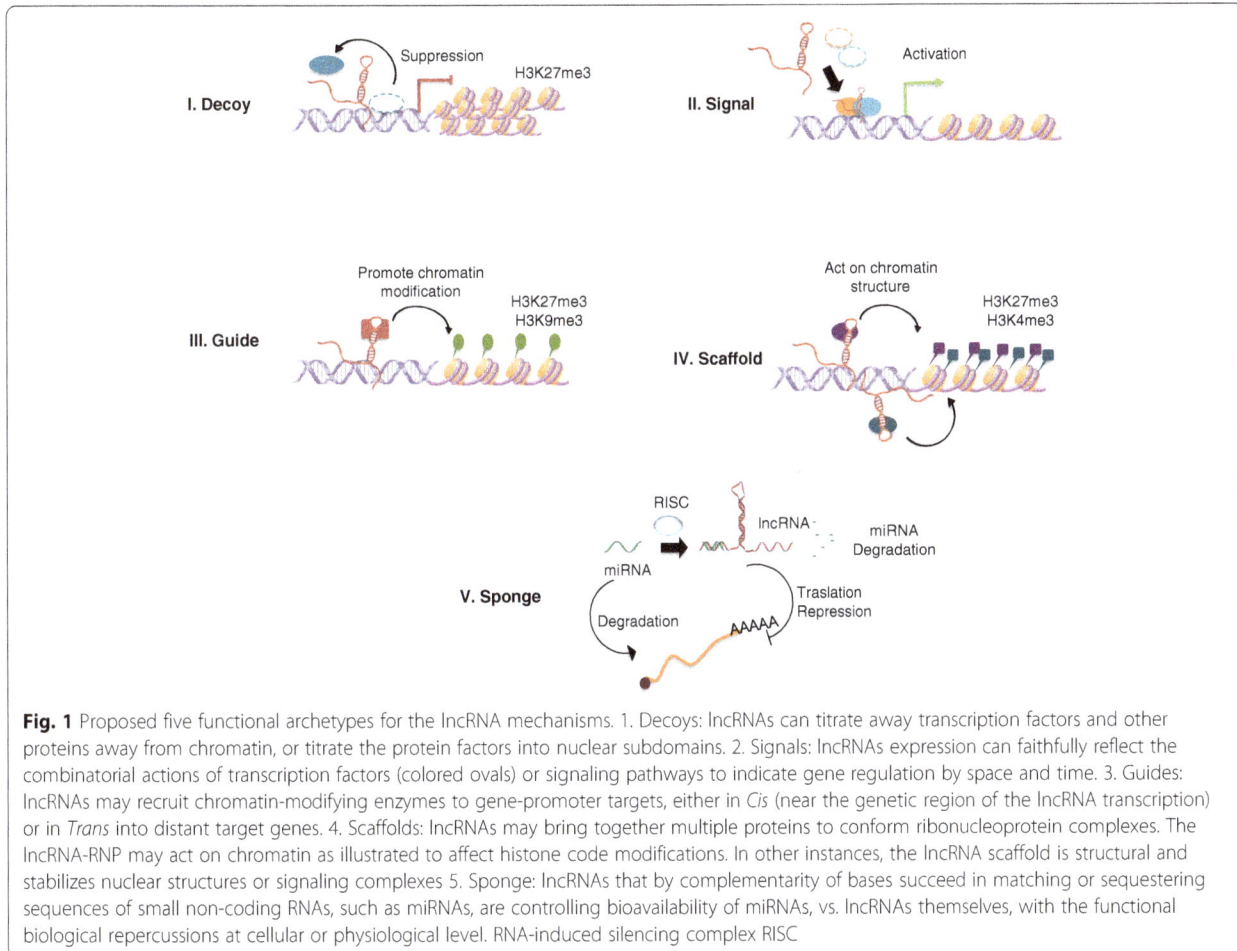

Fig. 1 Proposed five functional archetypes for the lncRNA mechanisms. 1. Decoys: lncRNAs can titrate away transcription factors and other proteins away from chromatin, or titrate the protein factors into nuclear subdomains. 2. Signals: lncRNAs expression can faithfully reflect the combinatorial actions of transcription factors (colored ovals) or signaling pathways to indicate gene regulation by space and time. 3. Guides: lncRNAs may recruit chromatin-modifying enzymes to gene-promoter targets, either in *Cis* (near the genetic region of the lncRNA transcription) or in *Trans* into distant target genes. 4. Scaffolds: lncRNAs may bring together multiple proteins to conform ribonucleoprotein complexes. The lncRNA-RNP may act on chromatin as illustrated to affect histone code modifications. In other instances, the lncRNA scaffold is structural and stabilizes nuclear structures or signaling complexes 5. Sponge: lncRNAs that by complementarity of bases succeed in matching or sequestering sequences of small non-coding RNAs, such as miRNAs, are controlling bioavailability of miRNAs, vs. lncRNAs themselves, with the functional biological repercussions at cellular or physiological level. RNA-induced silencing complex RISC

occurring in approximately 10% of patients [56]. Activating PIK3CA mutations are the most frequent mutations in TNBC. Other alterations in this pathway include loss of tumor suppressor phosphatases inositol polyphosphate 4-phosphatase type II (INPP4B), loss of phosphatase and tensin homolog (PTEN), AKT amplification, and AKT3 translocation [57–59]. In this regard, several studies have demonstrated the benefits of using serine/threonine kinase AKT inhibitors like ipatasertib in TNBC [37, 38, 60].

On the other hand, growth factor receptors are overexpressed in TNBC, including epidermal growth factor receptor (EGFR) and vascular endothelial growth factor receptor (VEGFR) [61–66]. Multiple signaling pathways, such as PI3K/AKT, mitogen-activated protein kinase (MAPK), and Wnt/β-catenin are activated by EGFR and, in turn, enhance proliferation, survival, invasion, and metastasis of cancer cells [67]. Expression of EGFR is frequently associated with TNBC and has been viewed as a promising therapeutic target. Unfortunately, the therapeutic efficacy of EGFR-targeting agents in BC has been disappointing [68, 69]. A recent report showed that combined treatment with lapatinib, a dual inhibitor of EGFR and ErbB2/HER2, and imatinib, a c-ABL inhibitor,

resulted in synergistic growth inhibition in a panel of EGFR/ErbB2-expressing BC cells, including the TNBC cell line MDAMB-468 [70].

Recently, studies on fibroblast growth factor receptor (FGFR) have shown that 9% of TNBC with FGFR1 (4%) and FGFR2 amplifications, treated with FGFR blockers like lucitanib (FGFR1-amplification) and JNJ-42756493 (FGFR translocation or FGFR activating mutation), provide clinical benefits [51, 71–73]. Approximately 10 to 15% of TNBC express the androgen receptor (AR), and several studies have reported pathological response benefits when targeting this receptor. Bicalutamide, enzalutamide, and orteronel are all oral non-steroidal anti-AR, on that the most recent clinical trials for TNBC are shown in Table 1 [72, 74–76].

As previously described, TNBC is a heterogeneous disease, and even though a high number of targeted therapies have been clinically tested, this has not yet translated into a substantial clinical benefit for TNBC patients. Hence, it is necessary to identify highly sensible biomarkers for a better stratification and treatment of these patients. Recently, long non-coding RNAs (lncRNAs) have been reported to drive many important

Table 1 The most recent clinical trials in TNBC patients in the search of therapeutic biomarkers for advanced disease

Clinical trial	Phase	Study groups	Indications	Therapeutic target
NCT02623972	II	Eribulin (Halaven®) by IV, for 4 cycles; followed by AC by IV, for 4 cycles	Advanced TNBC	Inhibitor of microtubule dynamics
NCT02120469	I	Everolimus (Afinitor®) by OA daily; eribulin mesylate (Halaven®) by IV twice every month	Metastatic TNBC	mTOR inhibitor
NCT02672475	I	Paclitaxel (Taxol®), by IV, weekly, 3 weeks on, 1 week off; Galunisertib (LY2157299), by OA, twice daily, 3 weeks on, 1 week off	Metastatic TNBC	Inhibitor of the TGF-β receptor I kinase
NCT02632071	I	ACY-1215 (ricolinostat), by OA, daily for 3 weeks on, 1 week off; nab-paclitaxel (Abraxane®), by IV, weekly for 3 weeks on, 1 week off	Advanced TNBC	HDAC6 blocker
NCT02393794	I–II	Romidepsin (Istodax®) by IV, twice every 3 weeks; cisplatin (Platinol®), by IV, every 3 weeks	TNBC or BRCA1 or BRCA2 mutation-associated locally recurrent or metastatic BC	HDAC inhibitor
NCT02425891	III	Experimental group: MPDL3280a (atezolizumab), by IV; nab-paclitaxel (Abraxane®), by IV Control group: placebo; nab-paclitaxel (Abraxane®), by IV	Locally advanced or metastatic TNBC	Anti-PD-L1
NCT02366949	I	Experimental group: BAY1217389, by OA, twice daily; paclitaxel (Taxol®) by IV, weekly Control group: paclitaxel (Taxol®) by IV, weekly	Advanced TNBC	MPS1
NCT02309177	I	Group 1 nab-paclitaxel, by IV, weekly for 3 weeks every month; nivolumab (Opdivo®), by IV, every 2 weeks, starting at 3 months; group 2 nab-paclitaxel, by IV, once every 3 weeks 28/02/2017 nivolumab (Opdivo®), by IV, every 3 weeks, starting at 3 months	HER2−, recurrent metastatic TNBC	Anti-PD-1
NCT02595320	II	Group 1: 1500 mg capecitabine (Xeloda®), by OA, twice daily, 1 week on, 1 week off; group 2: 1250 mg capecitabine (Xeloda®), by OA, twice daily, 2 weeks on, 1 week off	Metastatic TNBC	Alkylating agent; tumor-selective and tumor-activated cytotoxic agent
NCT02897375	I	Group 1: palbociclib (Ibrance®), by OA, daily (3 weeks on, 1 week off); cisplatin (Platinol®), by IV, once, monthly; group 2: palbociclib (Ibrance®), by OA, daily (3 weeks on, 1 week off); carboplatin (Paraplatin®), by IV, once, monthly	ER +, HER2− metastatic BC, advanced BC	CDK inhibitor
NCT00978250	II	FdCyd (5-fluoro-2′-deoxycytidine) and THU (tetrahydrouridine) by IV for 5 days per week for 2 weeks, followed by 2 weeks of no treatment	Advanced BC	FdCyd, a fluoropyrimidine nucleoside DNMT inhibitor, and THU; THU does not have any anticancer effects, but it can help keep the other drug
NCT02046421	I	Mifepristone by OA on days 0, 1, 7, and 8; carboplatin (Paraplatin) and gemcitabine hydrochloride (Gemzar) by IV on days 1 and 8	Advanced BC	GR antagonist
NCT02752685	II	Pembrolizumab (Keytruda®), by IV, every 3 weeks; nab-paclitaxel (Taxotere®), by IV, weekly, 2 weeks on 1 week off	HER2− metastatic BC	Anti PD-1
NCT02915744	III	Group 1: NKTR-102, by IV, once every 3 weeks, ongoing; group 2 treatment of physician's choice (eribulin/Halaven®, ixabepilone/Ixempra®, vinorelbine/Navelbine®, gemcitabine/Gemzar®, paclitaxel/Taxol®, docetaxel/Taxotere® or nab-paclitaxel/Abraxane®), by IV	Metastatic BC with brain metastases	Topoisomerase I inhibitor
NCT02929576	III	Group 1: Xtandi and Taxol, enzalutamide (Xtandi®), by OA, daily, ongoing, paclitaxel (Taxol®), by IV, weekly for 16 weeks; group 2: placebo and Taxol, placebo, by OA, daily, ongoing, paclitaxel (Taxol®), by IV, weekly for 16 weeks; group 3: Xtandi followed by Taxol, enzalutamide (Xtandi), by OA, daily, ongoing, followed by paclitaxel (Taxol®), by IV, weekly for 16 weeks	Advanced TNBC	Synthetic non-steroidal antiandrogen
NCT02163694	III	Group 1: experimental: veliparib by OA, on days 2 through 5, carboplatin (Paraplatin®) and paclitaxel (Taxol®) by IV, once every 3 weeks; group 2: control: placebo by OA on days 2 through 5, carboplatin and paclitaxel by IV, once every 3 weeks	Advanced HER2− BCr with BRCA1 or BRCA2 mutation	PARP inhibitor
NCT02187991	II	Group 1: paclitaxel (Taxol®), by IV, 3 times a month, ongoing; Group 2: paclitaxel (Taxol®), by IV, 3 times a month, ongoing, alisertib, by OA, 3 times a week, ongoing	ER+/HER2− or advanced TNBC	Aurora A kinase inhibitor

Table 1 The most recent clinical trials in TNBC patients in the search of therapeutic biomarkers for advanced disease (*Continued*)

Clinical trial	Phase	Study groups	Indications	Therapeutic target
NCT01990352	II	Doxil® (pegylated liposomal doxorubicin hydrochloride), by IV, every 3 weeks	Metastatic TNBC	Liposoma
NCT01999738	I	EC1456 by injection, twice a week on weeks 1 and 2 of every month	Metastatic TNBC	Injectable targeted SMDC consisting of folate (vitamin B9; a folate receptors agonist) covalently linked to the potent mitotic poison and cytotoxic agent, tubulysin B hydrazide (Tub-B-H, a tubulin polymerization inhibitor)
NCT0250064	I	BTP-114, by IV, once every 3 weeks, ongoing	Advanced TNBC with a BRCA 1/2 mutation	Albumin-binding cisplatin prodrug
NCT01802970	I	Anakinra (Kineret®) alone, by OA, for 2 weeks followed by: anakinra (Kineret®), by OA, nab-paclitaxel (Abraxane®) by IV weekly, for a maximum of 6 months	Advanced BC	IL-1 receptor antagonist, an anti-inflammatory
NCT02000882	II	BKM120 by OA daily; capecitabine by OA twice a day, for 2 weeks on, 1 week off, ongoing	TNBC with brain metastases	PI3K inhibitor
NCT02379247	I-II	BYL719, by OA, daily; nab-paclitaxel (Abraxane®) by IV, weekly for 3 out of every 4 weeks	Advanced HER2-negative BC	PI3K inhibitor
NCT02624700	II	Pemetrexed, by IV, every 2 weeks; sorafenib, by OA, twice daily for 5 days	Recurrent or metastatic TNBC	Small inhibitor of several tyrosine protein kinases, such as VEGFR, PDGFR, and Raf family kinases (more avidly C-Raf than B-Raf)
NCT02978716	II	Group 1: chemotherapy, only, gemcitabine (Gemzar®) and carboplatin (Paraplatin®), by IV, on days 1 and 8, ongoing; group 2: trilaciclib and chemotherapy, trilaciclib (G1T28), by IV, on days 1 and 8, ongoing, gemcitabine (Gemzar®) and carboplatin (Paraplatin®), by IV, on days 1 and 8, ongoing; group 3: trilaciclib and chemotherapy, trilaciclib (G1T28), by IV, on days 1, 2, 8, 9, ongoing, gemcitabine (Gemzar®) and carboplatin (Paraplatin®), by IV, on days 2 and 9, ongoing	Recurrent or metastatic TNBC	CDK4/6 inhibitor
NCT02753595	I-I	Eribulin mesylate (Halaven®), by IV, weekly (2 weeks on, 1 week off); PEGPH20, by IV, weekly (2 weeks on 1 week off)	HER2– metastatic BC	Pegylated recombinant human PH20 degrades hyaluronic acid (HA) coating tumor cells
NCT02762981	I-II	CORT125134, by OA, daily, ongoing; nab-paclitaxel (Abraxane®), by IV, weekly (3 weeks on 1 week off, ongoing	Advanced BC	GR antagonist

Intravenous IV, oral administration OA, AC Adriamycin® and Cytoxan®, mTOR mammalian target of rapamycin, HDAC6 histone deacetylase 6, BRCA1/2 breast cancer 1/2, PD-L1 programmed cell death ligand-1, MPS1 serine/threonine kinase monopolar spindle 1, HER2 human epidermal growth factor receptor 2, PD-1 programmed cell death receptor, ES+ estrogen receptor positive, CDK cyclin-dependent kinase, FdCyd 5-fluoro-2'-deoxycytidine, THU tetrahydrouridine, DNMT DNA methyltransferase, GR glucocorticoid receptor, PARP poly (ADP-ribose) polymerase, SMDC small molecule drug conjugate, IL1 Interleukin-1, PI3K phosphatidylinositol 3-kinase, VEGF vascular endothelial growth factor, PDGF-R platelet-derived growth factor receptors

cancer phenotypes through their interactions with other cellular macromolecules [77, 78]. To date, it has been strongly proposed that a deeper functional understanding of lncRNAs will provide novel insights into the molecular mechanism of cancer. As such, lncRNAs are likely to serve as the basis for many clinical applications in oncology [79], like potential biomarkers for diagnosis or therapy targets for clinical treatment of TNBC, as we discuss next.

lncRNAs: molecular mechanisms and potential therapeutic functionality

Protein-coding gene sequences represent a minority (less than 2%) of the human genome sequences; in contrast, the majority are represented by protein non-coding genome sequences, such as non-coding RNAs (ncRNAs) [80]. The ncRNAs can be divided into two categories: *house-keeping* ncRNAs (tRNA, rRNA, etc.) and *regulatory* ncRNAs (miRNA, lncRNA, piRNA, etc.) [81]. LncRNAs are regulatory ncRNAs with at least 200 nucleotides long (nt) that do not encode any protein [82].

Based on the genomic location sites of the lncRNA transcripts and their neighboring relation with the protein-coding genes, lncRNAs can be divided into five categories: (1) sense lncRNAs, which overlap one or more exons of transcripts on the same strand; (2) antisense lncRNAs, which overlap one or more exons of another transcript on the opposite strand; (3) bidirectional lncRNAs, which are located on the opposite strand from the neighboring exon whose transcription orientation has been identified at less than 1000 base pairs; (4) intronic lncRNAs, which are structurally located within another intron of another transcript; and (5) intergenic lncRNAs, which interact within the genomic interval between two genes [83]. In addition, many known lncRNAs have been identified *intracellularly* either within the cytosol and/or between the nuclear and cytoplasm compartments [84]. According to recent studies, the human transcriptome contains up to 16,000 lncRNAs, frequently spliced and polyadenylated, whose non-coding genes are mainly transcribed by the RNA polymerase II [85].

Raised evidence supports that lncRNAs have potential, diverse, and deep functional roles at the nucleus level, which include acting as a positive (activation) mechanism of the transcriptional regulation, as well as their involvement in the inactivation of epigenetic mechanisms (Eg., X-chromosome inactivation), heterochromatin conformation, telomere maintenance, and pluripotency capacity modulation and also have been seen to be involved in cancer development [86–88].

It has become increasingly important to link clinical correlation studies and experimental evidences, which has suggested that lncRNAs contribute to tumor promoting, progression, and metastasis for different malignant diseases through several cellular processes, ranging from transcriptional (cis/trans) and post-transcriptional regulation mechanisms in cell cycle distribution control and cell differentiation to epigenetic modification mechanisms [89–92]. LncRNAs modulate gene transcription by rearranging chromatin via chromosomal looping and by affecting the binding of transcription factors. LncRNAs also affect miRNA functions by controlling pre-mRNA splicing or as miRNA sponges. Recently, accumulating evidence indicates that there is aberrant expression of lncRNAs in many cancer types [93]. An increasing number of studies have demonstrated that a number of lncRNAs are not transcriptional noise, but have important functions, such as regulating gene expression at various molecular levels, including RNA, miRNA, DNA, and proteins, playing important roles in RNA translation and cytoplasmic protein trafficking [94]. Few studies like Yang et al. have focused on how lncRNA genes themselves are regulated by different transcripts activating regulatory regions of lncRNAs [95].

Other studies have indicated that altered expression levels of lncRNAs are associated with human diseases, including BC. Examples include the lncRNAs H19, HOTAIR (HOX transcript antisense RNA), and UCA1 (urothelial cancer associated 1, non-protein coding), which silence tumor suppressor genes. Likewise, lincRNA-p21 mediates global gene repression in the p53 response, while GAS5 plays a tumor suppressor role [96–100]. Another specific example is CYTOR (cytoskeleton regulator RNA), which plays a role in BC, regulating genes involved in the EGFR/mammalian target of the rapamycin pathway and is required for cell proliferation, cell migration, and cytoskeleton organization [101]. Other lncRNAs have been associated with drug resistance to standard BC treatment. Examples include ARA-lncRNA (adriamycin resistance associated), which provided novel insights into adriamycin resistance. Breast cancer antiestrogen resistance 4 (BCAR4) is related to tamoxifen resistance and could also sensitize BC cells to lapatinib. Lastly, CCAT2 (colon cancer-associated transcript 2) may be downregulated by chemotherapy with 5-FU, blocking different pathways involved with cell migration [102–105]. Other potential targeted lncRNA for breast cancer treatment include SPRY4-IT1 and PANDAR [8, 100]. However, recent studies have revealed that the dysregulation of lncRNAs that are known to be associated with human disease is often due to the aberrant expression of transcription factor inducers that could initiate oncogenic mechanisms by feedback complexes [8].

Recently, Lv et al. found lncRNAs as ANRIL, HIF1A-AS2, and UCA1 expression was significantly increased in plasma of patients with TNBC [106], suggesting their use as TNBC-specific diagnostic biomarkers and/or molecular prognostic predictors [106, 107].

LncRNAs in TNBC: biology and their potential therapeutic for clinical oncology

Non-coding sequences have a crucial participation for genetic expression regulation or modulation of several genes implicated in BC. However, it remains to be described a total pattern or profile expression of the long non-coding RNAs for the TNBC subgroup that could be implicated in the invasiveness malignity of these tumors.

First at all, Shen et al. identified 1758 lncRNAs and 1254 mRNAs with significant expression differences in TNBC vs. normal adjacent tissue based in microarray analysis [108]; subsequently, Yang et al. and other researcher groups have been working on the identification and validation of the differential expression of lncRNAs by RNA massive sequencing methods (RNA-seq) [9, 79], as well as, more recently single-cell RNA sequencing (scRNASeq) that allows the quantification of transcript expression profiles for individual cells in a cellular population of solid tumor [107, 109]. Following, on 2015,

Chen et al. discovered and validated a set of novel aberrant lncRNA profile expressed in TNBC, suggesting that deregulated lncRNA pattern may play a role in the developmental and progression of TNBC (Table 2).

An interesting study has suggested a lncRNA candidate named LINC00993, which is both considerably deregulated in TNBC and associated with the ER and ANKRD30A gene expression [110]. ANKRD30A (also known as NY-BR-1 or B726P) encodes a DNA-binding transcription factor previously detected in well-differentiated ER-positive and HER2-negative BC tumors [111]. Also, ANKRD30A has been identified as a BC antigen in disseminated tumor cells (DTCs), and is currently one of the most used DTC biomarkers, and a potential target for BC immunotherapy, so the correlated expression between lncRNA LINC00993 and ANKRD30A gene has supported strong evidence that ANKRD30A gene expression may be epigenetic-target of the lncRNA LINC00993; however, more studies are needed in this regard [112–114]. Some lncRNAs have been proposed as competitive endogenous RNA (ceRNA) for short non-coding RNA (miRNAs). LincRNA-RoR (regulator of reprogramming) is

Table 2 Main lncRNAs associated with triple-negative breast cancer

Author	lncRNA	Alteration in TNBC	Function/characteristics
Augoff et al. 2012 [127]	LOC554202	Upregulated	MIR31 host gene, regulates proliferation and migration in breast cancer cells and promotes hypermethylation of miR31 in TNBC
Chen et al. 2015 [110]	LINC00993	Upregulated	Associated with the expression of the estrogen receptor and the expression levels of ANKRD30A
	TCONS_I2_00002973	Upregulated	Associated with the expression of the estrogen receptor.
	TCONS_I2_00003939	Upregulated	Associated with the expression of the estrogen receptor.
	TCONS_I2_00002974	Upregulated	Associated with the expression of the estrogen receptor.
Eades et al. 2015 [118]	lincRNA-RoR	Upregulated	Prevents the core TFs from miRNA-mediated suppression in self-renewing human SC
Wang et al. 2015 [119]	HOTAIR	Upregulated	Regulates chromatin state. It is required for gene silencing of the HOXD locus by PRC2, highly expressed in metastatic breast cancers. High levels of expression in primary breast tumors are a significant predictor of subsequent metastasis and death
	MALAT1	Upregulated	Alternative splicing, nuclear organization, epigenetic modulating of gene expression, and a number of evidences indicate that MALAT1 also closely relate to various pathological processes, ranging from diabetes complications to cancer. It regulates the expression of metastasis-associated genes, with proliferation, motility, and apoptosis evasion
Lin et al. 2016 [10]	LINK-A (also known as LOC339535 and NR_015407)	Upregulated	Is an RNA of binding to kinases that phosphorylate HIF 1 alpha in different sites to the canonical ones in human cancer
	RMST	Downregulated	Tumor suppressor
Yang et al. 2016 [79]	LINC01234	Up/downregulated	Oncogene/tumor suppressor
Koduru et al. 2017 [9]	lnc-DNAJC16	Upregulated	Belonging to the DnaJ heat shock protein family, functions in protein translation, translocation and degradation
	lnc-PURA	Upregulated	It is a sequence-specific, multi-functional single-stranded-DNA/RNA-binding protein and RNA-binding protein which can act as a transcriptional activator and repressor

lncRNA, long non-coding RNA; ANKRD30A, Ankyrin repeat domain 30A; TFs, transcription factors; miRNA, microRNA; PRC2, polycomb repressive complex 2; HIF-1α, hypoxia-inducible factor 1 alpha; lincRNA-RoR, long intergenic non-protein coding RNA, regulator of reprogramming; HOTAIR, HOX transcript antisense RNA; MALAT1, metastasis-associated lung adenocarcinoma transcript 1; LINK-A, long intergenic noncoding RNA for kinase activation; RMST, rhabdomyosarcoma 2-associated transcript

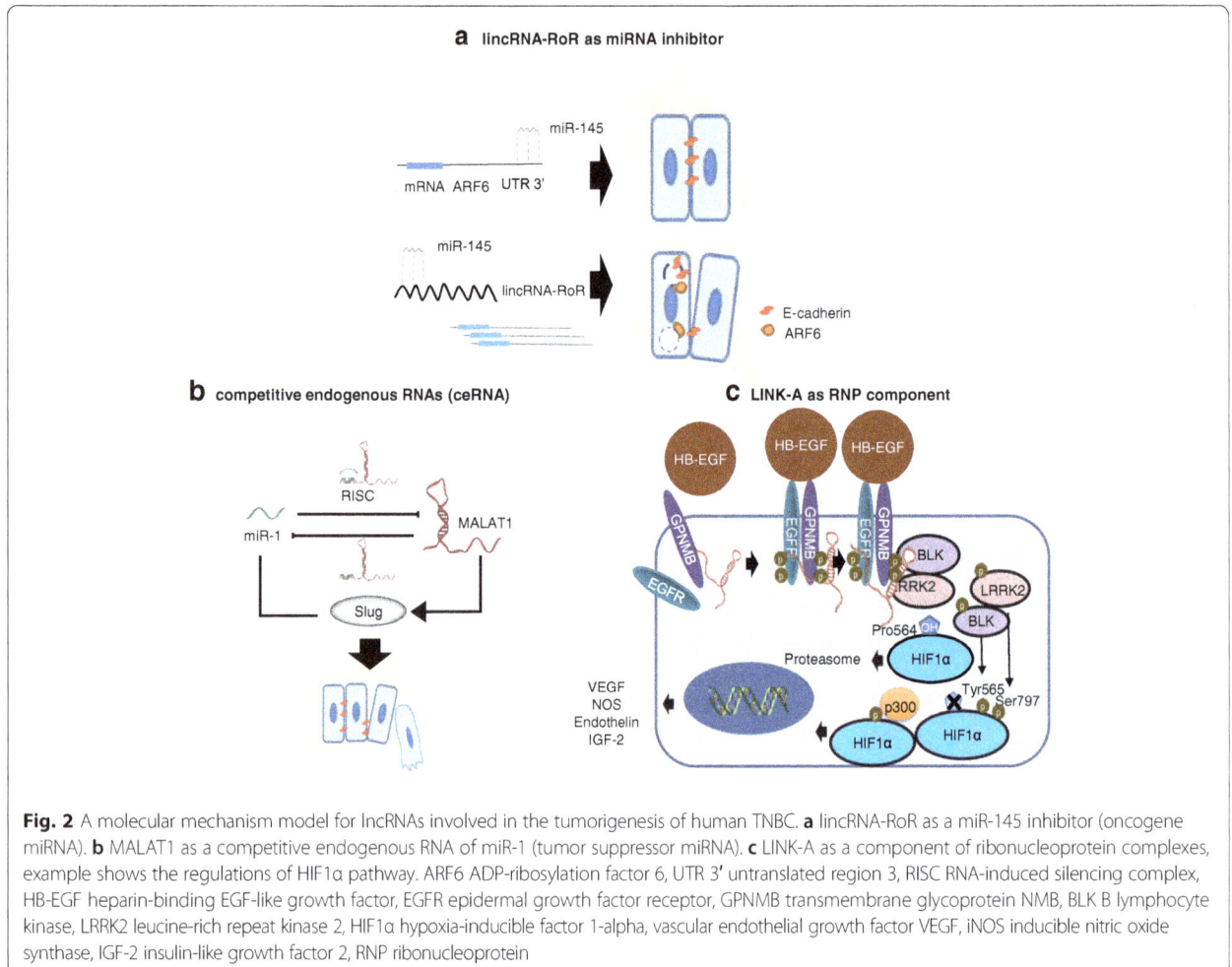

Fig. 2 A molecular mechanism model for lncRNAs involved in the tumorigenesis of human TNBC. **a** lincRNA-RoR as a miR-145 inhibitor (oncogene miRNA). **b** MALAT1 as a competitive endogenous RNA of miR-1 (tumor suppressor miRNA). **c** LINK-A as a component of ribonucleoprotein complexes, example shows the regulations of HIF1α pathway. ARF6 ADP-ribosylation factor 6, UTR 3′ untranslated region 3, RISC RNA-induced silencing complex, HB-EGF heparin-binding EGF-like growth factor, EGFR epidermal growth factor receptor, GPNMB transmembrane glycoprotein NMB, BLK B lymphocyte kinase, LRRK2 leucine-rich repeat kinase 2, HIF1α hypoxia-inducible factor 1-alpha, vascular endothelial growth factor VEGF, iNOS inducible nitric oxide synthase, IGF-2 insulin-like growth factor 2, RNP ribonucleoprotein

upregulated in pluripotent cells (shown in Fig. 2a) [115], where it functions as ceRNA for miR-145, thereby protecting pluripotency factors from miR-mediated silencing, leading to loss of mature miR-145 expression [116]. Recently, Eades et al. found that in TNBC, loss of miR-145 promotes tumor cell invasion. This is mediated through ARF6 overexpression, a protein implicated in tumor invasion through disturbance of cell-cell adhesion by endocytose E-cadherin. In this case, lincRNA-RoR generates a competitive inhibition of miR-145, which alters ARF6 expression. The authors also reported an overexpression of lincRNA-RoR in lymph node positive tumors of TNBC patients and reported the first ceRNA network in human cancer (shown in Fig. 2a) [117, 118].

The expression of other lncRNAs, like HOTAIR, has been shown to enhance the growth and metastasis in xenograft mammary tumors [97]. Wang et al. showed that HOTAIR expression is closely correlated with primary TNBC tumor tissues and demonstrated that HOTAIR expression is transcriptionally repressed by the combined treatment of lapatinib plus imatinib, the first inhibiting EGFR and ErbB2/HER2, and the second a

c-ABL inhibitor through β-catenin-binding sites LEF1/TCF4 [119]. In another study, Jin et al. showed that metastasis-associated lung adenocarcinoma transcript 1 (MALAT1) lncRNA exerts its oncogenic activity by interacting with miR-1. MALAT1 was found upregulated in TNBC tissues and is associated to tumor growth and metastasis, as well as poor overall survival. Downregulation of MALAT1 increased the expression of microRNA-1 (miR-1), while overexpression of miR-1 decreased MALAT1 expression. In this sense, MALAT1 exerted its function through the miR-1/slug axis and therefore MALAT1 may be a target for TNBC therapy (shown in Fig. 2b) [120]. Recently, Lin et al. showed that the long intergenic non-coding RNA for kinase activation (LINK-A) is critical for growth factor-induced normoxic signaling pathway by recruiting breast tumor kinase (BRK) activated together with leucine-rich repeat kinase 2 (LRRK2). The latter phosphorylates hypoxia-inducible factor 1-alpha (HIF1α) at Tyr565 and Ser797. The phosphorylation at Tyr565 inhibits hydroxylation at the adjacent Pro564, which prevents HIF1α degradation under normoxic conditions. Ser797 phosphorylation facilitates HIF1α-p300 interaction, leading to activation of HIF1α target genes upon heparin-binding EGF-like growth factor (HB-EGF) stimulation. Importantly, both LINK-A expression and activation of the LINK-A-mediated normoxic HIF1α signaling pathway could serve as a therapeutic strategy in TNBC (shown in Fig. 2c) [121]. Downregulation of lncRNAs has also been shown to be associated with worse clinical outcomes. Such is the case of rhabdomyosarcoma 2-associated transcript (RMST), which functions as an oncogene and whose expression has been correlated to a lower overall survival [79].

Potential lncRNAs as probable epigenetic biomarkers in TNBC

Nuclear lncRNAs may act as an epigenetic regulator or a guide by recruiting chromatin modification factors to cytogenetic locus, but particularly at gene regulatory/promoter sequences (shown in Fig. 1). As scaffold archetype, nuclear lncRNAs bring together multiple proteins to conform ribonucleoprotein (RNP) complexes. Such lncRNA-RNP complexes can either affect histone modifications or stabilize signaling complexes or nuclear structures [9], as decoy, signaling, and/or guide functional archetypes, as well (Fig. 1).

Recently, Rahman et al. have identified lncRNA lnc00673 (ERRLR01) as a marker of overall survival (OS) in BC patients. Specifically, ERRLR01 levels were

elevated in TNBC as compared with BC ERα-positive patients. LncRNA ERRLR01 expression levels were also inversely correlated with BC survival for all BC patients, suggesting that ERRLR01 is modulated by hormone signaling in BC [122]. Following this observation, Bamodu et al. showed that metastatic BC cell lines exhibited increased expression levels of lysine-specific demethylase 5B protein (KDM5B) and lncRNA MALAT1, suggesting a functional association. However KDM5B silencing in TNBC cells has been correlated with the upregulation of hsa-miR-448 and led to suppression of MALAT1 expression with a decreased migration, invasion, and clonogenic capacity in vitro, as well as poorer overall survival in vivo (shown in Fig. 3 a) [123]. On the other hand, some miRNAs (microRNAs) that control gene expression by post-transcriptional regulation have been shown to be transcribed as part of host genes. For example, miR-31 is a tumor suppressor-miRNA which is transcribed from the first intron of a host gene LOC554202, on human chromosome 9 [124]. On the other hand, some short non-coding RNA mediate oncogenic processes, such as miR-31, which regulates a group of pro-metastatic target genes, including WAVE3, RhoA, Radexin, and several integrin subunits that regulate key steps in the invasion metastasis cascade [125, 126]. Augoff et al. in 2012 identified a major CpG island upstream of the miR-31 locus, which also spans the first exon of LOC554202, suggesting an epigenetic regulation

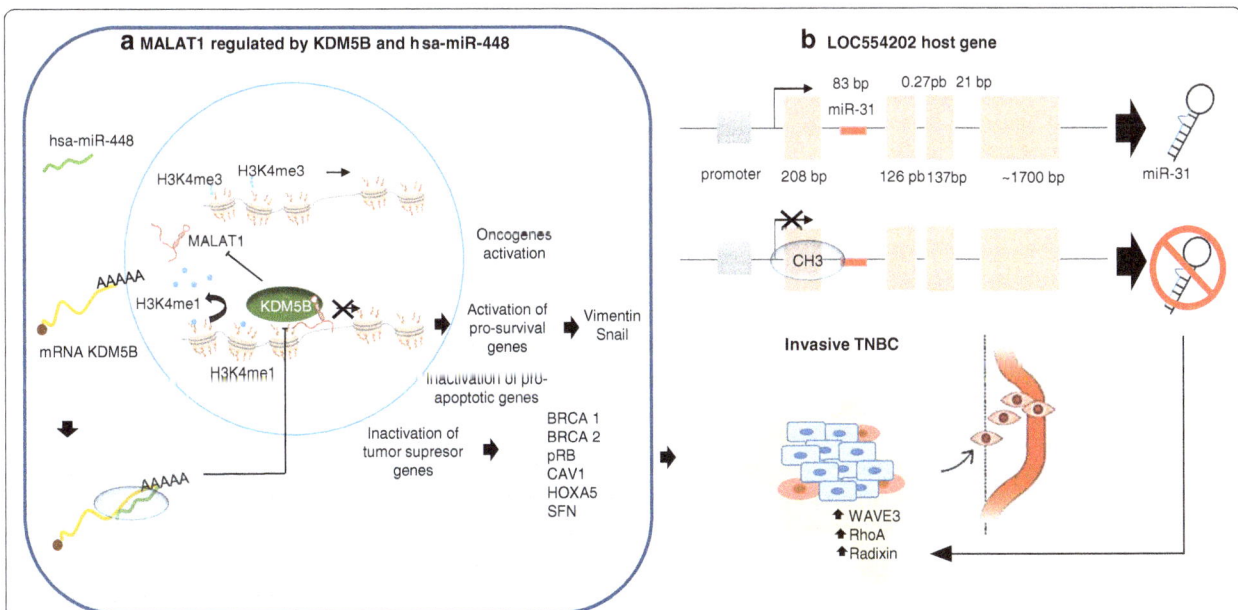

Fig. 3 Epigenetic implications of lncRNAs in the development of TNBC. a MALAT1 regulated by KDM5B and has-miR-448. b LOC554202 as a host gene of miR-31 (tumor suppressor miRNA), WAVE3 (WAS protein family member 3) KDM5B (lysine-specific demethylase 5B also known as histone demethylase JARID1B), H3K4me3 (trimethylation of lysine 4 on the histone H3 protein subunit), H3K4me1 (monomethylation of lysine 4 on the histone H3 protein subunit), hsa-miR-448 (also known miRNA448), BRCA1/2 (breast cancer 1/2), pRB (retinoblastoma protein), CAV 1 (caveolin 1) HOXA5 (Homeobox protein Hox-A5), SFN (Stratifin), CH3 (methyl group), and RhoA (Ras homolog gene family, member A)

by methylation of both miR31 and the host gene in basal TNBC compared to luminal BC cell lines (shown in Fig. 3 b) [127].

Perspectives: lncRNAs as potential therapeutic targets

As we have shown, lncRNAs play several roles in TNBC, but their biological participation is not yet fully understood. Some important advances have been reached, such as the study by Wang et al. which describes different expression patterns of lncRNAs in TNBC vs. non-cancer tissue. We believe that this opens new ideas for functional studies on lncRNAs that have not yet been totally defined as modulators of mRNA coding genes [119]. The lack of complete patterns impedes the development of new TNBC molecular targets, as well as, new-targeted drugs, which could specifically target functional lncRNAs.

However, it would be a fascinating and novel therapeutic strategy. On that recently, Xia et al. designed one oligonucleotide with some chemical modifications which improve its half-life in serum, this molecule antagonizes the function of one tumorigenic lncRNA named ASBEL [128]; in this regard, they have proposed it as a new field of research of potential therapeutic tools for the treatment of TNBC, also named gene therapy.

Notably, lncRNAs could be detected in human bodily fluids, acting as biomarkers. Chen et al. provided useful information for exploring potential therapeutic targets for TNBC [110]. Recently, studies have demonstrated that lncRNA expression could be regulated by conventional chemotherapy agents like tyrosine kinase receptors (TKRs) and non-TKRs by targeting multiple genes at the same time through unknown mechanisms [120]. More studies that strongly focus on molecular mechanisms are needed in order to improve our understanding of how these FDA-approved chemotherapeutic agents for malignant neoplasms exert regulatory action through epigenetic mechanisms on TNBC.

We also know the existence of lncRNA domains upon chromatin structure, where it plays a critical role in the development and/or progression of TNBC disease. Shen et al. explained that chromosome 1 and 10 are the major domains of dysregulation of lncRNAs and mRNA expression, both regulated by lncRNAs through an unknown mechanism [108]. Our research group suggests co-localization of lncRNAs that dictates oncogenic decisions during the development of aggressive TNBC. Several lncRNAs are implicated on hormonal resistance therapy [100]. While some platforms like Oncotype and MammaPrint help medical staff to better identify which patients will respond to standard chemotherapy and have a better prognosis, here, we take into consideration co-expressed mRNAs/lncRNAs that could identify

TNBC patients that could benefit from personalized pharmacological treatments. LncRNAs as biomarkers and their associated genetic-epigenetic and transcriptional mechanisms in co-expression patterns of mRNA coding genes open new insights for gene expression control, and epigenetic events that could explain pathophysiology and/or pharmacological actions for clinical diagnosis, treatment response, and prognosis of TNBC patients.

Conclusions

Perhaps we are approaching an era of personalized therapies for TNBC patients, as was initially idealized by Lehmann et al. who elucidated the TNBC heterogeneity [54, 129, 130]. These therapies, probably will aim to reduce the risk of recurrence and disease progression, as main TNBC tumors feature, as well as to develop more targeted and reduced toxic therapies for the six specific subtypes, previously described [130]. Theoretically, personalized treatments should improve stratification and timing of health care by utilizing biological information and biomarkers on the level of molecular disease pathways, genetics, proteomics, and metabolomics [131]. In this regard, it is imperative that we improve our understanding of biological processes such as epigenetic changes that occur by lncRNAs [132], considering lncRNA archetypes (shown in Fig. 1) for TNBC to reach that point, as a probable personalized epigenetic therapy. Efforts have been made in genomics to personalize the TNBC treatments that are currently oncological under use. This review has presented additional evidence that lncRNAs may work as diagnostic biomarkers and therapeutic targets in solid tumors, including BC and TNBC. However, their relative expression levels in various subtypes of human BC [133], particularly the TNBC subtype, remain to be determined [134].

Abbreviations

AC: Adriamycin® and Cytoxan®; ANKRD30A: Ankyrin repeat domain 30A; ARA-lncRNA: Adriamycin resistance associated; ARF6: ADP-ribosylation factor 6; BC: Breast cancer; BCAR4: Breast cancer antiestrogen resistance 4; BLK: B lymphocyte kinase; BRCA1/2: Breast cancer 1/2; BRK: Breast tumor kinase; CCAT2: Colon cancer-associated transcript 2; CDK: Cyclin-dependent kinase; ceRNA: Competitive endogenous RNA; CYTOR: Cytoskeleton regulator RNA; DFS: Disease-free survival; DNMT: DNA methyltransferase; DTCs: Disseminated tumor cells; EGFR: Epidermal growth factor receptor; EMA: European Medicines Agency; ER-α: Estrogen receptor alpha; ES+: Estrogen receptor positive; FDA: Food and Drug Administration; FdCyd: 5-Fluoro-2′-deoxycytidine; FGFR: Fibroblast growth factor receptor; GPNMB: Transmembrane glycoprotein NMB; GR: Glucocorticoid receptor; HB-EGF: Heparin-binding EGF-like growth factor; HDAC6: Histone deacetylase 6; HER2: Human epidermal growth factor receptor 2; HIF1α: Hypoxia-inducible factor 1-alpha; HOTAIR: HOX transcript antisense RNA; IGF-2: Insulin-like growth factor 2; IL1: Interleukin-1; iNOS: Inducible nitric oxide synthase; INPP4B: Inositol polyphosphate 4-phosphatase type II; IV: Intravenous; lincRNA-RoR: Long intergenic non-protein coding RNA regulator of reprogramming; LincRNA-RoR: Regulator of reprogramming; LINK-A: Long intergenic noncoding RNA for kinase activation; lncRNAs: Long noncoding ribonucleic acids; LRRK2: Leucine-rich repeat kinase 2; MALAT1: Metastasis-associated lung adenocarcinoma transcript 1; MAPK: Mitogen-activated protein kinase; miR-

1: MicroRNA-1; miR-31: Tumor suppressor miRNA; miRNA: MicroRNA; MPS1: Serine/threonine kinase monopolar spindle 1; mTOR: Mammalian target of rapamycin; NAC: Neoadjuvant chemotherapy; ncRNA: Non-coding RNA; OA: Oral administration; PARP: Poly (ADP-ribose) polymerase; pCR: Pathological complete response; PD-1: Programmed cell death receptor; PDGF-R: Platelet-derived growth factor receptors; PD-L1: Programmed cell death ligand-1; PI3K: Phosphatidylinositol 3-kinase; PR: Progesterone receptor; PRC2: Polycomb repressive complex 2; PTEN: Phosphatase and tensin homolog; RISC: RNA-induced silencing complex; RMST: Rhabdomyosarcoma 2-associated transcript; RNP: Ribonucleoprotein; SMDC: Small molecule drug conjugate; TFs: Transcription factors; THU: Tetrahydrouridine; TKRs: Tyrosine kinase receptors; TNBC: Triple-negative breast cancer; UCA1: Urothelial cancer associated 1 non-protein coding; UTR 3: Untranslated region 3'; VEGF: Vascular endothelial growth factor; VEGFR: Vascular endothelial growth factor receptor; WAVE3: WAS protein family member 3

Authors' contributions

All authors contributed to the conception of the article, writing, and revision of the final manuscript and agree on its submission to this journal.

Competing interests

The authors declare that they have no competing interests.

Author details

[1]Thoracic Oncology Unit and Laboratory of Personalized Medicine, Instituto Nacional de Cancerología (INCan), San Fernando #22, Section XVI, Tlalpan, 14080 Mexico City, Mexico. [2]Biomedical Science Doctorate Program, National Autonomous University of Mexico, Mexico City, Mexico. [3]Cancer Genomics Laboratory, INMEGEN, Mexico City, Mexico. [4]Biochemistry Department, Instituto Nacional de Ciencias Médicas y Nutrición Salvador Zubirán, Mexico D.F., Mexico. [5]Breast Oncology Department, National Cancer Institute of Mexico, Mexico City, Mexico. [6]Lung Diseases And Cancer Epigenomics Laboratory, Biomedicine Research Unit (UBIMED), Facultad de Estudios Superiores (FES) Iztacala, National University Autonomous of México (UNAM), Mexico City, Mexico. [7]Research Unit, National Institute of Respiratory Diseases (INER) "Ismael Cosío Villegas", Mexico City, Mexico.

References

1. Mortality, G. B. D., and Causes of Death, C. Global, regional, and national life expectancy, all-cause mortality, and cause-specific mortality for 249 causes of death, 1980–2015: a systematic analysis for the Global Burden of Disease Study 2015. Lancet. 2016;388:1459–544.
2. Siegel RL, Miller KD, Jemal A. Cancer statistics, 2017. CA Cancer J Clin. 2017; 67:7–30.
3. Senkus E, Kyriakides S, Ohno S, Penault-Llorca F, Poortmans P, Rutgers E, Zackrisson S, Cardoso F, Committee EG. Primary breast cancer: ESMO Clinical Practice Guidelines for diagnosis, treatment and follow-up. Ann Oncol. 2015;26(Suppl 5):v8–30.
4. Perou CM, Sorlie T, Eisen MB, van de Rijn M, Jeffrey SS, Rees CA, Pollack JR, Ross DT, Johnsen H, Akslen LA, Fluge O, Pergamenschikov A, Williams C, Zhu SX, Lonning PE, Borresen-Dale AL, Brown PO, Botstein D. Molecular portraits of human breast tumours. Nature. 2000;406:747–52.
5. Polyak K. Heterogeneity in breast cancer. J Clin Invest. 2011;121:3786–8.
6. Marusyk A, Almendro V, Polyak K. Intra-tumour heterogeneity: a looking glass for cancer? Nat Rev Cancer. 2012;12:323–34.
7. Martelotto LG, Ng CK, Piscuoglio S, Weigelt B, Reis-Filho JS. Breast cancer intra-tumor heterogeneity. Breast Cancer Res BCR. 2014;16:210.
8. Huarte M, Guttman M, Feldser D, Garber M, Koziol MJ, Kenzelmann-Broz D, Khalil AM, Zuk O, Amit I, Rabani M, Attardi LD, Regev A, Lander ES, Jacks T,

9. Rinn JL. A large intergenic noncoding RNA induced by p53 mediates global gene repression in the p53 response. Cell. 2010;142:409–19.
9. Koduru SV, Tiwari AK, Leberfinger A, Hazard SW, Kawasawa YI, Mahajan M, Ravnic DJ. A comprehensive NGS data analysis of differentially regulated miRNAs, piRNAs, lncRNAs and sn/snoRNAs in triple negative breast cancer. J Cancer. 2017;8:578–96.
10. Lin A, Li C, Xing Z, Hu Q, Liang K, Han L, Wang C, Hawke DH, Wang S, Zhang Y, Wei Y, Ma G, Park PK, Zhou J, Zhou Y, Hu Z, Zhou Y, Marks JR, Liang H, Hung M-C, Lin C, Yang L. The LINK-A lncRNA activates normoxic HIF1α signalling in triple-negative breast cancer. Nat Cell Biol. 2016;18:213.
11. Kong X, Liu W, Kong Y. Roles and expression profiles of long non-coding RNAs in triple-negative breast cancers. J Cell Mol Med. 2018;22:390–4.
12. Anders CK, Carey LA. Biology, metastatic patterns, and treatment of patients with triple-negative breast cancer. Clin Breast Cancer. 2009;9(Suppl 2):S73–81.
13. Anders C, Carey LA. Understanding and treating triple-negative breast cancer. Oncology. 2008;22:1233–9. discussion 1239–1240, 1243
14. Xie Y, Gou Q, Wang Q, Zhong X, Zheng H. The role of BRCA status on prognosis in patients with triple-negative breast cancer. Oncotarget. 2017;8:87151–62.
15. Couch FJ, Hart SN, Sharma P, Toland AE, Wang X, Miron P, Olson JE, Godwin AK, Pankratz VS, Olswold C, Slettedahl S, Hallberg E, Guidugli L, Davila JI, Beckmann MW, Janni W, Rack B, Ekici AB, Slamon DJ, Konstantopoulou I, Fostira F, Vratimos A, Fountzilas G, Pelttari LM, Tapper WJ, Durcan L, Cross SS, Pilarski R, Shapiro CL, Klemp J, Yao S, Garber J, Cox A, Brauch H, Ambrosone C, Nevanlinna H, Yannoukakos D, Slager SL, Vachon CM, Eccles DM, Fasching PA. Inherited mutations in 17 breast cancer susceptibility genes among a large triple-negative breast cancer cohort unselected for family history of breast cancer. J Clin Oncol. 2015;33:304–11.
16. Greenup R, Buchanan A, Lorizio W, Rhoads K, Chan S, Leedom T, King R, McLennan J, Crawford B, Kelly Marcom P, Shelley Hwang E. Prevalence of BRCA mutations among women with triple-negative breast cancer (TNBC) in a genetic counseling cohort. Ann Surg Oncol. 2013;20:3254–8.
17. Curtis C, Shah SP, Chin SF, Turashvili G, Rueda OM, Dunning MJ, Speed D, Lynch AG, Samarajiwa S, Yuan Y, Graf S, Ha G, Haffari G, Bashashati A, Russell R, McKinney S, Group, M, Langerod A, Green A, Provenzano E, Wishart G, Pinder S, Watson P, Markowetz F, Murphy L, Ellis I, Purushotham A, Borresen-Dale AL, Brenton JD, Tavare S, Caldas C, Aparicio S. The genomic and transcriptomic architecture of 2,000 breast tumours reveals novel subgroups. Nature. 2012;486:346–52.
18. Shah SP, Roth A, Goya R, Oloumi A, Ha G, Zhao Y, Turashvili G, Ding J, Tse K, Haffari G, Bashashati A, Prentice LM, Khattra J, Burleigh A, Yap D, Bernard V, McPherson A, Shumansky K, Crisan A, Giuliany R, Heravi-Moussavi A, Rosner J, Lai D, Birol I, Varhol R, Tam A, Dhalla N, Zeng T, Ma K, Chan SK, Griffith M, Moradian A, Cheng SW, Morin GB, Watson P, Gelmon K, Chia S, Chin SF, Curtis C, Rueda OM, Pharoah PD, Damaraju S, Mackey J, Hoon K, Harkins T, Tadigotla V, Sigaroudinia M, Gascard P, Tlsty T, Costello JF, Meyer IM, Eaves CJ, Wasserman WW, Jones S, Huntsman D, Hirst M, Caldas C, Marra MA, Aparicio S. The clonal and mutational evolution spectrum of primary triple-negative breast cancers. Nature. 2012;486:395–9.
19. Pal SK, Childs BH, Pegram M. Triple negative breast cancer: unmet medical needs. Breast Cancer Res Treat. 2011;125.627–36.
20. Cancer Genome Atlas N. Comprehensive molecular portraits of human breast tumours. Nature. 2012;490:61–70.
21. Rakha EA, Ellis IO. Triple-negative/basal-like breast cancer: review. Pathology. 2009;41:40–7.
22. Symmans WF, Peintinger F, Hatzis C, Rajan R, Kuerer H, Valero V, Assad L, Ponlecka A, Hennessy B, Green M, Buzdar AU, Singletary SE, Hortobagyi GN, Pusztai L. Measurement of residual breast cancer burden to predict survival after neoadjuvant chemotherapy. J Clin Oncol. 2007;25:4414–22.
23. Liedtke C, Mazouni C, Hess KR, Andre F, Tordai A, Mejia JA, Symmans WF, Gonzalez-Angulo AM, Hennessy B, Green M, Cristofanilli M, Hortobagyi GN, Pusztai L. Response to neoadjuvant therapy and long-term survival in patients with triple-negative breast cancer. J Clin Oncol. 2008;26:1275–81.
24. Foulkes WD, Smith IE, Reis-Filho JS. Triple-negative breast cancer. N Engl J Med. 2010;363:1938–48.
25. Lara-Medina F, Perez-Sanchez V, Saavedra-Perez D, Blake-Cerda M, Arce C, Motola-Kuba D, Villarreal-Garza C, Gonzalez-Angulo AM, Bargallo E, Aguilar JL, Mohar A, Arrieta O. Triple-negative breast cancer in Hispanic patients: high prevalence, poor prognosis, and association with menopausal status, body mass index, and parity. Cancer. 2011;117:3658–69.
26. Dent R, Trudeau M, Pritchard KI, Hanna WM, Kahn HK, Sawka CA, Lickley LA, Rawlinson E, Sun P, Narod SA. Triple-negative breast cancer: clinical features and patterns of recurrence. Clin Cancer Res. 2007;13:4429–34.

27. Ng CK, Schultheis AM, Bidard FC, Weigelt B, Reis-Filho JS. Breast cancer genomics from microarrays to massively parallel sequencing: paradigms and new insights. J Natl Cancer Inst. 2015;107 https://doi.org/10.1093/jnci/djv015.

28. Kandoth C, McLellan MD, Vandin F, Ye K, Niu B, Lu C, Xie M, Zhang Q, McMichael JF, Wyczalkowski MA, Leiserson MDM, Miller CA, Welch JS, Walter MJ, Wendl MC, Ley TJ, Wilson RK, Raphael BJ, Ding L. Mutational landscape and significance across 12 major cancer types. Nature. 2013;502:333–9.

29. Nik-Zainal S, Davies H, Staaf J, Ramakrishna M, Glodzik D, Zou X, Martincorena I, Alexandrov LB, Martin S, Wedge DC, Van Loo P, Ju YS, Smid M, Brinkman AB, Morganella S, Aure MR, Lingjaerde OC, Langerod A, Ringner M, Ahn SM, Boyault S, Brock JE, Broeks A, Butler A, Desmedt C, Dirix L, Dronov S, Fatima A, Foekens JA, Gerstung M, Hooijer GK, Jang SJ, Jones DR, Kim HY, King TA, Krishnamurthy S, Lee HJ, Lee JY, Li Y, McLaren S, Menzies A, Mustonen V, O'Meara S, Pauporte I, Pivot X, Purdie CA, Raine K, Ramakrishnan K, Rodriguez-Gonzalez FG, Romieu G, Sieuwerts AM, Simpson PT, Shepherd R, Stebbings L, Stefansson OA, Teague J, Tommasi S, Treilleux I, Van den Eynden GG, Vermeulen P, Vincent-Salomon A, Yates L, Caldas C, van't Veer L, Tutt A, Knappskog S, Tan BK, Jonkers J, Borg A, Ueno NT, Sotiriou C, Viari A, Futreal PA, Campbell PJ, Span PN, Van Laere S, Lakhani SR, Eyfjord JE, Thompson AM, Birney E, Stunnenberg HG, van de Vijver MJ, Martens JW, Borresen-Dale AL, Richardson AL, Kong G, Thomas G, Stratton MR. Landscape of somatic mutations in 560 breast cancer whole-genome sequences. Nature. 2016;534:47–54.

30. Gao Y, Jones A, Fasching PA, Ruebner M, Beckmann MW, Widschwendter M, Teschendorff AE. The integrative epigenomic-transcriptomic landscape of ER positive breast cancer. Clin Epigenetics. 2015;7:126.

31. Hicks J, Krasnitz A, Lakshmi B, Navin NE, Riggs M, Leibu E, Esposito D, Alexander J, Troge J, Grubor V, Yoon S, Wigler M, Ye K, Borresen-Dale AL, Naume B, Schlicting E, Norton L, Hagerstrom T, Skoog L, Auer G, Maner S, Lundin P, Zetterberg A. Novel patterns of genome rearrangement and their association with survival in breast cancer. Genome Res. 2006;16:1465–79.

32. Stefansson OA, Moran S, Gomez A, Sayols S, Arribas-Jorba C, Sandoval J, Hilmarsdottir H, Olafsdottir E, Tryggvadottir L, Jonasson JG, Eyfjord J, Esteller M. A DNA methylation-based definition of biologically distinct breast cancer subtypes. Mol Oncol. 2015;9:555–68.

33. Mathe A, Wong-Brown M, Locke WJ, Stirzaker C, Braye SG, Forbes JF, Clark SJ, Avery-Kiejda KA, Scott RJ. DNA methylation profile of triple negative breast cancer-specific genes comparing lymph node positive patients to lymph node negative patients. Sci Rep. 2016;6:33435.

34. Fatica A, Bozzoni I. Long non-coding RNAs: new players in cell differentiation and development. Nat Rev Genet. 2014;15:7–21.

35. Hauptman N, Glavac D. Long non-coding RNA in cancer. Int J Mol Sci. 2013;14:4655–69.

36. Esteller M. Non-coding RNAs in human disease. Nat Rev Genet. 2011;12:861–74.

37. Liu B, Sun L, Liu Q, Gong C, Yao Y, Lv X, Lin L, Yao H, Su F, Li D, Zeng M, Song E. A cytoplasmic NF-kappaB interacting long noncoding RNA blocks IkappaB phosphorylation and suppresses breast cancer metastasis. Cancer Cell. 2015;27:370–81.

38. Liu YR, Jiang YZ, Xu XE, Yu KD, Jin X, Hu X, Zuo WJ, Hao S, Wu J, Liu GY, Di GH, Li DQ, He XH, Hu WG, Shao ZM. Comprehensive transcriptome analysis identifies novel molecular subtypes and subtype-specific RNAs of triple-negative breast cancer. Breast Cancer Res BCR. 2016;18:33.

39. Cheetham SW, Gruhl F, Mattick JS, Dinger ME. Long noncoding RNAs and the genetics of cancer. Br J Cancer. 2013;108:2419–25.

40. Hon CC, Ramilowski JA, Harshbarger J, Bertin N, Rackham OJ, Gough J, Denisenko E, Schmeier S, Poulsen TM, Severin J, Lizio M, Kawaji H, Kasukawa T, Itoh M, Burroughs AM, Noma S, Djebali S, Alam T, Medvedeva YA, Testa AC, Lipovich L, Yip CW, Abugessaisa I, Mendez M, Hasegawa A, Tang D, Lassmann T, Heutink P, Babina M, Wells CA, Kojima S, Nakamura Y, Suzuki H, Daub CO, de Hoon MJ, Arner E, Hayashizaki Y, Carninci P, Forrest AR. An atlas of human long non-coding RNAs with accurate 5' ends. Nature. 2017;543:199–204.

41. Fedele P, Orlando L, Cinieri S. Targeting triple negative breast cancer with histone deacetylase inhibitors. Expert Opin Investig Drugs. 2017;26:1199–206.

42. Tsai M-C, Manor O, Wan Y, Mosammaparast N, Wang JK, Lan F, Shi Y, Segal E, Chang HY. Long noncoding RNA as modular scaffold of histone modification complexes. Science. 2010;329:689.

43. Kohler BA, Sherman RL, Howlader N, Jemal A, Ryerson AB, Henry KA, Boscoe FP, Cronin KA, Lake A, Noone AM, Henley SJ, Eheman CR, Anderson RN, Penberthy L. Annual report to the nation on the status of cancer, 1975-2011, featuring incidence of breast cancer subtypes by race/ethnicity, poverty, and state. J Natl Cancer Inst. 2015;107:djv048.

44. Coates, A. S., Winer, E. P., Goldhirsch, A., Gelber, R. D., Gnant, M., Piccart-Gebhart, M., Thurlimann, B., Senn, H. J., and Panel, M. Tailoring therapies—improving the management of early breast cancer: St Gallen International Expert Consensus on the Primary Therapy of Early Breast Cancer 2015. Ann Oncol. 2015;26:1533–46.

45. Cortazar P, Zhang L, Untch M, Mehta K, Costantino JP, Wolmark N, Bonnefoi H, Cameron D, Gianni L, Valagussa P, Swain SM, Prowell T, Loibl S, Wickerham DL, Bogaerts J, Baselga J, Perou C, Blumenthal G, Blohmer J, Mamounas EP, Bergh J, Semiglazov V, Justice R, Eidtmann H, Paik S, Piccart M, Sridhara R, Fasching PA, Slaets L, Tang S, Gerber B, Geyer CE Jr, Pazdur R, Ditsch N, Rastogi P, Eiermann W, von Minckwitz G. Pathological complete response and long-term clinical benefit in breast cancer: the CTNeoBC pooled analysis. Lancet. 2014;384:164–72.

46. Kaufmann, M., Hortobagyi, G. N., Goldhirsch, A., Scholl, S., Makris, A., Valagussa, P., Blohmer, J. U., Eiermann, W., Jackesz, R., Jonat, W., Lebeau, A., Loibl, S., Miller, W., Seeber, S., Semiglazov, V., Smith, R., Souchon, R., Stearns, V., Untch, M., and von Minckwitz, G. Recommendations from an international expert panel on the use of neoadjuvant (primary) systemic treatment of operable breast cancer: an update. J Clin Oncol. 2006; 24: 1940–1949.

47. Golshan M, Cirrincione CT, Sikov WM, Berry DA, Jasinski S, Weisberg TF, Somlo G, Hudis C, Winer E, Ollila DW, Alliance for Clinical Trials in, O. Impact of neoadjuvant chemotherapy in stage II-III triple negative breast cancer on eligibility for breast-conserving surgery and breast conservation rates: surgical results from CALGB 40603 (Alliance). Ann Surg. 2015;262:434–9. discussion 438–439

48. von Minckwitz G, Untch M, Blohmer JU, Costa SD, Eidtmann H, Fasching PA, Gerber B, Eiermann W, Hilfrich J, Huober J, Jackisch C, Kaufmann M, Konecny GE, Denkert C, Nekljudova V, Mehta K, Loibl S. Definition and impact of pathologic complete response on prognosis after neoadjuvant chemotherapy in various intrinsic breast cancer subtypes. J Clin Oncol. 2012;30:1796–804.

49. Tan DS, Marchio C, Jones RL, Savage K, Smith IE, Dowsett M, Reis-Filho JS. Triple negative breast cancer: molecular profiling and prognostic impact in adjuvant anthracycline-treated patients. Breast Cancer Res Treat. 2008;111:27–44.

50. Haffty BG, Yang Q, Reiss M, Kearney T, Higgins SA, Weidhaas J, Harris L, Hait W, Toppmeyer D. Locoregional relapse and distant metastasis in conservatively managed triple negative early-stage breast cancer. J Clin Oncol. 2006;24:5652–7.

51. Silver DP, Richardson AL, Eklund AC, Wang ZC, Szallasi Z, Li Q, Juul N, Leong CO, Calogrias D, Buraimoh A, Fatima A, Gelman RS, Ryan PD, Tung NM, De Nicolo A, Ganesan S, Miron A, Colin C, Sgroi DC, Ellisen LW, Winer EP, Garber JE. Efficacy of neoadjuvant Cisplatin in triple-negative breast cancer. J Clin Oncol. 2010;28:1145–53.

52. Byrski T, Huzarski T, Dent R, Marczyk E, Jasiowka M, Gronwald J, Jakubowicz J, Cybulski C, Wisniowski R, Godlewski D, Lubinski J, Narod SA. Pathologic complete response to neoadjuvant cisplatin in BRCA1-positive breast cancer patients. Breast Cancer Res Treat. 2014;147:401–5.

53. Andrew Tutt PE, Kilburn L, Gilett C, Pinder S, Abraham J, Barrett S, Barrett-Lee P, Chan S, Cheang M, Dowsett M, Fox L, Gazinska P, Grigoriadis A, Gutin A, Harper-Wynne C, Hatton M, Kernaghan S, Lanchbury J, Morden J, Owen J, Parikh J, Parker P, Rahman N, Roylance R, Shaw A, Smith I, Thompson R, Timms K, Tovey H, Wardley A, Wilson G, Harries M, Bliss J. The TNT trial: a randomized phase III trial of carboplatin (C) compared with docetaxel (D) for patients with metastatic or recurrent locally advanced triple negative or BRCA1/2 breast cancer (CRUK/07/012). Cancer Res. 2015;75:S3–01. AACR

54. Lehmann BD, Pietenpol JA, Tan AR. Triple-negative breast cancer: molecular subtypes and new targets for therapy. Am Soc Clin Oncol Educ Book. 2015: e31–9. https://doi.org/10.14694/EdBook_AM.2015.35.e31.

55. Robson M, Im SA, Senkus E, Xu B, Domchek SM, Masuda N, Delaloge S, Li W, Tung N, Armstrong A, Wu W, Goessl C, Runswick S, Conte P. Olaparib for metastatic breast cancer in patients with a germline BRCA mutation. N Engl J Med. 2017;377:523–33.

56. Stemke-Hale K, Gonzalez-Angulo AM, Lluch A, Neve RM, Kuo WL, Davies M, Carey M, Hu Z, Guan Y, Sahin A, Symmans WF, Pusztai L, Nolden LK, Horlings H, Berns K, Hung MC, van de Vijver MJ, Valero V, Gray JW, Bernards R, Mills GB, Hennessy BT. An integrative genomic and proteomic analysis of PIK3CA, PTEN, and AKT mutations in breast cancer. Cancer Res. 2008;68:6084–91.

57. Marty B, Maire V, Gravier E, Rigaill G, Vincent-Salomon A, Kappler M, Lebigot I, Djelti F, Tourdes A, Gestraud P, Hupe P, Barillot E, Cruzalegui F, Tucker GC, Stern MH, Thiery JP, Hickman JA, Dubois T. Frequent PTEN genomic alterations and activated phosphatidylinositol 3-kinase pathway in basal-like breast cancer cells. Breast Cancer Res BCR. 2008;10:R101.

58. Gewinner C, Wang ZC, Richardson A, Teruya-Feldstein J, Etemadmoghadam D, Bowtell D, Barretina J, Lin WM, Rameh L, Salmena L, Pandolfi PP, Cantley LC. Evidence that inositol polyphosphate 4-phosphatase type II is a tumor suppressor that inhibits PI3K signaling. Cancer Cell. 2009;16:115–25.

59. Banerji S, Cibulskis K, Rangel-Escareno C, Brown KK, Carter SL, Frederick AM, Lawrence MS, Sivachenko AY, Sougnez C, Zou L, Cortes ML, Fernandez-Lopez JC, Peng S, Ardlie KG, Auclair D, Bautista-Pina V, Duke F, Francis J, Jung J, Maffuz-Aziz A, Onofrio RC, Parkin M, Pho NH, Quintanar-Jurado V, Ramos AH, Rebollar-Vega R, Rodriguez-Cuevas S, Romero-Cordoba SL, Schumacher SE, Stransky N, Thompson KM, Uribe-Figueroa L, Baselga J, Beroukhim R, Polyak K, Sgroi DC, Richardson AL, Jimenez-Sanchez G, Lander ES, Gabriel SB, Garraway LA, Golub TR, Melendez-Zajgla J, Toker A, Getz G, Hidalgo-Miranda A, Meyerson M. Sequence analysis of mutations and translocations across breast cancer subtypes. Nature. 2012;486:405–9.

60. Isakoff SJ, J. C. B, Cervantes A, Soria J-C, Molife LR, Sanabria-Bohorquez SM, Punnoose EA, Jia S, Patel P, Saura C. Phase Ib dose-escalation study of an Akt inhibitor ipatasertib (Ipat) in combination with docetaxel (Doc) or paclitaxel (Pac) in patients (pts) with metastatic breast cancer (MBC). In: Thirty-seventh annual CTRC-AACR San Antonio breast cancer symposium, vol. 75. San Antonio, Texas; 2015. p. PC-12–02.

61. Baselga J, Gomez P, Greil R, Braga S, Climent MA, Wardley AM, Kaufman B, Stemmer SM, Pego A, Chan A, Goeminne JC, Graas MP, Kennedy MJ, Ciruelos Gil EM, Schneeweiss A, Zubel A, Groos J, Melezinkova H, Awada A. Randomized phase II study of the anti-epidermal growth factor receptor monoclonal antibody cetuximab with cisplatin versus cisplatin alone in patients with metastatic triple-negative breast cancer. J Clin Oncol. 2013;31:2586–92.

62. Carey LA, Rugo HS, Marcom PK, Mayer EL, Esteva FJ, Ma CX, Liu MC, Storniolo AM, Rimawi MF, Forero-Torres A, Wolff AC, Hobday TJ, Ivanova A, Chiu WK, Ferraro M, Burrows E, Bernard PS, Hoadley KA, Perou CM, Winer EP. TBCRC 001: randomized phase II study of cetuximab in combination with carboplatin in stage IV triple-negative breast cancer. J Clin Oncol. 2012; 30:2615–23.

63. Brufsky A, Valero V, Tiangco B, Dakhil S, Brize A, Rugo HS, Rivera R, Duenne A, Bousfoul N, Yardley DA. Second-line bevacizumab-containing therapy in patients with triple-negative breast cancer: subgroup analysis of the RIBBON-2 trial. Breast Cancer Res Treat. 2012;133:1067–75.

64. Miles DW, Dieras V, Cortes J, Duenne AA, Yi J, O'Shaughnessy J. First-line bevacizumab in combination with chemotherapy for HER2-negative metastatic breast cancer: pooled and subgroup analyses of data from 2447 patients. Ann Oncol. 2013;24:2773–80.

65. Cameron D, Brown J, Dent R, Jackisch C, Mackey J, Pivot X, Steger GG, Suter TM, Toi M, Parmar M, Laeufle R, Im YH, Romieu G, Harvey V, Lipatov O, Pienkowski T, Cottu P, Chan A, Im SA, Hall PS, Bubuteishvili-Pacaud L, Henschel V, Deurloo RJ, Pallaud C, Bell R. Adjuvant bevacizumab-containing therapy in triple-negative breast cancer (BEATRICE): primary results of a randomised, phase 3 trial. Lancet Oncol. 2013;14:933–42.

66. Ciardiello F, Tortora G. EGFR antagonists in cancer treatment. N Engl J Med. 2008;358:1160–74.

67. Corkery B, Crown J, Clynes M, O'Donovan N. Epidermal growth factor receptor as a potential therapeutic target in triple-negative breast cancer. Ann Oncol. 2009;20:862–7.

68. Finn RS, Press MF, Dering J, Arbushites M, Koehler M, Oliva C, Williams LS, Di Leo A. Estrogen receptor, progesterone receptor, human epidermal growth factor receptor 2 (HER2), and epidermal growth factor receptor expression and benefit from lapatinib in a randomized trial of paclitaxel with lapatinib or placebo as first-line treatment in HER2-negative or unknown metastatic breast cancer. J Clin Oncol. 2009;27:3908–15.

69. Lo YH, Ho PC, Zhao H, Wang SC. Inhibition of c-ABL sensitizes breast cancer cells to the dual ErbB receptor tyrosine kinase inhibitor lapatinib (GW572016). Anticancer Res. 2011;31:789–95.

70. Turner N, Lambros MB, Horlings HM, Pearson A, Sharpe R, Natrajan R, Geyer FC, van Kouwenhove M, Kreike B, Mackay A, Ashworth A, van de Vijver MJ, Reis-Filho JS. Integrative molecular profiling of triple negative breast cancers identifies amplicon drivers and potential therapeutic targets. Oncogene. 2010;29:2013–23.

71. Cerami E, Gao J, Dogrusoz U, Gross BE, Sumer SO, Aksoy BA, Jacobsen A, Byrne CJ, Heuer ML, Larsson E, Antipin Y, Reva B, Goldberg AP, Sander C, Schultz N. The cBio cancer genomics portal: an open platform for exploring multidimensional cancer genomics data. Cancer Discov. 2012;2:401–4.

72. Niemeier LA, Dabbs DJ, Beriwal S, Striebel JM, Bhargava R. Androgen receptor in breast cancer: expression in estrogen receptor-positive tumors and in estrogen receptor-negative tumors with apocrine differentiation. Modern Pathol. 2010;23:205–12.

73. Janssen Research & Development, L. A study to evaluate the safety, pharmacokinetics, and pharmacodynamics of JNJ-42756493 in patients with advanced or refractory solid tumors or lymphoma. 2016.

74. Gucalp A, Tolaney S, Isakoff SJ, Ingle JN, Liu MC, Carey LA, Blackwell K, Rugo H, Nabell L, Forero A, Stearns V, Doane AS, Danso M, Moynahan ME, Momen LF, Gonzalez JM, Akhtar A, Giri DD, Patil S, Feigin KN, Hudis CA, Traina TA, Translational Breast Cancer Research C. Phase II trial of bicalutamide in patients with androgen receptor-positive, estrogen receptor-negative metastatic breast cancer. Clin Cancer Res. 2013;19:5505–12.

75. Traina, J. C. C. P. S. A. A. H. U. I. C. T. M. E. B. J. L. S. D. A. Y. C. H. T. A. Stage 1 results from MDV3100-11: a 2-stage study of enzalutamide (ENZA), an androgen receptor (AR) inhibitor, in advanced AR+ triple-negative breast cancer (TNBC). Ann Oncol. 2015;26:iii6.

76. Yamaoka M, Hara T, Hitaka T, Kaku T, Takeuchi T, Takahashi J, Asahi S, Miki H, Tasaka A, Kusaka M. Orteronel (TAK-700), a novel non-steroidal 17,20-lyase inhibitor: effects on steroid synthesis in human and monkey adrenal cells and serum steroid levels in cynomolgus monkeys. J Steroid Biochem Mol Biol. 2012;129:115–28.

77. Huarte M. The emerging role of lncRNAs in cancer. Nat Med. 2015;21:1253–61.

78. Evans JR, Feng FY, Chinnaiyan AM. The bright side of dark matter: lncRNAs in cancer. J Clin Invest. 2016;126:2775–82.

79. Yang F, Liu YH, Dong SY, Yao ZH, Lv L, Ma RM, Dai XX, Wang J, Zhang XH, Wang OC. Co-expression networks revealed potential core lncRNAs in the triple-negative breast cancer. Gene. 2016;591:471–7.

80. Djebali S, Davis CA, Merkel A, Dobin A, Lassmann T, Mortazavi A, Tanzer A, Lagarde J, Lin W, Schlesinger F, Xue C, Marinov GK, Khatun J, Williams BA, Zaleski C, Rozowsky J, Roder M, Kokocinski F, Abdelhamid RF, Alioto T, Antoshechkin I, Baer MT, Bar NS, Batut P, Bell K, Bell I, Chakrabortty S, Chen X, Chrast J, Curado J, Derrien T, Drenkow J, Dumais E, Dumais J, Duttagupta R, Falconnet E, Fastuca M, Fejes-Toth K, Ferreira P, Foissac S, Fullwood MJ, Gao H, Gonzalez D, Gordon A, Gunawardena H, Howald C, Jha S, Johnson R, Kapranov P, King B, Kingswood C, Luo OJ, Park E, Persaud K, Preall JB, Ribeca P, Risk B, Robyr D, Sammeth M, Schaffer L, See LH, Shahab A, Skancke J, Suzuki AM, Takahashi H, Tilgner H, Trout D, Walters N, Wang H, Wrobel J, Yu Y, Ruan X, Hayashizaki Y, Harrow J, Gerstein M, Hubbard T, Reymond A, Antonarakis SE, Hannon G, Giddings MC, Ruan Y, Wold B, Carninci P, Guigo R, Gingeras TR. Landscape of transcription in human cells. Nature. 2012;489:101–8.

81. Sana J, Faltejskova P, Svoboda M, Slaby O. Novel classes of non-coding RNAs and cancer. J Transl Med. 2012;10:103.

82. Wilusz JE, Sunwoo H, Spector DL. Long noncoding RNAs: functional surprises from the RNA world. Genes Dev. 2009;23:1494–504.

83. Ponting CP, Oliver PL, Reik W. Evolution and functions of long noncoding RNAs. Cell. 2009;136:629–41.

84. Mercer TR, Mattick JS. Structure and function of long noncoding RNAs in epigenetic regulation. Nat Struct Mol Biol. 2013;20:300–7.

85. Derrien T, Johnson R, Bussotti G, Tanzer A, Djebali S, Tilgner H, Guernec G, Martin D, Merkel A, Knowles DG, Lagarde J, Veeravalli L, Ruan X, Ruan Y, Lassmann T, Carninci P, Brown JB, Lipovich L, Gonzalez JM, Thomas M, Davis CA, Shiekhattar R, Gingeras TR, Hubbard TJ, Notredame C, Harrow J, Guigo R. The GENCODE v7 catalog of human long noncoding RNAs: analysis of their gene structure, evolution, and expression. Genome Res. 2012;22:1775–89.

86. Morlando M, Ballarino M, Fatica A, Bozzoni I. The role of long noncoding RNAs in the epigenetic control of gene expression. ChemMedChem. 2014;9:505–10.

87. Vance KW, Ponting CP. Transcriptional regulatory functions of nuclear long noncoding RNAs. Trends Genet. 2014;30:348–55.

88. Gutschner T, Diederichs S. The hallmarks of cancer: a long non-coding RNA point of view. RNA Biol. 2012;9:703–19.

89. Zhao W, Luo J, Jiao S. Comprehensive characterization of cancer subtype associated long non-coding RNAs and their clinical implications. Sci Rep. 2014;4:6591.

90. Prensner JR, Iyer MK, Sahu A, Asangani IA, Cao Q, Patel L, Vergara IA, Davicioni E, Erho N, Ghadessi M, Jenkins RB, Triche TJ, Malik R, Bedenis R, McGregor N, Ma T, Chen W, Han S, Jing X, Cao X, Wang X, Chandler B, Yan W, Siddiqui J, Kunju LP, Dhanasekaran SM, Pienta KJ, Feng FY, Chinnaiyan AM. The long noncoding RNA SChLAP1 promotes aggressive prostate cancer and antagonizes the SWI/SNF complex. Nat Genet. 2013;45:1392–8.

91. Yuan JH, Yang F, Wang F, Ma JZ, Guo YJ, Tao QF, Liu F, Pan W, Wang TT, Zhou CC, Wang SB, Wang YZ, Yang Y, Yang N, Zhou WP, Yang GS, Sun SH.

A long noncoding RNA activated by TGF-beta promotes the invasion-metastasis cascade in hepatocellular carcinoma. Cancer Cell. 2014;25:666–81.

92. Prensner JR, Chinnaiyan AM. The emergence of lncRNAs in cancer biology. Cancer Discov. 2011;1:391–407.

93. Vikram R, Ramachandran R, Abdul KS. Functional significance of long non-coding RNAs in breast cancer. Breast Cancer. 2014;21:515–21.

94. Guo L, Zhao Y, Yang S, Zhang H, Wu Q, Chen F. An integrated evolutionary analysis of miRNA-lncRNA in mammals. Mol Biol Rep. 2014;41:201–7.

95. Yang X, Gao L, Guo X, Shi X, Wu H, Song F, Wang B. A network based method for analysis of lncRNA-disease associations and prediction of lncRNAs implicated in diseases. PLoS One. 2014;9:e87797.

96. Berteaux N, Lottin S, Monte D, Pinte S, Quatannens B, Coll J, Hondermarck H, Curgy JJ, Dugimont T, Adriaenssens E. H19 mRNA-like noncoding RNA promotes breast cancer cell proliferation through positive control by E2F1. J Biol Chem. 2005;280:29625–36.

97. Gupta RA, Shah N, Wang KC, Kim J, Horlings HM, Wong DJ, Tsai MC, Hung T, Argani P, Rinn JL, Wang Y, Brzoska P, Kong B, Li R, West RB, van de Vijver MJ, Sukumar S, Chang HY. Long non-coding RNA HOTAIR reprograms chromatin state to promote cancer metastasis. Nature. 2010;464:1071–6.

98. Huang J, Zhou N, Watabe K, Lu Z, Wu F, Xu M, Mo YY. Long non-coding RNA UCA1 promotes breast tumor growth by suppression of p27 (Kip1). Cell Death Dis. 2014;5:e1008.

99. Mourtada-Maarabouni M, Pickard MR, Hedge VL, Farzaneh F, Williams GT. GAS5, a non-protein-coding RNA, controls apoptosis and is downregulated in breast cancer. Oncogene. 2009;28:195–208.

100. Huarte M, Rinn JL. Large non-coding RNAs: missing links in cancer? Hum Mol Genet. 2010;19:R152–61.

101. Van Grembergen O, Bizet M, de Bony EJ, Calonne E, Putmans P, Brohee S, Olsen C, Guo M, Bontempi G, Sotiriou C, Defrance M, Fuks F. Portraying breast cancers with long noncoding RNAs. Sci Adv. 2016;2:e1600220.

102. Jiang M, Huang O, Xie Z, Wu S, Zhang X, Shen A, Liu H, Chen X, Wu J, Lou Y, Mao Y, Sun K, Hu S, Geng M, Shen K. A novel long non-coding RNA-ARA: adriamycin resistance-associated. Biochem Pharmacol. 2014;87:254–83.

103. Godinho M, Meijer D, Setyono-Han B, Dorssers LC, van Agthoven T. Characterization of BCAR4, a novel oncogene causing endocrine resistance in human breast cancer cells. J Cell Physiol. 2011;226:1741–9.

104. Godinho MF, Wulfkuhle JD, Look MP, Sieuwerts AM, Sleijfer S, Foekens JA, Petricoin EF 3rd, Dorssers LC, van Agthoven T. BCAR4 induces antioestrogen resistance but sensitises breast cancer to lapatinib. Br J Cancer. 2012;107:947–55.

105. Redis RS, Sieuwerts AM, Look MP, Tudoran O, Ivan C, Spizzo R, Zhang X, de Weerd V, Shimizu M, Ling H, Buiga R, Pop V, Irimie A, Fodde R, Bedrosian I, Martens JW, Foekens JA, Berindan-Neagoe I, Calin GA. CCAT2, a novel long non-coding RNA in breast cancer: expression study and clinical correlations. Oncotarget. 2013;4:1748–62.

106. Liu M, Xing LQ, Liu YJ. A three-long noncoding RNA signature as a diagnostic biomarker for differentiating between triple-negative and non-triple-negative breast cancers. Medicine. 2017;96:e6222.

107. Wang F, Dohogne Z, Yang J, Liu Y, Soibam B. Predictors of breast cancer cell types and their prognostic power in breast cancer patients. BMC Genomics. 2018;19:137.

108. Shen X, Xie B, Ma Z, Yu W, Wang W, Xu D, Yan X, Chen B, Yu L, Li J, Chen X, Ding K, Cao F. Identification of novel long non-coding RNAs in triple-negative breast cancer. Oncotarget. 2015;6:21730–9.

109. Chung W, Eum HH, Lee HO, Lee KM, Lee HB, Kim KT, Ryu HS, Kim S, Lee JE, Park YH, Kan Z, Han W, Park WY. Single-cell RNA-seq enables comprehensive tumour and immune cell profiling in primary breast cancer. Nat Commun. 2017;8:15081.

110. Chen C, Li Z, Yang Y, Xiang T, Song W, Liu S. Microarray expression profiling of dysregulated long non-coding RNAs in triple-negative breast cancer. Cancer Biol Ther. 2015;16:856–65.

111. Varga Z, Theurillat JP, Filonenko V, Sasse B, Odermatt B, Jungbluth AA, Chen YT, Old LJ, Knuth A, Jager D, Moch H. Preferential nuclear and cytoplasmic NY-BR-1 protein expression in primary breast cancer and lymph node metastases. Clin Cancer Res. 2006;12:2745–51.

112. Klein CA. Framework models of tumor dormancy from patient-derived observations. Curr Opin Genet Dev. 2011;21:42–9.

113. Lacroix M. Significance, detection and markers of disseminated breast cancer cells. Endocr Relat Cancer. 2006;13:1033–67.

114. Balafoutas D, zur Hausen A, Mayer S, Hirschfeld M, Jaeger M, Denschlag D, Gitsch G, Jungbluth A, Stickeler E. Cancer testis antigens and NY-BR-1

115. Loewer S, Cabili MN, Guttman M, Loh YH, Thomas K, Park IH, Garber M, Curran M, Onder T, Agarwal S, Manos PD, Datta S, Lander ES, Schlaeger TM, Daley GQ, Rinn JL. Large intergenic non-coding RNA-RoR modulates reprogramming of human induced pluripotent stem cells. Nat Genet. 2010; 42:1113–7.

116. Wang Y, Xu Z, Jiang J, Xu C, Kang J, Xiao L, Wu M, Xiong J, Guo X, Liu H. Endogenous miRNA sponge lincRNA-RoR regulates Oct4, Nanog, and Sox2 in human embryonic stem cell self-renewal. Dev Cell. 2013;25:69–80.

117. Hashimoto S, Onodera Y, Hashimoto A, Tanaka M, Hamaguchi M, Yamada A, Sabe H. Requirement for Arf6 in breast cancer invasive activities. Proc Natl Acad Sci U S A. 2004;101:6647–52.

118. Eades G, Wolfson B, Zhang Y, Li Q, Yao Y, Zhou Q. lincRNA-RoR and miR-145 regulate invasion in triple-negative breast cancer via targeting ARF6. Mol Cancer Res. 2015;13:330–8.

119. Wang YL, Overstreet AM, Chen MS, Wang J, Zhao HJ, Ho PC, Smith M, Wang SC. Combined inhibition of EGFR and c-ABL suppresses the growth of triple-negative breast cancer growth through inhibition of HOTAIR. Oncotarget. 2015;6:11150–61.

120. Jin C, Yan B, Lu Q, Lin Y, Ma L. Reciprocal regulation of Hsa-miR-1 and long noncoding RNA MALAT1 promotes triple-negative breast cancer development. Tumour Biol. 2016;37:7383–94.

121. Lin A, Li C, Xing Z, Hu Q, Liang K, Han L, Wang C, Hawke DH, Wang S, Zhang Y, Wei Y, Ma G, Park PK, Zhou J, Zhou Y, Hu Z, Zhou Y, Marks JR, Liang H, Hung MC, Lin C, Yang L. The LINK-A lncRNA activates normoxic HIF1alpha signalling in triple-negative breast cancer. Nat Cell Biol. 2016;18: 213–24.

122. Abdul-Rahman U, Gyorffy B, Adams BD. linc00673 (ERRLR01) is a prognostic indicator of overall survival in breast cancer. Transcription. 2017:1–13.

123. Bamodu OA, Huang WC, Lee WH, Wu A, Wang LS, Hsiao M, Yeh CT, Chao TY. Aberrant KDM5B expression promotes aggressive breast cancer through MALAT1 overexpression and downregulation of hsa-miR-448. BMC Cancer. 2016;16:160.

124. Corcoran DL, Pandit KV, Gordon B, Bhattacharjee A, Kaminski N, Benos PV. Features of mammalian microRNA promoters emerge from polymerase II chromatin immunoprecipitation data. PLoS One. 2009;4:e5279.

125. Sossey-Alaoui K, Downs-Kelly E, Das M, Izem L, Tubbs R, Plow EF. WAVE3, an actin remodeling protein, is regulated by the metastasis suppressor microRNA, miR-31, during the invasion-metastasis cascade. Int J Cancer. 2011;129:1331–43.

126. Valastyan S, Reinhardt F, Benaich N, Calogrias D, Szasz AM, Wang ZC, Brock JE, Richardson AL, Weinberg RA. A pleiotropically acting microRNA, miR-31, inhibits breast cancer metastasis. Cell. 2009;137:1032–46.

127. Augoff K, McCue B, Plow EF, Sossey-Alaoui K. miR-31 and its host gene lncRNA LOC554202 are regulated by promoter hypermethylation in triple-negative breast cancer. Mol Cancer. 2012;11:5.

128. Xia Y, Xiao X, Deng X, Zhang F, Zhang X, Hu Q, Sheng W. Targeting long non-coding RNA ASBEL with oligonucleotide antagonist for breast cancer therapy. Biochem Biophys Res Commun. 2017;489:386–92.

129. Perou CM. Molecular stratification of triple-negative breast cancers. Oncologist. 2010;15(Suppl 5):39–48.

130. Lehmann BD, Bauer JA, Chen X, Sanders ME, Chakravarthy AB, Shyr Y, Pietenpol JA. Identification of human triple-negative breast cancer subtypes and preclinical models for selection of targeted therapies. J Clin Invest. 2011;121:2750–67.

131. Schleidgen S, Klingler C, Bertram T, Rogowski WH, Marckmann G. What is personalized medicine: sharpening a vague term based on a systematic literature review. BMC Med Ethics. 2013;14:55.

132. Awada A, Vandone AM, Aftimos P. Personalized management of patients with solid cancers: moving from patient characteristics to tumor biology. Curr Opin Oncol. 2012;24:297–304.

133. Soudyab M, Iranpour M, Ghafouri-Fard S. The role of long non-coding RNAs in breast cancer. Arch Iranian Med. 2016;19:508–17.

134. Lv M, Xu P, Wu Y, Huang L, Li W, Lv S, Wu X, Zeng X, Shen R, Jia X, Yin Y, Gu Y, Yuan H, Xie H, Fu Z. LncRNAs as new biomarkers to differentiate triple negative breast cancer from non-triple negative breast cancer. Oncotarget. 2016;7:13047–59.

5

A panel of DNA methylation markers for the detection of prostate cancer from FV and DRE urine DNA

Igor Brikun[1], Deborah Nusskern[1,4], Andrew Decatus[2], Eric Harvey[3], Lin Li[2] and Diha Freije[1*] (iD)

Abstract

Background: Early screening for prostate cancer (PCA) remains controversial because of overdiagnosis and overtreatment of clinically insignificant cancers. Even though a number of diagnostic tests have been developed to improve on PSA testing, there remains a need for a more informative non-invasive test for PCA. The objective of this study is to identify a panel of DNA methylation markers suitable for a non-invasive diagnostic test from urine DNA collected following a digital rectal exam (DRE) and/or from first morning void (FV). A secondary objective is to determine if the cumulative methylation is indicative of biopsy findings.

Methods: DRE and FV urine samples were prospectively collected from 94 patients and analyzed using 24 methylation-specific quantitative PCR assays derived from 19 CpG islands. The methylation of individual markers and various combinations of markers was compared to biopsy results. A methylation threshold for cancer classification was determined using a target specificity of 70%. The average methylation and the number of positive markers were also compared to the result of the biopsy, and the area under the receiver operating characteristic curves (AUCs) were calculated.

Results: Methylation of all 19 markers was detected in FV and DRE DNAs. Combining the methylation of two or more markers improved on individual marker results. Using *6of19* methylated markers as the threshold for cancer classification yielded a specificity of 71% (95% CI, 0.57–0.86) from both DRE and FV and a sensitivity of 89% (95% CI, 0.79–0.97) from DRE and 94% (95% CI, 0.84–1.0) from FV. The negative predictive value at the 6of19 threshold was ≥ 90 for both DNA types.

Conclusions: PCA-specific methylation was detected in both FV and DRE DNA. There was no significant difference in diagnostic accuracy at the 6of19 threshold between DRE and FV urine DNA. The results support the development of a non-invasive diagnostic test to reduce unnecessary biopsies in men with elevated PSA. The test can also provide patients with personalized recommendations based on their own methylation profile.

Keywords: Prostate cancer, DNA methylation, Urine biomarker, Liquid biopsy, Circulating DNA

Background

Prostate cancer (PCA) remains the second leading cause of death from cancer in US men even though more men die with it than because of it [1, 2]. Over 25 years of prostate-specific antigen (PSA) testing uncovered the challenges of early screening for a heterogeneous and complex disease with a highly variable natural history. Early screening with the PSA advanced the lead time of

PCA diagnosis and treatment by 5 to 7 years with modest reduction in mortality observed mostly in European trials where PSA screening was not as routinely performed as in the USA [3–7]. The PSA lead time was not sufficient to significantly alter the mortality rates from prostate cancer but clinical studies showed a reduction in cancer progression for men who were screened and treated for PCA [8]. The modest benefits of early screening came at a significant cost of adverse effects and reduced quality of life [8–10]. Furthermore, PSA screening

* Correspondence: diha@eucliddiagnostics.com
[1]Euclid Diagnostics LLC, 9800 Connecticut Dr., Crown Point, IN 46307, USA
Full list of author information is available at the end of the article

significantly increased the incidence of PCA, possibly due to the overdiagnosis of indolent tumors [2].

The majority of men diagnosed with PCA do not require treatment, but differentiating between indolent and aggressive prostate cancer remains a challenge [11]. Several novel tests aimed at diagnosing clinically significant disease have been developed including the Prostate Cancer Antigen 3 (PCA3), the 4-Kallikrein Score, SelectMDX®, ExoDX®, the Michigan Prostate Score (MiPS), Oncotype DX, and the cell cycle progression score among others [12–18]. They are performed as secondary diagnostic tests for patients undergoing PCA screening to reduce the number of biopsies and/or reduce treatment for potentially insignificant tumors. Identifying patients with high-risk disease at the time of diagnosis remains a challenge [11]. Even patients diagnosed with low-grade cancer who opt for active surveillance (AS) require continued monitoring as one third progress within 5 years and one half require intervention within 10 years [8, 19–22]. There remains a clinical need for a non-invasive prostate cancer diagnostic test to overcome the limitations of PSA and assess an individual's risk of high-grade disease. Such a test will require a panel of cancer-specific markers that define a PCA molecular clock for pre-cancerous, indolent and potentially aggressive disease.

The hallmark of all cancers is the progressive acquisition of genomic aberrations. DNA methylation may be the most common involving hundreds if not thousands of CpG islands and can be detected in circulating DNA [23–26]. It is an ideal target for the early and non-invasive detection and monitoring of all cancers [27, 28]. Several studies have investigated the use of urine DNA methylation for PCA diagnosis using a small number of markers without achieving the accuracy needed for clinical adoption [29–32]. They also relied on a digital rectal exam (DRE) to enrich for prostate cells in urine samples, a process that is difficult to standardize. It was unclear if a DRE would be needed or if similar outcomes could be accomplished using first morning void (FV) urine samples. The advantage of using FV samples is the ability to collect multiple urine samples to reduce sampling errors associated with cell-free DNA (cfDNA) due to intra- and inter-day variation in cfDNA composition and concentration.

We undertook this study to identify a panel of markers suitable for PCA diagnosis from urine DNA and to determine if FV urine samples are an acceptable substitute for samples collected following DRE. In Brikun et al. [33], we presented evidence of extensive methylation in benign and cancerous biopsy cores of PCA patients. In the current study, we extend the methylation analysis to DNA isolated from DRE and FV urine samples.

At the start of the study, we aimed to identify a panel of markers that yields a specificity of ≥ 70% and a negative predictive value (NPV) of ≥ 90%. Prostate biopsies are an imperfect gold standard failing to diagnose up to a third of cancers on first biopsies [34, 35]. The 70% target specificity would correspond to a true specificity of over 90% had a true gold standard been available. The clinical utility and value of a urine-based PCA test depends heavily on reducing the number and cost of unnecessary biopsies, hence the target specificity and NPV. A high sensitivity would be required to achieve a negative predictive value ≥ 90%.

We selected for analysis 19 CpG islands associated with 18 genes that are methylated in prostate cancer (ADCY4, AOX1, APC, CXCL14, EPHX3, GFRA2, GSTP1, HEMK1, KIFC2, MOXD1, HOXA7, HOXB5, HOXD3 {2 islands}, HOXD9, HOXD10, NEUROG3, NODAL, and RASSF5). We developed 24 methylation-specific PCR (MS-qPCR) assays from the 19 selected markers and determined their methylation in DNA isolated from 154 urine samples obtained from 94 patients. The results show that the cumulative methylation of DRE or FV urine DNA can be used to help reduce the number of biopsies performed as a result of PSA screening. The ability to measure the methylation of a large number of markers without loss of specificity enables the development of a molecular clock for PCA to increase diagnostic lead time and to monitor disease progression in patients with potentially clinically insignificant tumors.

Results

Patient characteristics

Patients were classified as non-cancer if they had a negative biopsy (n = 52) and as cancer patients if the biopsy returned a positive finding regardless of Gleason score, the number of positive cores or volume of cancer (n = 42). All patients underwent transrectal ultrasound (TRUS)-guided 12-core biopsies. Patient demographics are shown in Table 1. The median Gleason score was 7 (range 1–10) and the median number of positive cores was 4 (range 1–12). Three patients who had a negative biopsy after urine collection were diagnosed with PCA within 2 years. They were included in the cancer group for the purpose of the statistical analysis.

DNA methylation in DRE and FV DNA

A binary presence (> 0) or absence (= 0) of methylation was used to determine the methylation status of a marker regardless of the amount of methylation detected in urine. Using a presence/absence of methylation limits any subjective interpretation of data to the analytical conditions used to assay marker methylation. Table 2 shows the estimated sensitivity and specificity of individual

Table 1 Patient demographics summarized in the overall population and by biopsy diagnosis

Variable		Cases (n = 42)	Controls (n = 52)	All (n = 94)
Age	n (%)	42 (100.0%)	50 (96.2%)	92 (97.8%)
	Median	66	64	65.5
	Mean (SD)	67.1 (7.1)	63.9 (7.6)	65.4 (7.5)
	Range	48–84	50–83	48–84
PSA	n (%)	40 (95%)	51 (98.1%)	91 (96.8%)
	Median	6.4	5.2	5.7
	Mean (SD)	7.1 (3.3)	5.6 (2.7)	6.3 (3.1)
	Range	3.26–18.92	0.63–14.9	0.63–18.92
Race	Alaskan Native	1 (2.4%)	0 (0.0%)	1 (1.1%)
	Asian	0 (0.0%)	1 (1.9%)	1 (1.1%)
	Black	4 (9.5%)	5 (9.6%)	9 (9.6%)
	Hispanic	1 (2.4%)	1 (1.9%)	2 (2.1%)
	White	36 (85.7%)	44 (84.6%)	80 (85.1%)
	Missing	0 (0.0%)	1 (1.9%)	1 (1.1%)
Urine samples	DRE and FV	28 (66.7%)	32 (61.5%)	60 (63.8%)
	DRE only	10 (23.8%)	17 (32.7%)	27 (28.7%)
	FV only	4 (9.5%)	3 (5.8%)	7 (7.4%)
Gleason score	n	39 (92.9%)	NA	
	Median	7		
	Range	6–10		
	=6	19 (45.2%)		
	7	8 (19%)		
	> 7	13 (30.9%)		
	Missing	3 (7.1%)		
Positive cores	n	39 (92.9%)	NA	
	Median	4		
	Range	1–12		
	≤ 3	19 (45.2%)		
	> 3	20 (47.6%)		
	Missing	3 (7.1%)		

The mean PSA for cases was calculated after excluding two outliers which were greater than two times the highest remaining PSA value from cases. All patients underwent 12-core TRUS biopsies. The number of positive cores is based on the histological examination of all 12 cores

PSA prostate-specific antigen, *SD* standard deviation, *DRE* digital rectal exam, *FV* first void, *NA* not applicable

markers in DRE and FV DNAs. For markers with two assays, results of individual and combined assays are shown.

Markers were recovered with variable frequencies from both DRE and FV. The observed sensitivities of individual assays ranged from 13 to 97% while specificities ranged from 57 to 100%. Combining the methylation information of markers with two assays showed improvement in sensitivity over individual assays without a significant loss in specificity. Several markers like HOXA7, HOXB5, and HOXD3b could be used individually to improve on PSA testing.

We had anticipated potentially excluding some markers due to constitutive methylation in cfDNA or equal methylation in cases and controls which would render them unsuitable for PCA diagnosis. However, none of the markers needed to be excluded. All markers were included in the statistical modeling.

Statistical modeling to select the best diagnostic marker combinations from DRE and FV urine DNA

Statistical modeling was performed to identify the best-performing marker combinations. A summary table for two modeling approaches (logitboost and elastic net) is shown in Additional file 1: Table S1. The mean area under the receiver operating characteristic (ROC) curves (AUCs) obtained with the various modeling approaches ranged from 0.71 to 0.91. The number of markers ranged from as few as one to as many as 17. Neither the age nor PSA added significantly to the outcome of modeling.

Statistical modeling identified a large number of candidate marker panels for validation. Markers HOXA7, HOXB5, and HOXD3b showed high out of sample diagnostic capability. One or more of these three markers were included in the best-performing models. Table 3 shows the results obtained on training and test sets using select models. Models with as few as two markers and as many as all 19 showed comparable AUCs.

To better illustrate the number of potential smaller panels that could be derived from the 19 markers, the area under the ROC curve (AUC) of all two, three, four, five, and six marker combinations was calculated based on the number of methylated markers (> 0 methylation level). Figure 1 is a graphical representation of AUCs for all two to six marker combinations. Increasing the number of markers showed incremental improvement in overall AUC values with the six-marker combinations outperforming the ≤ 5 marker combinations. The mean AUC increased for both DRE and FV with increasing marker numbers while the range of AUC values decreased. DRE DNA methylation outperformed FV DNA methylation for the 19 markers analyzed and resulted in higher mean AUC and smaller ranges for AUC values for all two, three, four, five, and six marker combinations. However, there were many marker combinations from FV DNAs with equivalent AUCs to the best-performing combinations from DRE.

Cumulative methylation in DRE and FV urine DNA from biopsy-positive and biopsy-negative patients

The total number of methylated markers was calculated for each DNA sample using the presence of methylation (> 0) to classify markers as positive. The median number of methylated markers in cases was 11 (range 2 to 19) in DRE and 9.5 (range 3 to 19) in FV. The median number of methylated markers in controls was 3 for both DRE

Table 2 Predictive performance of methylation status in individual assays based on urine samples from DRE ($n = 87$) and FV ($n = 67$)

Marker or assay	Sample	#Pos/#Cases	Sensitivity (95% CI)	#Neg/#Controls	Specificity (95% CI)
ADCY4	DRE	23/38	0.61 (0.45, 0.74)	38/49	0.78 (0.64, 0.87)
	FV	18/32	0.56 (0.39, 0.72)	24/35	0.69 (0.52, 0.81)
AOX1rc	DRE	27/38	0.71 (0.55, 0.83)	34/49	0.69 (0.55, 0.80)
	FV	14/32	0.44 (0.28, 0.61)	29/35	0.83 (0.67, 0.92)
APC2	DRE	10/38	0.26 (0.15, 0.42)	44/49	0.90 (0.78, 0.96)
	FV	4/32	0.13 (0.05, 0.28)	32/35	0.91 (0.78, 0.97)
CXCL14	DRE	8/38	0.21 (0.11, 0.36)	49/49	1.00 (0.93, 1.00)
	FV	9/32	0.28 (0.16, 0.45)	34/35	0.97 (0.85, 0.99)
CXCL14rc	DRE	6/38	0.16 (0.07, 0.30)	49/49	1.00 (0.93, 1.00)
	FV	4/32	0.13 (0.05, 0.28)	35/35	1.00 (0.90, 1.00)
CXCL14 Comb.	DRE	9/38	0.24 (0.13, 0.39)	49/49	1.00 (0.93, 1.00)
	FV	11/32	0.34 (0.20, 0.52)	34/35	0.97 (0.85, 0.99)
EPHX3	DRE	25/38	0.66 (0.50, 0.79)	35/49	0.71 (0.58, 0.82)
	FV	18/32	0.56 (0.39, 0.72)	24/35	0.69 (0.52, 0.81)
KIFC2	DRE	25/38	0.66 (0.50, 0.79)	38/49	0.78 (0.64, 0.87)
	FV	18/32	0.56 (0.39, 0.72)	28/35	0.80 (0.64, 0.90)
KIFC2rc	DRE	20/38	0.53 (0.37, 0.68)	42/49	0.86 (0.73, 0.93)
	FV	11/32	0.34 (0.20, 0.52)	32/35	0.91 (0.78, 0.97)
KIFC2 Comb.	DRE	30/38	0.79 (0.64, 0.89)	34/49	0.69 (0.55, 0.80)
	FV	21/32	0.66 (0.48, 0.80)	27/35	0.77 (0.61, 0.88)
GFRA2	DRE	17/38	0.45 (0.30, 0.60)	41/49	0.84 (0.71, 0.91)
	FV	13/32	0.41 (0.26, 0.58)	29/35	0.83 (0.67, 0.92)
GSTP1	DRE	18/38	0.47 (0.32, 0.63)	40/49	0.82 (0.69, 0.90)
	FV	15/32	0.47 (0.31, 0.64)	29/35	0.83 (0.67, 0.92)
HEMK1	DRE	15/38	0.39 (0.26, 0.55)	46/49	0.94 (0.83, 0.98)
	FV	8/32	0.25 (0.13, 0.42)	32/35	0.91 (0.78, 0.97)
HOXA7	DRE	32/38	0.84 (0.70, 0.93)	39/49	0.80 (0.66, 0.89)
	FV	21/32	0.66 (0.48, 0.80)	23/35	0.66 (0.49, 0.79)
HOXB5	DRE	29/38	0.76 (0.61, 0.87)	40/49	0.82 (0.69, 0.90)
	FV	23/32	0.72 (0.55, 0.84)	23/35	0.66 (0.49, 0.79)
HOXB5rc	DRE	27/38	0.71 (0.55, 0.83)	35/49	0.71 (0.58, 0.82)
	FV	22/32	0.69 (0.51, 0.82)	23/35	0.66 (0.49, 0.79)
HOXB5 Comb.	DRE	32/38	0.84 (0.70, 0.93)	29/49	0.59 (0.45, 0.72)
	FV	28/32	0.88 (0.72, 0.95)	20/35	0.57 (0.41, 0.72)
HOXD3a	DRE	19/38	0.50 (0.35, 0.65)	45/49	0.92 (0.81, 0.97)
	FV	15/32	0.47 (0.31, 0.64)	30/35	0.86 (0.71, 0.94)
HOXD3b	DRE	29/38	0.76 (0.61, 0.87)	37/49	0.76 (0.62, 0.85)
	FV	31/32	0.97 (0.84, 0.99)	21/35	0.60 (0.44, 0.74)
HOXD9	DRE	26/38	0.68 (0.53, 0.81)	29/49	0.59 (0.45, 0.72)
	FV	20/32	0.63 (0.45, 0.77)	25/35	0.71 (0.55, 0.84)
HOXD10	DRE	23/38	0.61 (0.45, 0.74)	42/49	0.86 (0.73, 0.93)
	FV	17/32	0.53 (0.36, 0.69)	27/35	0.77 (0.61, 0.88)
MOXD1	DRE	16/38	0.42 (0.28, 0.58)	41/49	0.84 (0.71, 0.91)
	FV	15/32	0.47 (0.31, 0.64)	32/35	0.91 (0.78, 0.97)

Table 2 Predictive performance of methylation status in individual assays based on urine samples from DRE (*n* = 87) and FV (*n* = 67) (*Continued*)

Marker or assay	Sample	#Pos/#Cases	Sensitivity (95% CI)	#Neg/#Controls	Specificity (95% CI)
NEUROG3	DRE	14/38	0.37 (0.23, 0.53)	42/49	0.86 (0.73, 0.93)
	FV	7/32	0.22 (0.11, 0.39)	33/35	0.94 (0.81, 0.98)
NODAL	DRE	24/38	0.63 (0.47, 0.77)	40/49	0.82 (0.69, 0.90)
	FV	16/32	0.50 (0.34, 0.66)	28/35	0.80 (0.64, 0.90)
NODALrc	DRE	20/38	0.53 (0.37, 0.68)	41/49	0.84 (0.71, 0.91)
	FV	10/32	0.31 (0.18, 0.49)	28/35	0.80 (0.64, 0.90)
NODAL Comb.	DRE	30/38	0.79 (0.64, 0.89)	35/49	0.71 (0.58, 0.82)
	FV	19/32	0.59 (0.42, 0.74)	24/35	0.69 (0.52, 0.81)
RASSF5	DRE	9/38	0.24 (0.13, 0.39)	46/49	0.94 (0.83, 0.98)
	FV	9/32	0.28 (0.16, 0.45)	35/35	1.00 (0.90, 1.00)
RASSF5rc	DRE	10/38	0.26 (0.15, 0.42)	43/49	0.88 (0.76, 0.94)
	FV	11/32	0.34 (0.20, 0.52)	30/35	0.86 (0.71, 0.94)
RASSF5 Comb.	DRE	17/38	0.45 (0.30, 0.60)	40/49	0.82 (0.69, 0.90)
	FV	19/32	0.59 (0.42, 0.74)	30/35	0.86 (0.71, 0.94)

The estimated sensitivity and specificity of individual assays and combined markers. The column #Pos/#cases shows the number of positive tests from cases and the total number of biopsy positive cases analyzed. Similarly, the column #Pos/#controls yields the number of negative tests from controls and the number of biopsy negative controls
CI confidence interval, *rc* reverse complement, *Comb.* combined results as described in the "Results" section

Table 3 Area under the receiver operating curves in training, test, and combined sets

	# of markers	Model	AUC/Train (25/58)[a]	AUC/Test (13/29)[a]	AUC/ALL (87)[b]
DRE	2	HOXA7, HOXB5	0.897	0.898	0.892
	3	HOXA7, HOXB5, HOXD3b	0.911	0.869	0.898
	4	HOXA7, HOXB5, HOXD3b, AOX1rc	0.915	0.875	0.91
	5	ADCY4, HOXA7, HOXB5, NODAL, MOXD1	0.89	0.909	0.9
	5	HOXA7, HOXD10, APC, GFRA2, KIFC2	0.892	0.886	0.888
	6	HOXA7, HOXB5, HOXD3b, HOXD9, GFRA2, AOX1rc	0.907	0.875	0.897
	7	HOXA7, HOXB5, HOXD3b, HOXD10, KIFC2, AOX1rc, HOXD3a	0.912	0.875	0.903
	8	ADCY4, HOXA7, HOXD3b, HOXB5, HOXD9, HOXD10, NODAL, KIFC2rc	0.891	0.847	0.876
	11	ADCY4, HOXA7, HOXB5, HOXD9, GSTP1, RASSF5, EPHX3, HEMK1rc, KIFC2, MOXD1, AOX1rc	0.916	0.949	0.925

	# of markers	Model	AUC/Train (20/45)[a]	AUC/Test (12/22)[a]	AUC/ALL (67)[b]
FV	2	HOXD3b, RASSF5	0.902	0.936	0.915
	3	HOXB5, HOXD3b, RASSF5	0.866	0.891	0.873
	3	HOXD3b, MOXD1, RASSF5	0.915	0.936	0.926
	4	ADCY4, HOXD3b, RASSF5, KIFC2	0.858	0.827	0.854
	6	HOXB5, HOXD3b, MOXD1, RASSF5, CXCL14, KIFC2	0.894	0.845	0.88
	8	ADCY4, HOXD3b, HOXD10, HOXD3a, MOXD1, RASSF5, CXCL14, GSTP1	0.902	0.882	0.895
	8	ADCY4, HOXB5, HOXD3b, HOXA7, HOXD9, HOXD3a, RASSF5, AOX1rc	0.824	0.891	0.846
	8	ADCY4, HOXA7, HOXD3b, HOXB5, HOXD9, HOXD10, NODAL, KIFC2rc	0.822	0.882	0.833

The AUCs for training and test sets as well as the combined (ALL) set for select model marker combinations and all 19 markers
[a]The numbers in the parentheses are the number of cases/total number of patients
[b]The number in the parentheses represents the combined training and test sets

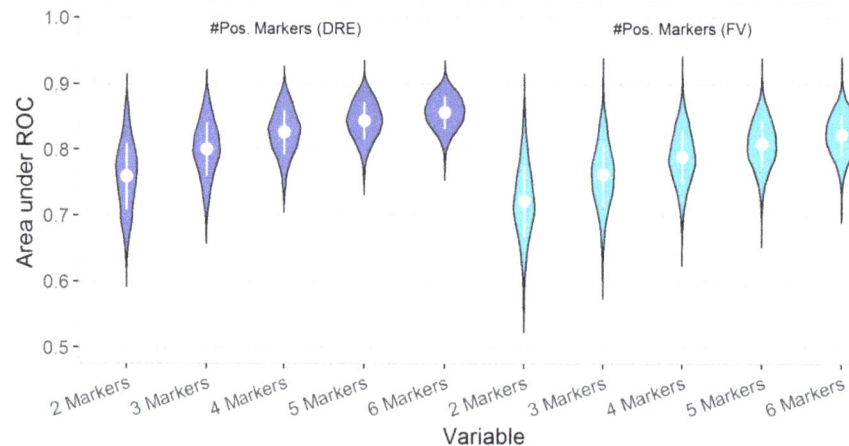

Fig. 1 Violin plot of AUCs obtained for two, three, four, five, and six marker combinations. Violin plots of the AUCs of all two to six marker combinations using as a variable the number of positive markers. The inner part of each note shows the mean ± 1 SD. As the number of markers increases, the AUC values increase and the range of AUC values decreases

and FV (range 0 to 11 for DRE and 0 to 12 for FV). Table 4 shows the sensitivity, specificity, positive predictive value (PPV), and negative predictive value (NPV) for the total number of methylated markers (*nof19*) at every threshold from 1 to 15 positive markers. For markers with two assays, only the combined data was used for the *nof19* calculations.

Using 6 out of 19 positive markers (*6of19*) as the threshold to refer a patient for a biopsy achieves the target specificity set at the start of the study. The negative predictive value for the *6of19* threshold was ≥ 0.90 for both DRE and FV with sensitivities of 0.89 for DRE and 0.94 for FV. As the methylation threshold increased, the positive predictive value of the number of methylated markers in urine DNA increased. The number of methylated markers in urine DNA can provide personalized diagnostic information that is not limited to a binary outcome to help inform subsequent clinical decisions.

The receiver operating characteristic (ROC) curve was calculated based on the number of methylated markers and the average methylation of all 19 markers in DRE and FV DNA. Figure 2 shows the individual ROC curves for the *nof19*, and average methylation and PSA for the DRE and the FV data. Urine DNA methylation yielded AUC values ranging from 0.87 in FV to 0.92 in DRE, a significant improvement over PSA.

Comparison of urine DNA methylation and Gleason score and tumor volume

The prostate cancer detected in positive biopsies (Gleason score, # of positive cores, tumor volume per core) varied widely between patients from a highly differentiated cancer focus in a single core (GS of 6, ≤1% tumor volume) to widespread, poorly differentiated cancer in multiple cores (GS of 8 to 10, up to 12 positive

cores and up to 100% tumor volume per core). Similarly, the number of methylated markers and the average methylation varied widely. Patients with positive biopsies were grouped based on UCSF-CAPRA risk scoring system into a low-risk group (Group 1: CAPRA score of 1 and 2) and an elevated risk group (Group 2: CAPRA score ≥ 3) [1]. Patients in Group 2 are expected to have an intermediate risk (CAPRA score of 3–5) except for five patients diagnosed with high-grade tumors (CAPRA score 6–9). Figure 3 shows the distribution of average urine DNA methylation and the number of positive markers for all three groups.

The minimum, mean, and maximum values obtained for the number of methylated markers and average methylation for each group are shown in Additional file 1: Table S2. The mean number of methylated markers and the average methylation differed significantly between cases and controls for both DRE and first void (Wilcoxon p values < 0.001 for both DNA types). Furthermore, both parameters differed significantly between Group 1 and 2 patients for DRE DNA (Wilcoxon p values < 0.001) but not for FV DNA (Wilcoxon p value of 0.898 and 0.446 respectively). Pearson's correlation coefficient between CAPRA grade and average methylation was 0.649 (95% CI, 0.403–0.808, p value < 0.001) for DRE DNA and 0.322 (95% CI, − 0.044–0.611, p value < 0.083) for FV DNA. Despite the small number of markers and the small number of patients, the correlation between grade and methylation supports further studies.

Comparison between the DRE and FV methylation results

Paired-sample analysis was performed on the 60 samples with both DRE and FV data. Thirty-two had a negative biopsy and 28 had a positive biopsy. Given the 60

Table 4 Predictive performance of the number of positive markers among the 19 markers

Marker	Sample type	#Pos/#Cases	Sensitivity (95% CI)	#Neg/#Controls	Specificity (95% CI)	PPV (95% CI)	NPV (95% CI)
≥ 1 of 19	DRE	38/38	1.00 (1.00, 1.00)	7/49	0.14 (0.06, 0.24)	0.47 (0.45, 0.51)	1.00 (1.00, 1.00)
	FV	32/32	1.00 (1.00, 1.00)	4/35	0.11 (0.03, 0.23)	0.51 (0.48, 0.54)	1.00 (1.00, 1.00)
≥ 2 of 19	DRE	38/38	1.00 (1.00, 1.00)	15/49	0.31 (0.18, 0.43)	0.53 (0.49, 0.58)	1.00 (1.00, 1.00)
	FV	32/32	1.00 (1.00, 1.00)	8/35	0.23 (0.11, 0.37)	0.54 (0.51, 0.59)	1.00 (1.00, 1.00)
≥ 3 of 19	DRE	37/38	0.97 (0.92, 1.00)	18/49	0.37 (0.24, 0.51)	0.54 (0.49, 0.60)	0.95 (0.83, 1.00)
	FV	32/32	1.00 (1.00, 1.00)	13/35	0.37 (0.23, 0.54)	0.59 (0.54, 0.67)	1.00 (1.00, 1.00)
≥ 4 of 19	DRE	36/38	0.95 (0.87, 1.00)	25/49	0.51 (0.38, 0.65)	0.60 (0.54, 0.68)	0.93 (0.82, 1.00)
	FV	31/32	0.97 (0.91, 1.00)	19/35	0.54 (0.37, 0.71)	0.66 (0.58, 0.74)	0.95 (0.85, 1.00)
≥ 5 of 19	DRE	36/38	0.95 (0.87, 1.00)	30/49	0.61 (0.47, 0.76)	0.65 (0.58, 0.74)	0.94 (0.85, 1.00)
	FV	31/32	0.97 (0.91, 1.00)	23/35	0.66 (0.51, 0.80)	0.72 (0.64, 0.82)	0.96 (0.88, 1.00)
≥ 6 of 19	DRE	34/38	0.89 (0.79, 0.97)	35/49	0.71 (0.59, 0.86)	0.71 (0.62, 0.82)	0.90 (0.81, 0.97)
	FV	30/32	0.94 (0.84, 1.00)	25/35	0.71 (0.57, 0.86)	0.75 (0.66, 0.86)	0.93 (0.83, 1.00)
≥ 7 of 19	DRE	32/38	0.84 (0.74, 0.95)	38/49	0.78 (0.65, 0.90)	0.74 (0.65, 0.87)	0.86 (0.78, 0.95)
	FV	26/32	0.81 (0.69, 0.94)	27/35	0.77 (0.63, 0.91)	0.76 (0.66, 0.89)	0.82 (0.71, 0.93)
≥ 8 of 19	DRE	30/38	0.79 (0.66, 0.92)	43/49	0.88 (0.78, 0.96)	0.83 (0.73, 0.94)	0.84 (0.76, 0.93)
	FV	21/32	0.66 (0.50, 0.81)	30/35	0.86 (0.74, 0.97)	0.81 (0.68, 0.95)	0.73 (0.64, 0.84)
≥ 9 of 19	DRE	28/38	0.74 (0.61, 0.87)	44/49	0.90 (0.82, 0.98)	0.85 (0.74, 0.97)	0.81 (0.74, 0.90)
	FV	19/32	0.59 (0.44, 0.75)	32/35	0.91 (0.83, 1.00)	0.86 (0.74, 1.00)	0.71 (0.63, 0.81)
≥ 10 of 19	DRE	27/38	0.71 (0.58, 0.84)	46/49	0.94 (0.86, 1.00)	0.90 (0.80, 1.00)	0.81 (0.74, 0.89)
	FV	16/32	0.50 (0.34, 0.66)	33/35	0.94 (0.86, 1.00)	0.89 (0.75, 1.00)	0.67 (0.61, 0.76)
≥ 11 of 19	DRE	22/38	0.58 (0.43, 0.74)	47/49	0.96 (0.90, 1.00)	0.92 (0.81, 1.00)	0.75 (0.69, 0.83)
	FV	12/32	0.38 (0.22, 0.53)	33/35	0.94 (0.86, 1.00)	0.86 (0.69, 1.00)	0.62 (0.57, 0.69)
≥ 12 of 19	DRE	13/38	0.34 (0.21, 0.50)	49/49	1.00 (1.00, 1.00)	1.00 (1.00, 1.00)	0.66 (0.62, 0.72)
	FV	9/32	0.28 (0.16, 0.44)	33/35	0.94 (0.86, 1.00)	0.82 (0.62, 1.00)	0.59 (0.54, 0.65)
≥ 13 of 19	DRE	11/38	0.29 (0.17, 0.45)	49/49	1.00 (1.00, 1.00)	1.00 (1.00, 1.00)	0.64 (0.61, 0.70)
	FV	7/32	0.22 (0.09, 0.38)	35/35	1.00 (1.00, 1.00)	1.00 (1.00, 1.00)	0.58 (0.55, 0.64)
≥ 14 of 19	DRE	9/38	0.24 (0.13, 0.37)	49/49	1.00 (1.00, 1.00)	1.00 (1.00, 1.00)	0.63 (0.60, 0.67)
	FV	5/32	0.16 (0.06, 0.28)	35/35	1.00 (1.00, 1.00)	1.00 (1.00, 1.00)	0.56 (0.54, 0.60)
≥ 15 of 19	DRE	7/38	0.18 (0.08, 0.32)	49/49	1.00 (1.00, 1.00)	1.00 (1.00, 1.00)	0.61 (0.58, 0.65)
	FV	3/32	0.09 (0.03, 0.22)	35/35	1.00 (1.00, 1.00)	1.00 (1.00, 1.00)	0.55 (0.53, 0.58)

The calculated sensitivity and specificity, positive predictive value (PPV), and negative predictive value (NPV) associated with *n* of 19 positive markers for DRE and FV urine samples. The column #Pos/#Cases shows the number of positive cases and the total number of cases. The column #Neg/#Controls shows the number of negative controls and the total number of controls. The numbers in the parentheses show the 95% confidence interval

samples, the FV 6of19 threshold has a sensitivity of 0.964 (95% CI, 0.896, 1.000) and a specificity of 0.688 (95% CI, 0.527, 0.848), and the DRE test has a sensitivity of 0.929 (95% CI, 0.833, 1.000) and a specificity of 0.688 (95% CI, 0.527, 0.848). There was no statistically significant difference between the observed sensitivities and specificities of the two tests (difference in sensitivity 0.035, *p* value = 1; difference in specificity 0.000, *p* value = 1).

The paired sample analysis was also performed to compare the methylation of individual markers in DRE and FV DNAs. Table 5 shows the observed within subject mean difference in methylation levels for individual markers for the 60 patients with both DRE and FV data.

The mean difference in methylation did not differ significantly between DRE and FV urine DNA for the majority of markers. Only markers AOX1, GFRA2, and NEUROG3 were better recovered from DRE samples ($p < 0.05$). The observed differences for these three markers are likely due to the position of the underlying assays within the CpG island.

Overall, 72% of patients had concordant diagnosis with all three tests and 82% had concordant diagnoses with FV and DRE urine methylation. Of the 28% of patients who had discordant diagnoses between the methylation results and biopsies, the majority had DNA methylation near but did not cross the threshold for one of the urine

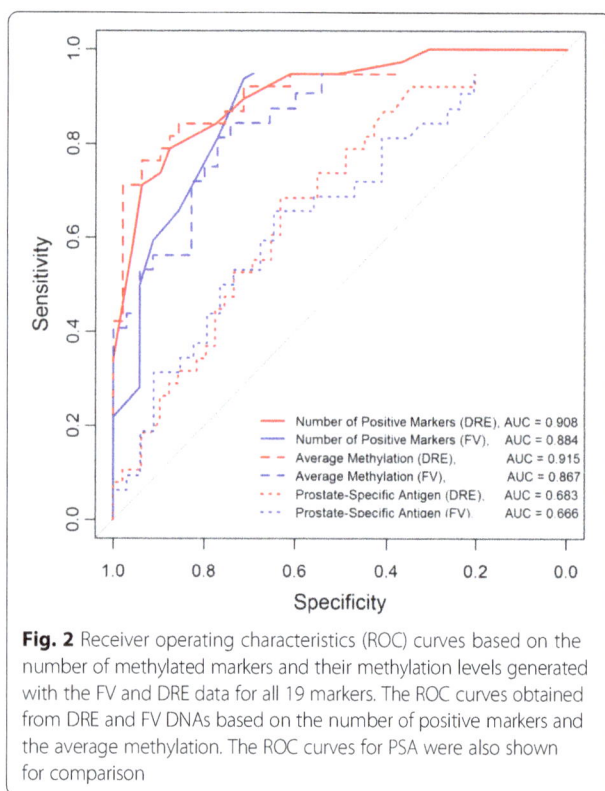

Fig. 2 Receiver operating characteristics (ROC) curves based on the number of methylated markers and their methylation levels generated with the FV and DRE data for all 19 markers. The ROC curves obtained from DRE and FV DNAs based on the number of positive markers and the average methylation. The ROC curves for PSA were also shown for comparison

samples or had a negative biopsy when both methylation tests were above the 6of19 threshold.

Discussion

This study shows that FV DNA methylation can be used as the basis of a non-invasive diagnostic test for PCA and yields comparable results to DRE DNA. The optimal threshold for PCA diagnosis based on target specificity ≥ 70% was *6of19* markers for both FV and DRE urine DNAs with FV slightly outperforming DRE at the 6of19 threshold. The diagnostic accuracy of a molecular test is critical when the purpose is to delay or eliminate biopsies aimed at the early diagnosis of cancer. Using the 6of19 threshold, the NPV obtained from DRE and FV was ≥ 90% with a PPV of > 70%. The urine DNA methylation test has the potential of significantly outperforming PSA and reducing the number of unnecessary biopsies.

The main challenge of using cell-free DNA (cfDNA) for diagnostic tests is the sampling error that is inherent to the DNA collection method. Genomic sequences are not equally represented in cfDNA. The use of DRE DNA was expected to reduce or eliminate the sampling error by enriching urine samples with prostate cells and/or DNA. The results of the five markers with two assays showed that interrogating the methylation of different portions of a CpG island improves the sensitivity of a marker without a significant loss of specificity from both

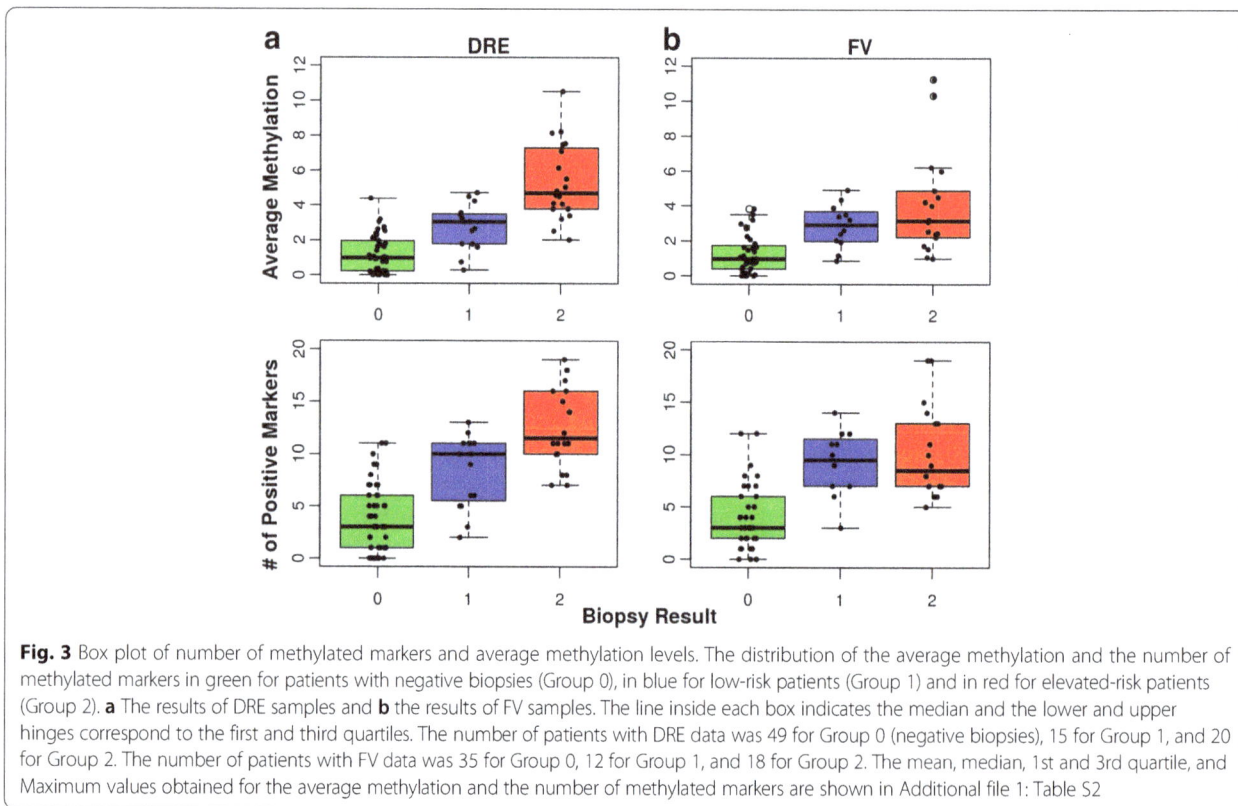

Fig. 3 Box plot of number of methylated markers and average methylation levels. The distribution of the average methylation and the number of methylated markers in green for patients with negative biopsies (Group 0), in blue for low-risk patients (Group 1) and in red for elevated-risk patients (Group 2). **a** The results of DRE samples and **b** the results of FV samples. The line inside each box indicates the median and the lower and upper hinges correspond to the first and third quartiles. The number of patients with DRE data was 49 for Group 0 (negative biopsies), 15 for Group 1, and 20 for Group 2. The number of patients with FV data was 35 for Group 0, 12 for Group 1, and 18 for Group 2. The mean, median, 1st and 3rd quartile, and Maximum values obtained for the average methylation and the number of methylated markers are shown in Additional file 1: Table S2

Table 5 Paired test of within subject mean difference in methylation of individual markers observed in DRE and FV samples ($N = 60$)

Marker	Mean difference	95% CI	p value
Average methylation	0.356	(− 0.074, 0.786)	0.103
# of positive markers	0.667	(− 0.421, 1.754)	0.225
ADCY4	0.748	(− 0.774, 2.269)	0.329
AOX1rc	1.788	(0.479, 3.098)	0.008
APC2	0.449	(− 0.175, 1.072)	0.155
CXCL14	− 0.140	(− 0.935, 0.655)	0.725
EPHX3	0.258	(− 1.013, 1.528)	0.686
KIFC2	1.133	(− 0.161, 2.426)	0.085
GFRA2	0.766	(0.134, 1.397)	0.018
GSTP1	0.501	(− 0.203, 1.204)	0.160
HEMK1rc	− 0.131	(− 1.124, 0.861)	0.792
HOXA7	0.360	(− 0.812, 1.531)	0.542
HOXB5	− 0.823	(− 2.148, 0.502)	0.219
HOXD10	0.493	(− 0.340, 1.325)	0.241
HOXD3a	0.218	(− 0.852, 1.288)	0.685
HOXD3b	− 0.797	(− 1.602, 0.008)	0.052
HOXD9	0.909	(− 0.378, 2.196)	0.163
MOXD1	0.067	(− 0.765, 0.899)	0.873
NEUROG3	1.159	(0.202, 2.116)	0.018
NODAL	− 0.500	(− 1.508, 0.508)	0.325
RASSF5	0.312	(− 0.575, 1.199)	0.484

The mean difference in individual marker methylation between DRE and FV DNA. Only markers AOX1, GFRA2, and NEUROG3 showed statistically significant differences ($p < 0.05$)

DRE and FV DNA. The use of DRE DNA was not sufficient to overcome the sampling error for these five markers. FV DNA may be a better choice because the ease of collecting and analyzing multiple urine samples can reduce the sampling error and increase the accuracy of the results. It may also be useful to include multiple assays for each marker in clinical trials to better understand the recovery of the marker from urine DNA and to select the best-performing assays for the final test.

Paired samples analysis showed that there was no significant difference in the recovery of the majority of markers from DRE and FV DNA with the exception of AOX1, GFRA2, and NEUROG3 which were better recovered from DRE DNA. The poorer performance of these markers in FV may be a reflection of the poor representation of the assayed portion of the CpG island in FV DNA. Cancer-derived cfDNA may not be randomly fragmented and/or the stability of DNA sequences in circulation may vary leading to poorer recovery of some genomic sequences in FV DNA. The performance of these three markers in FV DNA may improve if additional assays interrogating the methylation of a different portion of the CpG island are analyzed.

Statistical modeling identified many potential models that would yield comparable results for a diagnostic test with binary outcome. Increasing the number of markers analyzed from two to six resulted in more marker combinations yielding comparable outcomes. Larger marker panels may outperform panels with two or three markers because they better compensate for the sampling errors of liquid biopsies. PSA and age were included in the statistical modeling but the small number of patients prevented meaningful correlations with methylation levels. The inclusion of the age of patients and PSA in larger studies would be important given the wide range of patients' age, PSA levels, and biopsy results at the time of diagnosis.

How many markers are necessary for a PCA diagnostic test and which ones to choose will depend on the purpose of the test and the clinical utility and value needed to justify clinical adoption. A diagnostic test for patients with elevated PSA can easily be accomplished using 6 to 12 markers. Ideally, the panel will include markers that are indicative of the Gleason score and the tumor volume. Predictive and prognostic tests and tests to monitor the progression of cancer in patients on active surveillance or following treatment will require larger targeted panels.

The methylation of the 19 marker panel in DRE DNA was better at identifying patients with elevated risk for significant cancer (higher volumes and higher Gleason scores) than FV DNA. The potential enrichment of DRE samples with cells derived from the prostate may have improved the recovery of all 19 markers. Other markers or assays may perform better in FV DNA. Alternatively, the FV results may better reflect the steady state release of DNA from tumor cells and may provide additional information about the underlying cancer. The average methylation outperformed the number of methylated markers at differentiating between patients with low and elevated risk for significant disease. It is possible that including the level of methylation reduces potential analytical errors from incomplete DNA deamination which is inherent to the bisulfite conversion method. The analytical detection methods can be further optimized when validation studies are performed and absolute quantitation of methylation markers can be used to further improve the accuracy of the test. It is not known if the level of methylation observed for individual markers in urine DNA is directly proportional to the level of methylation observed in the prostate. Correlation of urine and biopsy DNA methylation during validation studies will help identify the most representative markers for the clinical test.

The markers used for this study were selected based on analytical conditions, i.e., they could be analyzed under the same bisulfite conditions. DNA methylation affects a large number of markers in cancer and other tissues. The recovery of cancer-specific markers from cfDNA is not well understood. It was not clear at the start of the study how well a panel of 19 DNA methylation markers would perform in FV or DRE urine. This study shows that DNA methylation could be detected in the urine of patients diagnosed with small well-differentiated tumors. It makes it likely that larger panels could be successfully analyzed and correlated to the aberrant methylation of the prostate tissue.

The true potential of using DNA methylation for a non-invasive PCA diagnostic test can be inferred from Table 4. The likelihood of a positive biopsy increases with increasing number of positive markers. The test can provide patients with personalized recommendations based on their own methylation signature. Once predictive and prognostic markers are added to the panel, the urine methylation score can be added to current PCA risk calculators. Patients with positive methylation tests may be able to delay treatment and potentially biopsies in favor of active surveillance if the methylation profile indicates insignificant tumors.

PCA3 and other PCA molecular tests can potentially reduce overtreatment of insignificant cancers. However, they are limited in their utility because they aim to identify patients with higher-grade disease. The diagnostic lead time afforded by PSA was not sufficient to eliminate PCA-specific mortality [3–8] and molecular tests that are secondary to PSA will have the same limitation. There remains a need for an early PCA diagnostic test that can increase the PSA lead time as well as measure the rate of PCA progression so only patients with fast-growing tumors are treated. The results of this study show that DNA methylation markers could potentially form the basis of such diagnostic tests. A true early PCA detection test would require markers that are methylated early during tumorigenesis. Currently, there is limited information regarding the temporal acquisition of methylation events in PCA. Extensive studies of urine, biopsy, and tumor DNAs will need to be performed in order to develop a true early PCA diagnostic panel.

The results of this study were not compared to other urine PCA methylation studies because of differences in the analytical conditions used to assay markers. To enable future comparisons, we included full details of the assays and conditions used in this study.

Urine DNA recovery varied widely between patients from as little as 25 ng to over a microgram. A minimum DNA yield will need to be established for inclusion in validation studies. Based on our results, the amount will likely be around 1.5 ng/ml of urine.

The assays developed for the 19 markers are semi-quantitative because they relied on a limited amplification of multiplexed markers for detection. The impact of PCR amplification on copy number will likely vary between markers. No exogenous or contrived DNA control can truly replicate urine DNA. External controls provide general guidelines to determine assay conditions and verify that they are performed reproducibly during data collection. Ultimately, the only true controls for assay validations are urine DNAs from the population under study. The assay validations performed on cancer cell line DNAs support their use for the urine methylation test. Additional assay validations will be needed when more accurate quantitation of markers is required. Alternative methods that do not involve PCR amplification could also be used for marker detection to further improve quantitation of DNA methylation.

Conclusion

The study shows that the methylation of 19 CpG islands in FV and DRE urine DNA obtained from patients undergoing screening for PCA can be used to develop a non-invasive test for PCA diagnosis. Using 6 of 19 positive markers as the threshold to recommend a biopsy would reduce unnecessary biopsies performed because of elevated PSA. There was no difference in the diagnostic outcome at the 6of19 threshold between DRE and FV urine DNAs. Several markers such as HOXD3 and HOXA7 showed good diagnostic accuracy and can be used individually as secondary diagnostic tests for men referred for a biopsy. However, combining the methylation information of multiple markers improves diagnostic accuracy. Furthermore, the total number of methylated markers and the average methylation recovered from DRE urine samples differed significantly between patients with low and elevated risk for clinically significant disease.

Methods
Urine collection and DNA preparation
Urine samples were collected under an IRB protocol approved by Western Institutional Review Board (WIRB, study # 1139453, Puyallup, WA) from two urology clinics in Poughkeepsie, NY, and Toledo, OH. All patients signed an informed consent form prior to sample collection. Urine samples were collected prospectively from 106 patients who were recommended a prostate biopsy due to suspicion of cancer. The majority of patients had elevated PSA. Each patient was asked to provide two urine samples, one following a DRE and a second first morning void (FV) sample collected at home within 6 weeks of the DRE sample collection. Biopsy results were not available for 12 patients because they either opted not to undergo a biopsy after urine collection or the biopsy results were not available.

The urine samples were shipped to the lab without associated clinical information. The marker data was collected blindly. Urine samples were collected using the AssayAssure® urine preservative (Fisher Scientific). The volume varied between 20 and 90 ml. The entire urine sample was centrifuged at 2500 rpm for 10 min at room temperature. The sediment and the supernatant were stored separately at − 80 °C until processed. DNA was extracted from both urine fractions. Fifteen milliliters of the supernatant were concentrated using Amicon Ultra 30 15-ml columns (Millipore) to < 500 μl and mixed with a 500 μl of lysis buffer (4.0 M guanidium isocyanate, 1% triton X-100, 10 mM Tris pH 8.0, 1 mM EDTA, 10 μg per ml proteinase K), incubated at 50 °C for 1 h followed by chloroform extraction and isopropanol precipitation. The DNA was isolated from the sediment by resuspending the pellet directly in lysis buffer and following the protocol used for the supernatant extraction.

DNA was quantitated with the Qubit fluorometer (Life Technologies, Grand Island, NY) using a DNA quantitation kit (Life Technologies, Kit # Q32854). Samples with less than 20 ng of DNA were excluded from analysis. The recovery of DNA varied significantly between samples and ranged from less than 20 ng to over a microgram. For some patients, we isolated DNA from a larger volume to obtain sufficient amount for analysis. We used a fixed amount of DNA (10 ng) for each bisulfite conversion reaction regardless of yield. DNA was recovered from 87 (out of 94) DRE samples and 67 (out of 75) FV samples. The lower number of FV samples was due to poor patient compliance with the FV collection before biopsy. No urine samples were collected after the biopsy.

All DNAs were methylated in vitro at AluI and HaeIII sites according to manufacturer's protocol (New England Biolabs) in preparation for bisulfite conversion. The cancer cell lines DU145 (ATCC HTB-81D, prostate cancer), PC3 (ATCC CRL-1435D, prostate cancer), CCRF-CEM (ATCC CCL-119, leukemia), and COLO-205 (ATCC CCL-222, colon cancer) were used as controls. DNAs and cell lines were obtained from ATCC.

Bisulfite conversion and primary PCR amplification

The CpG island sequences are shown in Additional file 2. The assays were designed from portions of the CpG islands that allowed for the selection of two primary amplification primers, a Taqman hydrolysis probe, and at least two amplification primers. The primary amplification primers were separated by < 200 bp and preferably contained no CpGs or at most a single CpG dinucleotide. The Taqman hydrolysis probe contained at least three CpGs and the PCR amplification primers preferably contained two or more CpGs. The conditions of the bisulfite conversion and subsequent amplifications were optimized for 10 ng of input DNA. The length of

the bisulfite treatment was determined blindly using a training set of 10 urine DNAs selected from the urine samples collected for this study. Three or more bisulfite time points were performed on 10 ng of the training set DNAs to select the best conditions for the deamination of individual markers as well as groups of markers. Markers were grouped into two bisulfite conditions, (14 min at 70 °C and 42 min at 80 °C) based on the results obtained with the training set. Ten nanograms of urine DNA (a mix of sediment and supernatant DNA) were used for each bisulfite reaction. The bisulfite conversion, DNA recovery, and amplification were as described [33]. The length of treatment used for the analysis of each assay is shown in Additional file 3: Table S4. DNAs were bisulfite treated in batches of 24 which included control DNAs (AluI and HaeIII methylated DNA from cancer cell lines, white blood cell DNA, and fully methylated CCL-119 DNA). Following bisulfite treatment and desulfonation, the DNA was eluted in 35 μl of water and 5 μl was used for primary amplifications. None of the cancer cell line DNAs were methylated at all markers.

To verify the recovery of DNA following bisulfite, two control assays were added to the primary amplification multiplexes, one for NSD1, an imprinted gene that is normally methylated in all DNA for the 14 min bisulfite and a second for the HOXD9 gene for the 42 min bisulfite. The imprinted promoter assay was used to verify the recovery of amplifiable DNA through all marker detection steps from urine collection to MS-qPCR amplification. The HOXD9 promoter is methylated in PCA but the unmethylated copy can still be detected after a 42 min bisulfite treatment using degenerate primers. The primers for the NSD1 gene were specific for the methylated copy. The primer sequences are shown in Additional file 3: Table S4.

Biomarker panel

The panel of markers is composed of 19 CpG islands associated with 18 genes. The list of CpG islands and chromosomal coordinates are listed in Additional file 3: Table S3. The sequences are listed in Additional file 2. A subset of the markers were previously analyzed in prostate biopsy tissues (HOXB5, HOXD9, ADCY4, KIFC2, HEMK1, NEUROG3, CXCL14, RASSF5, GFRA2, MOXD1, APC, and GSTP1 [33]). Several markers (NODAL, HOXA7, HOXD3a, HOXD3b, and HOXD10) were selected based on the authors' unpublished data and were methylated in 50% to over 85% of tumors. AOX1 and EPHX3 were selected based on published data [36–38]. Two CpG islands associated with the HOXD3 gene are separated by a few KB and flank a region previously associated with prostate cancer and were treated as two separate markers [38]. In total, 24 assays were analyzed from 19 CpG islands on 87 DRE and 67 FV DNAs. Two assays were generated from five markers (CXCL14, HOXB5, KIFC2, NODAL, and RASSF5), one from the forward strand and one from the reverse. Some of the marker assays described in Brikun et al. [33] were modified to shorten the amplicon when possible or were redesigned from a different portion of the CpG island or from the reverse compliment (rc) sequence if needed. All probes, primers, and assay conditions are listed in Additional file 3: Table S4.

Assay validation and detection

DNA methylation was analyzed using nested methylation-specific quantitative PCR (MS-qPCR).

Taqman hydrolysis probes were labeled with FAM and quenched with BHQ1 (Biosearch Technologies, Petaluma, CA). Unlabeled primers were obtained from Biosearch Technologies or Eurofins Genomics. The primers selected for the multiplex amplification were neutral (no CGs) or degenerate (at CGs) and were designed to amplify all templates regardless of methylation. Primers were also degenerate at positions of in vitro methylation. The secondary MS-qPCR reactions were not multiplexed.

To validate the MS-qPCR assays, DNA from cancer cell lines, white blood cells, and CCL-119 methylated with SssI methyltransferase (NEB) were serially diluted and bisulfite converted in duplicate for 42 min at 80 °C or for 14 min at 70 °C. Input DNA ranged between 0.625 ng (~ 300 genomic copies) and 20 ng (~ 6000 copies). All DNAs were methylated in vitro using AluI and HaeIII methyl transferases (NEB) prior to deamination. The bisulfite converted DNA was first amplified with four primer multiplexes (M1, M4, M5, M6 as listed in Additional file 3: Table S4) to generate templates for the MS-qPCR as follows: 5 µl of the bisulfite-treated DNA were subjected to 23 cycles of 95 °C for 15 s, 58 °C for 45 s, 72 °C for 45 s using the manufacturer's supplied buffer (adjusted to 2.5 mM MgCl$_2$) and dNTPs, one unit of Takara Taq polymerase HS (Takara Bio), and 200 nM of each primer in the multiplex. For the imprinted gene, 50 nM of each primer was used in the primer mix. The amplified DNA was diluted with 300 µl of H$_2$O. Four microliters were used as input for the nested qPCR reactions.

MS-qPCR reactions were performed in duplicate for 32 cycles using the manufacturer's supplied buffer and dNTPs supplemented with 1.0 mM MgCl$_2$ (2.5 mM total), 0.5 unit of Takara Taq polymerase HS, 0.66 µM forward primer (same orientation as the probe), 1.3 µM reverse primer and 0.5 to 1 µM of the probe (labeled with FAM, Biosearch Technologies) on an Illumina Eco qPCR Real-Time PCR system (Illumina, San Diego, CA). The reaction conditions for all assays were 32 cycles of

95 °C for 15 s, 68 °C for 20 s, and 64 °C for 20 s. Urine DNA was analyzed using the same conditions. Marker analysis was performed blindly without access to clinical data.

The limit of detection of individual assays from cancer cell line DNAs ranged between 0.625 and 2.5 ng of cancer cell line DNA. All markers failed to amplify from 10 ng of white blood cell DNA. On average, each doubling of bisulfite DNA amount resulted in a decrease of Cq value between 1 and 1.5. For this study, we did not exclude any Cq values obtained from urine DNA which means all analytical errors produced under the assay conditions used during this study were included in the data analyzed.

DNA control reactions were performed on an Eppendorf Mastercycler using 4 µl of the diluted primary multiplex PCR for 35 cycles of 95 °C for 20 s, 60 °C for 20 s, and 72 °C for 45 s using the manufacturer's supplied buffer and dNTPs with 1.5 mM MgCl$_2$, 0.5 unit of Takara Taq polymerase HS, and 1.0 mM of forward and reverse primers. The amplified DNA was separated on an acrylamide gel to verify the amplification of the control fragment.

For five CpG islands (RASSF5, NODAL, KIFC2, HOXB5 and CXCL14), two assays were developed to determine if the recovery of a marker from urine DNAs might be improved by interrogating the methylation of different portions of the CpG island. Data for these markers were merged using the highest methylation level detected when both assays were positive. All fragments of a CpG island are not necessarily recovered from urine DNA in a comparable copy number. The highest methylation level detected for each marker was used because it more accurately reflects its methylation status.

Data collection

The data was tabulated using the Eco Study application provided with the Illumina ECO Real-Time PCR system. The range of Cq values obtained during assay optimizations was not used to eliminate Cq values higher than the limit of detection because cancer cell line DNAs are not valid controls for circulating DNA. Urine DNA differs from cancer cell line DNA in its representation, fragmentation pattern, and potentially its deamination rate. The limit of detection for marker assays will need to be calculated from urine DNA when larger studies are performed. A cutoff of 32 for the Cq was used as the upper limit for a positive reaction for all markers. A higher Cq represents a lower number of methylated copies in the sample. The data was further transformed by subtracting the Cq values from 32 (except for the 0 data points) to generate an increasing range of values from 0 (no amplification) to 15 (highest level of amplification, lowest Cq). The data was used directly for statistical analysis with no further manipulations.

Statistical analysis

Each subject in the study had at least one type of urine sample (DRE or FV) collected. Subject characteristics were summarized within the cases and within the controls, respectively. The cases are defined as the subjects with positive diagnosis of prostate cancer based on biopsy, and the controls are defined as those with negative diagnosis. Arithmetic means or medians and standard deviations were summarized for continuous characteristics, and frequency and percentage were calculated for categorical characteristics. Characteristics such as Gleason score and positive cores are applicable only for cases and were summarized at both continuous and dichotomized levels. The following statistical analyses were performed for both DRE and FV samples (and DRE and FV combined) unless otherwise specified.

Sensitivity and specificity associated with the presence of individual methylation markers or their assays were computed using the observed proportion of individuals with positive markers conditional upon diagnosis status, and their 95% confidence intervals were also provided.

Similarly, sensitivity, specificity, negative, and positive predictive values and their 95% confidence intervals were calculated for each of the possible number of positive markers among the 19 markers and for various thresholds for the average methylation. The average methylation for each DNA sample was calculated by adding the values obtained for all 19 assays and dividing by 19. Box plots were generated by diagnosis status for both the number of positive markers and the average methylation levels of the 19 markers.

Multi-marker modeling was performed using machine learning algorithms including logit boost and elastic net [39, 40]. Methylation markers and clinical variables such as age and PSA were subject to variable selection by the algorithms. The optimal models were determined using a fivefold cross-validation approach. The top-performing models were ranked based on the area under the ROC curve (AUC) or Youden's Index in the test sets. The average AUC in the test sets of selected top models was then reported for comparison. The AUC of the average methylation of the 19 markers was also calculated. In addition, a best subset procedure was also employed to search for top-performing models given the number of markers. A training set (approximately 2/3 of the data) and a test set were used.

The AUCs of all possible combinations of one to six markers were calculated based on the number of positive markers. Using all available data, violin plots (with mean and standard deviation) of the AUC of all combinations of two, three, four, five, or six markers were generated. ROC curves were plotted for the 19 markers based on either average methylation or the number of positive markers. ROC curve for PSA was also plotted for comparison.

The average number of positive markers by patient grading group was compared using the Wilcoxon rank-sum test. Grading groups of grade 0, 1, or 2 and the group combining grades 1 and 2 were considered. Similar analysis was performed to compare the means of average methylation by grading group.

A paired-sample analysis was performed on the samples with both DRE and FV data to compare the DRE 6of19 test and the FV 6of19 test. The difference in sensitivity, the difference in specificity, and corresponding 95% confidence intervals between the DRE and FV tests were calculated. An exact binomial test was used to test for differences in sensitivity and specificity of the two binary diagnostic tests [41].

All statistical analyses were performed using R with version 3.3.0 (https://cran.r-project.org), and the R package "pROC" with version 1.10.0 was used for AUC calculation. Additional calculations were performed using SAS 9.4.

Abbreviations

ATCC: American Tissue Culture Collection; AUC: Area under the ROC curve; CpG: 5'-Deoxycytosine-phosphate-deoxyguanosine-3'; DRE: Digital rectal exam; FV: First morning void; MS-qPCR: Methylation-specific quantitative polymerase chain reaction; PCA: Prostate cancer; PSA: Prostate-specific antigen; ROC: Receiver operating characteristic; SD: Standard deviation

Acknowledgements

We would like to thank Drs Daniel Murtagh (Toledo, OH) and Evan Goldfisher (Poughkeepsie, NY) for the collection of urine samples and Drs Ena Bromley and Clint Dart for critical review of the manuscript.

Funding

The study was funded in part by grant R43CA165444 from NCI. Additional funding was from private sources. The funding institutions were not involved in the design and execution of the study or the decision to publish.

Authors' contributions

IB contributed to study design, data collection, and manuscript preparation. DN contributed to the marker assay design, data collection, and statistical analysis. AD, LL, and EH contributed to the statistical analysis and manuscript preparation. DF contributed to the study design, data collection, statistical analysis, and manuscript preparation. All authors read and approved the final manuscript.

Competing interests

IB and DF are members and employees of Euclid Diagnostics LLC. DN is a member of Euclid Diagnostics. IB, DN, and DF have patent applications covering some of the markers in this study. LL, AD, and EH declare that they have no competing interests.

Author details

[1]Euclid Diagnostics LLC, 9800 Connecticut Dr., Crown Point, IN 46307, USA. [2]BioStat Solutions Inc., 5280 Corporate Dr., Suite C200, Frederick, MD 21703, USA. [3]Health Decisions Inc., 2510 Meridian Parkway, Durham, NC 27713, USA. [4]Present Address: Luminex Corporation, 4088 Commercial Ave, Northbrook, IL 60062, USA.

References

1. Cooperberg MR, Broering JM, Carroll PR. Risk assessment for prostate cancer metastasis and mortality at the time of diagnosis. JNCI J Natl Cancer Inst. 2009;101:878–87.
2. Pishgar F, Ebrahimi H, Moghaddam SS, Fitzmaurice C, Amini E. Global, Regional and National Burden of Prostate Cancer, 1990–2015: Results from the global burden of disease study 2015. J Urol. 2018;199:1224–32.
3. de Koning HJ, Gulati R, Moss SM, Hugosson J, Pinsky PF, Berg CD, et al. The efficacy of prostate-specific antigen screening: impact of key components in the ERSPC and PLCO trials. Cancer. 2018;124:1197–206.
4. Draisma G, Boer R, Otto SJ, van der Cruijsen IW, Damhuis RAM, Schröder FH, et al. Lead times and overdetection due to prostate-specific antigen screening: estimates from the European randomized study of screening for prostate Cancer. J Natl Cancer Inst. 2003;95:868–78.
5. Finne P, Fallah M, Hakama M, Ciatto S, Hugosson J, de Koning H, et al. Lead-time in the European randomised study of screening for prostate cancer. Eur J Cancer. 2010;46:3102–8.
6. Hayes JH, Barry MJ. Screening for prostate cancer with the prostate-specific antigen test: a review of current evidence. JAMA. 2014;311:1143–9.
7. Schröder FH, Hugosson J, Roobol MJ, Tammela TLJ, Zappa M, Nelen V, et al. Screening and prostate cancer mortality: results of the European randomised study of screening for prostate cancer (ERSPC) at 13 years of follow-up. Lancet. 2014;384:2027–35.
8. Hamdy FC, Donovan JL, Lane JA, Mason M, Metcalfe C, Holding P, et al. 10-year outcomes after monitoring, surgery, or radiotherapy for localized prostate cancer. N Engl J Med. 2016;375:1415–24.
9. Gulati R, Inoue LYT, Gore JL, Katcher J, Etzioni R. Individualized estimates of overdiagnosis in screen-detected prostate cancer. J Natl Cancer Inst. 2014; 106(2):djt367.
10. Loeb S, Bjurlin M, Nicholson J, Tammela TL, Penson D, Carter HB, et al. Overdiagnosis and overtreatment of prostate cancer. Eur Urol. 2014;65:1046–55.
11. Chang AJ, Autio KA, Roach M, Scher HI. "High-risk" prostate cancer: classification and therapy. Nat Rev Clin Oncol. 2014;11:308–23.
12. Carlsson S, Assel M, Sjoberg D, Ulmert D, Hugosson J, Lilja H, et al. Influence of blood prostate specific antigen levels at age 60 on benefits and harms of prostate cancer screening: population based cohort study. BMJ. 2014;g2296:348.
13. Carlsson SV, Roobol MJ. Improving the evaluation and diagnosis of clinically significant prostate cancer in 2017. Curr Opin Urol. 2017;27:198–204.
14. Cuzick J, Stone S, Fisher G, Yang ZH, North BV, Berney DM, et al. Validation of an RNA cell cycle progression score for predicting death from prostate cancer in a conservatively managed needle biopsy cohort. Br J Cancer. 2015;113:382–9.
15. Hendriks RJ, van der Leest MMG, Dijkstra S, Barentsz JO, Van Criekinge W, Hulsbergen-van de Kaa CA, et al. A urinary biomarker-based risk score correlates with multiparametric MRI for prostate cancer detection. Prostate. 2017;77:1401–7.
16. Klein EA, Cooperberg MR, Magi-Galluzzi C, Simko JP, Falzarano SM, Maddala T, et al. A 17-gene assay to predict prostate cancer aggressiveness in the context of Gleason grade heterogeneity, tumor multifocality, and biopsy undersampling. Eur Urol. 2014;66:550–60.
17. Kretschmer A, Tilki D. Biomarkers in prostate cancer - current clinical utility and future perspectives. Crit Rev Oncol Hematol. 2017;120:180–93.
18. McKiernan J, Donovan MJ, O'Neill V, Bentink S, Noerholm M, Belzer S, et al. A novel urine exosome gene expression assay to predict high-grade prostate cancer at initial biopsy. JAMA Oncol. 2016;2:882–9.
19. Garisto JD, Klotz L. Active surveillance for prostate cancer: how to do it right. Oncol (Williston Park). 2017;31:333–40. 345
20. Klotz L. Active surveillance for low-risk prostate cancer. Curr Opin Urol. 2017; 27:225–30.
21. Romero-Otero J, Garcia-Gómez B, Duarte-Ojeda JM, Rodriguez-Antolín A, Vilaseca A, Carlsson SV, et al. Active surveillance for prostate cancer. Int J Urol. 2016;23:211–8.
22. Saad F. Active surveillance in prostate cancer: how far should we go? JAMA Oncol. 2015;1:340–1.
23. Cree IA, Uttley L, Buckley Woods H, Kikuchi H, Reiman A, Harnan S, et al. The evidence base for circulating tumour DNA blood-based biomarkers for the early detection of cancer: a systematic mapping review. BMC Cancer. 2017;17:697.
24. Leygo C, Williams M, Jin HC, Chan MWY, Chu WK, Grusch M, et al. DNA methylation as a noninvasive epigenetic biomarker for the detection of cancer. Dis Markers. 2017;3726595:2017.
25. Payne SR, Serth J, Schostak M, Kamradt J, Strauss A, Thelen P, et al. DNA methylation biomarkers of prostate cancer: confirmation of candidates and evidence urine is the most sensitive body fluid for non-invasive detection. Prostate. 2009;69:1257–69.
26. Wu T, Giovannucci E, Welge J, Mallick P, Tang W-Y, Ho S-M. Measurement of GSTP1 promoter methylation in body fluids may complement PSA screening: a meta-analysis. Br J Cancer. 2011;105:65–73.
27. Blute ML, Damaschke NA, Jarrard DF. The epigenetics of PCA diagnosis and prognosis: update on clinical applications. Curr Opin Urol. 2015;25:83–8.
28. Geybels MS, Wright JL, Bibikova M, Klotzle B, Fan J-B, Zhao S, et al. Epigenetic signature of Gleason score and prostate cancer recurrence after radical prostatectomy. Clin Epigenetics. 2016;8:97.
29. Baden J, Adams S, Astacio T, Jones J, Markiewicz J, Painter J, et al. Predicting prostate biopsy result in men with prostate specific antigen 2.0 to 10.0 ng/ml using an investigational prostate cancer methylation assay. J Urol. 2011; 186:2101–6.
30. Baden J, Green G, Painter J, Curtin K, Markiewicz J, Jones J, et al. Multicenter evaluation of an investigational prostate cancer methylation assay. J Urol. 2009;182:1186–93.
31. Enokida H, Shiina H, Urakami S, Igawa M, Ogishima T, Li L-C, et al. Multigene methylation analysis for detection and staging of prostate cancer. Clin Cancer Res. 2005;11:6582–8.
32. Gonzalgo ML, Pavlovich CP, Lee SM, Nelson WG. Prostate cancer detection by GSTP1 methylation analysis of postbiopsy urine specimens. Clin Cancer Res. 2003;9:2673–7.
33. Brikun I, Nusskern D, Gillen D, Lynn A, Murtagh D, Feczko J, et al. A panel of DNA methylation markers reveals extensive methylation in histologically benign prostate biopsy cores from cancer patients. Biomark Res. 2014;2:25.
34. Djavan B, Ravery V, Zlotta A, Dobronski P, Dobrovits M, Fakhari M, et al. Prospective evaluation of prostate cancer detected on biopsies 1, 2, 3 and 4: when should we stop? J Urol. 2001;166:1679–83.
35. Djavan B, Mazal P, Zlotta A, Wammack R, Ravery V, Remzi M, et al. Pathological features of prostate cancer detected on initial and repeat prostate biopsy: results of the prospective European prostate cancer detection study. Prostate. 2001;47:111–7.
36. Geybels MS, Zhao S, Wong C-J, Bibikova M, Klotzle B, Wu M, et al. Epigenomic profiling of DNA methylation in paired prostate cancer versus adjacent benign tissue. Prostate. 2015;75:1941–50.
37. Haldrup C, Mundbjerg K, Vestergaard EM, Lamy P, Wild P, Schulz WA, et al. DNA methylation signatures for prediction of biochemical recurrence after radical prostatectomy of clinically localized prostate cancer. J Clin Oncol. 2013;31:3250–8.
38. Stott-Miller M, Zhao S, Wright JL, Kolb S, Bibikova M, Klotzle B, et al. Validation study of genes with hypermethylated promoter regions associated with prostate cancer recurrence. Cancer Epidemiol Biomark Prev. 2014;23(7):1331–9.
39. Friedman J, Hastie T, Tibshirani R. Additive logistic regression: a statistical view of boosting (with discussion and a rejoinder by the authors). Ann Stat. 2000;28(2):337–407.
40. Zou H, Hastie T. Regularization and variable selection via the elastic net. J R Stat Soc Ser B Stat Methodol. 2005;67(2):301–20.
41. Zhou X, Obuchowski N, McClish D. Statistical methods in diagnostic medicine. Wiley Series in Probability and Statistics. 2nd ed. Hoboken: Wiley; 2011.

6

DNA methylation and socioeconomic status in a Mexican-American birth cohort

Eric S. Coker[1,2*], Robert Gunier[1,2], Karen Huen[1,3], Nina Holland[1,3] and Brenda Eskenazi[1,2]

Abstract

Background: Maternal social environmental stressors during pregnancy are associated with adverse birth and child developmental outcomes, and epigenetics has been proposed as a possible mechanism for such relationships.

Methods: In a Mexican-American birth cohort of 241 maternal-infant pairs, cord blood samples were measured for repeat element DNA methylation (*LINE-1* and *Alu*). Linear mixed effects regression was used to model associations between indicators of the social environment (low household income and education, neighborhood-level characteristics) and repeat element methylation. Results from a dietary questionnaire were also used to assess the interaction between maternal diet quality and the social environment on markers of repeat element DNA methylation.

Results: After adjusting for confounders, living in the most impoverished neighborhoods was associated with higher cord blood LINE-1 methylation ($\beta = 0.78$, 95%CI 0.06, 1.50, $p = 0.03$). No other neighborhood-, household-, or individual-level socioeconomic indicators were significantly associated with repeat element methylation. We observed a statistical trend showing that positive association between neighborhood poverty and LINE-1 methylation was strongest in cord blood of infants whose mothers reported better diet quality during pregnancy ($p_{interaction} = 0.12$).

Conclusion: Our findings indicate a small yet unexpected positive association between neighborhood-level poverty during pregnancy and methylation of repetitive element DNA in infant cord blood and that this association is possibly modified by diet quality during pregnancy. However, our null findings for other adverse SES indicators do not provide strong evidence for an adverse association between early-life socioeconomic environment and repeat element DNA methylation in infants.

Keywords: Diet, Epigenetics, Methylation, Repeat element, Social adversity, Socioeconomic status

Background

Social disadvantage in early-life can adversely affect child development as evidenced by the higher rates of preterm birth and low birth weight, asthma, and poorer cognitive function of children from economically impoverished families and neighborhoods [1–10]. While the precise mechanisms by which social disadvantage affects child health is not fully understood, it has been hypothesized that maternal exposure to social stressors during pregnancy, such as poverty, may alter the offspring's epigenome [11, 12].

DNA methylation, which is the attachment of methyl groups primarily at CpG sites, is an example of an epigenetic modification that can regulate gene expression [13,

14], with methylation of repetitive elements being one commonly studied epigenetic marker. Repetitive elements make up approximately half of the human genome and include retrotransposable elements like long and short interspersed nuclear elements (LINEs and SINEs, respectively). Of the LINEs and SINES, the LINE-1 and Alu elements are the most abundant, together representing nearly a third of the human genome [15]. Although previously referred to as markers of global methylation, recent studies have demonstrated that LINE-1 and Alu methylation do not correlate well with global genomic methylation content [16, 17], are not correlated with each other [18, 19], and each represents distinct and important components of the epigenome [17, 20].

In the present study, we focus on perinatal LINE-1 and Alu methylation related to the maternal socioeconomic environment because previous epidemiological

* Correspondence: escoker@gmail.com
[1]Center for Environmental Research and Children's Health (CERCH), School of Public Health, University of California, Berkeley, CA, USA
[2]Berkeley, USA
Full list of author information is available at the end of the article

studies suggest associations with social and environmental stressors on LINE-1 and Alu methylation in both children and in adults. Both human and animal studies indicate hypomethylation or high copy numbers of LINE-1 or SINE elements in relation to stress or psychiatric disorders [21–25]. DNA methylation of LINE-1 and Alu elements have also been associated with environmental pollutant exposures (both hypomethylation and hypermethylation) [26–31], diet and nutrition [32–34], and other lifestyle factors [31, 35]. These relationships may have biological relevance since hypomethylation of repetitive elements may affect genomic instability and later disease states [36, 37].

Few studies have examined the relationships between early-life socioeconomic disadvantage and methylation in newborn blood or placental tissue. A birth cohort study conducted in New York [38] found no association between maternal education during pregnancy and global DNA methylation measured by immunoassay in infant cord blood, while another study in Rhode Island found maternal socioeconomic disadvantage, including lower education level, to be related to placental hypomethylation of the HSD11B2 gene (that may affect maternal cortisol exposure in the infant) [39]. Meanwhile, a birth cohort study from North Carolina found that lower maternal education and household income were associated with hypomethylation of IGF2 and H19 imprinted genes but there was no association with other genes (MEG3 and NNAT) [40]. In a separate analysis in this same North Carolina cohort, authors observed an opposite and significant association with neighborhood socioeconomic status (SES) for MEG3 (hypermethylation) [41]. Finally, a birth cohort study from China [42] measured DNA methylation at several hundred CpG sites and found that lower maternal SES was associated with older epigenetic age using a novel 'epigenetic clock' method. However, repeat element methylation in infants has yet to be examined in relation to socioeconomic status.

Maternal nutrition may be an important co-exposure to consider in the context of socioeconomic disadvantage because neighborhood food environments and poverty level [43–45], and maternal socioeconomic status and nutrition [46–48] have been associated with each other. In addition, prenatal nutrition is associated with changes in DNA methylation [32, 33, 49, 50]. For example, prospective studies have found that supplementation with methyl donors during pregnancy, such as folate, was associated with hypermethylation of LINE-1 elements in cord and maternal blood [34, 49, 51]. In a Dutch population, epigenetic changes (hyper- or hypo methylation depending on the gene) have been observed with prenatal famine exposure in a time of great social stress (World War II) and these changes have been retained into adulthood along with modifications of the imprinted genes that were preserved

for several generations of offspring [52, 53]. Thus, it appears plausible that good maternal diet during pregnancy may protect against the adverse effects of social adversity on the newborn epigenome.

In our study, we used a multi-level analysis to investigate associations between indicators of maternal socioeconomic status and DNA methylation of LINE-1 and Alu repeat elements in cord blood of infants who participated in the Center for Health Assessment of Mothers and Children of Salinas (CHAMACOS), a birth cohort study of predominantly economically disadvantaged Mexican-American farmworker families. We hypothesized that maternal socioeconomic status (SES) at the individual, household, and neighborhood level will influence the newborn epigenome as measured by LINE-1 and Alu repeat elements and that maternal diet quality will modify this association.

Methods
Study population
Pregnant women were recruited from six community health clinics in the Salinas Valley, California (1999–2000) and were eligible for the CHAMACOS study if they were at least 18 years of age, less than 20 weeks gestation, spoke Spanish or English, were eligible for low income health insurance, and were planning to deliver at the local public hospital. There were 601 women enrolled of whom 526 delivered a live singleton infant. Cord blood samples were collected at the time of delivery, of which 241 had sufficient DNA to analyze methylation of LINE-1 and Alu repeats and cell composition estimates. There were no significant differences in sociodemographic characteristics or important health behaviors (e.g., smoking) between the mothers of children who were included and those who were not included in these analyses (data not shown).

Socioeconomic disadvantage and maternal diet during pregnancy
Women were interviewed to collect individual- and household-level indicators of SES and other demographic information (e.g., age and race). Maternal interviews occurred twice during pregnancy at ~ 13 and ~ 26 weeks gestation, and all interviews were administered in English or Spanish by trained bilingual interviewers.

Individual- and household-level variables
We obtained information on maternal education and household income, and the number of people living in the home at the first interview. Mother's education was constructed into three categories (≤ 6th grade, 7–12th grade, and ≥ high school), while household poverty income ratio variables were classified into quartiles for analysis. Household poverty income ratio was computed by combining information on the reported household income and the

number of people supported by that income and then dividing these values by the year 2000 US Census poverty threshold values for the number of people living in the household [54]. Hence, a poverty income ratio < 1 entails that the household is below the poverty line and conversely a poverty income ratio ≥ 1 entails that the household is above the poverty line.

Neighborhood-level variables

Census tract data were obtained for the year 2000 from the US Census Bureau. We examined sociodemographic measures for the census tract the woman lived in including: percent of homes below the poverty line, median household income, and percent of people that completed high school within census tracts. Each neighborhood SES variable was categorized into quartiles for analysis.

Dietary intake during pregnancy

Information regarding dietary and nutritional supplement intake were ascertained at the second prenatal interview (~ 26 weeks gestation) [54]. Briefly, we used a validated 72-item food-frequency questionnaire (FFQ) that was developed for Spanish-speaking populations [55, 56]. The FFQ collected information on typical food intake such as frequency and portion sizes for specific food items. We converted food and vitamin supplement intake into average daily energy and nutrient intake as set out by United States Department of Agriculture Nutrient Database for Standard Reference [57]. With data from the FFQ, we determined maternal diet quality, using the Diet Quality Index for Pregnancy (DQI-P) [58]. The original DQI-P comprises eight different components of dietary intake; however, we had data for seven of these components (we were not able to include the component for the number of meals and snacks per day). The seven components assessed the adequacy of intake grains, fruits, and vegetables; the intake of fat as a proportion of all energy intake; and the adequacy of specific nutrient intake of folate, iron, and calcium. A higher DQI-P score is indicative of better diet quality while a lower score is indicative of poorer diet quality. For greater details on how these data were collected and DQI-P values were derived, see Harley et al. 2006 [54].

DNA methylation in cord blood

Umbilical cord blood samples were collected at the delivery room. Samples were centrifuged and divided into serum and clot and stored at − 80 °C [59]. DNA were isolated from clots with a QIAamp Blood DNA Maxi kit (Qiagen, Inc., Santa Clarita, CA, USA) (further details described in Holland et al. 2006) [59]. For bisulfite conversion of 500 ng of DNA, we used EpiTect Bisulfite Conversion Kits (Qiagen, Germantown, MD, USA). Bisulfite converted samples were then eluted into 20 μL Elution buffer. To confirm complete bisulfite conversion, we calculated the proportion

of cytosine at the first non-CpG site, considering proportions over 7% as an indicator of incomplete bisulfite conversion. Cytosine proportions for the non-CpG site in individual samples reflective of incomplete bisulfite conversion ranged from 0.1 to 4.2% (mean = 1.5%), confirming excellent conversion efficiency for the majority of samples (99%) [26]. Pyrosequencing of PCR-amplified and bisulfite-treated DNA samples was used to determine LINE-1 and Alu methylation levels, using the Pyromark Q96MD System (Qiagen). Methylation of LINE-1 and Alu (%5-mC [%5-methylated cytosine]) was calculated at each of the four known CpG sites and for each triplicate analysis of each participant sample using Pyro Q-CpG Software (Qiagen) [60, 61]. Details of bisulfite pyrosequencing of Alu and LINE-1 methylation have been described by previous studies [60, 62].

A combination of QA/QC approaches was used to reduce technical and batch sources of variability. We included a no template control (NTC) in addition to unmethylated, partially methylated, and completely methylated genomic DNA. Intraplate repeats of samples were also randomly distributed across plates. We ran all sample plates on the same day in order to limit batch variability. All coefficients of variation for repeat measures and intraplate coefficients of variation were in acceptable ranges (≤ 5%) [26], and all isolated DNA samples had 260/280 ratios > 1.6.

Covariates

Covariates were selected for fully adjusted models based on the literature [26, 51, 63–65] and a directed acyclic graph (DAG) (Additional file 1: Figure S1). For all models, confounders included maternal age at delivery, the number of years living in the USA (≤ 1 year, 2–5 years, 6–10 years, 11–24 years, and entire life), maternal smoking during pregnancy, maternal diet quality during pregnancy (DQI-P), and maternal urinary phthalate concentrations of monobenzyl phthalate (MBzP) during pregnancy. Maternal age was obtained during the baseline interview as was tobacco smoking status during pregnancy. In a previous work, we showed that prenatal exposure to urinary MBzP (a phthalate metabolite) was inversely associated with LINE-1 methylation [26] and that indicators of maternal SES were moderately to highly correlated with urinary MBzP [66]. Maternal urinary MBzP concentrations were determined for pregnancy by collecting maternal urine at each prenatal interview and measured by on-line solid phase extraction coupled with isotope dilution-high-performance liquid chromatography-electrospray ionization-tandem mass spectrometry at the Center for Disease Control and Prevention [67]. The two measurements were averaged to derive an overall pregnancy average concentration. We used log-transformed values of MBzP in the regression analyses. Cell composition was controlled for in sensitivity analyses. Cell composition estimation was performed using a recently validated reference database of nucleated cord blood cell types [68, 69]. Cell types included CD8T, CD4T, Natural killer, B lymphocytes, Monocytes, Granulocytes, and nucleated red blood cells.

Statistical analysis

Summary statistics were computed for all study covariates, exposures of interest, and basic study population characteristics. Linear mixed effects regression was used to detect associations between LINE-1 and Alu DNA methylation in cord blood and indicators of the social environment at the individual, household, and neighborhood levels, and for maternal diet quality during pregnancy (DQI-P). Continuous SES indicator variables (percent below poverty, median household income, percent with a high school education, and poverty income ratio) were modeled in separate analyses as continuous and in quartiles (to account for potential non-linearity). We then explored whether SES associations with repeat element methylation were modified by prenatal maternal diet quality. Consistent with our previous work [26, 27], we ran mixed effects models with a random effect for repeat analyses (triplicate) of DNA methylation to account for correlation within subject and a separate random effect for methylation sites (four CpG sites analyzed for both LINE-1 and Alu assays) to account for site-specific correlation. In our main analyses looking at socioeconomic indicators and diet quality, we implemented three separate mixed effects models. In model 1, we only controlled for random effects to estimate crude associations between exposures of interest and methylation. In model 2 we adjusted for maternal factors including smoking during pregnancy, age at delivery, MBzP urinary concentrations, and diet quality. Model 3 was a sensitivity analysis, where we adjusted for cell type estimates since methylation is likely to be dependent on cell type. Finally, to test for interaction between diet quality and measures of socioeconomic disadvantage, we applied interaction terms between each categorical socioeconomic indicator variable and DQI-P (diet quality, modeled continuous), adjusting for all other covariates in model 2. For illustrative purposes and to display interaction effects, we consider stratified analyses by DQI-P quintiles. All summary statistics and regression models were analyzed with R statistical software (version 3. 2.4) using the *lmer* function (lmerTest, version 2.0–32) for linear mixed effects regression models. A p value < 0.05 and < 0.1 were considered statistically significant and marginally significant, respectively, for main effects. Since there are simultaneous tests when assessing for interaction between a categorical variable (e.g., quantiles) and another variable, we applied a partial sum of squares F test (*anova* command in R) in order to report on p values for the diet quality (significance-level at $p_{interaction} < 0.05$). In addition to p values, we also qualitatively assessed the heterogeneity in effect sizes when stratifying by quintiles of diet quality. In

order to take advantage of the complete data on the study outcomes, missing values on the covariates included in the regression models were imputed using factorial analysis for mixed data on both continuous and categorical variables (R package: *missMDA*). The percent missing for the three imputed covariates were as follows: $< 1\%$ ($N = 1$) on maternal MBzP concentration, $< 1\%$ ($N = 1$) on maternal age, and 5% ($N = 13$) on DQI-P.

Results

Maternal and infant characteristics included in our analysis are presented in Table 1. Newborns were evenly split between males (49.8%) and females (50.2%) with mean gestation length and birth weight of 39 weeks and 3467 g, respectively. Most of the mothers were Latina (96%) with an average maternal age at delivery of 26 years. Mean pre-pregnancy BMI was 26.5 kg/m^2, with the majority of mothers classified as either overweight (37%) or obese (20%) prior to pregnancy.

Individual-level socioeconomic disadvantage (Table 1) and household-level socioeconomic disadvantage (Table 2) was severe in the study population. A majority of mothers have less than a high school degree (79%) and live in households with a poverty income ratio < 1 (70%). Neighborhood socioeconomic disadvantage was similarly high, with a tract-level median of $34, 211 for median household income and median percentages of 24% for household poverty and 73% without a high school education. Correlations between maternal- or household- and neighborhood-level socioeconomic class indicators were generally weak although mostly in the anticipated directions (Additional file 1: Figure S2). Of all the study covariates included in adjusted regression models, MBzP and the number of years living in the USA exhibited the strongest correlations with the SES variables of interest for this study ($r = -0.27$ to 0.30). Maternal smoking was only weakly correlated with household-level poverty income ratio ($r = 0.10$) and income ($r = 0.06$), moderately correlated with the number of years living in the USA ($r = 0.27$), and moderately correlated with neighborhood SES (range $r = -0.23$, 0.22).

DNA methylation: LINE-1 and Alu

Average LINE-1 methylation was 78.9 (%5-mC) (95%CI 78.7, 79.1). As much as 11% (chi-squared test p value < 0.05) of the overall variance in LINE-1 methylation was explained by differences between CpG sites (suggesting significant level 2 CpG site effects). LINE-1 methylation levels were also slightly higher in boys compared to girls ($p = 0.03$), marginally lower in low birth weight infants compared to normal weight infants ($p = 0.06$), but there was no association between preterm infants and LINE-1 methylation. The summary statistics for LINE-1 methylation, stratified by quantiles of the SES indicators, are

Table 1 Summary statistics of participating infants and mothers, CHAMACOS (n = 241 mother-infant dyads)

	All
Infant	
Preterm birth, N (%)	
Yes	13 (5.4)
No	228 (94.6)
Low birth weight, N (%)	
Yes	7 (2.9)
No	234 (97.1)
Mother	
Age at pregnancy, years (M ± SD)	25.8 ± 5.3
Pre-pregnancy body mass index, kg/m^2 (M ± SD)	26.5 ± 5.0
Race/ethnicity, N (%)	
Latino	232 (96.2)
White	5 (2.1)
Other	4 (1.7)
Educational attainment, N (%)	
< 6th grade	98 (40.7)
7–12 grade	92 (38.2)
≥ High school	51 (21.1)
Country of birth, N (%)	
U.S.	32 (13.3)
Mexico	205 (85.1)
Central America/other	4 (1.7)
Years spent living in the U.S., N (%)	
< =1 year	61 (25.3)
2–5 years	70 (29.0)
6–10 years	48 (19.9)
11–24 years	34 (14.1)
Entire life (18–32 years)	28 (11.6)
Diet quality index during pregnancy (M ± SD)	44.90 ± 9.66
Urinary MBzP[a], μg/L (IQR[b])	9.5 (4.7, 17.8)

[a]Median urinary concentration, limit of detection is 0.3 μg/L
[b]*IQR* interquartile range

Table 2 Summary statistics of SES at the household and census tract level, CHAMACOS (n = 241)

SES indicators	
Household	Median (IQR)
Income, monthly ($)	375.2 (281.4, 562.8)
Poverty income ratio	0.98 (0.65, 1.20)
Neighborhood (census tracts)	Median (IQR)
Household income, yearly ($)	34211 (31910, 41354)
% of household below poverty	23.50 (19.38, 27.54)
% of people with no high school diploma	72.80 (50.10, 75.34)

presented in Table 3. Average Alu methylation was 25.3 (%5-mC) (95%CI 25.1, 25.5) and clustering of methylation levels by CpG site. There were no significant differences in Alu methylation levels between boys and girls or by preterm or low birth weight of the infant. Confirming our previous work, maternal urinary MBzP consistently resulted in a statistically significant linear negative association with LINE-1 methylation (model 2). Interestingly, fewer years spent living in the USA (≤ 1 year and 2–5 years) consistently had significantly higher LINE-1 methylation compared to those who lived their entire life in the USA.

Associations of SES and DNA methylation

The summary statistics for LINE-1 methylation, stratified by the different SES categories, are presented in Additional file 1: Table S1. There were no significant differences in LINE-1 methylation by neighborhood income levels or by neighborhood educational attainment, in both crude (model 1) and adjusted (model 2) analyses (Table 4). Living in the highest poverty neighborhood quartile was significantly associated with higher LINE-1 methylation compared to living in the lowest poverty neighborhood quartile (adjusted $\beta = 0.78$, 95%CI: 0.06, 1.50, $p = 0.03$). There was a lack of a linear trend ($p = 0.51$) for increasing neighborhood poverty quartiles and methylation. We found no statistically significant differences in LINE-1 methylation by individual- or household-level SES (Table 4) in crude or adjusted models. Although after adjustment, the second household income quartile and second poverty income ratio quartile were marginally associated with higher methylation compared to the highest SES quartile categories (p-value = 0.05 and 0.06, respectively). After controlling for estimated cell type proportions (Model 3, Table 4), the neighborhood-level poverty association with LINE-1 methylation strengthened slightly ($\beta = 0.88$, $p - 0.02$), but the household-level SES variables attenuated substantially and were no longer marginally associated after controlling for cell type proportions. No significant associations of socioeconomic indicators were observed with Alu methylation (Additional file 1: Table S1).

Diet quality during pregnancy, SES, and LINE-1 methylation

Diet quality index during pregnancy (DQI-P) was positively, albeit non-significantly, associated with LINE-1 methylation in crude and adjusted models ($p_{adjusted} = 0.19$) (Table 4). Including an interaction term between neighborhood poverty quartiles and DQI-P indicated a statistical trend towards interaction ($p_{interaction} = 0.12$). In Fig. 1a, we present the adjusted regression coefficients for each poverty quartiles on LINE-1 methylation when the regression analyses are stratified by DQI-P quintiles. We observed that in the highest quintile of DQI-P

Table 3 Mean LINE-1% methylation overall and stratified by SES indicator categories and years living in the USA

SES indicators	LINE-1% mean methylation (95% CI)
Overall	78.9 (78.7, 79.1)
Maternal-level	
Educational attainment	
< 6th grade	78.8 (78.5, 79.1)
7th–12th grade	79.2 (78.8, 79.4)
≥ High school	78.7 (78.3, 79.2)
Household-level	
Monthly income quartiles	
1st quartile ($37–$225)	78.7 (78.3, 79.2)
2nd quartile ($281–$375)	79.1 (78.8, 79.4)
3rd quartile ($438–$563)	78.8 (78.4, 79.2)
4th quartile ($583–$1750)	78.7 (78.1, 79.2)
Poverty income ratio quartiles	
1st quartile (0.13–0.65)	78.8 (78.4, 79.2)
2nd quartile (0.71–0.98)	79.1 (78.8, 79.5)
3rd quartile (1.01–1.21)	78.9 (78.8, 79.3)
4th quartile (1.30–2.40)	78.7 (78.2, 79.1)
Neighborhood (census tract)-level	
Median household income quartiles	
1st quartile ($24,896–$31910)	78.9 (78.6, 79.2)
2nd quartile ($31,989–$34593)	78.7 (78.2, 79.2)
3rd quartile ($34,848–$40856)	78.9 (78.5, 79.4)
4th quartile ($41,354–$77272)	79.0 (78.6, 79.4)
Percent below poverty quartiles	
1st quartile (2.8–18.2)	78.7 (78.3, 79.1)
2nd quartile (19.0–22.3)	79.0 (78.6, 79.4)
3rd quartile (23.5–27.5)	78.7 (78.4, 79.0)
4th quartile (27.7–34.2)	79.8 (79.1, 80.4)
Percent without a highschool education quartiles	
1st quartile (13.7–50.1)	78.9 (78.5, 79.3)
2nd quartile (51.4–71.4)	79.1 (78.7, 79.5)
3rd quartile (72.5–75.3)	78.6 (78.2, 79.0)
4th quartile (78.7–87.0)	78.9 (78.6, 79.3)
Years living in the USA ("acculturation")	
< =1 year	79.2 (78.6, 79.7)
2–5 years	79.3 (78.9, 79.8)
6–10 years	78.8 (78.4, 79.8)
11–24 years	78.8 (78.4, 79.2)
Entire life (18–32 years)	78.4 (77.8, 78.9)

(best diet quality), the adjusted mean LINE-1 methylation was higher by 2.6% in the highest quartile of neighborhood poverty compared with the lowest poverty quartile. Conversely, in the lower DQI-P quintiles (poorer diet quality), there was either no differences in LINE-1 methylation or lower methylation with increasing neighborhood poverty quartiles compared to the lowest poverty quartile. When neighborhood poverty is modeled as a continuous variable along with an interaction term with DQI-P, this statistical trend strengthened ($p_{interaction}$ = 0.06). As shown in Fig. 1b, at very low levels of maternal diet quality, there is a negative exposure-response relationship between neighborhood poverty and LINE-1 methylation, and conversely, at high levels of maternal diet quality, there is a positive exposure-response relationship between neighborhood poverty and LINE-1 methylation. In Fig. 1c, the relationship between neighborhood poverty and LINE-1 methylation is significant only at very high levels of maternal diet quality. There was no evidence for interaction between other indicators of SES and diet quality on LINE-1 methylation ($p_{interaction}$ > 0.2 in all cases). Finally, we did not observe any differences in Alu methylation by diet (Additional file 1: Table S2) or by combination of diet and SES indicators ($p_{interaction}$ > 0.2 in all cases).

Discussion

In the CHAMACOS cohort, we observed a small but statistically significant association between the prenatal socioeconomic environment and DNA methylation of LINE-1 repeat elements in infant cord blood. Specifically, only higher neighborhood poverty was significantly associated with LINE-1 hypermethylation and this association was possibly moderated by the quality of maternal diet during pregnancy.

As already discussed in the introduction, previous studies relating to epigenetic markers with maternal SES or neighborhood SES indicators during pregnancy vary by methodology, design, and findings. For instance, a cohort study in NY that examined the relationship between maternal SES and global DNA methylation in infant cord blood found no associations [38]. Our findings also show a null association between maternal education and LINE-1 methylation but a positive relationship with neighborhood poverty. The NY study, however, did not consider neighborhood SES indicators. Furthermore, they used a measure of global methylation measured by immunoassay while our pyrosequencing analysis presented here focused on repetitive element methylation that does not necessarily correlate with global methylation.

Prenatal neighborhood-level poverty and individual-level poverty have each been associated with adverse developmental outcomes such as low birth weight and preterm birth [70]. In our study, we only observed an epigenetic association with neighborhood poverty. The precise mechanisms of neighborhood effects on health or epigenetic changes are not clear. Such neighborhood effects possibly result from the sustained and combined exposures to multiple adverse social and

Table 4 Results from linear regression mixed effects (LMER) models of crude and adjusted associations between maternal, household, and neighborhood indicators of SES and diet quality index and LINE-1 DNA methylation

Socioeconomic status indicators	Model 1[a]		Model 2[b]		Model 3[c]	
	β (95% CI)	p value	aβ (95% CI)	p value	aβ (95% CI)	p value
Household income						
1st quartile ($37–$225)	0.05 (−0.59, 0.70)	0.88	0.08 (−0.59, 0.75)	0.82	−0.18 (−0.87, 0.52)	0.62
2nd quartile ($281–$375)	0.46 (−0.13, 1.04)	0.12	0.60 (−0.01, 1.21)	0.05	0.18 (−0.48, 0.83)	0.60
3rd quartile ($438–$563)	0.14 (−0.52, 0.80)	0.68	0.20 (−0.46, 0.86)	0.56	−0.07 (−0.75, 0.60)	0.84
4th quartile ($583–$1750)	Reference		Reference		Reference	
Household poverty income ratio						
1st quartile (0.13–0.65)	0.07 (−0.49, 0.63)	0.80	0.12 (−0.45, 0.69)	0.68	−0.18 (−0.78, 0.41)	0.54
2nd quartile (0.71–0.98)	0.08 (−0.12, 1.01)	0.09	0.53 (−0.03, 1.08)	0.07	0.15 (−0.45, 0.75)	0.62
3rd quartile (1.01–1.21)	0.45 (−0.42, 0.82)	0.56	0.21 (−0.43, 0.85)	0.52	−0.13 (−0.78, 0.53)	0.71
4th quartile (1.30–2.40)	Reference		Reference		Reference	
Maternal education						
< = 6th grade	0.04 (−0.46, 0.53)	0.89	−0.09 (−0.65, 0.47)	0.75	−0.03 (−0.60, 0.54)	0.92
7–12th grade	0.39 (−0.12, 0.90)	0.13	0.33 (−0.20, 0.86)	0.22	0.35 (−0.18, 0.89)	0.20
> =Highschool	Reference		Reference			
% Households below poverty (CT)						
1st quartile (2.8–18.2)	Reference		Reference		Reference	
2nd quartile (19.0–22.3)	0.26 (−0.27, 0.80)	0.34	0.24 (−0.31, 0.78)	0.39	0.31 (−0.26, 0.85)	0.30
3rd quartile (23.5–27.5)	−0.01 (−0.49, 0.47)	0.97	−0.11 (−0.61, 0.39)	0.68	−0.04 (−0.47, 0.54)	0.89
4th quartile (27.7–34.2)	1.03 (0.33, 1.73)	0.004	0.78 (0.06, 1.50)	0.03	0.88 (0.14, 1.64)	0.02
Median household income (CT)						
1st quartile ($24,896–$31910)	−0.05 (−0.53, 0.43)	0.84	−0.03 (−0.58, 0.53)	0.93	−0.02 (−0.58, 0.53)	0.94
2nd quartile ($31,989–$34593)	−0.26 (−0.84, 0.32)	0.39	−0.40 (−0.93, 0.13)	0.14	−0.48 (−1.01, 0.05)	0.08
3rd quartile ($34,848–$40856)	0.02 (−0.61, 0.57)	0.94	−0.12 (−0.66, 0.42)	0.66	−0.01 (−0.55, 0.53)	0.98
4th quartile ($41,354–$77272)	Reference		Reference		Reference	
% No highschool education (CT)						
1st quartile (13.7–50.1)	Reference		Reference		Reference	
2nd quartile (51.4–71.4)	0.16 (−0.38, 0.70)	0.55	0.07 (−0.49, 0.63)	0.81	0.08 (−0.48, 0.64)	0.77
3rd quartile (72.5–75.3)	−0.33 (−0.84, 0.19)	0.21	−0.30 (−0.84, 0.24)	0.28	−0.33 (−0.87, 0.22)	0.24
4th Quartile (78.7–87.0)	−0.02 (−0.50, 0.54)	0.94	−0.10 (−0.66, 0.46)	0.72	0.04 (−0.53, 0.60)	0.90
Diet quality index	0.020 (−0.008, 0.032)	0.24	0.13 (−0.06, 0.32)[d]	0.19	0.08 (−0.12, 0.27)[d]	0.44

[a]Model 1: random effect for position and individual only
[b]Model 2: random effect for position and individual, maternal smoking during pregnancy, maternal age, diet quality during pregnancy, years living in the USA for the mother, and prenatal MBzP exposure
[c]Model 3: random effect for position and individual, maternal smoking during pregnancy, maternal age, diet quality during pregnancy, years living in the USA for the mother, prenatal MBzP exposure, and cell estimate proportions
[d]Neighborhood poverty included as a covariate due to evidence of confounding by neighborhood poverty. Diet quality index was Z standardized so that continuous variables were on similar scales

physical individual-level risk factors that may be experienced by individuals living in impoverished neighborhoods. The multiple social and physical risk factors can include low access to healthy foods [71] and health care, mental stress associated with violence and social isolation, higher exposure to environmental pollutants, and built environments that promote unhealthy behaviors [72]. Thus, one possible explanation behind our observing only neighborhood effects, rather than individual-level effects in our study, could be related to this concept of sustained and combined stressors tied to neighborhood SES, while a single parameter of individual socioeconomic adversity is unable to capture this accumulation of combined social, physical, and economic stressors. Additionally, our null findings for maternal-level and household-level socioeconomic indicators may be related to a relative homogeneity in low SES among the CHAMACOS participants.

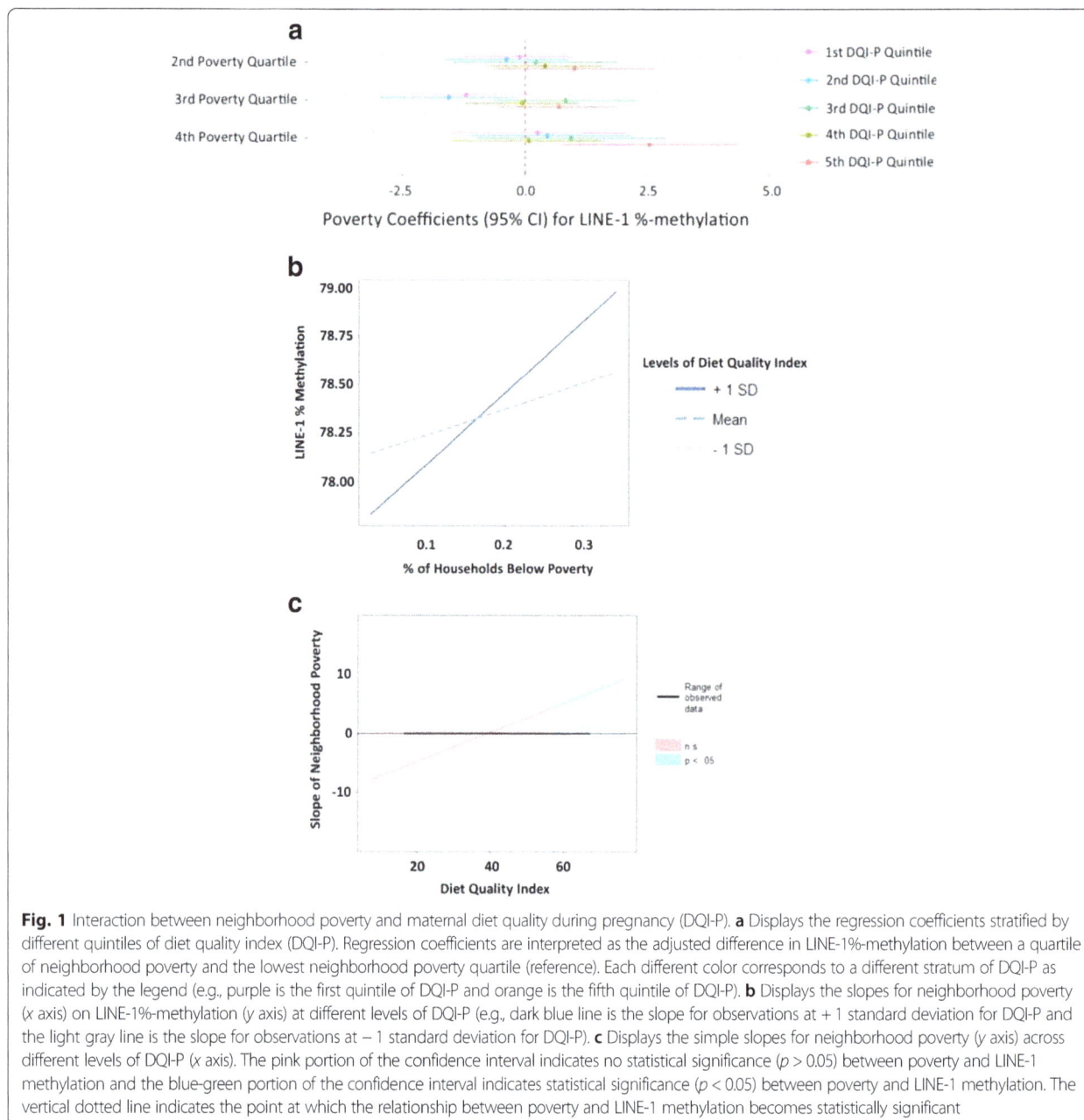

Fig. 1 Interaction between neighborhood poverty and maternal diet quality during pregnancy (DQI-P). **a** Displays the regression coefficients stratified by different quintiles of diet quality index (DQI-P). Regression coefficients are interpreted as the adjusted difference in LINE-1%-methylation between a quartile of neighborhood poverty and the lowest neighborhood poverty quartile (reference). Each different color corresponds to a different stratum of DQI-P as indicated by the legend (e.g., purple is the first quintile of DQI-P and orange is the fifth quintile of DQI-P). **b** Displays the slopes for neighborhood poverty (x axis) on LINE-1%-methylation (y axis) at different levels of DQI-P (e.g., dark blue line is the slope for observations at + 1 standard deviation for DQI-P and the light gray line is the slope for observations at − 1 standard deviation for DQI-P). **c** Displays the simple slopes for neighborhood poverty (y axis) across different levels of DQI-P (x axis). The pink portion of the confidence interval indicates no statistical significance (p > 0.05) between poverty and LINE-1 methylation and the blue-green portion of the confidence interval indicates statistical significance (p < 0.05) between poverty and LINE-1 methylation. The vertical dotted line indicates the point at which the relationship between poverty and LINE-1 methylation becomes statistically significant

Since neighborhood poverty has typically been associated with greater exposure to maternal stress as well as adverse developmental outcomes in previous studies, it may appear counterintuitive that the children of CHAMACOS mothers living in higher poverty neighborhoods during pregnancy are observed to have higher LINE-1 methylation in cord blood, relative to lower poverty neighborhoods. Unexpected observation of protective social adversity effects in utero is not unfounded however. The prenatal LINE-1 hypermethylation observed in our study could reflect an adaptive response to maternal stress cues that is intended to influence the development of a phenotype that is adapted to coping with a similarly stressful environment later in life [73]. In other words, hypermethylation of LINE-1 may be a response to stress that could make the individual more resilient to similar stressful events in the future. For instance, the timing of elevated maternal anxiety during pregnancy and related prenatal exposure to higher levels of cortisol in utero has been shown to be protective of mental health and neurodevelopment in infancy [74], and newborn DNA methylation has been linked with infant cortisol response (glucocorticoid receptor gene methylation) [75] and infant neurodevelopment (LINE-1 methylation) [76]. A potential adaptive phenomenon with LINE-1 hypermethylation has also been reported in a military service personnel with post-traumatic stress disorder [21].

Further, a positive association between higher neighborhood poverty and LINE-1 methylation was primarily seen in the cord blood of infants from CHAMACOS mothers who had the highest quality dietary patterns during pregnancy (Fig. 1a). This finding of the potentially moderating epigenetic effects between neighborhood poverty and maternal diet quality lends some support to the hypothesis that maternal diet may supply "epi-nutrients" that influence epigenetic effects from exposure to stressors in utero [77]. In addition, other studies suggest that neighborhood poverty and nutrition, and their health effects, may be closely linked. Neighborhood-level disadvantage has been associated with poorer diet quality [78], poorer nutritional status [79], and higher hair cortisol levels (an indicator of chronic stress), while better diet among those with lower SES has been shown to be protective against inflammatory [80] and poor mental health outcomes [81, 82]. Future studies should measure maternal diet quality or nutritional status when considering neighborhood SES or maternal stress effects on infant epigenetics in order to assess the potential moderating role of maternal diet.

While no human studies have used a diet quality index to investigate associations with epigenetic changes, some researchers have investigated associations of specific nutrients as well as eating disorders during pregnancy in relation to repeat element methylation. One human study [65] found that choline intake during pregnancy was significantly and inversely related to cord blood LINE-1 methylation in boys but positively associated with LINE-1 methylation in girls (albeit non-significant). Another human study reported that folate supplementation was inversely related with cord blood LINE-1 methylation [51]. A recent study [83] found that maternal eating disorders (restrictive, purging, binge eating, binge-purge) during pregnancy were associated with hypomethylation in infant cord blood, possibly related to lower calorie intake. Our finding of a positive association (albeit statistically insignificant) between better diet quality during pregnancy and repeat element methylation also supports the role of maternal diet as a determinant of infant methylation levels.

Although the consideration of SES at multiple levels (individual, household, and neighborhood) is an important strength of our study because each level may act independent of one another [84], it does not implicate any specific environmental stressors related to area poverty. In addition to the socioeconomic indicators we considered, other factors potentially may contribute to differential LINE-1 and Alu methylation such as prenatal exposures to persistent organic pollutants [27] and other chemicals [85], or other relevant biologic measures (e.g., BMI or cortisol levels [23]). Some of these effects have been assessed in previously published CHAMACOS studies [26, 27] and do not appear to be confounders in

the current analyses. Although the homogeneity of the CHAMACOS population in the Salinas Valley, California is another potential limitation of our study, it is also a strength in that there is less likely to be uncontrolled confounding due to other factors. To make our findings more generalizable, additional studies in other ethnic and SES cohorts are warranted. It will be important to also further explore potential influence of maternal nutrition on associations between the socioeconomic status and DNA methylation.

Conclusions

We observed a modest but statistically significant association between neighborhood-level poverty and LINE-1 repeat element methylation in newborns, and the direction of this relationship appears to be modified by maternal diet during pregnancy. This finding implies that maternal diet may have a moderating effect on the association between neighborhood poverty and repeat element DNA methylation and that future epigenetic studies investigating the prenatal effects of social class should consider maternal diet as a potential moderator of neighborhood socioeconomic effects on epigenetics.

Abbreviations
BMI: Body mass index; CHAMACOS: Center for Health Assessment of Mothers and Children of Salinas; DAG: Directed acyclic graph; DQI-P: Diet Quality Index for Pregnancy; FFQ: Food-frequency questionnaire; LINEs: Long interspersed nuclear elements; MBzP: Monobenzyl phthalate; SES: Socioeconomic status; SINEs: Short interspersed nuclear elements

Acknowledgements
We are grateful to the numerous laboratory and field staff and participants of the CHAMACOS study for their contributions.

Funding
This publication was made possible by grants from the National Institute of Environmental Health Science (NIEHS) [P01 ES009605, R01 ES021369, R01 ES023067], from the US Environmental Protection Agency (EPA)[R82670901, and RD83451301], the National Institutes of Health (NIH) [UG3OD023356], Health Resources and Services Administration (HRSA) [T76MC00002], and a grant support from The JPB Foundation through the JPB Research Network on Toxic Stress, a project of the Center on the Developing Child at Harvard University.
Its contents are solely the responsibility of the authors and do not necessarily represent the official views of NIEHS, EPA, HRSA, or JPB Foundation.

Authors' contributions
EC analyzed and interpreted the participant data regarding the study finding and wrote the first draft of the manuscript. RG assisted with the conception and design of the data analysis and contributed to the writing and editing of the manuscript. KH assisted with the design of the data analysis, performed laboratory epigenetics analyses, and contributed to the writing and editing of the manuscript. NH assisted with the design of the data analysis and oversaw the epigenetics laboratory procedures, and contributed significantly to the writing and editing of the manuscript. BE designed and oversaw the collection of all aspects of the study data, assisted with the design of the data analysis, and contributed significantly to the writing and editing of the manuscript. All authors read and approved the final manuscript.

Competing interests
The authors declare that they have no competing interests.

Author details
[1]Center for Environmental Research and Children's Health (CERCH), School of Public Health, University of California, Berkeley, CA, USA. [2]Berkeley, USA. [3]Richmond, USA.

References
1.   Earnshaw VA, Rosenthal L, Lewis JB, Stasko EC, Tobin JN, Lewis TT, et al. Maternal experiences with everyday discrimination and infant birth weight: a test of mediators and moderators among young, urban women of color. Ann Behav Med. 2013;45:13–23.
2.   Finch BK. Socioeconomic gradients and low birth-weight: empirical and policy considerations: socioeconomic gradients and low birth-weight. Health Serv Res. 2003;38:1819–42.
3.   Nepomnyaschy L. Socioeconomic gradients in infant health across race and ethnicity. Matern Child Health J. 2009;13:720–31.
4.   Silvestrin S, da Silva CH, Hirakata VN, AAS G, Silveira PP, Goldani MZ. Maternal education level and low birth weight: a meta-analysis. J Pediatr. 2013;89:339–45.
5.   Cerdá M, Buka SL, Rich-Edwards JW. Neighborhood influences on the association between maternal age and birthweight: a multilevel investigation of age-related disparities in health. Soc Sci Med. 2008;66:2048–60.
6.   Alhusen JL, Bower KM, Epstein E, Sharps P. Racial discrimination and adverse birth outcomes: an integrative review. J Midwifery Womens Health. 2016;61:707–20.
7.   Blumenshine P, Egerter S, Barclay CJ, Cubbin C, Braveman PA. Socioeconomic disparities in adverse birth outcomes. Am J Prev Med. 2010;39:263–72.
8.   Mutambudzi M, Meyer JD, Warren N, Reisine S. Effects of psychosocial characteristics of work on pregnancy outcomes: a critical review. Women Health. 2011;51:279–97.
9.   Littleton HL, Bye K, Buck K, Amacker A. Psychosocial stress during pregnancy and perinatal outcomes: a meta-analytic review. J Psychosom Obstet Gynaecol. 2010;31:219–28.
10. Vuong B, Odero G, Rozbacher S, Stevenson M, Kereliuk SM, Pereira TJ, et al. Exposure to gestational diabetes mellitus induces neuroinflammation, derangement of hippocampal neurons, and cognitive changes in rat offspring. J Neuroinflammation. 2017;14:80.
11. Wallack L, Thornburg K. Developmental origins, epigenetics, and equity: moving upstream. Matern Child Health J. 2016;20:935–40.
12. Meaney MJ. Epigenetics and the biological definition of gene x environment interactions. Child Dev. 2010;81:41–79.
13. NIH. Epigenomics Fact Sheet. Natl. Hum. Genome Res. Inst. NHGRI. 2016 [cited 2017 Sep 12]. Available from: https://www.genome.gov/27532724/Epigenomics-Fact-Sheet
14. Notterman DA, Mitchell C. Epigenetics and understanding the impact of social determinants of health. Pediatr Clin N Am. 2015;62:1227–40.
15. Wilhelm-Benartzi CS, Houseman EA, Maccani MA, Poage GM, Koestler DC, Langevin SM, et al. In utero exposures, infant growth, and DNA methylation of repetitive elements and developmentally related genes in human placenta. Environ Health Perspect. 2011;120:296–302.
16. Wang L, Wang F, Guan J, Le J, Wu L, Zou J, et al. Relation between hypomethylation of long interspersed nucleotide elements and risk of neural tube defects. Am J Clin Nutr. 2010;91:1359–67.
17. Price EM, Cotton AM, Peñaherrera MS, McFadden DE, Kobor MS, Robinson W. Different measures of "genome-wide" DNA methylation exhibit unique properties in placental and somatic tissues. Epigenetics. 2012;7:652–63.
18. Hou L, Wang H, Sartori S, Gawron A, Lissowska J, Bollati V, et al. Blood leukocyte DNA hypomethylation and gastric cancer risk in a high-risk Polish population. Int J Cancer. 2010;127:1866–74.
19. Gao Y, Baccarelli A, Shu XO, Ji B-T, Yu K, Tarantini L, et al. Blood leukocyte Alu and LINE-1 methylation and gastric cancer risk in the Shanghai Women's Health Study. Br J Cancer. 2012;106:585–91.
20. Alexeeff SE, Baccarelli AA, Halonen J, Coull BA, Wright RO, Tarantini L, et al. Association between blood pressure and DNA methylation of retrotransposons and pro-inflammatory genes. Int J Epidemiol. 2013;42:270–80.
21. Rusiecki JA, Chen L, Srikantan V, Zhang L, Yan L, Polin ML, et al. DNA methylation in repetitive elements and post-traumatic stress disorder: a case-control study of US military service members. Epigenomics. 2012;4:29–40.
22. Nätt D, Thorsell A. Stress-induced transposon reactivation: a mediator or an estimator of allostatic load? Environ Epigenetics. 2016;2:dvw015.
23. Nätt D, Johansson I, Faresjö T, Ludvigsson J, Thorsell A. High cortisol in 5-year-old children causes loss of DNA methylation in SINE retrotransposons: a possible role for ZNF263 in stress-related diseases. Clin Epigenetics. 2015 [cited 2018 Mar 7];7. Available from: http://www.clinicalepigeneticsjournal.com/content/7/1/91
24. Hunter RG, Gagnidze K, McEwen BS, Pfaff DW. Stress and the dynamic genome: steroids, epigenetics, and the transposome: fig. 1. Proc Natl Acad Sci 2015;112:6828–6833.
25. Bundo M, Toyoshima M, Okada Y, Akamatsu W, Ueda J, Nemoto-Miyauchi T, et al. Increased L1 retrotransposition in the neuronal genome in schizophrenia. Neuron. 2014;81:306–13.
26. Huen K, Calafat AM, Bradman A, Yousefi P, Eskenazi B, Holland N. Maternal phthalate exposure during pregnancy is associated with DNA methylation of LINE-1 and Alu repetitive elements in Mexican-American children. Environ Res. 2016;148:55–62.
27. Huen K, Yousefi P, Bradman A, Yan L, Harley KG, Kogut K, et al. Effects of age, sex, and persistent organic pollutants on DNA methylation in children: DNA methylation in children. Environ Mol Mutagen. 2014;55:209–22.
28. Watkins DJ, Wellenius GA, Butler RA, Bartell SM, Fletcher T, Kelsey KT. Associations between serum perfluoroalkyl acids and LINE-1 DNA methylation. Environ Int. 2014;63:71–6.
29. Bellavia A, Urch B, Speck M, Brook RD, Scott JA, Albetti B, et al. DNA hypomethylation, ambient particulate matter, and increased blood pressure: findings from controlled human exposure experiments. J Am Heart Assoc. 2013;2:e000212–2.
30. Lee MH, Cho ER, Lim J, Jee SH. Association between serum persistent organic pollutants and DNA methylation in Korean adults. Environ Res. 2017;158:333–41.
31. Tajuddin SM, Amaral AFS, Fernández AF, Rodríguez-Rodero S, Rodríguez RM, Moore LE, et al. Genetic and Non-genetic Predictors of LINE-1 Methylation in Leukocyte DNA. Environ Health Perspect. 2013 [cited 2017 Nov 3]; Available from: http://ehp.niehs.nih.gov/1206068/
32. van Dijk SJ, Zhou J, Peters TJ, Buckley M, Sutcliffe B, Oytam Y, et al. Effect of prenatal DHA supplementation on the infant epigenome: results from a randomized controlled trial. Clin Epigenetics. 2016 [cited 2017 Aug 3];8. Available from: http://clinicalepigeneticsjournal.biomedcentral.com/articles/10.1186/s13148-016-0281-7
33. Devi S, Mukhopadhyay A, Dwarkanath P, Thomas T, Crasta J, Thomas A, et al. Combined vitamin B-12 and balanced protein-energy supplementation affect homocysteine remethylation in the methionine cycle in pregnant South Indian women of low vitamin B-12 status. J Nutr. 2017;147:1094–103.
34. Pauwels S, Ghosh M, Duca RC, Bekaert B, Freson K, Huybrechts I, et al. Dietary and supplemental maternal methyl-group donor intake and cord blood DNA methylation. Epigenetics. 2017;12:1–10.
35. Searles NS, Harvey C, Butler RA, Nelson HH, Farin FM, Longstreth WT, et al. LINE-1 DNA methylation, smoking and risk of Parkinson's disease. J Park Dis. 2012;2:303–8.
36. Ayarpadikannan S, Kim H-S. The impact of transposable elements in genome evolution and genetic instability and their implications in various diseases. Genomics Inform. 2014;12:98.
37. Su J, Shao X, Liu H, Liu S, Wu Q, Zhang Y. Genome-wide dynamic changes of DNA methylation of repetitive elements in human embryonic stem cells and fetal fibroblasts. Genomics. 2012;99:10–7.
38. Herbstman JB, Wang S, Perera FP, Lederman SA, Vishnevetsky J, Rundle AG, et al. Predictors and consequences of global DNA methylation in cord blood and at three years. PLoS One. 2013;8:e72824. El-Maarri O, editor
39. Marsit CJ, Maccani MA, Padbury JF, Lester BM. Placental 11-beta hydroxysteroid dehydrogenase methylation is associated with newborn growth and a measure of neurobehavioral outcome. PLoS One. 2012;7: e33794. Oudejans C, editor
40. King K, Murphy S, Hoyo C. Epigenetic regulation of newborns' imprinted genes related to gestational growth: patterning by parental race/ethnicity and maternal socioeconomic status. J Epidemiol Community Health. 2015;69:639–47.
41. King KE, Kane JB, Scarbrough P, Hoyo C, Murphy SK. Neighborhood and family environment of expectant mothers may influence prenatal programming of adult cancer risk: discussion and an illustrative DNA methylation example. Biodemography Soc Biol. 2016;62:87–104.

42. Javed R, Chen W, Lin F, Liang H. Infant's DNA methylation age at birth and epigenetic aging accelerators. Biomed Res Int. 2016;2016:1–10.

43. Krukowski RA, West DS, Harvey-Berino J, Elaine PT. Neighborhood impact on healthy food availability and pricing in food stores. J Community Health. 2010;35:315–20.

44. Laraia B. Proximity of supermarkets is positively associated with diet quality index for pregnancy. Prev Med. 2004;39:869–75.

45. Larson NI, Story MT, Nelson MC. Neighborhood environments. Am J Prev Med. 2009;36:74–81. e10

46. McLeod ER, Campbell KJ, Hesketh KD. Nutrition knowledge: a mediator between socioeconomic position and diet quality in Australian first-time mothers. J Am Diet Assoc. 2011;111:696–704.

47. Darmon N, Drewnowski A. Contribution of food prices and diet cost to socioeconomic disparities in diet quality and health: a systematic review and analysis. Nutr Rev. 2015;73:643–60.

48. Tarasuk V, McIntyre L, Li J. Low-income women's dietary intakes are sensitive to the depletion of household resources in one month. J Nutr. 2007;137:1980–7.

49. Pauwels S, Ghosh M, Duca RC, Bekaert B, Freson K, Huybrechts I, et al. Maternal intake of methyl-group donors affects DNA methylation of metabolic genes in infants. Clin Epigenetics [Internet]. 2017 [cited 2017 Aug 3];9. Available from: http://clinicalepigeneticsjournal.biomedcentral.com/articles/10.1186/s13148-017-0321-y

50. McCullough LE, Miller EE, Mendez MA, Murtha AP, Murphy SK, Hoyo C. Maternal B vitamins: effects on offspring weight and DNA methylation at genomically imprinted domains. Clin Epigenetics [Internet]. 2016 [cited 2017 Aug 3];8. Available from: http://www.clinicalepigeneticsjournal.com/content/8/1/8

51. Haggarty P, Hoad G, Campbell DM, Horgan GW, Piyathilake C, McNeill G. Folate in pregnancy and imprinted gene and repeat element methylation in the offspring. Am J Clin Nutr. 2013;97:94–9.

52. Heijmans BT, Tobi EW, Stein AD, Putter H, Blauw GJ, Susser ES, et al. Persistent epigenetic differences associated with prenatal exposure to famine in humans. Proc Natl Acad Sci. 2008;105:17046–9.

53. Tobi EW, Lumey LH, Talens RP, Kremer D, Putter H, Stein AD, et al. DNA methylation differences after exposure to prenatal famine are common and timing- and sex-specific. Hum Mol Genet. 2009;18:4046–53.

54. Harley K, Eskenazi B. Time in the United States, social support and health behaviors during pregnancy among women of Mexican descent. Soc Sci Med. 2006;62:3048–61.

55. Block G, Woods M, Potosky A, Clifford C. Validation of a self-administered diet history questionnaire using multiple diet records. J Clin Epidemiol. 1990;43:1327–35.

56. Block G, Thompson FE, Hartman AM, Larkin FA, Guire KE. Comparison of two dietary questionnaires validated against multiple dietary records collected during a 1-year period. J Am Diet Assoc. 1992;92:686–93.

57. U.S. Department of Agriculture Agricultural Research Service. USDA National Nutrient Database for standard reference, release 13. Bethesda: U.S. Department of Agriculture; 1999.

58. Bodnar LM, Siega-Riz AM. A diet quality index for pregnancy detects variation in diet and differences by sociodemographic factors. Public Health Nutr. 2002;5:801–9.

59. Holland N, Furlong C, Bastaki M, Richter R, Bradman A, Huen K, et al. Paraoxonase polymorphisms, haplotypes, and enzyme activity in Latino mothers and newborns. Environ Health Perspect. 2006;114:985–91.

60. Yang AS. A simple method for estimating global DNA methylation using bisulfite PCR of repetitive DNA elements. Nucleic Acids Res. 2004;32:38e–38.

61. Royo JL, Hidalgo M, Ruiz A. Pyrosequencing protocol using a universal biotinylated primer for mutation detection and SNP genotyping. Nat Protoc. 2007;2:1734–9.

62. Bollati V, Baccarelli A, Hou L, Bonzini M, Fustinoni S, Cavallo D, et al. Changes in DNA methylation patterns in subjects exposed to low-dose benzene. Cancer Res. 2007;67:876–80.

63. Michels KB, Harris HR, Barault L. Birthweight, maternal weight trajectories and global DNA methylation of LINE-1 repetitive elements. PLoS One. 2011; 6:e25254. Fugmann SD, editor

64. Burris HH, Rifas-Shiman SL, Baccarelli A, Tarantini L, Boeke CE, Kleinman K, et al. Associations of LINE-1 DNA methylation with preterm birth in a prospective cohort study. J Dev Orig Health Dis. 2012;3:173–81.

65. Boeke CE, Baccarelli A, Kleinman KP, Burris HH, Litonjua AA, Rifas-Shiman SL, et al. Gestational intake of methyl donors and global LINE-1 DNA methylation in maternal and cord blood: prospective results from a folate-replete population. Epigenetics. 2012;7:253–60.

66. Holland N, Huen K, Tran V, Street K, Nguyen B, Bradman A, et al. Urinary phthalate metabolites and biomarkers of oxidative stress in a Mexican-American cohort: variability in early and late pregnancy. Toxics. 2016;4:7.

67. Silva MJ, Samandar E, Preau JL, Reidy JA, Needham LL, Calafat AM. Quantification of 22 phthalate metabolites in human urine. J Chromatogr B Analyt Technol Biomed Life Sci. 2007;860:106–12.

68. Cardenas A, Allard C, Doyon M, Houseman EA, Bakulski KM, Perron P, et al. Validation of a DNA methylation reference panel for the estimation of nucleated cells types in cord blood. Epigenetics. 2016;11:773–9.

69. Bakulski KM, Feinberg JI, Andrews SV, Yang J, Brown S, L McKenney S, et al. DNA methylation of cord blood cell types: applications for mixed cell birth studies. Epigenetics. 2016;11:354–62.

70. Metcalfe A, Lail P, Ghali WA, Sauve RS. The association between neighbourhoods and adverse birth outcomes: a systematic review and meta-analysis of multi-level studies. Paediatr Perinat Epidemiol. 2011;25:236–45.

71. Merlo J. Multilevel analytical approaches in social epidemiology: measures of health variation compared with traditional measures of association. J Epidemiol Community Health. 2003;57:550–2.

72. Olden K, Olden HA, Lin Y-S. The role of the epigenome in translating neighborhood disadvantage into health disparities. Curr Environ Health Rep. 2015;2:163–70.

73. Bateson P, Gluckman P, Hanson M. The biology of developmental plasticity and the predictive adaptive response hypothesis: developmental plasticity and the PAR response. J Physiol. 2014;592:2357–68.

74. Davis EP, Sandman CA. The timing of prenatal exposure to maternal cortisol and psychosocial stress is associated with human infant cognitive development. Child Dev. 2010;81:131–48.

75. Oberlander TF, Weinberg J, Papsdorf M, Grunau R, Misri S, Devlin AM. Prenatal exposure to maternal depression, neonatal methylation of human glucocorticoid receptor gene (NR3C1) and infant cortisol stress responses. Epigenetics. 2008;3:97–106.

76. Lee J, Kalia V, Perera F, Herbstman J, Li T, Nie J, et al. Prenatal airborne polycyclic aromatic hydrocarbon exposure, LINE1 methylation and child development in a Chinese cohort. Environ Int. 2017;99:315–20.

77. Mazzio EA, Soliman KFA. Epigenetics and nutritional environmental signals. Integr Comp Biol. 2014;54:21–30.

78. Keita AD, Casazza K, Thomas O, Fernandez JR. Neighborhood-level disadvantage is associated with reduced dietary quality in children. J Am Diet Assoc. 2009;109:1612–6.

79. Stimpson JP, Nash AC, Ju H, Eschbach K. Neighborhood deprivation is associated with lower levels of serum carotenoids among adults participating in the Third National Health and Nutrition Examination Survey. J Am Diet Assoc. 2007;107:1895–902.

80. Kuczmarski MF, Cremer Sees A, Hotchkiss L, Cotugna N, Evans MK, Zonderman AB. Higher healthy eating Index-2005 scores associated with reduced symptoms of depression in an urban population: findings from the Healthy Aging in Neighborhoods of Diversity Across the Life Span (HANDLS) study. J Am Diet Assoc. 2010;110:383–9.

81. Molendijk M, Molero P, Ortuño Sánchez-Pedreño F, Van der Does W, Angel M-GM. Diet quality and depression risk: a systematic review and dose-response meta-analysis of prospective studies. J Affect Disord. 2018;226:346–54.

82. Marx W, Moseley G, Berk M, Jacka F. Nutritional psychiatry: the present state of the evidence. Proc Nutr Soc. 2017;1–10.

83. Kazmi N, Gaunt TR, Relton C, Micali N. Maternal eating disorders affect offspring cord blood DNA methylation: a prospective study. Clin Epigenetics [Internet]. 2017 [cited 2017 Nov 9];9. Available from: http://clinicalepigeneticsjournal.biomedcentral.com/articles/10.1186/s13148-017-0418-3

84. Ellen IG, Mijanovich T, Dillman K-N. Neighborhood effects on health: exploring the links and assessing the evidence. J Urban Aff. 2001;23:391–408.

85. Hossain K, Suzuki T, Hasibuzzaman MM, Islam MS, Rahman A, Paul SK, et al. Chronic exposure to arsenic, LINE-1 hypomethylation, and blood pressure: a cross-sectional study in Bangladesh. Environ Health [Internet]. 2017 [cited 2018 Mar 14];16. Available from: http://ehjournal.biomedcentral.com/articles/10.1186/s12940-017-0231-7

7

Dysregulation and prognostic potential of 5-methylcytosine (5mC), 5-hydroxymethylcytosine (5hmC), 5-formylcytosine (5fC), and 5-carboxylcytosine (5caC) levels in prostate cancer

Tine Maj Storebjerg[1,2,3], Siri H. Strand[3], Søren Høyer[2], Anne-Sofie Lynnerup[1,2,3], Michael Borre[1], Torben F. Ørntoft[3] and Karina D. Sørensen[3*] (iD)

Abstract

Background: Prognostic tools for prostate cancer (PC) are inadequate and new molecular biomarkers may improve risk stratification. The epigenetic mark 5-hydroxymethylcytosine (5hmC) has recently been proposed as a novel candidate prognostic biomarker in several malignancies including PC. 5hmC is an oxidized derivative of 5-methylcytosine (5mC) and can be further oxidized to 5-formylcytosine (5fC) and 5-carboxylcytosine (5caC). The present study is the first to investigate the biomarker potential in PC for all four DNA methylation marks in parallel. Thus, we determined 5mC, 5hmC, 5fC, and 5caC levels in non-malignant (NM) and PC tissue samples from a large radical prostatectomy (RP) patient cohort ($n = 546$) by immunohistochemical (IHC) analysis of serial sections of a tissue microarray. Possible associations between methylation marks, routine clinicopathological parameters, *ERG* status, and biochemical recurrence (BCR) after RP were investigated.

Results: 5mC and 5hmC levels were significantly reduced in PC compared to NM prostate tissue samples ($p \leq 0.027$) due to a global loss of both marks specifically in *ERG*− PCs. 5fC levels were significantly increased in *ERG*+ PCs ($p = 0.004$), whereas 5caC levels were elevated in both *ERG*− and *ERG*+ PCs compared with NM prostate tissue samples ($p \leq 0.019$). Positive correlations were observed between 5mC, 5fC, and 5caC levels in both NM and PC tissues ($p < 0.001$), while 5hmC levels were only weakly positively correlated to 5mC in the PC subset ($p = 0.030$). There were no significant associations between 5mC, 5fC, or *ERG* status and time to BCR in this RP cohort. In contrast, high 5hmC levels were associated with BCR in *ERG*− PCs ($p = 0.043$), while high 5caC levels were associated with favorable prognosis in *ERG* + PCs ($p = 0.011$) and were borderline significantly associated with worse prognosis in *ERG*− PCs ($p = 0.058$). Moreover, a combined high-5hmC/high-5caC score was a significant adverse predictor of post-operative BCR beyond routine clinicopathological variables in *ERG*− PCs (hazard ratio 3.18 (1.54–6.56), $p = 0.002$, multivariate Cox regression).

Conclusions: This is the first comprehensive study of 5mC, 5hmC, 5fC, and 5caC levels in PC and the first report of a significant prognostic potential for 5caC in PC.

Keywords: Prostate cancer, Prognosis, Biomarker, Epigenetics, Immunohistochemistry, 5-methylcytosine, 5-hydroxymethylcytosine, 5-formylcytosine, 5-carboxylcytosine, ERG

* Correspondence: kdso@clin.au.dk
[3]Department of Molecular Medicine, Aarhus University Hospital, Aarhus, Denmark
Full list of author information is available at the end of the article

Background

Prostate cancer (PC) is the most commonly diagnosed non-cutaneous malignancy among men in Europe and the USA [1], and approximately 1.6 million men were diagnosed worldwide in 2015 [2]. PC represents a heterogeneous group of cancers, ranging from indolent (clinically insignificant) to highly aggressive tumors with potential lethal outcome. Currently, serum prostate-specific antigen (PSA), Gleason score (GS), and TNM stage represent the best available prognostic tools for newly diagnosed PC, but are inadequate at predicting exact outcomes for individual patients. Novel prognostic biomarkers are needed to accurately identify aggressive PCs and focus active treatment (radical prostatectomy, RP) towards these patients, while avoiding unnecessary surgery and treatment-associated side effects in men with indolent PC.

The most frequently occurring genetic alterations in PC are genomic fusions between the Transmembrane protease, serine 2 (*TMPRSS2*) gene, and the ETS-related transcription factor gene (*ERG*), which are present in approximately half of all primary PCs and lead to *ERG* overexpression [3]. Several studies have investigated the prognostic value of *TMPRSS2:ERG* fusion status in early stage PC, but have shown conflicting results [4, 5]. In contrast, DNA methylation changes have shown promising prognostic potential [6–8].

Methylation on the 5-carbon position of cytosine (5-methylcytosine, 5mC) in CpG-dinucleotides is a well-characterized epigenetic mark involved in regulation of gene expression and chromatin structure. Cancer cells are characterized by aberrant hypermethylation of promoter-associated CpG islands, which is closely linked with transcriptional silencing of, e.g., tumor-suppressor genes, as well as by genome-wide DNA hypomethylation (i.e., global loss of 5mC) that is associated with chromosomal instability and activation of oncogenes [9–11].

Methylation of CpG-dinucleotides (5mC) is catalyzed by DNA methyltransferases (DNMTs) and can be erased by a family of α-ketoglutarate-dependent dioxygenases, named ten-eleven translocation (TET) proteins, through sequential oxidation of 5mC to 5-hydroxymethylcytosine (5hmC), 5-formylcytosine (5fC), and finally 5-carboxylcytosine (5caC) [12]. Subsequently, 5fC and 5caC are converted to unmethylated cytosine through base excision repair, completing the demethylation process [13–15].

Although tissue and cell-type specific variations occur, it has been estimated that ~ 5% of all cytosines in the genome of mammalian cells are marked as 5mC and less than 1% as 5hmC, while 5fC and 5caC are 10–1000-fold less abundant than 5hmC [12, 16]. Accordingly, it has been proposed that 5fC and 5caC may simply be short-lived intermediates in the active demethylation process, while 5hmC is likely to represent an independent epigenetic mark. Consistent with this, different chromatin-binding proteins have been shown to bind to 5mC and 5hmC, respectively, indicating distinct roles for 5mC and 5hmC in epigenomic regulation [17]. Some proteins, however, seem to bind specifically to 5fC or 5caC, suggesting possible independent epigenetic signaling functions for these marks as well [18, 19].

So far, the vast majority of epigenetic biomarker discovery studies have focused exclusively on 5mC and have not distinguished between 5mC and other less abundant DNA methylation marks. Yet, accumulating evidence suggests that global loss of 5hmC is an epigenetic hallmark of cancer, including PC [14, 20]. Indeed, a series of recent studies found reduced levels of 5hmC in glioma, colorectal, breast, liver, lung, pancreatic, and prostate cancer, as compared to corresponding normal tissues [14, 20, 21]. Furthermore, low 5hmC levels have been associated with poor outcome in glioma [22, 23], lung [24], cervical [25], breast [26], ovarian [27], and gastric [28] cancer, but with good prognosis in AML [29]. Moreover, by immunohistochemical (IHC) analysis of a tissue microarray (TMA) based on a large RP cohort, we recently demonstrated reduced 5hmC levels in *ERG* negative (*ERG*–) PCs [30]. We also observed that high 5hmC immunoreactivity was significantly associated with post-operative biochemical recurrence (BCR) in *ERG*– but not in *ERG* positive (*ERG+)* PCs [30]. Although 5hmC levels have been subject to increasing scrutiny in recent years, only one study has investigated the possible dysregulation of 5caC levels in cancer [21], and no previous studies have investigated 5fC nor 5caC in PC.

In the present study, we determined the global levels of all four DNA methylation marks (5mC, 5hmC, 5fC, and 5caC) in parallel, through IHC staining of serial sections of a large PC tissue microarray (TMA) [30] consisting of malignant cores from 546 RP patients, compared with > 300 matched adjacent non-malignant (NM) prostate tissue samples. We systematically investigated possible correlations between the four DNA methylation marks, *ERG* status, and routine clinicopathological parameters, and assessed the prognostic potential of each mark using post-operative BCR as clinical endpoint.

Methods

Tissue microarray

A TMA was generated using paraffin-embedded formalin-fixed RP tissue samples from 552 patients [30], who underwent curatively intended RP for histologically verified clinically localized PC at the Department of Urology, Aarhus University Hospital, Denmark, between 2001 and 2009. All PC specimens were re-graded by an expert uropathologist (SH) according to the 2014

International Society of Urological Pathology criteria for Gleason score [31].

Patients provided written informed consent and were followed passively until May 2015 with a mean/median clinical follow-up time of 82.9/80.0 months. By this time, six cases had withdrawn consent, leaving 546 PC patients eligible for IHC analysis on the TMA (for clinical characteristics see Table 1). For analyses of IHC scores (see below), another 88 patients were excluded because they had received either pre/post-operative endocrine or radiation treatment, had less than 3 months follow-up, or suffered BCR ≤ 3 months after RP. Details on the inclusion/exclusion process according to REMARK criteria are given in Additional files 1, 2, 3, 4, 5, and 6: Figures S1–S2, and clinicopathological data for the final patient sets used for biomarker evaluation are presented in Additional files 7, 8, 9, and 10: Tables S1A-D. The study was approved by the local scientific ethical committee and by the Danish Data Protection Agency.

IHC staining

Immunohistochemical staining for *ERG* and 5hmC has been previously described for this TMA [30]. Here, IHC staining for 5mC, 5fC, and 5caC was performed on serial sections of the same TMA, using the Benchmark XT fully automated stainer (Ventana). Slicing and heating was performed manually. TMA tissue sections (2.5 μm) were deparaffinized followed by endogenous peroxidase blocking using TBS/H_2O_2. Epitopes were retrieved using TEG pH 9.00 (5mC) or citrate pH 6.00 (5fC and 5caC) buffer. Subsequently, primary antibodies for 5mC, 5fC, and 5caC were applied (for details, see Additional file 11: Table S2). Secondary staining was performed with Horse Radish Peroxidase (HRP) conjugated rabbit secondary antibody (Envision, Cat. No. K4003, Dako), except for 5mC, which was detected by HRP conjugated mouse secondary antibody (Envision, Cat. No. K4001, Dako). Colorimetric signals were detected using diaminobenzidine (DAB), and sections were counterstained with hematoxylin for microscopic evaluation.

IHC evaluation

Immunoreactivity for 5mC, 5fC, and 5caC was evaluated by two independent observers (SH and TMS) using the Pannoramic Viewer software (3DHISTECH, Hungary). A numerical IHC score was given for each core, based on the antibody staining intensity in the nuclei of malignant or NM prostate epithelial cells, respectively (0, no-weak; 1, moderate; 2, strong; see Figs. 1, 2, 3, and 4 for representative images). As some cores had changed status from malignant to NM or vice-versa from one TMA

section to the next, we carefully re-evaluated the PC/NM status of every core during IHC scoring. In addition, some cores were lost during TMA processing. In total, malignant cores from 344, 367, 281, and 351 PC patients could be evaluated for 5mC, 5hmC, 5fC, and 5caC immunoreactivity, respectively (Additional file 1: Figure S1; Additional file 7, 8, 9, and 10: Tables S1A–D). NM tissue samples could be evaluated from 328 (5mC), 293 (5hmC), 259 (5fC), and 311 (5caC) patients in total (Additional file 2: Figure S2).

For 5hmC and *ERG*, we used immunohistochemistry scores from neighboring sections of the exact same TMA from a previous study [30]. In the present study, all patients for whom at least one malignant or at least one NM core could be evaluated for each methylation mark were included in the final analyses, which for 5hmC resulted in a moderately larger patient set ($n = 367$) than in our previous work ($n = 311$) [30]. For patients with multiple PC/NM cores that could be evaluated for each antibody, we calculated a mean IHC score for each tissue type for each patient (< 1, weak; = 1, moderate; > 1, strong). Positive *ERG* immunoreactivity was used as a proxy for *ERG* fusion status [32]. As described previously [30], a PC patient was considered *ERG*+ if nuclear *ERG* immunoreactivity was detected in at least one malignant core from that patient, and otherwise as *ERG*−.

Statistical methods

All statistical analyses were performed using Stata IC version 14 (StataCorp, College Station TX, USA). p values < 0.05 were considered significant. Associations between methylation marks and clinicopathological characteristics were evaluated by two-sided chi^2 tests. Spearman's rank correlation coefficients were used to assess correlations between 5mC, 5hmC, 5fC, and 5caC levels in patients where all four marks could be evaluated.

Uni- and multivariate Cox regression analyses and Kaplan-Meier analyses were used to test the prognostic value of *ERG*, 5mC, 5hmC, 5fC, and 5caC, using BCR (defined as PSA ≥ 0.2 ng/ml in two consecutive measurements after RP) as clinical endpoint. For recurrence-free survival analyses, patients were censored at their last clinical follow-up. Statistical significance in Kaplan-Meier analysis was evaluated using 2-sided log-rank tests. Predictive accuracy was estimated using Harrell's C-index [33].

For analysis of methylation marks as dichotomized variables, we used mean IHC score ≤ 1 vs. > 1 as cut-point. To evaluate the prognostic value of a combination of 5hmC score and 5caC score, we divided patients into three subgroups: low (5hmC ≤ 1 and 5caC ≤ 1), moderate (5hmC ≤ 1 and 5caC > 1, or 5hmC > 1 and 5caC ≤ 1), and high (5hmC > 1 and 5caC > 1).

Table 1 Clinical characteristics

	546 RP patients included on TMA
Age at RP (years), median (range)	63 (34–76)
Pathological GS	
< 7, n (%)	229 (41.9)
≥ 7, n (%)	317 (58.1)
Pathological T stage	
≤pT2c, n (%)	363 (66.5)
≥pT3a, n (%)	182 (33.3)
Unknown, n (%)	1 (0.2)
Preoperative PSA	
PSA ≤ 10 ng/ml, n (%)	222 (40.7)
PSA > 10 ng/ml, n (%)	324 (59.3)
Surgical margin status	
Negative, n (%)	366 (67.0)
Positive, n (%)	175 (32.1)
Unknown, n (%)	5 (0.9)
Follow-up (months), median (range)	80 (12–158)
BCR	
No, n (%)	310 (56.8)
Yes, n (%)	236 (43.2)

	PC	NM
5mC (IHC), n (%)		
Total	344	328
Score < 1	–	3 (0.8)
Score = 1	160 (34.9)	126 (35.7)
Score > 1	184 (40.2)	199 (56.4)
Not determined	114 (24.9)	25 (7.1)
5hmC (IHC), n (%)		
Total	367	293
Score < 1	27 (5.9)	8 (2.5)
Score = 1	153 (33.4)	111 (34.0)
Score > 1	187 (40.8)	174 (53.4)
Not determined	91 (19.9)	33 (10.1)
5fC (IHC), n (%)		
Total	281	259
Score < 1	155 (33.8)	163 (50.6)
Score = 1	65 (14.2)	50 (15.5)
Score > 1	61 (13.3)	46 (14.3)
Not determined	177 (38.6)	63 (19.6)
5caC (IHC), n (%)		
Total	351	311
Score < 1	102 (22.2)	146 (41.4)
Score = 1	96 (21.0)	60 (17.0)
Score > 1	153 (33.4)	105 (29.7)
Not determined	107 (23.4)	42 (11.9)

Table 1 Clinical characteristics *(Continued)*

ERG (IHC), n (%)		
Total	433	NA
ERG–	205 (44.8)	NA
ERG+	228 (49.8)	NA
Not determined	25 (5.4)	NA

Clinical data for the 546 RP patients analyzed on the TMA and distribution of IHC staining scores for each antibody in NM and PC tissue samples, respectively
NA not applicable

Results

Methylation levels in PC compared with NM specimens

By IHC staining of a TMA from a large RP cohort ($n = 546$; Table 1), we assessed the levels of DNA methylation marks 5mC, 5hmC, 5fC, and 5caC. Nuclear staining intensity in NM and PC epithelial cells, respectively, was scored as 0 (weak staining), 1 (moderate staining), or 2 (strong staining) (Figs. 1, 2, 3, and 4).

Staining for 5mC could be evaluated in 344 PC and 328 NM specimens (Table 1). We found that 5mC levels were moderately, but statistically significantly reduced in PC compared with NM tissue samples ($p = 0.027$; chi^2 test; Fig. 5a). The reduction in 5mC levels was specific for *ERG* – PCs ($p < 0.001$; chi^2 test; Fig. 5a), while 5mC levels were similar in *ERG+* PCs and NM samples ($p = 0.360$; chi^2 test; Fig. 5a). The significant decrease of 5mC staining observed in *ERG–* PC (Fig. 5a) was also confirmed by a paired analysis of 107 patients for whom matched NM and *ERG–* PC samples with 5mC score were available (data not shown). Specifically, 38% (41/107) of these patients had an altered 5mC score in the *ERG–* PC sample, most of which were reduced (71%; 29/41 patients) compared to the matched NM sample.

Staining for 5hmC could be evaluated in 367 PC and 293 NM specimens (Table 1). For the full RP cohort, we observed a significant reduction of 5hmC staining in PC compared with NM tissue samples ($p = 0.010$; chi^2 test; Fig. 5b). This was explained by a global loss of 5hmC specifically in *ERG–* PCs ($p < 0.001$; chi^2 test; Fig. 5b), whereas 5hmC levels were similar in *ERG+* PC and NM samples ($p = 0.582$; chi^2 test; Fig. 5b), consistent with our previous report [30]. The significant decrease of 5hmC staining observed in *ERG–* PC (Fig. 5b) was also corroborated by a paired analysis of 107 patients for whom matched NM and *ERG–* PC samples with 5hmC score were available. Here, 42% (45/107) displayed an altered 5hmC score in the *ERG–* PC sample, the majority of which were reduced (78%; 35/45 patients) as compared to the matched NM sample.

5fC levels could be evaluated in 281 PC and 259 NM specimens (Table 1). There were no significant differences in 5fC levels in the full PC set compared with NM tissue samples ($p = 0.185$; chi^2 test; Fig. 5c), nor in *ERG-* PCs

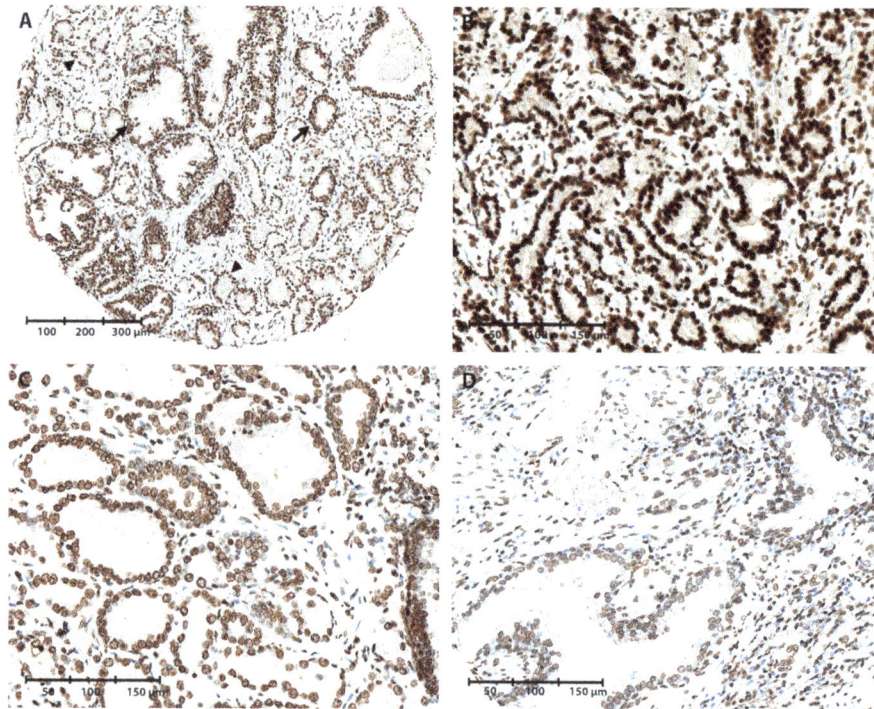

Fig. 1 Representative images of 5mC immunoreactivity in malignant and non-malignant prostate tissue samples. **a** TMA core containing both malignant and NM prostate glands, illustrating reduced 5mC levels in malignant (IHC score = 1, arrowheads) compared to NM (IHC score = 2, arrows) glands. **b** Strong 5mC staining in a malignant core (IHC score = 2). **c** Moderate 5mC staining in a malignant core (IHC score = 1). **d** Weak 5mC staining in a NM core (IHC score = 0)

compared with NM samples ($p = 0.305$; chi^2 test; Fig. 5c). However, *ERG+* PCs displayed significantly higher 5fC scores than NM prostate tissue samples ($p = 0.004$; chi^2 test; Fig. 5c). A similar pattern was seen in a paired analysis of 83 patients for whom matched NM and *ERG+* PC samples with 5fC score were available (data not shown). Specifically, 47% (39/83) of these patients had a changed 5fC score in the *ERG+* PC sample, most of which went up (54%; 21/39 patients) as compared to the matched NM sample, together also indicating some interpatient variation for 5fC.

Finally, 5caC immunoreactivity could be evaluated in 351 PC and 311 NM specimens (Table 1) and was significantly stronger in PC tissue samples ($p < 0.001$; chi^2 test; Fig. 5d). Elevated 5caC levels were seen both in *ERG–* PCs ($p = 0.019$; chi^2 test; Fig. 5d) and was even more pronounced in *ERG+* PCs ($p < 0.001$; chi^2 test; Fig. 5d), as compared to NM samples. This was confirmed in a paired analysis of 113 patients for whom matched NM and *ERG–* PC samples with 5caC scores were available (data not shown). Here, 46% (52/113) of the patients had an altered 5caC score in the matched *ERG–* PC sample, the majority of which were increased (65%; 34/52 patients). Likewise, a paired analysis of 128 patients for whom matched NM and *ERG+* PC samples

with 5caC scores were available (data not shown) showed that 52% (66/128) of the patients had an altered 5caC score in the paired *ERG+* PC sample, most of which went up (79%; 52/66 patients).

In summary, we observed a significant reduction of 5mC and 5hmC levels in *ERG–* but not in *ERG+* PCs, compared to NM prostate tissue samples. In addition, 5fC levels were moderately increased in *ERG+* but not in *ERG–* PCs, whereas 5caC levels were elevated in both *ERG–* and *ERG+* PCs. These findings were also corroborated by paired analyses of the subset of patients for whom matched NM and PC samples could be evaluated and scored.

Furthermore, based on immunoreactivity scores for 232 PC and 209 NM specimens that could be evaluated for all four DNA methylation marks, we observed moderate positive correlations between 5mC, 5fC, and 5caC levels in both PC and NM samples (Spearman's correlations: rho 0.43–0.53, $p < 0.001$; Additional file 12: Table S3). In contrast, 5hmC levels were weakly positively correlated only to 5mC and only in the PC subset (rho 0.14; $p = 0.030$; Additional file 12: Table S3). These results are consistent with previous reports, suggesting that 5hmC is an independent epigenetic mark [17, 34, 35].

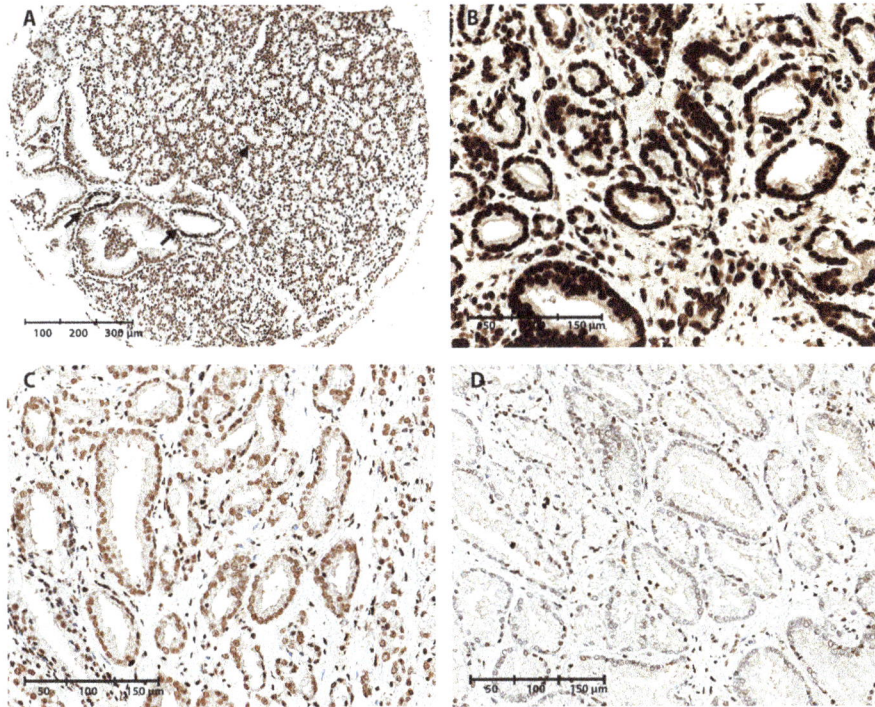

Fig. 2 Representative images of 5hmC immunoreactivity in malignant and non-malignant prostate tissue samples. **a** TMA core containing both malignant and NM prostate glands, illustrating reduced 5hmC levels in malignant (IHC score = 1, arrowheads) compared to NM glands (IHC score = 2, arrows). **b** Strong 5hmC staining in a malignant core (IHC score = 2). **c** Moderate 5hmC staining in a malignant core (IHC score = 1). **d** Weak 5hmC staining in malignant core (IHC score = 0)

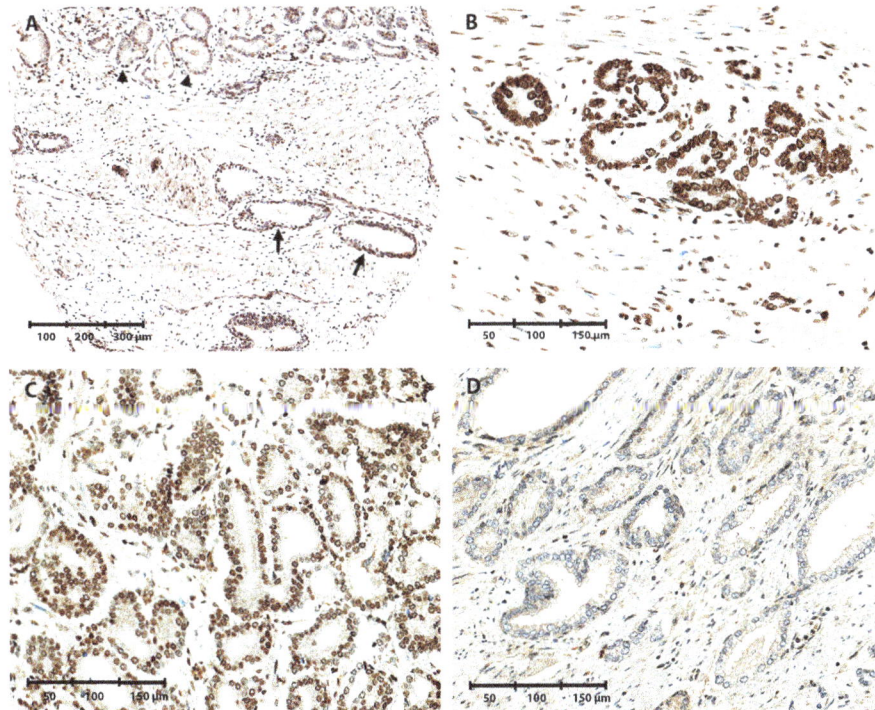

Fig. 3 Representative images of 5fC immunoreactivity in malignant and non-malignant prostate tissue samples. **a** TMA core containing both malignant (IHC score = 0, arrowheads), and NM (IHC score = 0, arrows) glands. **b** Strong 5fC staining in a malignant core (IHC score = 2). **c** Moderate 5fC staining in a malignant core (IHC score = 1). **d** Weak 5fC staining in a malignant core (IHC score = 0)

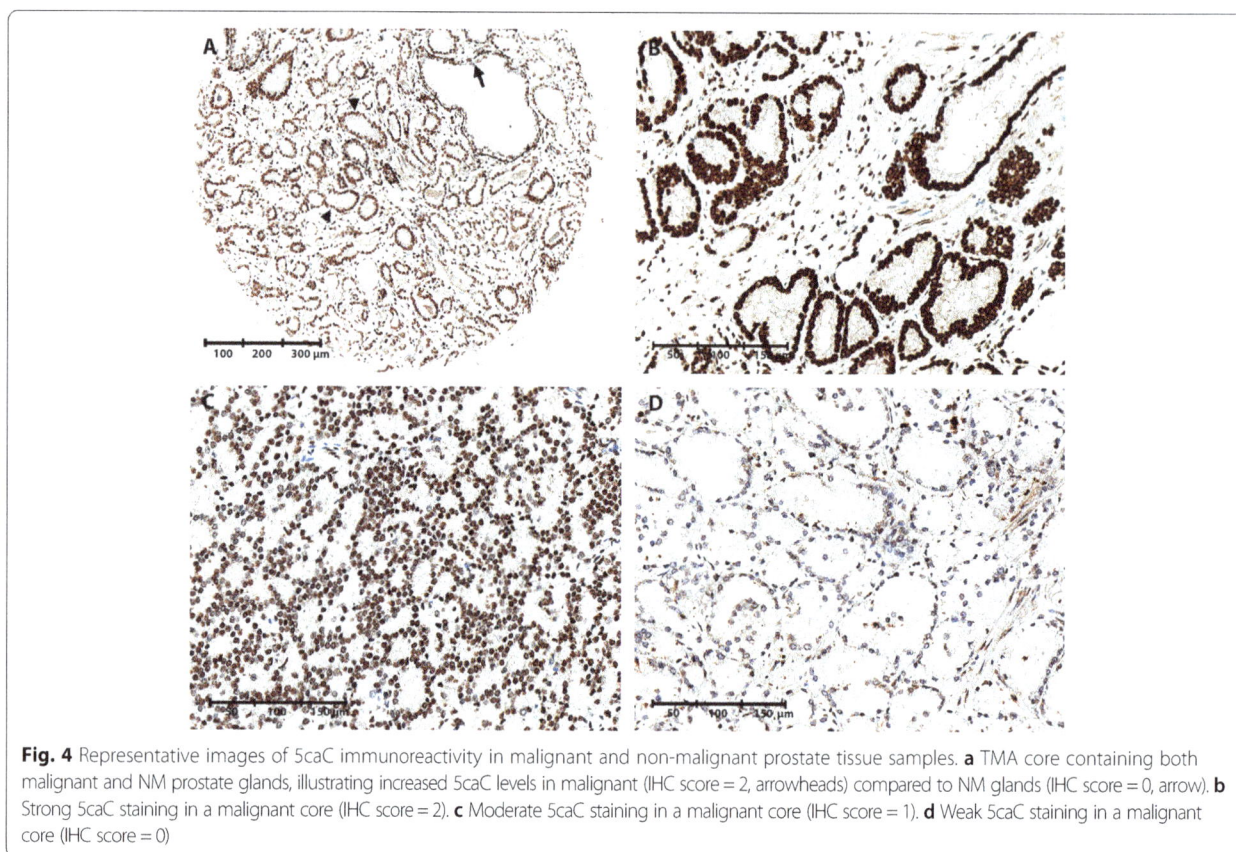

Fig. 4 Representative images of 5caC immunoreactivity in malignant and non-malignant prostate tissue samples. **a** TMA core containing both malignant and NM prostate glands, illustrating increased 5caC levels in malignant (IHC score = 2, arrowheads) compared to NM glands (IHC score = 0, arrow). **b** Strong 5caC staining in a malignant core (IHC score = 2). **c** Moderate 5caC staining in a malignant core (IHC score = 1). **d** Weak 5caC staining in a malignant core (IHC score = 0)

Association of 5mC, 5hmC, 5fC, and 5caC levels with clinicopathological parameters

Next, we investigated possible correlations between IHC scores for the four DNA methylation marks in PC tissue samples and key clinicopathological parameters associated with tumor aggressiveness, i.e., GS, pathological tumor (pT) stage, preoperative PSA level, surgical margin (SM) status, and BCR status.

5mC levels were not significantly associated with any of the clinicopathological parameters in the full PC patient set ($p \geq 0.122$; chi^2 test; Additional file 3: Figure S3A). We also found no significant correlations in ERG– ($p \geq 0.495$; Additional file 3: Figure S3B) or in ERG+ PCs ($p \geq 0.150$, Additional file 3: Figure S3C), except that a higher 5mC score was weakly associated with higher GS in the ERG+ PC subgroup ($p = 0.045$; Additional file 3: Figure S3C).

Strong 5hmC staining was significantly associated with post-operative BCR in the full PC cohort ($p = 0.038$; Additional file 4: Figure S4A), but not with any of the routine clinicopathological variables ($p \geq 0.317$; Additional file 4: Figure S4A). Similarly, in ERG– PCs, strong 5hmC staining was associated with BCR ($p = 0.015$) and advanced pT stage ($p = 0.001$) (Additional file 4: Figure S4B). There were no other significant correlations

in the ERG– nor in the ERG+ subset ($p \geq 0.146$; chi^2 test; Additional file 4: Figure S4B, C). In summary, high 5hmC levels were associated with adverse clinical parameters in ERG– PCs, consistent with our previous findings for a smaller subset of this cohort [30].

In the full PC set, as well as in the ERG+ PC subset, stronger 5fC staining was significantly associated with low pT stage (<pT3; $p = 0.023/p = 0.019$) and low BCR risk ($p = 0.049/p = 0.019$), but not with any other clinical parameters (Additional file 5: Figure S5A and C). In contrast, there were no significant correlations in ERG– PCs ($p \geq 0.227$; Fig. 6b). Thus, high 5fC levels may be associated with favorable prognosis in ERG+ PCs.

In the full PC set, stronger 5caC staining was significantly associated with low pT stage ($p = 0.004$) and low pre-operative PSA ($p = 0.019$; Additional file 6: Figure S6A). Similarly, in ERG+ PCs, stronger 5caC staining was associated with low pre-operative PSA ($p = 0.006$), low pT stage ($p < 0.001$), and low BCR risk ($p = 0.019$; Additional file 6: Figure S6C). However, in ERG– PCs, stronger 5caC staining was associated with higher GS ($p = 0.012$; Additional file 6: Figure S6B). These results suggest that high 5caC levels may be associated with less aggressive disease in ERG+ PC, but with more aggressive disease in ERG– PCs.

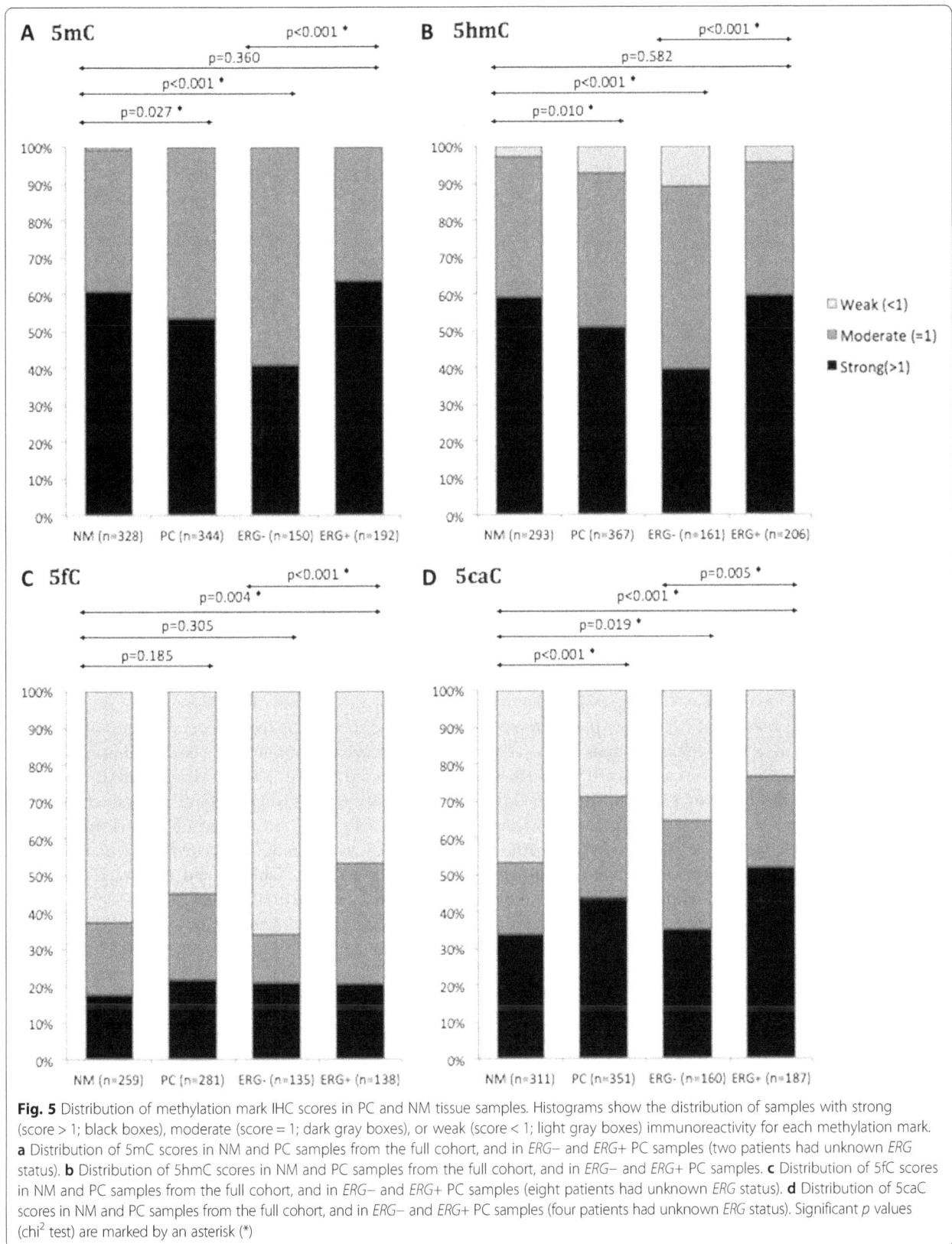

Fig. 5 Distribution of methylation mark IHC scores in PC and NM tissue samples. Histograms show the distribution of samples with strong (score > 1; black boxes), moderate (score = 1; dark gray boxes), or weak (score < 1; light gray boxes) immunoreactivity for each methylation mark. **a** Distribution of 5mC scores in NM and PC samples from the full cohort, and in *ERG−* and *ERG+* PC samples (two patients had unknown *ERG* status). **b** Distribution of 5hmC scores in NM and PC samples from the full cohort, and in *ERG−* and *ERG+* PC samples. **c** Distribution of 5fC scores in NM and PC samples from the full cohort, and in *ERG−* and *ERG+* PC samples (eight patients had unknown *ERG* status). **d** Distribution of 5caC scores in NM and PC samples from the full cohort, and in *ERG−* and *ERG+* PC samples (four patients had unknown *ERG* status). Significant *p* values (chi^2 test) are marked by an asterisk (*)

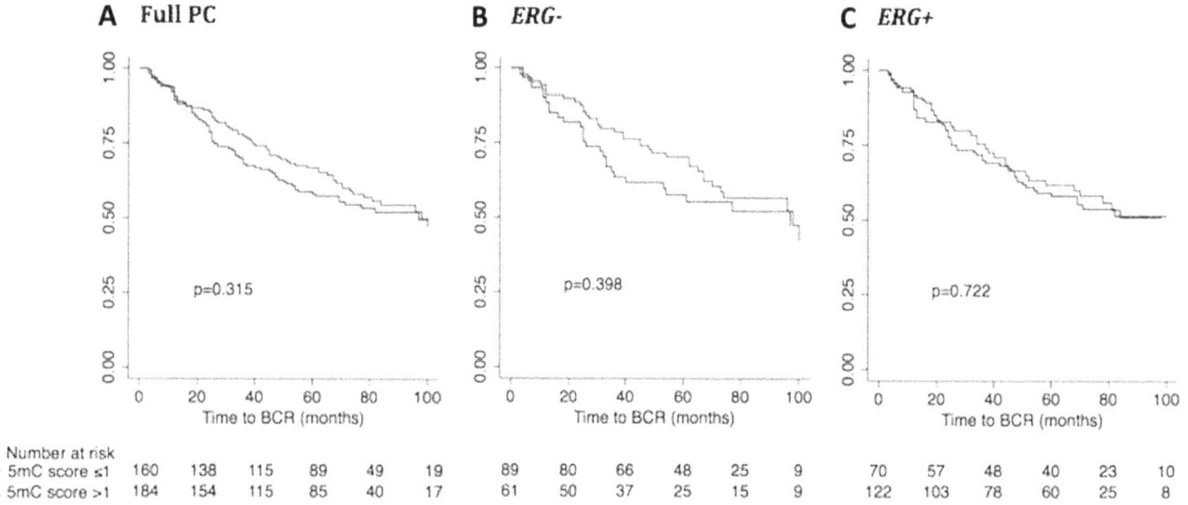

Fig. 6 Kaplan-Meier analysis: Association between 5mC score and time to BCR after RP. The prognostic value of 5mC score was evaluated through Kaplan-Meier analysis using time to BCR after RP as the clinical endpoint. Patients with low 5mC score (≤ 1; blue curves) were compared with patients with high 5mC score (> 1; red curves) in (**a**) the full PC patient set, **b** the *ERG–* PC subset, and **c** the *ERG+* PC subset. The number of patients in each subgroup are listed at the bottom and *p* values for 2-sided log-rank tests are given for each panel. No significant differences were observed

Prognostic value of DNA methylation levels in PC

To evaluate the potential prognostic value of 5mC, 5hmC, 5fC, and 5caC levels, we used time to BCR after RP as the clinical endpoint.

In the full RP cohort, there were no significant correlations between 5mC immunoreactivity in PC tissue samples and time to BCR in univariate Cox regression analysis (5mC *continuous/dichotomized* variable: $p = 0.834/p = 0.318$; Table 2) or in Kaplan-Meier analysis ($p = 0.315$; Fig. 6a). 5mC staining was also not significantly associated with time to BCR in the *ERG–* or *ERG+* subgroup in Cox regression analysis ($p ≥ 0.401$; Table 2) or in Kaplan-Meier analysis ($p ≥ 0.398$; Fig. 6b, c). All established clinicopathological prognostic parameters (high PSA, high GS, positive SM status, and advanced pT stage) were significantly associated with shorter time to BCR in this RP patient set ($p < 0.001$, Additional file 13: Table S4), indicating that it

is a representative cohort. Furthermore, *ERG* status did not predict time to BCR in our RP cohort ($p = 0.840$; Additional file 13: Table S4), consistent with other studies [36, 37].

In accordance with our previous work [30], high 5hmC levels were significantly associated with shorter BCR time in the full PC patient set in univariate (continuous: $p = 0.045$; Table 2) and multivariate Cox regression analysis (continuous: $p = 0.026$; Additional file 14: Table S5), as well as in Kaplan-Meier analysis ($p = 0.036$; log-rank test; Fig. 7a). The significant association was specific to the *ERG–* PC subgroup, where high 5hmC scores were significantly associated with BCR in both univariate ($p = 0.043$; Table 2) and multivariate Cox regression analysis ($p = 0.042$; Additional file 14: Table S5) as well as in Kaplan-Meier analysis ($p = 0.007$; Fig. 7b), but not in *ERG+* PCs ($p = 0.537$; Table 2; $p = 0.805$;

Table 2 Univariate Cox regression analysis of BCR-free survival for 5mC, 5hmC, 5fC, and 5caC score

Variable	Full PC patient set			*ERG-* PC patient subset			*ERG+* PC patient set		
	HR (95% CI)	*p* value	C-index	HR (95% CI)	*p* value	C-index	HR (95% CI)	*p* value	C-index
5mC score (cont.)	1.04 (0.72–1.50)	0.834	0.51	1.26 (0.69–2.28)	0.454	0.54	0.88 (0.54–1.43)	0.599	0.52
5mC score (dich.)	1.18 (0.85–1.62)	0.318	0.53	1.23 (0.76–2.00)	0.401	0.54	1.08 (0.70–1.69)	0.723	0.51
5hmC score (cont.)	1.37 (1.01–1.87)	*0.045*	0.55	1.62 (1.02–2.57)	*0.043*	0.59	1.14 (0.75–1.75)	0.537	0.51
5hmC score (dich.)	1.40 (1.02–1.92)	*0.038*	0.55	1.93 (1.19–3.14)	*0.008*	0.60	1.05 (0.69–1.61)	0.805	0.50
5fC score (cont.)	0.94 (0.73–1.20)	0.613	0.51	1.10 (0.78–1.56)	0.583	0.53	0.75 (0.52–1.09)	0.130	0.55
5fC score (dich.)	1.02 (0.67–1.56)	0.926	0.50	1.38 (0.77–2.49)	0.282	0.54	0.67 (0.34–1.33)	0.253	0.53
5caC score (cont.)	0.91 (0.73–1.14)	0.419	0.53	1.21 (0.86–1.71)	0.277	0.54	0.68 (0.51–0.92)	*0.011*	0.60
5caC score (dich.)	1.01 (0.73–1.40)	0.966	0.49	1.61 (0.98–2.63)	0.058	0.56	0.62 (0.40–0.97)	*0.034*	0.57

Significant *p* values are highlighted in italics

HR hazard ratio, *CI* confidence interval, *C-index* Harrell's C-index

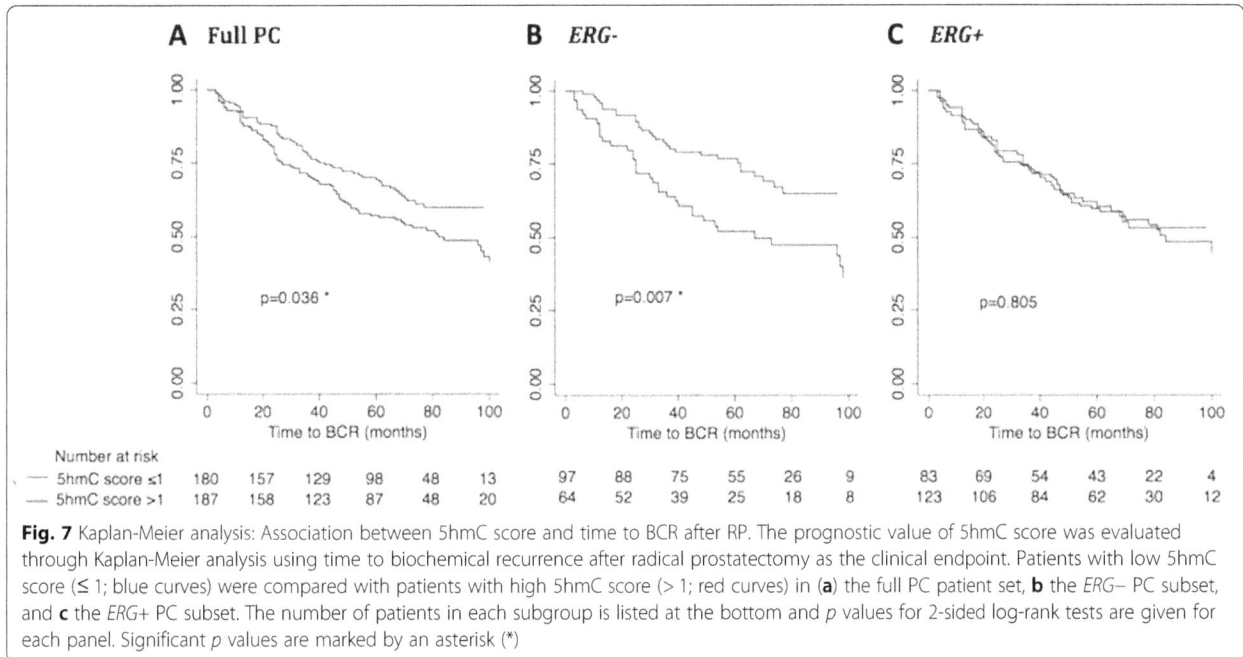

Fig. 7 Kaplan-Meier analysis: Association between 5hmC score and time to BCR after RP. The prognostic value of 5hmC score was evaluated through Kaplan-Meier analysis using time to biochemical recurrence after radical prostatectomy as the clinical endpoint. Patients with low 5hmC score (≤ 1; blue curves) were compared with patients with high 5hmC score (> 1; red curves) in (**a**) the full PC patient set, **b** the *ERG–* PC subset, and **c** the *ERG+* PC subset. The number of patients in each subgroup is listed at the bottom and *p* values for 2-sided log-rank tests are given for each panel. Significant *p* values are marked by an asterisk (*)

Fig. 7c). We obtained similar results when 5hmC was analyzed as a dichotomized variable by Cox regression in both the full PC set and in the *ERG* stratified subsets (Table 2 and Additional file 15: Table S6).

For 5fC, we observed no significant correlation with time to BCR in univariate Cox regression analysis (5fC continuous/dichotomized: $p = 0.613/p = 0.926$, Table 2) or in Kaplan Meier analysis ($p = 0.926$; Fig. 8a) in the full PC patient set, and also not after stratification for *ERG* status (*ERG–/ERG+: $p \geq 0.282/$

$p \geq 0.130$, Additional file 11: Table S2; and $p = 0.278/p = 0.248$, Fig. 8b, c). Accordingly, multivariate Cox regression analyses were not performed for 5fC (Additional file 16: Table S7).

For 5caC, we found no significant correlation with time to BCR in the full patient set in univariate Cox regression analysis (continuous/dichotomized: $p = 0.419/p = 0.966$; Table 2) or in Kaplan-Meier analysis ($p = 0.966$; Fig. 9a). Likewise, in *ERG–* PCs, there was no significant correlation between time to BCR when 5caC score was analyzed

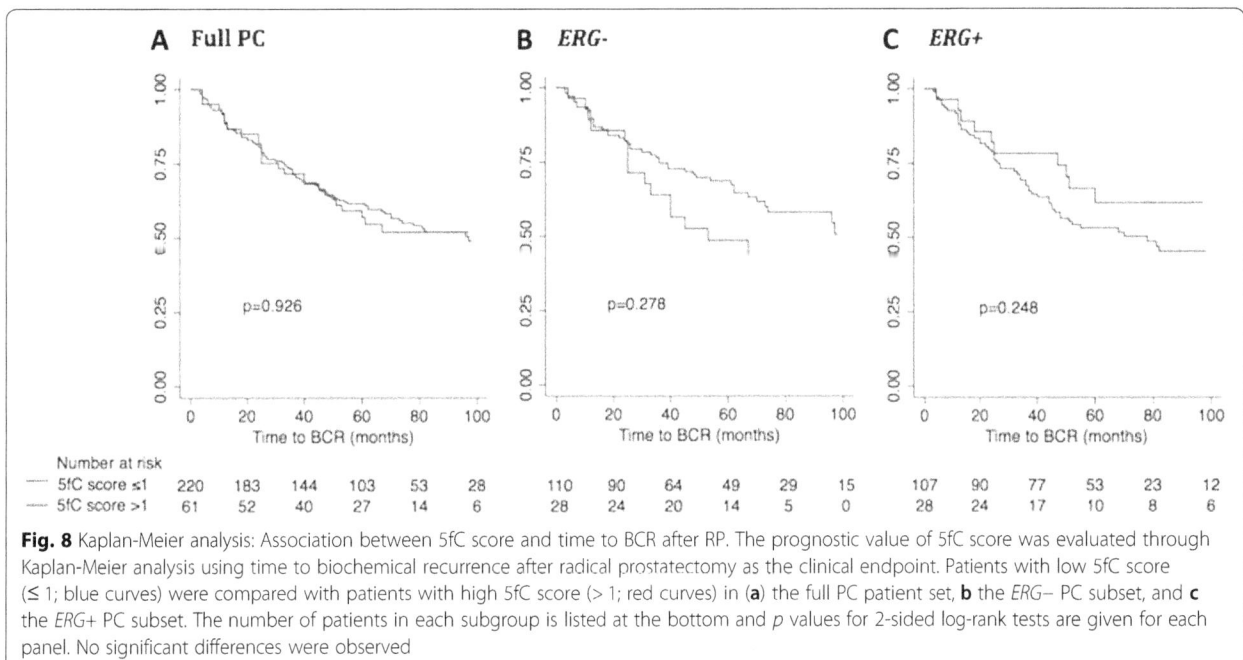

Fig. 8 Kaplan-Meier analysis: Association between 5fC score and time to BCR after RP. The prognostic value of 5fC score was evaluated through Kaplan-Meier analysis using time to biochemical recurrence after radical prostatectomy as the clinical endpoint. Patients with low 5fC score (≤ 1; blue curves) were compared with patients with high 5fC score (> 1; red curves) in (**a**) the full PC patient set, **b** the *ERG–* PC subset, and **c** the *ERG+* PC subset. The number of patients in each subgroup is listed at the bottom and *p* values for 2-sided log-rank tests are given for each panel. No significant differences were observed

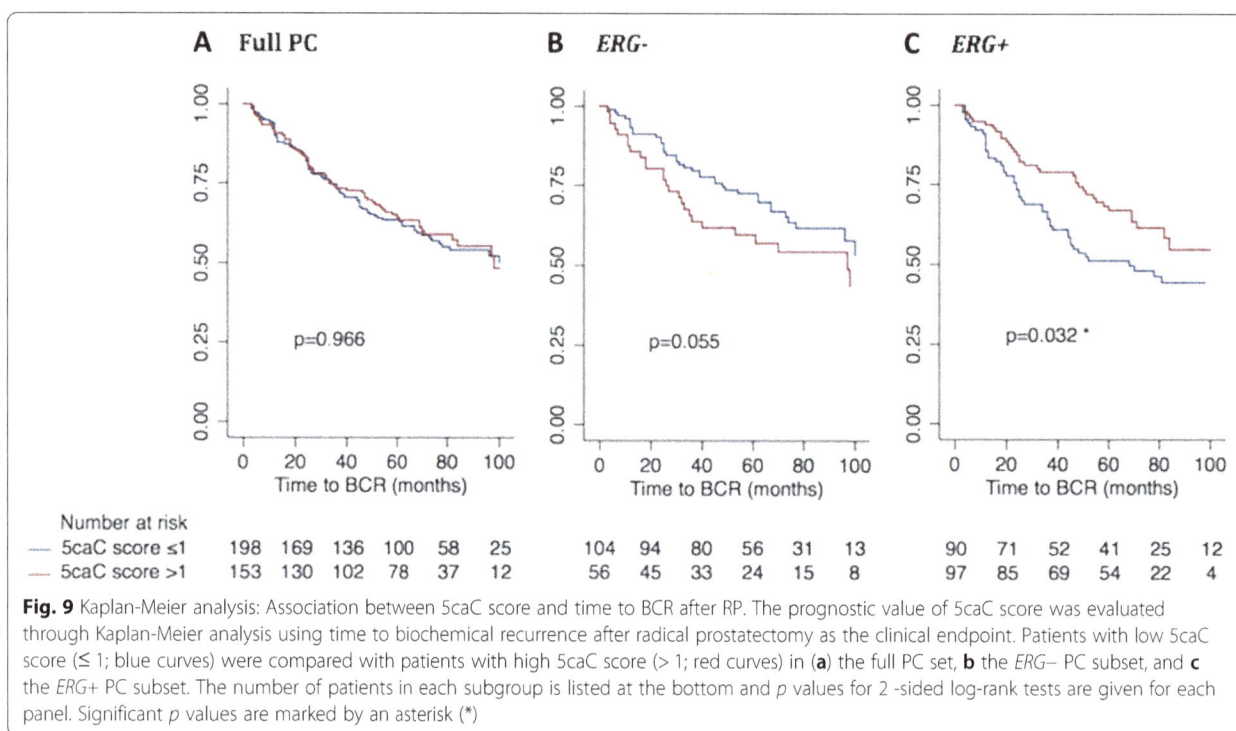

Fig. 9 Kaplan-Meier analysis: Association between 5caC score and time to BCR after RP. The prognostic value of 5caC score was evaluated through Kaplan-Meier analysis using time to biochemical recurrence after radical prostatectomy as the clinical endpoint. Patients with low 5caC score (≤ 1; blue curves) were compared with patients with high 5caC score (> 1; red curves) in (**a**) the full PC set, **b** the ERG– PC subset, and **c** the ERG+ PC subset. The number of patients in each subgroup is listed at the bottom and p values for 2 -sided log-rank tests are given for each panel. Significant p values are marked by an asterisk (*)

as a continuous variable ($p = 0.277$; Table 2), although a high 5caC score was borderline significantly associated with BCR when analyzed as a dichotomized variable in univariate Cox regression ($p = 0.058$; Table 2) and Kaplan-Meier analyses ($p = 0.055$; log-rank test; Fig. 9b). In contrast, in ERG+ PCs, a low 5caC score (continuous and dichotomized) was significantly associated with early BCR in univariate Cox regression ($p = 0.011$/$p = 0.034$, Table 2) as well as in Kaplan-Meier analysis ($p = 0.032$; log-rank test; Fig. 9c). However, 5caC did not remain significant in multivariate Cox regression analysis after adjustment for routine clinicopathological parameters (5caC continuous/dichotomized: $p = 0.299$/$p = 0.182$; Additional file 17: Table S8/Additional file 18: Table S9).

In summary, high levels of 5hmC were significantly associated with shorter time to BCR in ERG– PCs, consistent with our previous report [30]. Additionally, in the present study, we found that high 5caC levels were significantly associated with favorable prognosis after RP in ERG + PCs, but were borderline significantly associated with poor prognosis in ERG– PCs. Finally, 5mC and 5fC did not show significant prognostic value in our RP cohort.

Prognostic potential in ERG– PC for a combined 5hmC/5caC score

To investigate whether a 5hmC/5caC dual-marker panel could improve prognostic performance in ERG– PCs, three patient subgroups were defined: low (5hmC ≤ 1 and 5caC ≤ 1), moderate (5hmC ≤ 1 and 5caC > 1, or

5hmC > 1 and 5caC ≤ 1), and high 5hmC/5caC score (5hmC > 1 and 5caC > 1).

In ERG– PCs, a high 5hmC/5caC score was significantly associated with poor BCR-free survival in Kaplan-Meier analysis (low vs. high: $p = 0.002$; log-rank test; Fig. 10) and in univariate Cox regression analysis (low vs. high: hazard ration (HR) (95% confidence interval (CI)): 2.99 (1.49–6.02); $p = 0.002$; Table 3). Moreover, a high 5hmC/5caC score remained significant also after adjustment for routine clinical variables in multivariate Cox regression analysis (low vs. high: HR (95%CI): 2.48 (1.20–5.13); $p = 0.014$; Table 3). We used Harrell's C-index to estimate predictive accuracy. In the final model, Harrell's C-index improved from 0.69 to 0.75 when adding 5hmC/5caC score to a multivariate model based only on clinicopathological factors (Table 3). Similar analyses in the full PC patient set and in the ERG+ PC subgroup, respectively, showed no significant associations between 5hmC/5caC score and time to BCR (data not shown). To the best of our knowledge, this is the first report to demonstrate a significant association between 5caC levels and PC outcome.

Discussion
The present study is the first comprehensive investigation of 5mC, 5hmC, 5fC, and 5caC levels in PC. Based on IHC analysis of serial sections of a large tissue microarray, including NM and PC tissue samples from more than 500 RP patients, we observed

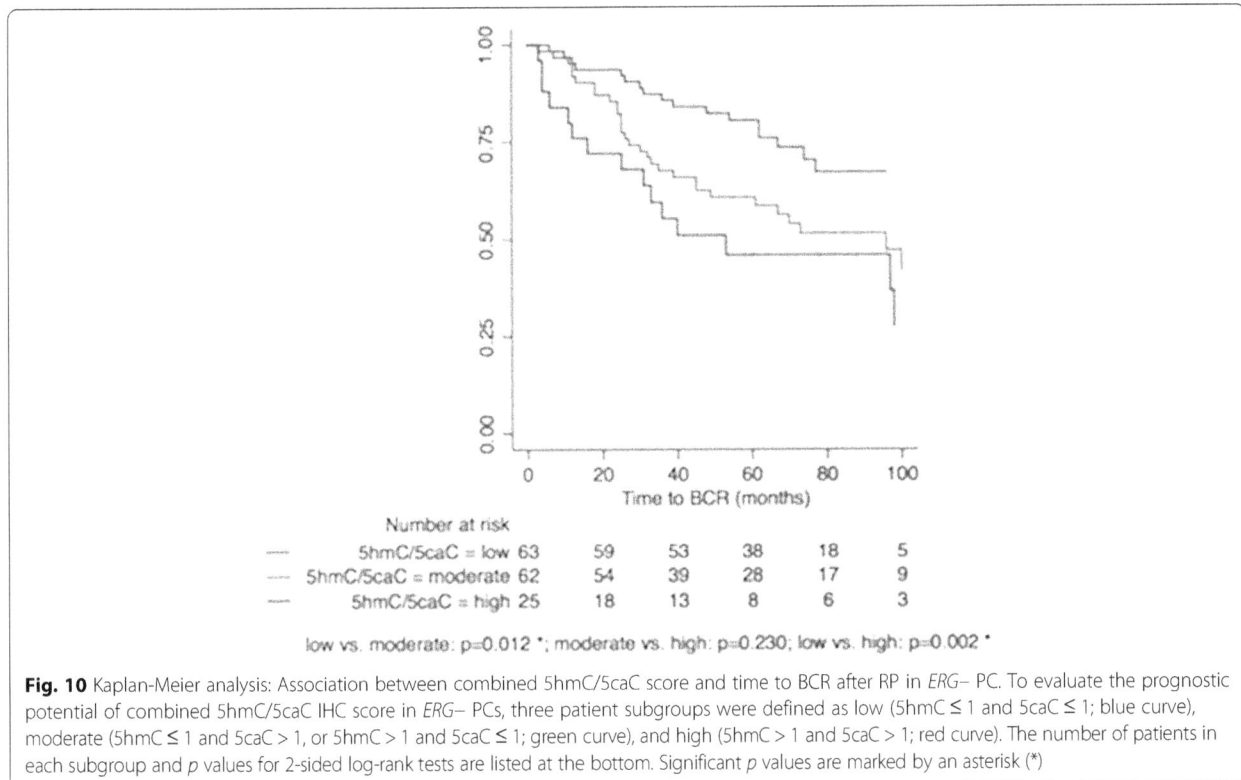

Fig. 10 Kaplan-Meier analysis: Association between combined 5hmC/5caC score and time to BCR after RP in *ERG−* PC. To evaluate the prognostic potential of combined 5hmC/5caC IHC score in *ERG−* PCs, three patient subgroups were defined as low (5hmC ≤ 1 and 5caC ≤ 1; blue curve), moderate (5hmC ≤ 1 and 5caC > 1, or 5hmC > 1 and 5caC ≤ 1; green curve), and high (5hmC > 1 and 5caC > 1; red curve). The number of patients in each subgroup and *p* values for 2-sided log-rank tests are listed at the bottom. Significant *p* values are marked by an asterisk (*)

significantly reduced levels of 5mC and 5hmC particularly in *ERG−* PCs. Furthermore, we found that 5fC levels were significantly increased in *ERG+* PCs, whereas 5caC levels were significantly elevated in both *ERG+* and *ERG−* PCs, as compared to NM prostate tissue samples. In addition, we observed significant positive correlations between the global levels of 5mC, 5fC, and 5caC in both NM and PC tissue samples, whereas 5hmC levels were weakly positively correlated only to 5mC levels and only in the PC subset.

Moreover, high 5hmC levels were associated with poor BCR-free survival in *ERG−* PCs, consistent with our earlier findings for a smaller subset of patients in this RP cohort [30]. While there were no significant associations between 5mC, 5fC, or *ERG* status and BCR-free survival in our RP cohort, we found that high 5caC levels were significantly associated with favorable prognosis in *ERG+* PCs, while at the same time being borderline significantly associated with poor prognosis in *ERG−* PCs. Moreover, in *ERG−*

Table 3 Prognostic value of combined 5hmC/5caC IHC score in *ERG−* PC

ERG− PC patient subset (*n* = 150, 64 BCR)

Variable	Univariate			Multivariate[a]		Multivariate[b]			
	HR (95% CI)	p value	C-index	HR (95% CI)	p value	HR (95% CI)	p value	C-index[c]	C-index[d]
5hmC/5caC (low vs. moderate)	2.06 (1.14–3.72)	*0.017*	0.62	1.79 (0.98–3.28)	0.057	–	–	0.75	–
5hmC/5caC (low vs. high)	2.99 (1.49–6.02)	*0.002*	0.62	2.48 (1.20–5.13)	*0.014*	3.18 (1.54–6.56)	*0.002*		–
Pre-op. PSA (≤ 10 vs. > 10 ng/ml)	2.65 (1.47–4.76)	*0.001*	0.60	2.79 (1.52–5.12)	*0.001*	4.22 (1.67–10.65)	*0.002*		0.69
Gleason score (< 7 vs. ≥ 7)	2.18 (1.27–3.72)	*0.005*	0.59	1.61 (0.88–2.94)	0.123	–	–		
Surgical margin (neg. vs. pos.)	2.63 (1.63–4.22)	*< 0.001*	0.61	2.04 (1.17–3.56)	*0.012*	4.17 (2.02–8.63)	*< 0.001*		
Tumor stage (≤pT2c vs. ≥pT3a)	2.55 (1.59–4.11)	*< 0.001*	0.61	1.70 (0.98–2.95)	0.060	–	–		

Univariate and multivariate Cox regression analyses of time to BCR using a combined 5hmC/5caC IHC score (low: 5hmC ≤ 1 and 5caC ≤ 1; moderate: 5hmC ≤ 1 and 5caC > 1, or 5hmC > 1 and 5caC ≤ 1; high: 5hmC > 1 and 5caC > 1)

Significant *p* values are highlighted in italics

[a]Global multivariate model including all parameters

[b]Final multivariate model including only significant variables

[c]Harrell's C-index for final model including 5hmC/5caC

[d]Harrell's C-index for final model excluding 5hmC/5caC

PCs, a combined high-5hmC/high-5caC score was a significant adverse predictor of post-operative BCR beyond routine clinicopathological variables.

Our current findings for 5mC and 5hmC immunoreactivity patterns in PC compared to NM prostate tissues confirm and expand on previous reports of global DNA methylation loss in PC as well as in other malignancies [38]. Consistent with our results, two previous small-scale studies observed reduced 5mC immunoreactivity in PC tissue samples based on analysis of 48 NM vs. 48 PC [39] and 10 NM vs. 14 PC samples [20], respectively. Similarly, two earlier small-scale studies reported that 5hmC levels were reduced in PC tissue samples based on IHC analyses of 10 NM vs. 30 PC [20] and 11 NM vs. 11 PC [14] samples, respectively. However, as opposed to our present study, none of these earlier studies [14, 20, 39] distinguished clearly between 5mC and 5hmC, while also stratifying for *ERG* fusion status. We have recently reported that 5hmC immunoreactivity levels were reduced particularly in *ERG–* PCs, based on analysis of smaller subset of patients from this RP cohort [30]. Here, we confirmed these results and extended our analyses to three additional DNA methylation marks (5mC, 5fC and 5caC), while also stratifying for *ERG* status.

The present study is the first to describe 5fC and 5caC immunoreactivity patterns in NM and PC tissue samples. We found that 5fC levels were significantly elevated in *ERG+* PCs, while 5caC levels were significantly increased in both *ERG+* and *ERG–* PCs. It has previously been reported that global 5caC levels are increased in breast cancer and glioma compared to their corresponding normal tissues [21], together indicating that global 5caC alterations are associated with malignant transformation in multiple cancer types. However, future studies are needed to investigate this in more detail. Furthermore, to fully understand the epigenetic reprogramming mechanisms associated with PC development and progression, such future studies should include not only an assessment of the global levels of 5caC and 5fC in NM and PCs (*ERG+* vs. *ERG–*), but should also map the genome-wide distribution of these marks as compared to 5mC and 5hmC, ideally at single-base resolution. Moreover, since reactive oxygen species and hypoxia can induce TET expression [40–42], it cannot be excluded that variable levels of tumor hypoxia may have affected the levels of 5hmC, 5fC, and/or 5caC observed in our study. Thus, further studies are needed to investigate the possible associations between hypoxia and TET-dependent epigenetic marks in PC, but is considered beyond the scope of the present work.

We are the first to demonstrate significant positive correlations between matching 5mC, 5fC, and 5caC global levels in both PC and NM samples. For 5hmC, we observed only a weak positive correlation with 5mC, which is consistent with several previous reports, suggesting that 5hmC is an independent epigenetic mark, while 5fC and 5caC are more likely to be short-lived intermediates in the active demethylation processes [17, 20, 34, 35]. Yet, our correlation analysis results are also consistent with the possibility that 5fC and/or 5caC hold independent regulatory roles, as suggested by the identification of proteins that bind specifically to 5fC or 5caC [18, 19, 43]. It has also been reported that 5fC can be stably detected in vivo, favoring a possible biological role for 5fC beyond that of a demethylation intermediate [44]. Likewise, the significant prognostic value demonstrated for 5caC in the present study might be interpreted in favor of a possible independent regulatory role for this mark. Further studies are needed to investigate this, but are beyond the scope of the current work.

We assessed the prognostic potential of 5mC, 5hmC, 5fC, and 5caC in a large RP cohort using BCR-free survival as the clinical endpoint. There was no significant association between 5mC immunoreactivity and BCR in this RP cohort, also not after stratification for *ERG* status. This is in accordance with results from an earlier small-scale study that also found no prognostic value for 5mC immunoreactivity in PC ($n = 48$) [39]. In contrast, global loss of 5mC has been associated with poor prognosis in tongue squamous cell carcinoma [45], while increased 5mC levels in myelodysplastic syndrome have been linked with a worse prognosis [46].

Consistent with our previous results for a smaller subset of patients in this RP cohort [30], we found that high 5hmC levels were significantly associated with shorter BCR-free survival in *ERG–* PCs. Likewise, high levels of 5hmC have previously been associated with poor prognosis in AML [29]. Conversely, in several other cancers, including esophageal squamous cell carcinoma [47], diffuse astrocytoma [22], NSCLC [24], cervical squamous cell carcinoma [25], gastric cancer [28], and malignant melanoma [48], poor prognosis has been associated with low 5hmC immunoreactivity. Disease-specific differences may likely reflect that phenotypic effects of epigenetic deregulation are influenced not only by the global level of specific DNA methylation marks, but also by their genomic distribution in any given cell type.

The potential prognostic value of 5fC or 5caC has not previously been evaluated in relation to cancer in general or to PC in particular. Here, we found no significant associations between 5fC immunoreactivity and BCR-free survival in our RP cohort. In contrast, high 5caC levels were significantly associated with favorable outcome in *ERG+* PCs, while at the same time being borderline significantly associated with poor prognosis in *ERG–* PCs. In addition, we found that the combination of high 5hmC and high 5caC score in *ERG–* PCs were significantly associated with shorter BCR-free survival and thereby considerably worse prognosis (HR > 3) after adjustment for routine clinicopathological factors. Although further validation is needed, this suggests that a 5hmC/5caC dual-marker panel has the potential to help improve risk stratification for this patient subset. Better and more accurate risk stratification is crucial for PC patient management, as it could be used to guide more individualized treatment decisions in the future.

There are some limitations to the present study. First, our analyses were restricted to patients who underwent RP for clinically localized PC. Accordingly, conclusions cannot necessarily be transferred to PC patients with advanced/metastatic disease. Nevertheless, it is considered to be a strength of the current study that our results are based on a large consecutive and representative RP cohort from one clinical center with clinical annotation and follow-up information available for all patients. Furthermore, our study was based on IHC staining, which only allows assessment of global 5mC, 5hmC, 5fC, and 5caC levels. Thus, future studies are needed to map the genome-wide distribution of these marks at single-base resolution in NM and PC tissue samples. We did not apply multiple testing correction to the statistical analyses, as each methylation mark was analyzed individually. However, the main results (prognostic value of 5hmC score in *ERG*– PC and of 5caC score in *ERG*+ PC; Table 2) would also have remained significant after correction for multiple testing, even if using the most stringent Bonferroni correction method.

Another possible limitation is the use of BCR as endpoint for prognostic biomarker evaluation, as BCR is known to be only a surrogate for PC aggressiveness. However, due to the slow-growing nature of PC, we did not have sufficient numbers of events for metastatic progression and/or PC-specific mortality analyses. Moreover, as we did not have access to primary and secondary Gleason grades from all patients, our prognostic analyses did not distinguish Gleason 3 + 4 vs. 4 + 3, although these are generally accepted as separate risk groups in the clinic. Finally, our study was restricted to one large RP cohort from Denmark and further independent validation is needed. Future validation studies should include multiple large PC patient cohorts with full clinical annotation, long clinical follow-up, and representing different ethnic populations.

Conclusions

To the best of our knowledge, this is the first study to analyze 5fC and 5caC immunoreactivity patterns in NM and PC tissue samples as well as the first report to demonstrate a significant association between 5caC levels and PC outcome. The results from our parallel IHC analyses of 5mC, 5hmC, 5fC, and 5caC in NM and PC tissue samples from more than 500 RP patients support the notion that epigenetic deregulation is a molecular hallmark of PC, and furthermore suggest that PC-associated epigenetic reprogramming differs between *ERG*+ and *ERG*– PCs. Future studies are warranted to further investigate this.

Additional files

Additional file 1: Figure S1. Flow chart illustrating the sample inclusion/exclusion process in malignant cores. A) 5mC score. B) 5hmC score. **C)** 5fC score. D) 5caC score. N, number of patients. (PNG 931 kb)

Additional file 2: Figure S2. Flow chart illustrating the sample inclusion/exclusion process in NM cores. A) 5mC score. B) 5hmC score. C) 5fC score. D) 5caC score. N, number of patients. (PNG 1027 kb)

Additional file 3: Figure S3. Correlations between 5mC score and clinicopathological parameters. A) In the full PC set ($n = 344$), B) in *ERG*– PC ($n = 150$), and C) in *ERG*+ PC ($n = 192$). Significant p values (chi^2 test) are marked by an asterisk (*). (JPG 392 kb)

Additional file 4: Figure S4. Correlations between 5hmC score and clinicopathological parameters. A) In the full PC set ($n = 367$), B) in *ERG*– PCs ($n = 161$), and C) in *ERG*+ PCs ($n = 206$). Significant p values (chi^2 test) are marked by an asterisk (*). (JPG 406 kb)

Additional file 5: Figure S5. Correlations between 5fC score and clinicopathological parameters. A) In the full PC set ($n = 281$), B) in *ERG*– PC ($n = 135$), and C) in *ERG*+ PC ($n = 138$). Significant p values (chi^2 test) are marked by an asterisk (*). (JPG 407 kb)

Additional file 6: Figure S6. Correlations between 5caC score and clinicopathological parameters. A) In the full PC set ($n = 351$), B) in *ERG*– PC ($n = 160$), and C) in *ERG*+ PC ($n = 187$). Significant p values (chi^2 test) are marked by an asterisk (*). (JPG 415 kb)

Additional file 7: Table S1A. Clinical characteristics for PC patients represented on the TMA. Data for RP patients for whom a 5mC score could be evaluated in malignant cores. Two PC specimens had unknown *ERG* status. (DOCX 15 kb)

Additional file 8: Table S1B. Clinical characteristics for PC patients represented on the TMA. Data for RP patients for whom a 5hmC score could be evaluated in malignant cores. (DOCX 15 kb)

Additional file 9: Table S1C. Clinical characteristics for PC patients represented on the TMA. Data for RP patients for whom a 5fC score could be evaluated in malignant cores. Eight PC specimens had unknown *ERG* status. (DOCX 15 kb)

Additional file 10: Table S1D. Clinical characteristics for PC patients represented on the TMA. Data for RP patients for whom a 5caC score could be evaluated in malignant cores. Four PC specimens had unknown *ERG* status. (DOCX 15 kb)

Additional file 11: Table S2. Details for the antibodies used for IHC (DOCX 14 kb)

Additional file 12: Table S3. Correlation between the methylation marks in PC and NM specimens. Correlation between the methylation marks in PC ($n = 232$) and NM ($n = 209$) specimens evaluated with Spearman's rank correlation coefficient (rho, ρ) based on mean IHC scores. Significant p values are highlighted in bold. (DOCX 14 kb)

Additional file 13: Table S4. 5mC score (continuous and dichotomized) in univariate Cox regression analysis of BCR-free survival. Significant p values are highlighted in bold. (DOCX 16 kb)

Additional file 14: Table S5. 5hmC score (continuous) in univariate and multivariate Cox regression analysis of BCR-free survival. (DOCX 18 kb)

Additional file 15: Table S6. 5hmC score (dichotomized) in univariate and multivariate Cox regression analysis of BCR-free survival. (DOCX 19 kb)

Additional file 16: Table S7. 5fC score (continuous and dichotomized) in univariate Cox regression analysis of BCR-free survival. (DOCX 15 kb)

Additional file 17: Table S8. 5caC score (continuous) in univariate and multivariate Cox regression analysis of BCR-free survival. (DOCX 16 kb)

Additional file 18: Table S9. 5caC score (dichotomized) in univariate and multivariate Cox regression analysis of BCR-free survival. (DOCX 20 kb)

Abbreviations
5caC: 5-carboxylcytosine; 5fC: 5-formylcytosine; 5hmC: 5-hydroxymethylcytosine; 5mC: 5-methylcytosine; BCR: Biochemical recurrence; CI: Confidence interval; DAB: Diaminobenzidine; DNMTs: DNA methyltransferases; ERG: ETS-related gene; ERG+: ERG positive; ERG–: ERG negative; GS: Gleason score; HR: Hazard ratio; HRP: Horse radish peroxidase; IHC: Immunohistochemistry; NM: Adjacent non-malignant; PC: Prostate cancer; PSA: Prostate-specific antigen; pT stage: Pathological tumor stage; RP: Radical prostatectomy; SM: Surgical margin; TET: Ten-eleven translocation; TMA: Tissue microarray; TMPRSS2: Transmembrane protease, serine 2

Acknowledgements
Excellent technical assistance from Pamela Celis, Kristina Bang Christensen, Kristina Lystlund Lauridsen, Jameela Safi, and Susanne Skou Jensen is gratefully acknowledged. The Danish Cancer Biobank is acknowledged for guidance on storage and handling of tissue samples.

Funding
This work was supported by the Danish Strategic Research Council (Innovation Fund Denmark), The Danish Cancer Society, The Velux Foundation, Tømmerhandler Vilhelm Bangs Fond, Grosserer L.F. Foghts Fond, Købmand Sven Hansen og Hustru Ina Hansens Fond, Direktør Emil C. Hertz og Hustru Inger Hertz' Fond, Grosserer Georg Bjørkner og hustru Ellen Bjørkners Fond, Fonden 1870, and Tømrermester Jørgen Holm og Hustru Elisa f. Hansens Mindelegat.

Authors' contributions
KDS, SHS, and TMS designed the study. ASL and SH constructed the tissue microarray. TMA scoring was done by SHS, ASL, SH, and TMS. TMS performed all the statistical analyses under supervision from KDS. MB and TFØ contributed to the acquisition and interpretation of the data. The manuscript was written by TMS, SHS, and KDS. All authors read and approved the final manuscript.

Author details
[1]Department of Urology, Aarhus University Hospital, Aarhus, Denmark. [2]Department of Pathology, Aarhus University Hospital, Aarhus, Denmark. [3]Department of Molecular Medicine, Aarhus University Hospital, Aarhus, Denmark.

References
1. Ferlay J, Steliarova-Foucher E, Lortet-Tieulent J, Rosso S, Coebergh JW, Comber H, et al. Cancer incidence and mortality patterns in Europe: estimates for 40 countries in 2012. Eur J Cancer. 2013;49:1374–403.
2. Fitzmaurice C, Allen C, Barber RM, Barregard L, Bhutta ZA, Brenner H, et al. Global, regional, and national cancer incidence, mortality, years of life lost, years lived with disability, and disability-adjusted life-years for 32 cancer groups, 1990 to 2015: a systematic analysis for the global burden of disease study. JAMA Oncol. 2017;3(4):524–548.
3. Network CGAR. The molecular taxonomy of primary prostate cancer. Cell. 2015;163:1011–25.
4. Bostrom PJ, Bjartell AS, Catto JW, Eggener SE, Lilja H, Loeb S, et al. Genomic predictors of outcome in prostate cancer. Eur Urol. 2015;68:1033–44.
5. Abou-Ouf H, Zhao L, Bismar TA. ERG expression in prostate cancer: biological relevance and clinical implication. J Cancer Res Clin Oncol. 2016;142:1781–93.
6. Strand SH, Switnicki M, Moller M, Haldrup C, Storebjerg TM, Hedegaard J, et al. RHCG and TCAF1 promoter hypermethylation predicts biochemical recurrence in prostate cancer patients treated by radical prostatectomy. Oncotarget. 2017;8:5774–88.
7. Strand SH, Orntoft TF, Sorensen KD. Prognostic DNA methylation markers for prostate cancer. Int J Mol Sci. 2014;15:16544–76.
8. Haldrup C, Mundbjerg K, Vestergaard EM, Lamy P, Wild P, Schulz WA, et al. DNA methylation signatures for prediction of biochemical recurrence after radical prostatectomy of clinically localized prostate cancer. J Clin Oncol. 2013;31:3250–8.
9. Sandoval J, Esteller M. Cancer epigenomics: beyond genomics. Curr Opin Genet Dev. 2012;22:50–5.
10. Esteller M. Epigenetics in cancer. N Engl J Med. 2008;358:1148–59.
11. Guibert S, Weber M. Functions of DNA methylation and hydroxymethylation in mammalian development. Curr Top Dev Biol. 2013;104:47–83.
12. Ito S, Shen L, Dai Q, Wu SC, Collins LB, Swenberg JA, et al. Tet proteins can convert 5-methylcytosine to 5-formylcytosine and 5-carboxylcytosine. Science. 2011;333:1300–3.
13. Tahiliani M, Koh KP, Shen Y, Pastor WA, Bandukwala H, Brudno Y, et al. Conversion of 5-methylcytosine to 5-hydroxymethylcytosine in mammalian DNA by MLL partner TET1. Science. 2009;324:930–5.
14. Yang H, Liu Y, Bai F, Zhang JY, Ma SH, Liu J, et al. Tumor development is associated with decrease of TET gene expression and 5-methylcytosine hydroxylation. Oncogene. 2013;32:663–9.
15. Rodger EJ, Chatterjee A, Morison IM. 5-hydroxymethylcytosine: a potential therapeutic target in cancer. Epigenomics. 2014;6:503–14.
16. Song CX, Yi C, He C. Mapping recently identified nucleotide variants in the genome and transcriptome. Nat Biotechnol. 2012;30:1107–16.
17. Song CX, He C. Potential functional roles of DNA demethylation intermediates. Trends Biochem Sci. 2013;38:480–4.
18. Spruijt CG, Gnerlich F, Smits AH, Pfaffeneder T, Jansen PW, Bauer C, et al. Dynamic readers for 5-(hydroxy)methylcytosine and its oxidized derivatives. Cell. 2013;152:1146–59.
19. Iurlaro M, Ficz G, Oxley D, Raiber EA, Bachman M, Booth MJ, et al. A screen for hydroxymethylcytosine and formylcytosine binding proteins suggests functions in transcription and chromatin regulation. Genome Biol. 2013;14:R119.
20. Haffner MC, Chaux A, Meeker AK, Esopi DM, Gerber J, Pellakuru LG, et al. Global 5-hydroxymethylcytosine content is significantly reduced in tissue stem/progenitor cell compartments and in human cancers. Oncotarget. 2011;2:627–37.
21. Eleftheriou M, Pascual AJ, Wheldon LM, Perry C, Abakir A, Arora A, et al. 5-Carboxylcytosine levels are elevated in human breast cancers and gliomas. Clin Epigenetics. 2015;7:88.
22. Zhang F, Liu Y, Zhang Z, Li J, Wan Y, Zhang L, et al. 5-hydroxymethylcytosine loss is associated with poor prognosis for patients with WHO grade II diffuse astrocytomas. Sci Rep. 2016;6:20882.
23. Orr BA, Haffner MC, Nelson WG, Yegnasubramanian S, Eberhart CG. Decreased 5-hydroxymethylcytosine is associated with neural progenitor phenotype in normal brain and shorter survival in malignant glioma. PLoS One. 2012;7:e41036.
24. Liao Y, Gu J, Wu Y, Long X, Ge DI, Xu J, et al. Low level of 5-Hydroxymethylcytosine predicts poor prognosis in non-small cell lung cancer. Oncol Lett. 2016;11:3753–60.
25. Zhang LY, Han CS, Li PL, Zhang XC. 5-Hydroxymethylcytosine expression is associated with poor survival in cervical squamous cell carcinoma. Jpn J Clin Oncol. 2016;46:427–34.
26. Tsai KW, Li GC, Chen CH, Yeh MH, Huang JS, Tseng HH, et al. Reduction of global 5-hydroxymethylcytosine is a poor prognostic factor in breast cancer patients, especially for an ER/PR-negative subtype. Breast Cancer Res Treat. 2015;153:219–34.
27. Zhang LY, Li PL, Wang TZ, Zhang XC. Prognostic values of 5-hmC, 5-mC and TET2 in epithelial ovarian cancer. Arch Gynecol Obstet. 2015;292:891–7.
28. Yang Q, Wu K, Ji M, Jin W, He N, Shi B, et al. Decreased 5-hydroxymethylcytosine (5-hmC) is an independent poor prognostic factor in gastric cancer patients. J Biomed Nanotechnol. 2013;9:1607–16.
29. Kroeze LI, Aslanyan MG, van Rooij A, Koorenhof-Scheele TN, Massop M, Carell T, et al. Characterization of acute myeloid leukemia based on levels of global hydroxymethylation. Blood. 2014;124:1110–8.
30. Strand SH, Hoyer S, Lynnerup AS, Haldrup C, Storebjerg TM, Borre M, et al. High levels of 5-hydroxymethylcytosine (5hmC) is an adverse predictor of biochemical recurrence after prostatectomy in ERG-negative prostate cancer. Clin Epigenetics. 2015;7:111.

31. Epstein JI, Egevad L, Amin MB, Delahunt B, Srigley JR, Humphrey PA. The 2014 International Society of Urological Pathology (ISUP) consensus conference on Gleason grading of prostatic carcinoma: definition of grading patterns and proposal for a new grading system. Am J Surg Pathol. 2016;40:244–52.

32. Park K, Tomlins SA, Mudaliar KM, Chiu YL, Esgueva R, Mehra R, et al. Antibody-based detection of ERG rearrangement-positive prostate cancer. Neoplasia. 2010;12:590–8.

33. Harrell FE Jr, Califf RM, Pryor DB, Lee KL, Rosati RA. Evaluating the yield of medical tests. Jama. 1982;247:2543–6.

34. Yildirim O, Li R, Hung JH, Chen PB, Dong X, Ee LS, et al. Mbd3/NURD complex regulates expression of 5-hydroxymethylcytosine marked genes in embryonic stem cells. Cell. 2011;147:1498–510.

35. Shen L, Zhang Y. 5-Hydroxymethylcytosine: generation, fate, and genomic distribution. Curr Opin Cell Biol. 2013;25:289–96.

36. Pettersson A, Graff RE, Bauer SR, Pitt MJ, Lis RT, Stack EC, et al. The TMPRSS2: ERG rearrangement, ERG expression, and prostate cancer outcomes: a cohort study and meta-analysis. Cancer Epidemiol Biomark Prev. 2012;21:1497–509.

37. Hoogland AM, Jenster G, van Weerden WM, Trapman J, van der Kwast T, Roobol MJ, et al. ERG immunohistochemistry is not predictive for PSA recurrence, local recurrence or overall survival after radical prostatectomy for prostate cancer. Mod Pathol. 2012;25:471–9.

38. Taberlay PC, Jones PA. DNA methylation and cancer. Prog Drug Res. 2011;67:1–23.

39. Yang B, Sun H, Lin W, Hou W, Li H, Zhang L, et al. Evaluation of global DNA hypomethylation in human prostate cancer and prostatic intraepithelial neoplasm tissues by immunohistochemistry. Urol Oncol. 2013;31:628–34.

40. Iurlaro M, McInroy GR, Burgess HE, Dean W, Raiber EA, Bachman M, et al. In vivo genome-wide profiling reveals a tissue-specific role for 5-formylcytosine. Genome Biol. 2016;17:141.

41. Bachman M, Uribe-Lewis S, Yang X, Burgess HE, Iurlaro M, Reik W, et al. 5-Formylcytosine can be a stable DNA modification in mammals. Nat Chem Biol. 2015;11:555–7.

42. Kang KA, Piao MJ, Kim KC, Kang HK, Chang WY, Park IC, et al. Epigenetic modification of Nrf2 in 5-fluorouracil-resistant colon cancer cells: involvement of TET-dependent DNA demethylation. Cell Death Dis. 2014;5:e1183.

43. Mariani CJ, Vasanthakumar A, Madzo J, Yesilkanal A, Bhagat T, Yu Y, et al. TET1-mediated hydroxymethylation facilitates hypoxic gene induction in neuroblastoma. Cell Rep. 2014;7:1343–52.

44. Tsai YP, Chen HF, Chen SY, Cheng WC, Wang HW, Shen ZJ, et al. TET1 regulates hypoxia-induced epithelial-mesenchymal transition by acting as a co-activator. Genome Biol. 2014;15:513.

45. Chen HC, Yang CM, Cheng JT, Tsai KW, Fu TY, Liou HH, et al. Global DNA hypomethylation is associated with the development and poor prognosis of tongue squamous cell carcinoma. J Oral Pathol Med. 2016;45:409–17.

46. Poloni A, Goteri G, Zizzi A, Serrani F, Trappolini S, Costantini B, et al. Prognostic role of immunohistochemical analysis of 5 mc in myelodysplastic syndromes. Eur J Haematol. 2013;91:219–27.

47. Shi X, Yu Y, Luo M, Zhang Z, Shi S, Feng X, et al. Loss of 5-Hydroxymethylcytosine is an independent unfavorable prognostic factor for esophageal squamous cell carcinoma. PLoS One. 2016;11:e0153100.

48. Saldanha G, Joshi K, Lawes K, Bamford M, Moosa F, Teo KW, et al. 5-Hydroxymethylcytosine is an independent predictor of survival in malignant melanoma. Mod Pathol. 2017;30:60–8.

8

Differentially methylated regions in T cells identify kidney transplant patients at risk for de novo skin cancer

Fleur S. Peters[1]*[iD], Annemiek M. A. Peeters[1], Pooja R. Mandaviya[2], Joyce B. J. van Meurs[2], Leo J. Hofland[3], Jacqueline van de Wetering[1], Michiel G. H. Betjes[1], Carla C. Baan[1] and Karin Boer[1]

Abstract

Background: Cutaneous squamous cell carcinoma (cSCC) occurs 65–200 times more in immunosuppressed organ transplant patients than in the general population. T cells, which are targeted by the given immunosuppressive drugs, are involved in anti-tumor immune surveillance and are functionally regulated by DNA methylation. Prior to kidney transplantation, we aim to discover differentially methylated regions (DMRs) in T cells involved in de novo post-transplant cSCC development.

Methods: We matched 27 kidney transplant patients with a future de novo cSCC after transplantation to 27 kidney transplant patients without cSCC and studied genome-wide DNA methylation of T cells prior to transplantation. From 11 out of the 27 cSCC patients, the DNA methylation of T cells after transplantation was also examined to assess stability of the observed differences in DNA methylation. Raw methylation values obtained with the 450k array were confirmed with pyrosequencing.

Results: We found 16 DMRs between patients with a future cSCC and those who do not develop this complication after transplantation. The majority of the DMRs were located in regulatory genomic regions such as flanking bivalent transcription start sites and bivalent enhancer regions, and most of the DMRs contained CpG islands. Examples of genes annotated to the DMRs are *ZNF577*, coding for a zinc-finger protein, and *FLOT1*, coding for a protein involved in T cell migration. The longitudinal analysis revealed that DNA methylation of 9 DMRs changed significantly after transplantation. DNA methylation of 5 out of 16 DMRs was relatively stable, with a variation in beta-value lower than 0.05 for at least 50% of the CpG sites within that region.

Conclusions: This is the first study demonstrating that DNA methylation of T cells from patients with a future de novo post-transplant cSCC is different from patients without cSCC. These results were obtained before transplantation, a clinically relevant time point for cSCC risk assessment. Several DNA methylation profiles remained relatively stable after transplantation, concluding that these are minimally affected by the transplantation and possibly have a lasting effect on post-transplant cSCC development.

Keywords: DNA methylation, T lymphocytes, Epigenetics, Cutaneous squamous cell carcinoma, Non-melanoma skin cancer, Solid organ transplantation

* Correspondence: f.s.peters@erasmusmc.nl
[1]Nephrology and Transplantation, Department of Internal Medicine, Rotterdam Transplant Group, Erasmus MC, Erasmus University Medical Center, Rotterdam, The Netherlands
Full list of author information is available at the end of the article

Background

The risk of developing cancer is markedly higher in organ transplant patients than in the general population [1]. The most common cancer in transplant patients is non-melanoma skin cancer whereby cutaneous squamous cell carcinoma (cSCC) occurs most frequently [2], with an increased risk of 65–200 fold [2–4]. Not only the incidence of cSCC increases after organ transplantation, the skin cancer also behaves more aggressively. Transplant patients experience more metastasis and more recurrence of the cSCC: 70% of the patients develop a subsequent skin cancer within 5 years [5, 6]. Identification of transplant patients at increased risk for cSCC may allow early intervention and will improve the quality of life for these patients.

Transplant patients are at high risk for cSCC because of their impaired immune system due to lifelong immunosuppressive therapy [7–9]. Immunosuppressive drugs used after organ transplantation suppress T cell activity [10]. T cells are an important cell type for anti-tumor immune surveillance (CD8+), but can also provide a more immune-tolerant environment for the tumor (regulatory T cells) [11, 12]. Carroll et al. [13] showed that high numbers of peripheral regulatory CD4 +FOXP3+ cells predicted the development of a new cSCC in kidney transplant patients who had a previous cSCC. Also the presence of CD8+CD57[hi] cells, a phenotype associated with T cell senescence, was shown to predict development of a subsequent cSCC in kidney transplant patients [14]. These studies both predicted recurrence of the cSCC; tools to predict de novo cSCC after transplantation are currently unavailable.

Considering the recurrent nature of cSCC and the increased incidence in immunocompromised transplant patients, we hypothesized that there is a systemic defect in patients who will develop cSCC due to an altered state of T cell function. Such an altered state of T cell function is a well-known consequence of loss of kidney function [15]. T cell function is determined by the chromatin state of its DNA, which is a combination of epigenetic features such as DNA methylation, DNA accessibility, histone modifications, and RNA expression [16, 17]. DNA methylation is an important epigenetic regulator of cellular function [18, 19], and high methylation in the transcription start site (TSS) of a gene is in most cases associated with transcriptional silencing of the corresponding gene [20].

Differential DNA methylation between transplant patients with or without a future post-transplant cSCC might provide insight in the pathogenesis of cSCC. However, DNA methylation is a dynamic feature and significantly influenced by the environment [21]. After kidney transplantation, immunosuppressive therapy is given and the metabolic complications associated with loss of kidney function largely disappear. Therefore, it can be expected that changes in DNA methylation will occur and this may also affect any DNA methylation profiles identifying patients at risk for de novo post-transplant cSCC. By comparing these DNA methylation profiles before and after transplantation, the extent of their functional effect on post-transplant cSCC development could be assessed.

In this retrospective study, we aimed to identify kidney transplant patients at risk for de novo post-transplant cSCC by studying genome-wide DNA methylation of T cells. We analyzed samples collected before transplantation and compared patients with a future de novo post-transplant cSCC to patients without cSCC. Highly enriched T cell populations were isolated from these patients and genome-wide DNA methylation was measured. We then searched for differentially methylated regions (DMRs) by comparing the future cSCC patients' methylation profiles to the non-cSCC profiles. For a subset of cSCC patients, a post-transplantation sample was available which enabled us to compare DNA methylation before and after transplantation. A technical validation of the raw methylation values on the array was performed with pyrosequencing.

Methods
Patient samples

Anonymized biobank samples were used in this study; this approach had been approved by the local ethical committee (MEC-2015-642). Kidney transplant patients with a future post-transplant cSCC were matched to kidney transplant patients who have not developed an cSCC based on gender, age (± 2 years), ethnicity, cytomegalovirus (CMV) status, and availability of biobank material. We included patients with at least one cSCC after transplantation and patients with cSCC in situ (Bowen's disease). Patients with a previous kidney transplantation or another donor organ such as liver, heart, or lung were excluded, as well as patients with a history of malignancy prior to transplantation. Non-cSCC patients with actinic keratosis, a pre-cancerous lesion, were excluded.

The patient cohort consisted of 27 cSCC patients and 27 non-cSCC patients who had been transplanted between 1997 and 2014. No statistical differences were found between the clinical characteristics of the cSCC and non-cSCC patients; however, after cell sorting, the composition of CD4+ and CD8+ T cells significantly differed between the cSCC and non-cSCC patients (Table 1). One cSCC patient had received immunosuppressive drugs prior to an AB0-incompatible transplantation.

From 11 cSCC patients, material collected after transplantation was available for a longitudinal analysis; characteristics of this subset of patients are given in Table 2. The post-transplantation samples were collected based

Table 1 Patient characteristics

	cSCC	Non-cSCC	
	$N = 27$	$N = 27$	
Age (years)[a]	61.7 (27–77)	61.3 (27–77)	$p = 0.802$
Gender (male)	19 (70.4%)	19 (70.4%)	$p = 1$
Years between Tx and first cSCC[a]	5.4 (0.9–12.5)	–	–
CMV status			$p = 0.46$
Negative	12 (44.4%)	9 (33.3%)	
Positive	15 (55.6%)	17 (63.0%)	
Unknown	–	1 (3.7%)	
Dialysis pre-transplantation			$p = 0.783$
Yes	16 (59.3%)	15 (55.6%)	
No	11 (40.7%)	12 (44.4%)	
ESRD diagnosis			$p = 0.058$
Polycystic kidney	6 (22.2%)	1 (3.7%)	
Hypertension	6 (22.2%)	3 (11.1%)	
Diabetic nefropathy	1 (3.7%)	6 (22.2%)	
Glomerulonefritis	3 (11.1%)	6 (22.2%)	
Other	11 (40.7%)	11 (40.7%)	
% CD3[a]	97.4 (92.4–99.5)	98.0 (95.1–99.5)	$p = 0.225$
% CD4[a]	73.0 (45.1–91.4)	60.3 (34.8–80.7)	$p = 0.000$
% CD8[a]	20.7 (5.8–46.2)	32.8 (14.8–60.6)	$p = 0.000$

[a]Median and range

cSCC cutaneous squamous cell carcinoma, *CMV* cytomegalovirus, *ESDR* end-stage renal disease

Table 2 Patient characteristics longitudinal analysis

	$N = 11$
Age at Tx (years)[a]	65.4 (47–75)
Gender (male)	8 (72.7%)
Years between Tx and first cSCC[a]	2.6 (1.1–11.5)
Years between Tx and post-Tx sample[a]	2.1 (0.3–13.0)
CMV acceptor	
Negative	4 (36.4%)
Positive	7 (63.6%)
CMV donor	
Negative	7 (63.6%)
Positive	4 (36.4%)
HLA mismatches[a]	2 (0–6)
Type of immunosuppression directly after transplantation	
Corticosteroids	10 (90.9%)
Tacrolimus	10 (90.9%)
MMF	10 (90.9%)
Cyclosporine	1 (9.1%)
Sirolimus	1 (9.1%)
Basiliximab induction	3 (27.3%)
ATG induction	1 (9.1%)
ESRD diagnosis	
Polycystic kidney	5 (45.5%)
Hypertension	1 (9.1%)
Other	5 (45.5%)
Dialysis pre-transplantation	
Yes	8 (72.7%)
No	3 (27.3%)

[a]Median and range

cSCC cutaneous squamous cell carcinoma, *CMV* cytomegalovirus, *ESDR* end-stage renal disease

on the availability of biobank material and are therefore at different time points after transplantation (Table 3). Three of the post-transplant samples were taken after the diagnosis of the first cSCC. All of these patients received treatment, patient "p1" was treated with a topical chemotherapeutic agent 5-fluorouacil, patient "p2" was treated with photodynamic therapy and surgical excision, and patient "p4" was treated with a surgical excision.

Peripheral blood mononuclear cells (PBMCs) were isolated by density gradient centrifugation using standard Ficoll-Paque procedures (GE Healthcare, Chicago, IL, US). Isolated PBMCs were stored at – 140 °C until further use. T cells were isolated from the PBMCs using fluorescence-activated cell sorting (FACS) by the BD FACSAria™ ll (BD Biosciences, San Jose, CA, US). PBMCs were stained with anti-CD3 Brilliant Violet 510 (Biolegend, San Diego, CA, US), anti-CD4 Pacific Blue (BD Biosciences), and anti-CD8 APC-cy7 (BD Biosciences), and to exclude non-viable cells, 7AAD PerCP (BD Biosciences) was used. After cell sorting, the purities were > 92% for CD3+ cells; samples below 90% were excluded for further analysis.

Before isolating DNA from the T cells, all patient samples were randomized to minimize batch effects. DNA was isolated using the QIAamp DNA Micro kit (Qiagen,

Venlo, The Netherlands) according to the manufacturer's protocol. Purity and concentration of the isolated DNA was assessed with the NanoDrop ND-8000 (Isogen Life Science, Utrecht, The Netherlands). DNA degradation was determined by gel electrophoresis; none of the samples showed significant degradation.

DNA methylation microarrays

To generate genome-wide DNA methylation data, 500 ng of genomic DNA was treated with sodium-bisulfite to induce methylation-dependent changes in the DNA sequence, using the EZ DNA Methylation kit (Zymo Research, Irvine, CA, US). DNA was then hybridized on Infinium HumanMethylation450 arrays (Illumina, San Diego, CA, USA) according to the manufacturer's protocol, and IDAT files were generated by the iScan BeadChip scanner (Illumina).

Table 3 Time points longitudinal analysis

Patient	Time after Tx (y)	Time between Tx and first cSCC (y)	Comment
p1	13.0	11.0	Material obtained after diagnosis of first cSCC
p2	7.7	4.1	Material obtained after diagnosis of first cSCC
p3	6.9	7.7	
p4	3.4	2.4	Material obtained after diagnosis of first cSCC
p5	0.9	4.7	
p6	2.1	2.6	
p7	0.3	1.6	
p8	1.1	2.0	
p9	1.1	1.1	
p10	0.6	2.2	
p11	5.0	11.5	

Tx transplantation, *cSCC* cutaneous squamous cell carcinoma, *y* years

Data quality was examined using the MethylAid R package [22, 23]. All samples passed the five quality controls performed using the default MethylAid thresholds. Probes with a detection p value > 0.01 were removed from the dataset as well as probes containing single nucleotide polymorphisms. Since our patient population was a mixture of male and female, all probes on the sex chromosomes were also removed. A between-array normalization was applied to the type I and type II probes separately using the DASEN method within the wateRmelon Bioconductor R package [23–25]. The methylation level for each cytosine-phosphate-guanine (CpG) site was calculated as the ratio of the methylated probe intensity and the overall intensity. This is presented as a beta-value, a value between 0 (unmethylated) and 1 (fully methylated). After the quality controls and normalization, beta-values of 423,289 CpG sites remained for further analysis. Both the raw and normalized data are available via the NCBI Gene Expression Omnibus (GEO) database with accession number GSE103911.

Data analysis DNA methylation microarrays

To identify DNA methylation differences between the future cSCC and non-cSCC patients, we fitted a linear mixed effect model using the lme4 R package [26]. The fixed effects included age, percentage CD4, percentage CD8, and CMV status. %CD4 and %CD8 were included in the model because we found that the composition was different between the cSCC and non-cSCC patients after cell sorting (Table 1). Array IDs were included as a random effect to account for technical variation between the arrays. Single site-specific p values were obtained and these p values together with the genomic location of

the CpG sites were used as input into comb-p [27] to find differentially methylated regions (DMRs).

Comb-p is a command-line tool based on a python library to spatially correlate p values [27]. Since DNA methylation at adjacent CpG sites is correlated, it strengthens the data to study regions that are differentially methylated instead of single sites [28, 29]. Comb-p calculates a weighted correlation between the p values from the single CpG site-specific analysis and combines adjacent p values based on this correlation. A sliding window of 500 base pair (bp) was used, and the seed was set at $p < 0.01$. It then performs a false discovery rate (FDR) adjustment to this new correlation adjusted p values, finds regions of enrichment at an FDR cut off of 0.05, and assigns significance to those regions. Multiple testing correction in this analysis is done using a Šidák correction (Šidák < 0.05) [30]. The resulting DMRs were annotated to ROADMAP reference data of primary CD3+ cells [16] to determine the CpG island content and the chromatin state of the DMRs.

Longitudinal analysis

For 11 cSCC patients (Tables 2 and 3), we compared DNA methylation values of the DMRs before and after transplantation. A paired statistical analysis was done per region. To improve clarity, only those CpG sites within a DMR with a Δbeta-value larger than 0.05 (5% methylation) were used for detailed graphical representation and the patients were evenly divided in four time segments after transplantation. The CpG sites within a region that increased or decreased less than 0.05 in beta-value per patient were considered stable in time.

Technical validation

Performing methylation arrays for a risk assessment is not easily applicable to clinical practice due to high costs and labor-intensive workflow. Therefore, we tested whether we could obtain the same methylation values with bisulfite pyrosequencing, an easy technique to quantitatively measure single-site DNA methylation [31]. CpG sites within the DMRs 2 and 3 were analyzed in the same DNA samples that were used for the array analysis. Of 10 patients, a mixture of cSCC and non-cSCC patients, 200 ng genomic DNA was bisulfite converted using the EZ DNA Methylation-Direct kit (Zymo Research) according to the manufacturer's protocol. The bisulfite-treated DNA was then amplified by polymerase chain reaction (PCR) using the Pyromark PCR kit (Qiagen). Primers for PCR and pyrosequencing were designed using PyroMark Assay Design 2.0 software (Qiagen). The PCR primers, melting temperatures, and amplicon sizes for the different PCR products can be found in Additional file 1 together with the specific PCR programs for each DMR.

After confirming the amplicon size by gel electrophoresis, the PCR products were sequenced using a PyroMark Q24 pyrosequencer (Qiagen). Minor adjustments were made to the manufacturer's protocol: to immobilize the PCR product 1 μL Streptadivin Sepharose High Performance Beads (GE Healthcare) was used per sequence reaction and annealing of the sequence primers was done for 3 min at 80 °C. The sequence primers were added at a concentration of 10 μM. Human high and low methylated DNA (EpigenDx, Hopkinton, MA, USA) were used as controls. DNA methylation percentages were calculated by PyroMark Q24 software (Qiagen).

Statistical analysis

Differences in characteristics between the future cSCC and non-cSCC patients were statistically tested using SPSS version 21.0 (IBM Corp., Armonk, NY, US). The Mann-Whitney U test was used for the continuous variables and χ^2 test for the categorical variables. Data processing and statistical analysis of all the microarray data was done in RStudio version 1.0.136 (Rstudio Inc., Boston, MA, US) with R version 3.2.5 [24]. Cohen's D was calculated on the residuals of the linear mixed effect model by the formula $D = (\text{mean}_{cSCC} - \text{mean}_{\text{non-cSCC}})/\text{sd}_{\text{pooled}}$ in R. Analysis of the differences between methylation in pre-transplantation and post-transplantation samples was done using a paired Wilcoxon ranked sum test using R. Correlation between the DNA methylation levels quantified by pyrosequencing and the beta-values of the Illumina 450k arrays was calculated using Spearman's rank correlation coefficient using SPSS. All

statistical tests were two-tailed, and a $p < 0.05$ was considered statistically significant.

Results
Differentially methylated regions

To identify DMRs in T cells between patients who will develop cSCC after kidney transplantation and those without cSSC, we analyzed genome-wide DNA methylation of kidney transplant patients before transplantation. After cell sorting the T cells, we observed a difference in CD4/CD8 composition between the future cSCC and non-cSCC patients' T cells. The future cSCC patients had a higher percentage of CD4+ cells than the non-cSCC patients ($p < 0.001$; Table 1). For this reason, we included the percentage CD4+ and CD8+ in the linear mixed model as covariates, thereby avoiding potentially biased results with respect to the differences in DNA methylation. None of the single-site p values passed the multiple testing correction (Additional file 2: Figure S1); therefore, we continued to DMR analysis.

We found 16 regions significantly differentially methylated between the future cSCC and non-cSCC patients. In Table 4, the genes annotated to the DMRs, the genomic location of the DMRs according to the hg19 genome build (UCSC Genome Browser), and the number of array probes within the regions are presented, and the gene functions are shortly described. Also the Cohen's D is presented per region which is a measure for effect size taking into account the standard deviation in the two groups. Out of the 16 DMRs, 5

Table 4 Resulting differentially methylated regions of the pre-transplantation analysis

	Genomic location (hg19)	Length DMR (bp)	No. of probes	Regional p value	Cohen's D	DMR state
1	chr19:4531638-4531962	324	4	$3.57 \cdot 10^{-11}$	0.95	Hyper
2	chr5:63461216-63461931	715	10	$5.51 \cdot 10^{-10}$	−0.54	Hypo
3	chr3:44753865-44754399	534	11	$8.18 \cdot 10^{-10}$	−0.60	Hypo
4	chr2:3699195-3699564	369	5	$9.35 \cdot 10^{-10}$	0.81	Hyper
5	chr6:168197177-168197700	523	6	$6.54 \cdot 10^{-9}$	−0.68	Hypo
6	chr4:165898666-165898968	302	8	$1.49 \cdot 10^{-8}$	0.54	Hyper
7	chr5:140305947-140306459	512	10	$2.38 \cdot 10^{-8}$	−0.53	Hypo
8	chr2:177014555-177015126	571	12	$4.35 \cdot 10^{-8}$	0.41	Hyper
9	chr1:185703201-185703689	488	12	$1.89 \cdot 10^{-7}$	−0.42	Hypo
10	chr6:30698584-30698988	404	11	$2.90 \cdot 10^{-7}$	−0.48	Hypo
11	chr19:52391078-52391606	528	12	$6.59 \cdot 10^{-7}$	0.58	Hyper
12	chr8:54164051-54164443	392	8	$1.20 \cdot 10^{-6}$	−0.48	Hypo
13	chr7:51539131-51539584	453	5	$1.61 \cdot 10^{-6}$	−0.64	Hypo
14	chr6:88757302-88757704	402	6	$1.80 \cdot 10^{-6}$	−0.55	Hypo
15	chr2:74875227-74875549	322	8	$1.45 \cdot 10^{-6}$	−0.47	Hypo
16	chr8:96085385-96085690	305	3	$1.22 \cdot 10^{-5}$	−0.74	Hypo

DMR differentially methylated region, *chr* chromosome, *bp* base pair

were hyper methylated and 11 were hypo methylated in the future cSCC patients.

Genomic characteristics of the DMRs

Since CpG islands are often found near transcription start sites (TSS) and are involved in transcription initiation [32], methylation of CpG islands could have a downstream effect on gene activity. Together with the cell-type-specific chromatin state of the DNA, this could indicate the biological function of a genomic region. In Fig. 1a, the CpG island content is depicted for all regions together and the individual DMRs separately; the array content is given as reference. The 16 DMRs are enriched for CpG islands, slightly less CpG sites are within the shores (< 2 kb flanking CpG islands), and CpG sites within shelves (< 2 kb flanking shores) are absent in these DMRs. For the

chromatin state, we annotated the CpG probes within each DMR to ROADMAP epigenomics reference data of primary T cells using the 15-state model [16] (Fig. 1b). Although this might not be an accurate representation of the chromatin state within the T cells we analyzed, it does provide a general perspective on functional and primary T cell-specific characteristics of the genomic region where the DMRs are located. The chromatin states "flanking bivalent TSS/enh" and "bivalent enhancer" are enriched in our results; also 7 out of the 16 DMRs are within repressed or weakly repressed polycomb which is a slight enrichment compared to the array content.

DNA methylation of the DMRs after transplantation

To study whether DNA methylation of the 16 DMRs changed after transplantation, we compared beta-values

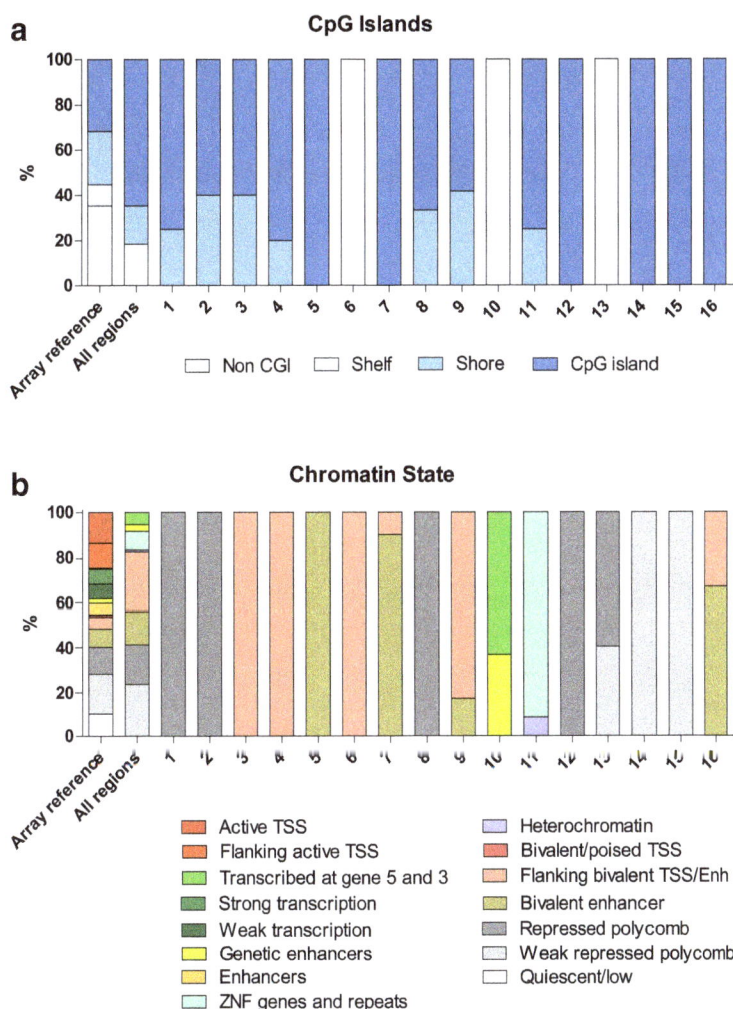

Fig. 1 The genomic characteristics of the CpG sites within each DMR. **a** CpG island content for all regions together and the individual DMRs separately, the array content is given as reference. The color represents the CpG island content of each CpG site within that region according to the legend below the graph. **b** Primary T cell-specific chromatin state according to the 15-state model of the ROADMAP epigenomics reference data [16] for all regions together and the individual DMRs separately, the array content is given as reference. The color represents the primary T cell-specific chromatin state of the CpG sites within that region according to the legend below the graph

of 11 cSCC patients before and after transplantation. Figure 2a shows the mean difference in beta-value which is an average of all CpG sites per region for all 11 patients together. Overall mean beta-value increased after transplantation. In most regions, there were CpG sites that increased and CpG sites that decreased, therefore showing a mean difference close to zero. All differences in beta-value per DMR and per patient can be found in Additional file 2: Figure S2. A paired Wilcoxon ranked sum test per region resulted in 9 regions that were significantly different after transplantation, after a Bonferroni multiple testing correction (Table 5).

All CpG sites showed variation within all patients; therefore, to reduce noise and improve clarity, we considered a CpG site that increased or decreased less than 0.05 in beta-value stable. None of the DMRs were 100% stable in time (Fig. 2b); however, some regions showed more stability than others. DMRs 1, 5, 9, 14, and 16 showed at least 50% stable CpG sites whereas in DMRs 4, 11, and 13, none of the sites were stable in time. A

more detailed graphical representation of the changes in beta-value per region, per patient, and in time can be found in Additional file 2: Figure S3.

We also analyzed the mean methylation differences per patient to examine a possible relationship with time after transplantation and with time to clinical onset of the cSCC (Table 3). These mean differences were relatively small in 5 out of 11 patients (Δbeta-value < 0.01) (Fig. 3). Mean methylation differences were not significantly correlated to the time between transplantation and clinical onset of cSCC ($p = 0.46$), nor to time after transplantation ($p = 0.50$), nor to time between post-transplant sample and the clinical onset of cSCC ($p = 0.09$).

Technical validation

To confirm the raw beta-values obtained with the 450k array, we performed pyrosequencing analysis of two DMRs (six CpG sites) on the same DNA samples that were analyzed on the array. The DNA methylation values obtained with pyrosequencing were slightly lower

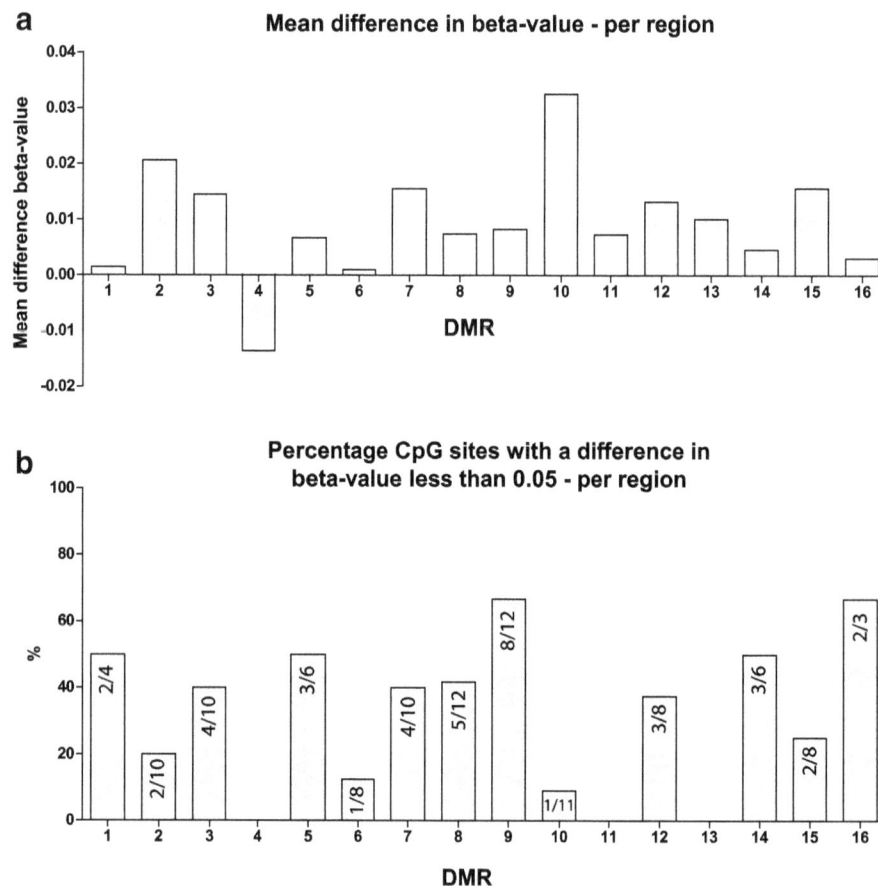

Fig. 2 Stability of the 16 DMRs. **a** Mean difference in beta-value per region between pre-transplant and post-transplant samples. The difference is calculated per CpG site for each individual patient and is then averaged over all CpG sites per region for all 11 cSCC patients together. **b** Percentage of CpG sites that show a Δbeta-value of less than 0.05 presented per region. The numbers within each bar represent the number of stable CpG sites from the total sites within that region

Table 5 Results of statistical tests between pre-transplant and post-transplant beta-values per region

DMR	p value	Bonferroni correction
1	0.87	
2	$1.83 \cdot 10^{-6}$	$2.92 \cdot 10^{-5}$
3	$2.03 \cdot 10^{-5}$	$3.25 \cdot 10^{-4}$
4	0.002	0.038
5	0.082	
6	0.55	
7	$8.09 \cdot 10^{-8}$	$1.29 \cdot 10^{-6}$
8	0.002	0.033
9	$1.51 \cdot 10^{-5}$	$2.41 \cdot 10^{-4}$
10	$3.71 \cdot 10^{-13}$	$5.93 \cdot 10^{-12}$
11	0.028	
12	$9.42 \cdot 10^{-5}$	0.002
13	0.14	
14	0.32	
15	$5.48 \cdot 10^{-5}$	$8.78 \cdot 10^{-4}$
16	0.33	

than the beta-values obtained with the arrays; this was a consistent deviation across all samples (Fig. 4). There was a strong correlation between the results obtained with the two different techniques; the two sites within DMR 2 had a Spearman correlation coefficient (r) of 0.95 ($p < 0.0001$) and the four sites within DMR 3 had an r of 0.88 ($p < 0.0001$).

Discussion

Our results demonstrate that the T cells of patients with a future post-transplant cSCC have different DNA methylation profiles compared to the T cells of kidney transplant patients without cSCC. To our knowledge, this is the first study to show DNA methylation

differences in peripheral T cells between patients who develop a post-transplant cSCC and those who do not develop cSCC. In addition, we were able to obtain these results at a clinically relevant time point, before transplantation. The retrospective nature of this study allowed us to carefully match the future cSCC patients to non-cSCC patients and examine the DNA methylation within a highly enriched T cell population.

The observed differences in DNA methylation are predominantly located in CpG islands and bivalent enhancer regions (Fig. 1). Since these are both regulatory genomic regions, it is likely that these differences have a downstream effect in T cells and that differential DNA methylation within these regions could affect T cell function. However, the effect of differential methylation at enhancer regions is difficult to assess since enhancers can regulate genes at large distances in the genome [33]. RNA sequencing would reveal any distal gene regulation by these enhancers; however, that was outside the scope of this study. Here, we focus on the genes that were annotated solely on the basis of close proximity to the DMR.

Out of the 16 DMRs, a few could be associated to cancer by studying literature. Even though these studies were not performed in T cells but mostly in the tumor tissue itself, we can speculate on a possible relationship with post-transplant cSCC development. An example is DMR 11 (annotated to *ZNF577*) which was hypermethylated in our future cSCC patients and showed to be hypermethylated in SCC and adenocarcinoma of the lungs [34]. In addition, an inverse correlation between *ZNF577* gene expression and its DNA methylation was found [35]. DMR 10, which was situated within the actively transcribed gene *FLOT1*, was hypo methylated in our cSCC patients. At first sight, it is an interesting gene due to its involvement in migration of hematopoietic cells [36] and it showed to promote invasion and metastasis of several SCC subtypes when overexpressed [37,

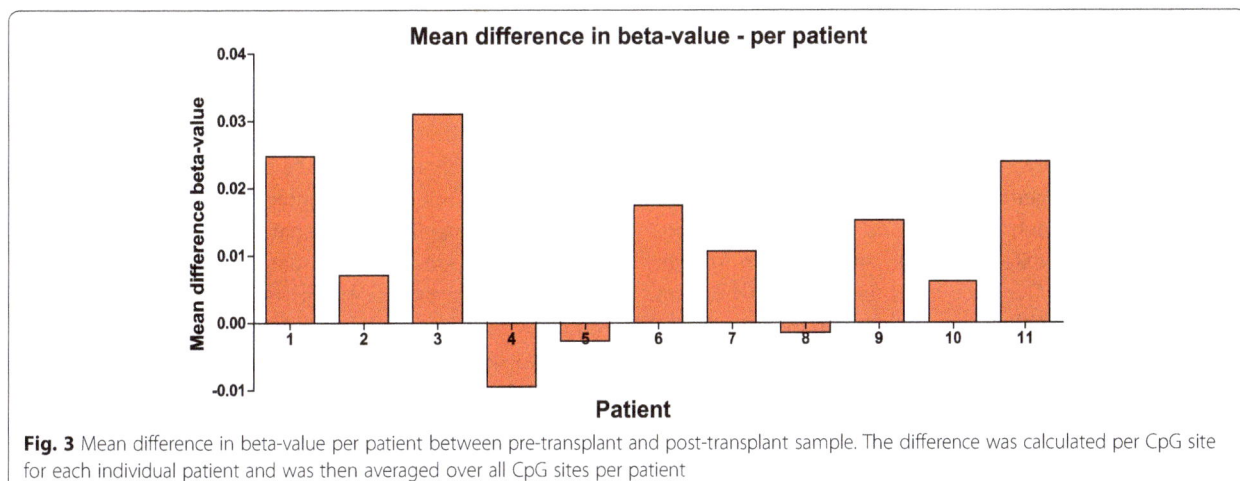

Fig. 3 Mean difference in beta-value per patient between pre-transplant and post-transplant sample. The difference was calculated per CpG site for each individual patient and was then averaged over all CpG sites per patient

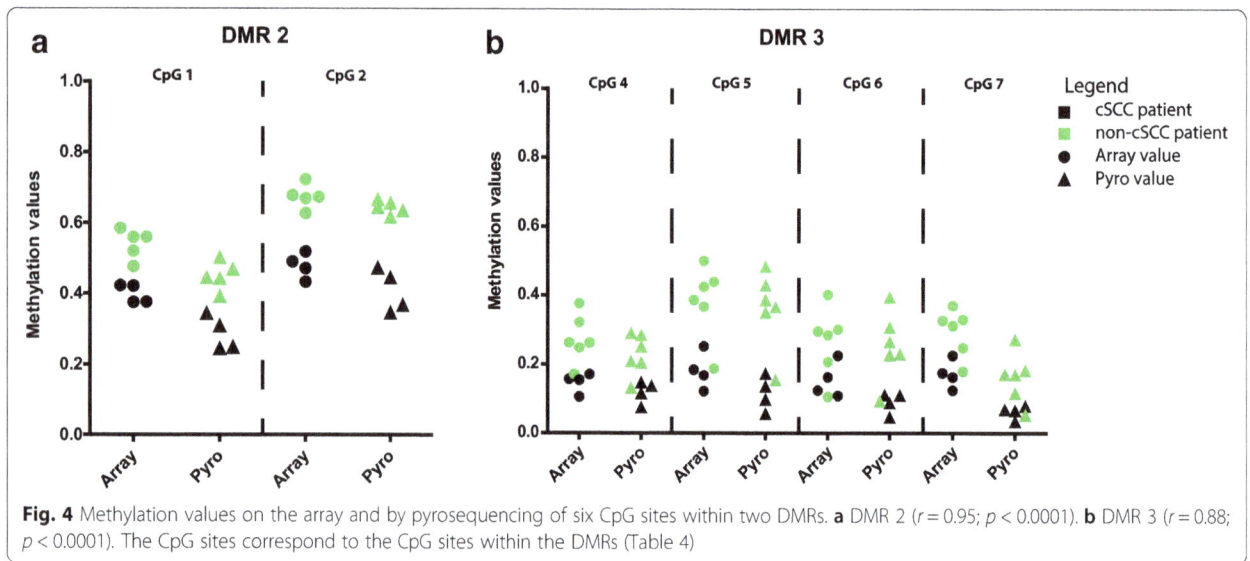

Fig. 4 Methylation values on the array and by pyrosequencing of six CpG sites within two DMRs. **a** DMR 2 ($r = 0.95$; $p < 0.0001$). **b** DMR 3 ($r = 0.88$; $p < 0.0001$). The CpG sites correspond to the CpG sites within the DMRs (Table 4)

38]. However, in the longitudinal analysis, this was the most varying region (Table 5) with the majority of CpG sites increasing in DNA methylation after transplantation (Additional file 2: Figure S2J). This suggests that this region is greatly influenced by transplantation and it remains unsure how this differential methylation at time of transplantation could affect post-transplant cSCC development.

A kidney transplantation is a procedure with major health effects for an end-stage renal disease (ESRD) patient, and these effects influence DNA methylation. Several studies have shown that blood DNA methylation is associated to kidney function [39, 40]. In addition to that, we showed in a previous study that DNA methylation of T cells can also be modulated by the immunosuppressive medication that kidney transplant patients receive after transplantation [41]. We therefore expected variation between the pre-transplant and post-transplant DNA methylation values in the longitudinal analysis. Indeed, we see that beta-values were significantly different in 9 of the 16 DMRs (Table 4). More interestingly, all but one region increased in mean DNA methylation after transplantation (Fig. 2). This could be a general effect of the transplantation and is in line with findings by Boer et al. [42] showing increased DNA methylation at the *PD1* and *IFNγ* gene 3 months after transplantation.

To determine which regions could have a lasting effect on post-transplant cSCC development, we examined stability of the 16 DMRs after transplantation and considered the CpG sites that stayed within a Δbeta-value of 0.05 stable. DMRs 1, 5, 14, and 16 have 50% or more stable CpG sites and were also not significantly different in a paired statistical analysis (Table 4), suggesting that these differential methylation profiles might have a prolonged effect after transplantation. Considering the

possibility of distal gene regulation by these DMRs, their functional effect could be determined by a genome-wide RNA and protein analysis within these T cells. Additionally, to overcome the variability in sampling time points within this study, a prospective study with sampling at regular intervals after transplantation would further assess stability of these DMRs and their function in post-transplant cSCC development.

The development of post-transplant cSCC is the result of a series of events involving different risk factors [2]. Known examples are age, skin type, gender, and possibly immune phenotype [43]. After cell sorting the T cells, we found significantly higher percentages of CD4+ T cells and consequently lower percentages of CD8+ T cells in the future cSCC patients (Table 1). This suggests that an altered CD4/CD8 ratio might be another risk factor for post-transplant cSCC. There is no consensus in literature on the CD4/CD8 ratio in relation to post-transplant cancer development. In contrast to our findings Thibaudin et al. [44] found, over a 10-year observation period, consistently lower counts of CD4+ T cells in patients with future post-transplant malignancy. Although this was not evident at time of transplantation but occurred thereafter. Whereas Bottomley et al. [14] found no significant difference in CD4+ T cell and CD8 + T cell counts or percentages between cSCC and non-cSCC kidney transplant patients.

The relative small sample size in this study is a consequence of selective matching and availability of biobank material. This combined with the single-center design of the study leads to cautious interpretation of the findings. Moreover, we acknowledge that patient pairs can never be perfectly matched. Since we are studying T cells and not skin tissue, where the differences between healthy and malignant tissue are much larger, it was expected that the differences would be subtle. Despite these limitations, the results of this study are a promising first step towards early risk assessment for post-transplant cSCC. To assess the clinical value of these findings, a validation in a different and larger cohort of transplant patients is necessary in addition to our technical validation [45, 46].

Conclusion

The findings presented here demonstrate the potential of studying DNA methylation of the T cells to identify kidney transplant patients at risk for de novo post-transplant cSCC [47]. We showed that there were systemic differences between future cSCC and non-cSCC patients prior to transplantation. A longitudinal analysis showed that several DNA methylation profiles remained relatively stable after transplantation, suggesting a lasting effect on the development of de novo cSCC after transplantation. In the future, identification of patients at increased risk for post-transplant cSCC before transplantation will allow for early clinical interventions such as regular visits to the dermatologist and stricter lifestyle advice to the patient to minimize additional sun exposure [48]. Ultimately, it may lead to adjustment of the immunosuppressive load but this remains a fine balance between reducing the risk for cancer and causing irreversible damage to the allograft.

Abbreviations
bp: Base pair; CMV: Cytomegalovirus; CpG: Cytosine-phosphate-guanine; cSCC: Cutaneous squamous cell carcinoma; DMR: Differentially methylated region; ESRD: End-stage renal disease; PBMC: Peripheral blood mononuclear cells; PCR: Polymerase chain reaction; TSS: Transcription start site; Tx: Transplantation

Acknowledgements
The authors would like to thank R. Kraaijeveld and W. Verschoor for performing all the FACS sorting experiments and M. Verbiest for performing the microarray experiments.

Authors' contributions
FP contributed to designing, performing, and analyzing the experiments; interpreting the results; and writing of the manuscript. AP performed the experiments. PM performed the data analysis. JM and LH provided the analytical tools. MB contributed to interpreting the results and reviewing the manuscript. CB and KB both contributed to designing the experiments, interpreting the results, and writing of the manuscript. All authors read and approved the final manuscript.

Competing interests
The authors declare that they have no competing interests.

Author details
[1]Neprology and Transplantation, Department of Internal Medicine, Rotterdam Transplant Group, Erasmus MC, Erasmus University Medical Center, Rotterdam, The Netherlands. [2]Department of Internal Medicine, Erasmus MC, Erasmus University Medical Center, Rotterdam, The Netherlands. [3]Endocrinology, Department of Internal Medicine, Erasmus MC, Erasmus University Medical Center, Rotterdam, The Netherlands.

References
1. van de Wetering J, Roodnat JI, Hemke AC, Hoitsma AJ, Weimar W. Patient survival after the diagnosis of cancer in renal transplant recipients: a nested case-control study. Transplantation. 2010;90(12):1542–6.
2. Euvrard S, Kanitakis J, Claudy A. Skin cancers after organ transplantation. N Engl J Med. 2003;348(17):1681–91.
3. Hartevelt MM, Bavinck JN, Kootte AM, Vermeer BJ, Vandenbroucke JP. Incidence of skin cancer after renal transplantation in The Netherlands. Transplantation. 1990;49(3):506–9.
4. Krynitz B, Edgren G, Lindelof B, Baecklund E, Brattstrom C, Wilczek H, Smedby KE. Risk of skin cancer and other malignancies in kidney, liver, heart and lung transplant recipients 1970 to 2008—a Swedish population-based study. Int J Cancer. 2013;132(6):1429–38.
5. Euvrard S, Kanitakis J, Decullier E, Butnaru AC, Lefrançois N, Boissonnat P, Sebbag L, Garnier J-L, Pouteil-Noble C, Cahen R, et al. Subsequent skin cancers in kidney and heart transplant recipients after the first squamous cell carcinoma. Transplantation. 2006;81(8):1093–100.
6. Wisgerhof HC, Edelbroek JR, de Fijter JW, Haasnoot GW, Claas FH, Willemze R, Bavinck JN. Subsequent squamous- and basal-cell carcinomas in kidney-transplant recipients after the first skin cancer: cumulative incidence and risk factors. Transplantation. 2010;89(10):1231–8.
7. Coghill AE, Johnson LG, Berg D, Resler AJ, Leca N, Madeleine MM. Immunosuppressive medications and squamous cell skin carcinoma: nested case-control study within the skin cancer after organ transplant (SCOT) cohort. Am J Transplant. 2016;16(2):565–73.
8. Rangwala S, Tsai KY. Roles of the immune system in skin Cancer. Br J Dermatol. 2011;165(5):953–65.
9. Ingvar A, Smedby KE, Lindelof B, Fernberg P, Bellocco R, Tufveson G, Hoglund P, Adami J. Immunosuppressive treatment after solid organ transplantation and risk of post-transplant cutaneous squamous cell carcinoma. Nephrol Dial Transplant. 2010;25(8):2764–71.
10. Halloran PF. Immunosuppressive drugs for kidney transplantation. N Engl J Med. 2004;351(26):2715–29.
11. Gajewski TF, Schreiber H, Fu Y-X. Innate and adaptive immune cells in the tumor microenvironment. Nat Immunol. 2013;14(10):1014–22.
12. Clark RA, Huang SJ, Murphy GF, Mollet IG, Hijnen D, Muthukuru M, Schanbacher CF, Edwards V, Miller DM, Kim JE, et al. Human squamous cell carcinomas evade the immune response by down-regulation of vascular E-selectin and recruitment of regulatory T cells. J Exp Med. 2008;205(10):2221–34.
13. Carroll RP, Segundo DS, Hollowood K, Marafioti T, Clark TG, Harden PN, Wood KJ. Immune phenotype predicts risk for posttransplantation squamous cell carcinoma. J Am Soc Nephrol. 2010;21(4):713–22.
14. Bottomley MJ, Harden PN, Wood KJ. CD8+ immunosenescence predicts post-transplant cutaneous squamous cell carcinoma in high-risk patients. J Am Soc Nephrol. 2016;27(5):1505–15.
15. Betjes MG. Immune cell dysfunction and inflammation in end-stage renal disease. Nat Rev Nephrol. 2013;9(5):255–65.
16. Roadmap Epigenomics C, Kundaje A, Meuleman W, Ernst J, Bilenky M, Yen A, Heravi-Moussavi A, Kheradpour P, Zhang Z, Wang J, et al. Integrative analysis of 111 reference human epigenomes. Nature. 2015;518(7539):317–30.
17. Putiri EL, Robertson KD. Epigenetic mechanisms and genome stability. Clin Epigenetics. 2011;2(2):299–314.
18. Suarez-Alvarez B, Rodriguez RM, Fraga MF, López-Larrea C. DNA methylation: a promising landscape for immune system-related diseases. Trends Genet. 2012;28(10):506–14.
19. Wilson CB, Rowell E, Sekimata M. Epigenetic control of T-helper-cell differentiation. Nat Rev Immunol. 2009;9(2):91–105.
20. Suzuki MM, Bird A. DNA methylation landscapes: provocative insights from epigenomics. Nat Rev Genet. 2008;9(6):465–76.

21. Feil R, Fraga MF. Epigenetics and the environment: emerging patterns and implications. Nat Rev Genet. 2012;13(2):97–109.

22. van Iterson M, Tobi EW, Slieker RC, den Hollander W, Luijk R, Slagboom PE, Heijmans BT. MethylAid: visual and interactive quality control of large Illumina 450k datasets. Bioinformatics. 2014;30(23):3435–7.

23. Huber W, Carey VJ, Gentleman R, Anders S, Carlson M, Carvalho BS, Bravo HC, Davis S, Gatto L, Girke T, et al. Orchestrating high-throughput genomic analysis with Bioconductor. Nat Methods. 2015;12(2):115–21.

24. RCoreTeam. R: a language and environment for statistical computing. *Vienna: R Foundation for Statistical Computing;* 2016.

25. Pidsley R, Y Wong CC, Volta M, Lunnon K, Mill J, Schalkwyk LC. A data-driven approach to preprocessing Illumina 450K methylation array data. BMC Genomics. 2013;14:293.

26. Bates D, Mächler M, Bolker B, Walker S. Fitting linear mixed-effects models using lme4. J Stat Softw. 2015;67(1):48.

27. Pedersen BS, Schwartz DA, Yang IV, Kechris KJ. Comb-p: software for combining, analyzing, grouping and correcting spatially correlated P-values. Bioinformatics. 2012;28(22):2986–8.

28. Bock C, Walter J, Paulsen M, Lengauer T. Inter-individual variation of DNA methylation and its implications for large-scale epigenome mapping. Nucleic Acids Res. 2008;36(10):e55.

29. Talens RP, Boomsma DI, Tobi EW, Kremer D, Jukema JW, Willemsen G, Putter H, Slagboom PE, Heijmans BT. Variation, patterns, and temporal stability of DNA methylation: considerations for epigenetic epidemiology. FASEB J. 2010;24(9):3135–44.

30. Šidák Z. Rectangular confidence regions for the means of multivariate normal distributions. J Am Stat Assoc. 1967;62(318):626–33.

31. Tost J, Gut IG. DNA methylation analysis by pyrosequencing. Nat Protoc. 2007;2(9):2265–75.

32. Deaton AM, Bird A. CpG islands and the regulation of transcription. Genes Dev. 2011;25(10):1010–22.

33. Stadhouders R, van den Heuvel A, Kolovos P, Jorna R, Leslie K, Grosveld F, Soler E. Transcription regulation by distal enhancers: who's in the loop? Transcription. 2012;3(4):181–6.

34. Rauch TA, Wang Z, Wu X, Kernstine KH, Riggs AD, Pfeifer GP. DNA methylation biomarkers for lung cancer. Tumor Biol. 2012;33(2):287–96.

35. Crujeiras AB, Diaz-Lagares A, Stefansson OA, Macias-Gonzalez M, Sandoval J, Cueva J, Lopez-Lopez R, Moran S, Jonasson JG, Tryggvadottir L, et al. Obesity and menopause modify the epigenomic profile of breast cancer. Endocr Relat Cancer. 2017;24(7):351–63.

36. Rajendran L, Beckmann J, Magenau A, Boneberg EM, Gaus K, Viola A, Giebel B, Illges H. Flotillins are involved in the polarization of primitive and mature hematopoietic cells. PLoS One. 2009;4(12):e8290.

37. Cao S, Cui Y, Xiao H, Mai M, Wang C, Xie S, Yang J, Wu S, Li J, Song L, et al. Upregulation of flotillin-1 promotes invasion and metastasis by activating TGF-β signaling in nasopharyngeal carcinoma. Oncotarget. 2016;7(4):4252–64.

38. Song L, Gong H, Lin C, Wang C, Liu L, Wu J, Li M, Li J. Flotillin-1 promotes tumor necrosis factor-alpha receptor signaling and activation of NF-kappaB in esophageal squamous cell carcinoma cells. Gastroenterology. 2012;143(4): 995–1005. e1012

39. Chu AY, Tin A, Schlosser P, Ko Y-A, Qiu C, Yao C, Joehanes R, Grams ME, Liang L, Gluck CA, et al. Epigenome-wide association studies identify DNA methylation associated with kidney function. Nat Commun. 2017;8(1):1286.

40. Smyth LJ, McKay GJ, Maxwell AP, McKnight AJ. DNA hypermethylation and DNA hypomethylation is present at different loci in chronic kidney disease. Epigenetics. 2013;9(3):366–76.

41. Peters FS, Peeters AMA, Hofland LJ, Betjes MGH, Boer K, Baan CC. Interferon-gamma DNA methylation is affected by mycophenolic acid but not by tacrolimus after T-cell activation. Front Immunol. 2017;8:822.

42. Boer K, de Wit LEA, Peters FS, Hesselink DA, Hofland LJ, Betjes MGH, Looman CWN, Baan CC. Variations in DNA methylation of interferon gamma and programmed death 1 in allograft rejection after kidney transplantation. Clin Epigenetics. 2016;8:116.

43. Sherston SN, Carroll RP, Harden PN, Wood KJ. Predictors of cancer risk in the long-term solid-organ transplant recipient. Transplantation. 2014;97(6):605–11.

44. Thibaudin D, Alamartine E, Mariat C, Absi L, Berthoux F. Long-term kinetic of T-lymphocyte subsets in kidney-transplant recipients: influence of anti–T-cell antibodies and association with posttransplant malignancies. Transplantation. 2005;80(10):1514–7.

45. Kurian SM, Whisenant T, Mas V, Heilman R, Abecassis M, Salomon DR, Moss A, Kaplan B. Biomarker guidelines for high-dimensional genomic studies in transplantation: adding method to the madness. Transplantation. 2017; 101(3):457–63.

46. Naesens M, Anglicheau D. Precision transplant medicine: biomarkers to the rescue. J Am Soc Nephrol. 2018;29(1):24–34.

47. Peters FS, Manintveld OC, Betjes MG, Baan CC, Boer K. Clinical potential of DNA methylation in organ transplantation. J Heart Lung Transplant. 2016; 35(7):843–50.

48. Ulrich C, Degen A, Patel MJ, Stockfleth E. Sunscreens in organ transplant patients. Nephrol Dial Transplant. 2008;23(6):1805–8.

9

Increased *BDNF* methylation in saliva, but not blood, of patients with borderline personality disorder

Mara Thomas[1,2], Nora Knoblich[1], Annalena Wallisch[1], Katarzyna Glowacz[1], Julia Becker-Sadzio[1], Friederike Gundel[1], Christof Brückmann[1] and Vanessa Nieratschker[1*]

Abstract

Background: The importance of epigenetic alterations in psychiatric disorders is increasingly acknowledged and the use of DNA methylation patterns as markers of disease is a topic of ongoing investigation. Recent studies suggest that patients suffering from Borderline Personality Disorder (BPD) display differential DNA methylation of various genes relevant for neuropsychiatric conditions. For example, several studies report differential methylation in the promoter region of the brain-derived neurotrophic factor gene (*BDNF*) in blood. However, little is known about *BDNF* methylation in other tissues.

Results: In the present study, we analyzed DNA methylation of the *BDNF* IV promoter in saliva and blood of 41 BPD patients and 41 matched healthy controls and found significant hypermethylation in the BPD patient's saliva, but not blood. Further, we report that *BDNF* methylation in saliva of BPD patients significantly decreased after a 12-week psychotherapeutic intervention.

Conclusions: Providing a direct comparison of *BDNF* methylation in blood and saliva of the same individuals, our results demonstrate the importance of choice of tissue for the study of DNA methylation. In addition, they indicate a better suitability of saliva for the study of differential *BDNF* methylation in BPD patients. Further, our data appear to indicate a reversal of disease-specific alterations in *BDNF* methylation in response to psychotherapy, though further experiments are necessary to validate these results and determine the specificity of the effect.

Keywords: Epigenetics, Saliva, DNA methylation, BPD, DBT, Biomarker, Treatment outcome, BDNF

Background

Borderline personality disorder (BPD) is a severe mental disorder that is characterized by instability in affect, interpersonal relationships, and self-image, in addition to impulsivity, fear of abandonment, anger, and self-mutilating behavior [1]. The estimated lifetime prevalence of BPD is 1.6–5.9%, as estimated by two large nonclinical surveys in the USA [2, 3]. However, despite its high prevalence, the pathogenesis and underlying biological mechanisms of BPD are not fully understood. According to the biosocial developmental model of BPD proposed by M. Linehan in 1993, the susceptibility for the disorder is enhanced by an early emotional vulnerability, which is then potentiated across the life span. Initial vulnerability is mainly caused by environmental risk factors such as childhood abuse or neglect. The estimated contribution of genetic factors to the disorder is in the range of 42–68% [4, 5], while environmental factors account for the remaining variance.

Recent evidence indicates that the interplay of environmental and genetic factors in the development of psychiatric disorders is partially mediated by epigenetic regulation [6, 7]. Epigenetic modifications induce changes in gene expression without altering the DNA sequence. One of the most prominent and best studied epigenetic mechanisms is DNA methylation, a covalent modification of cytosine in a cytosine-guanine-dimer (CpG site). Although DNA methylation is generally described as a silencing epigenetic mark, it is increasingly acknowledged that its effect

* Correspondence: vanessa.nieratschker@med.uni-tuebingen.de
[1]Department of Psychiatry and Psychotherapy, University Hospital Tübingen, Calwerstr. 14, 72076 Tübingen, Germany
Full list of author information is available at the end of the article

on gene expression is context-dependent. Hence, it may induce silencing of a gene, when found within its promoter region, but enhance expression, when found in the gene body [8, 9]. The degree of DNA methylation at a specific locus is determined by the underlying DNA sequence [10] and is to some extent dynamically regulated by DNA methyltransferase enzymes. As these act in response to environmental stimuli [11], DNA methylation provides the cell with a way to adapt to changes in the environment [12] and is an ideal candidate mechanism for studying the interplay of genetic and environmental signals on disease development [13]. A major challenge in epigenetic research is the cell type and tissue specificity of DNA methylation [14]. As access to brain tissue is limited, the great majority of epigenetic studies in psychiatry are conducted with blood as surrogate tissue [15].

In line with this, DNA methylation signatures have been analyzed in the peripheral blood of several BPD patient cohorts. Using targeted approaches aimed at well-known psychiatric candidate genes, epigenetic dysregulation in the blood of BPD patients has been reported e.g., for the serotonin receptor 2A (HTR2A), the monoamine oxidase A and B (MAOA and MAOB), the soluble catechol-o-methyltransferase (S-COMT), the glucocorticoid receptor (GR/NR3C1) (all reported by [16]), and the brain-derived neurotrophic factor (BDNF) [17]. Further, hypothesis-free epigenome-wide studies revealed a number of novel candidate genes to be differentially methylated in patients suffering from BPD [18, 19]. However, the findings for most of the above-mentioned studies are not fully consistent with each other, and their significance yet remains to be determined by replication in independent cohorts. For the role of BDNF methylation in BPD, support is already available from a study conducted by Thaler et al. [20], showing that increased BDNF methylation in patients with bulimic eating behavior is particularly prominent when associated with comorbid BPD. In addition, Thaler et al. and Perroud et al. [17] had found an association of BDNF methylation with childhood trauma. In line with these findings, several independent studies report a link between BDNF methylation, stress, and trauma [21–23]. Here, the most convincing evidence is available for animal models of early-life stress (ELS) [24–26]. For example, Roth et al. [26] report increased methylation of the BDNF gene in the prefrontal cortex of rats exposed to abusive mothers. In humans, post-traumatic stress disorder in combat veterans [22] and exposure to domestic violence in women [21] have been associated with increased BDNF methylation in peripheral blood. Further, a recent study found that DNA methylation within the BDNF gene moderates the association between childhood trauma and depressive symptoms [23]. It is hypothesized that the link between BDNF and psychological stress is mediated via

the crosstalk of neurotrophin and glucocorticoid pathways [27], as BDNF signaling is a target of the glucocorticoid stress response [28]. Hence, the high prevalence of ELS among patients with BPD [29] makes it difficult to disentangle its effects on DNA methylation from BPD-specific effects. Another confounder for epidemiologic studies of BDNF methylation is smoking. Next to its reported global effects on DNA methylation [30, 31], there is evidence for the association of prenatal smoke exposure with changes in offspring BDNF methylation and expression [32]. These alterations may be long-lasting and promote vulnerability to psychiatric disease later in life, as suggested by human [33] and animal studies [34, 35]. With regard to direct effects of smoking on BDNF expression, most studies indicate increased peripheral BDNF protein in smokers as compared to non-smokers [36–38], but there are no reports of altered BDNF methylation.

Adding even further to the difficulty of studying BPD-specific effects, BDNF methylation was also found associated with a broad range of psychiatric symptoms and disorders other than BPD, such as bipolar disorder [39, 40], depression [41], schizophrenia [42], and suicidality [43, 44] (reviewed in [45, 46]). The ubiquitous role of BDNF methylation in psychiatry is presumably caused by the broad expression of the BDNF protein in the brain, its importance in learning and memory [47] and its key regulating function in neuronal differentiation, and neurite and synaptic growth [48]. BDNF promoter hypermethylation, as reported in the vast majority of studies, should lead to a decreased expression of the protein. Indeed, this is what independent studies of patient cohorts report for depression [49, 50], bipolar disorder [39, 51], schizophrenia [52] and, most interestingly, also for BPD [53] (for general review see [54]). In addition, an increasing number of studies suggest that antidepressant and mood-stabilizing substances increase BDNF expression in the blood [55–57] and brain [58, 59]. In line with this, D'Addario et al. [39] reported that mood-stabilizing medication decreases BDNF exon I promoter methylation. These findings provide further indication that low BDNF expression plays a role in the pathophysiology of BPD.

In 2013, Perroud et al. reported that psychotherapeutic treatment alone (dialectical behavior therapy) leads to a reversion of the initially increased DNA methylation of BDNF promoter I and IV in BPD patients [17]. The effect was specific for those patients that had responded with significant alleviation of symptoms to the therapy [17]. This indicates that BDNF methylation may serve as biomarker for symptom severity in BPD patients and as an indicator of treatment success. Epigenetic biomarker have already been proposed as both predictors and correlates of symptom improvement in PTSD patients [60] and would also be highly desirable for BPD patients, where they could pave the way towards personalized treatment. In addition to *BDNF* methylation, DNA methylation of *APBA3* (amyloid beta A4 precursor protein-binding family A member 3) and *MCF2* (oncogene MCF2) has recently been proposed as blood-based biomarker for BPD patients. In this case, methylation at the respective genes was proposed as predictor of therapy response [61].

However, recent evidence indicates that saliva might be a superior surrogate tissue to blood for the study of DNA methylation in psychiatric disorders. Cross-tissue comparisons show that saliva mirrors methylation levels in the brain to a greater extent than blood does [62]. This was explicitly shown for a number of CpG sites within *BDNF* [63], even though the explanatory power of the respective study is limited as data on the brain tissue did not originate from the same study cohort from which blood and saliva was sampled. In addition, salivary biomarkers display a much more convenient, non-invasive, and safe method for studying DNA methylation alterations. As such, saliva-based epigenetic biomarkers are universally applicable in in- and out-patient settings.

So far, differential *BDNF* methylation initially found in blood [39, 41], was confirmed to be also present in saliva for bipolar disorder [64], anxiety and depression [65, 66], but has not been investigated for BPD yet. For that reason, we assessed *BDNF* promoter IV methylation in both saliva and blood from the same BPD patients, thereby enabling a direct comparison of methylation levels in both tissues. Further, since Perroud et al. [17] had reported that dialectical behavior therapy (DBT), one of the most frequently applied psychotherapeutic intervention for BPD patients [67], leads to a decrease of previously elevated *BDNF* methylation levels in BPD patients, we sought to replicate this finding by reassessing the blood and salivary *BDNF* methylation in a subsample of patients after a 12-week DBT.

Results
Study population
BPD patients and healthy controls did not differ significantly in age, sex, and alcohol consumption. However, there were significantly more habitual smokers in the group of BPD patients (see Table 1 for details). Further, 85.36% of all BPD patients were under current psychopharmacological medication at the time of sampling, as opposed to 0% in the healthy control group. BPD patients scored significantly higher in the BSL23 (Borderline Symptom List 23), SCL90R (Symptom Checklist-90-revised), and Childhood Trauma Questionnaire (CTQ).

Table 1 Comparison of BPD patient and healthy control cohorts

	BPD patients (T1)	Healthy controls	p value
N	41	41	
Age	30.4 ± 8.6	30.7 ± 9.3	n.s.
Proportion of women (%)	85.36%	85.36%	n.s.
Proportion of individuals who are			
Habitual smokers	53.65%	9.76%	< 0.001
Habitual drinkers	85.37%	95.12%	n.s.
Under current medication*	85.36%	0%	< 0.001
Psychiatric questionnaires			
GSI score (SCL90R)	2.1 ± 0.54	0.27 ± 0.24	< 0.001
PST score (SCL90R)	69.88 ± 9.15	17.8 ± 13	< 0.001
BSL23 total score	2.48 ± 0.76	0.17 ± 0.23	< 0.001
CTQ total score	62.9 ± 24.4	33.93 ± 8.47	< 0.001

Age and results from self-administered psychiatric questionnaires are displayed as mean ± standard deviation. p values derive from statistical analysis with independent *t* test or chi-square test for comparison of percentages
*Psychopharmacological medication only
n.s. not significant (p value > 0.05)

Higher *BDNF* IV promoter methylation levels in saliva, but not blood, of BPD patients as compared to healthy controls

In saliva samples, DNA methylation was significantly higher in BPD patients than in healthy controls at all four analyzed CpG sites within the *BDNF* IV promoter ($p < 0.001$ for all sites, Fig. 1, see Table 2 for details). Further, the average methylation level calculated from all analyzed sites was higher in BPD patients than in healthy controls (M = 6.9%, SE = 0.19 vs. M = 4.3%, SE = 0.20, M = mean, SE = standard error). This difference, – 2.6%, 95% CI [– 3.163, – 2.061] was significant (t (80) = – 9.431, p value = 1.26×10^{-14}) and represented a large effect (Cohen's d = 2.1). These differences between BPD patients and healthy controls were also significant after including smoking behavior and experience of ELS as covariates into a general linear model to predict DNA methylation (b = 2.33, SE = 0.38, 95% CI [1.571, 3.058], β = 0.65, t (78) = 6.123, p value = 3.46×10^{-8} for average methylation). Neither covariate had a significant influence on DNA methylation in the model for any of the analyzed CpG sites (see Additional file 1: Table S2, for detailed results) and their addition to the model resulted in an average change in estimate (CIE) of 3.4% (smoking) and 10.2% (ELS). In DNA isolated from whole blood, *BDNF* methylation levels did not differ significantly between BPD patients and healthy controls neither for single CpG sites, nor for the average calculated from all sites (patient average 9.0% vs. healthy controls average 8.9%, detailed data in Additional file 1: Table S1). In line with this, multiple

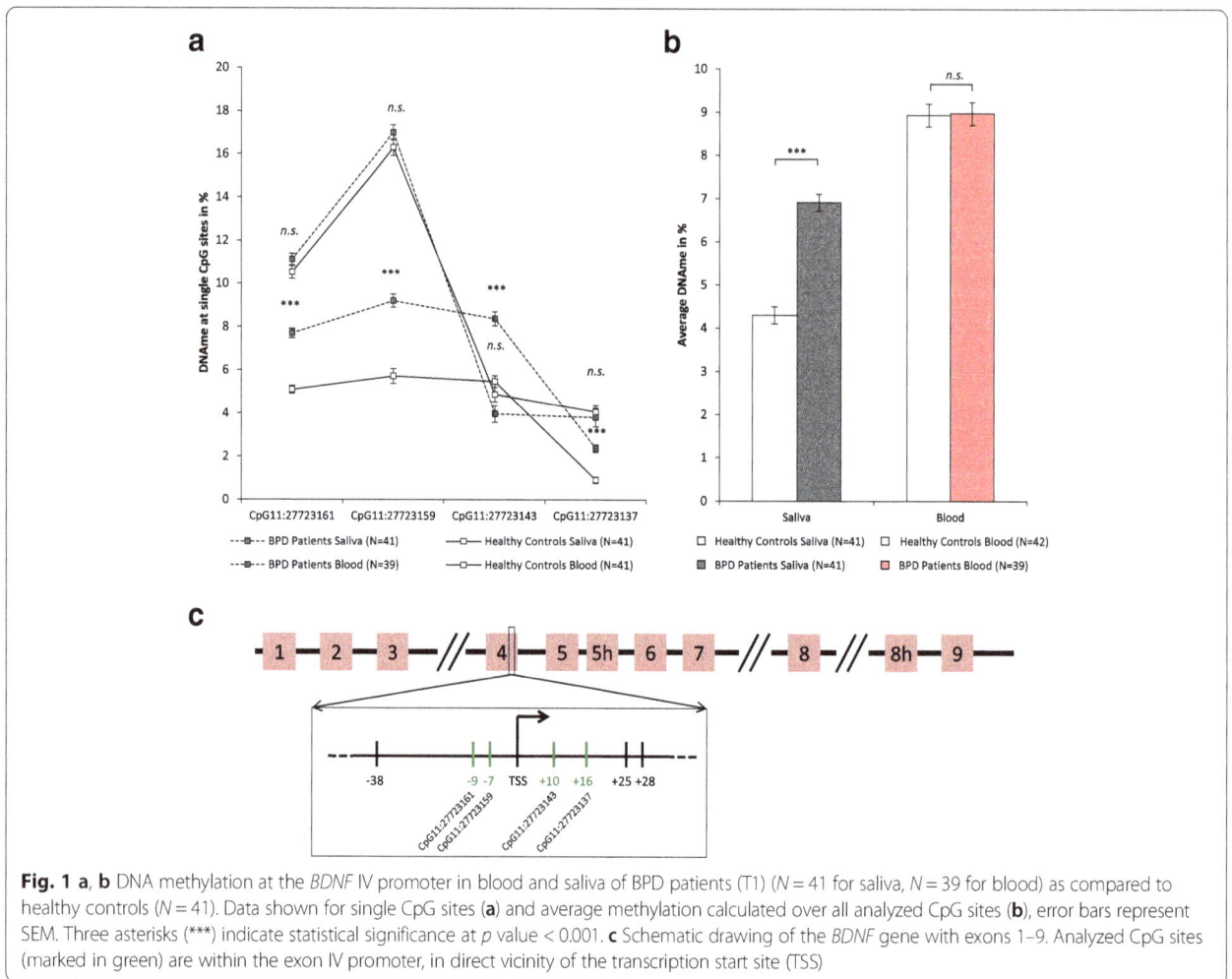

Fig. 1 a, b DNA methylation at the *BDNF* IV promoter in blood and saliva of BPD patients (T1) (*N* = 41 for saliva, *N* = 39 for blood) as compared to healthy controls (*N* = 41). Data shown for single CpG sites (**a**) and average methylation calculated over all analyzed CpG sites (**b**), error bars represent SEM. Three asterisks (***) indicate statistical significance at *p* value < 0.001. **c** Schematic drawing of the *BDNF* gene with exons 1–9. Analyzed CpG sites (marked in green) are within the exon IV promoter, in direct vicinity of the transcription start site (TSS)

regression analysis showed no effect of group, smoking, or ELS on the blood DNA methylation at all analyzed CpG sites (see Additional file 1: Table S2 for detailed results).

No correlation between the blood and salivary *BDNF* IV methylation

We compared *BDNF* IV promoter methylation in the saliva and blood of patients and controls and did neither find any significant correlation (Pearson's correlation coefficient) in the combined cohort (*N* = 80) nor in the BPD patient cohort alone (*N* = 39). In the healthy cohort

(*N* = 41), CpG11:27723143 and the average methylation were significantly but weakly correlated between both tissues (CpG11:27723143: *r* = 0.33, *p* = 0.035, 95% CI [0.088, 0.515]; average methylation: *r* = 0.33, *p* = 0.036, 95% CI [0.096, 0.574]) (Fig. 2, see Additional file 1: Table S4 for all data).

Decrease of salivary DNA methylation levels in BPD patients following psychotherapeutic intervention

Following psychotherapeutic intervention, patients (*N* = 26) showed a significant reduction in general and BPD-specific

Table 2 Statistics for the comparison of saliva *BDNF* methylation in BPD patients and healthy controls

CpG site	Mean difference	CI lower	CI upper	*p* value	Cohen's *d*
CpG11:27723161	− 2.6	− 3.181	− 2.047	3.966×10^{-14}	2.1
CpG11:27723159	− 3.5	− 4.392	− 2.556	6.637×10^{-10}	1.7
CpG11:27723143	− 2.9	− 3.725	− 2.064	9.387×10^{-9}	0.9
CpG11:27723137	− 1.5	− 1.922	− 1.007	1.110×10^{-8}	1.5
Average	− 2.6	− 3.163	− 2.061	1.255×10^{-14}	2.1

Results of independent *t* test for salivary *BDNF* IV promoter methylation in BPD patients (T1) and healthy controls. Results shown for individual CpG sites and average calculated from all sites

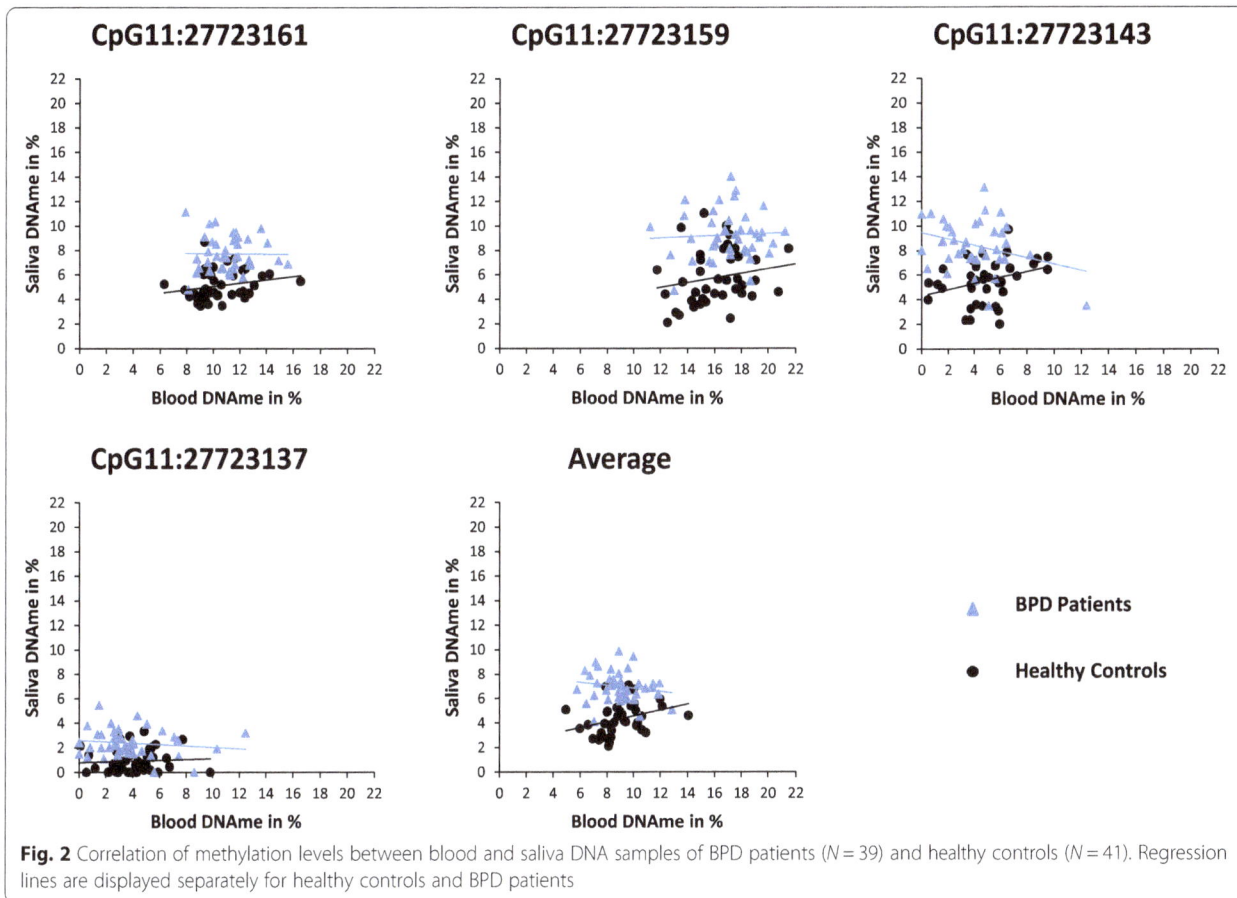

Fig. 2 Correlation of methylation levels between blood and saliva DNA samples of BPD patients (*N* = 39) and healthy controls (*N* = 41). Regression lines are displayed separately for healthy controls and BPD patients

psychiatric symptoms, as assessed by SCL90R and BSL23, respectively (Table 3).

After treatment, salivary DNA methylation at *BDNF* IV promoter decreased at all analyzed CpG sites (Fig. 3a–c, Table 4), though the effect was significant only for CpG11: 27723161, CpG11:27723143, and the average calculated from all sites, where *BDNF* methylation decreased from 7.2 to 6.5% (mean difference = − 0.7%, SE = 0.33, 95% CI [− 1.370,-0.019], *t* (25) = − 2.118, *p* value = 0.044, Cohen's *d* = 0.4). Analysis of changes in individual patients revealed that DNA methylation levels remained unchanged (difference less than 0.5%) in seven out of 26 patients. Of the remaining 19 patients, 14 showed decreased, and five increased methylation levels. However, the observed change in DNA methylation did not correlate with

Table 3 Psychiatric symptoms of BPD patients before and after DBT

	Before treatment	After treatment	*p* value
GSI score (SCL90R)	2.03 ± 0.46	1.49 ± 0.67	< 0.001
PST score (SCL90R)	69.0 ± 8.79	59.31 ± 14.29	0.001
BSL23 total score	2.29 ± 0.75	1.86 ± 0.77	0.012

Results from self-administered psychiatric questionnaires of 26 BPD patients before and after 12-week psychotherapeutic treatment (DBT) as means ± standard deviation. *p* values derive from statistical analysis with *t* test for paired samples

symptom reduction in individual patients (Additional file 1: Table S5). Blood DNA methylation did not change from T1 to T2, neither for single CpG sites nor for the average calculated from all sites (8.7% vs. 8.6%, mean difference = − 0.1%, SE = 0.48, 95% CI [− 1.124,0.860], *t* (22) = − 0.276, *p* value = 0.785) (Fig. 3d–f, Additional file 1: Table S3).

Discussion

We assessed *BDNF* IV promoter methylation in blood and saliva of the same individuals and found no correlation between the tissues. This has been reported previously [63], even though there is evidence for a correlation between blood and saliva methylation on a genome-wide level [62].

When comparing *BDNF* methylation in BPD patients and healthy controls, we unexpectedly did not find differences in DNA extracted from blood, as had previously been reported [17] (Table 5). One reason for this discrepancy might be that Perroud et al. [17] had analyzed the average methylation level calculated from a longer section of the *BDNF* IV promoter and did not report individual CpG methylation. Therefore, our assay might not have covered the relevant CpG sites. Further, the different methods used for DNA methylation analysis (high resolution melt analysis in [17] vs. pyrosequencing

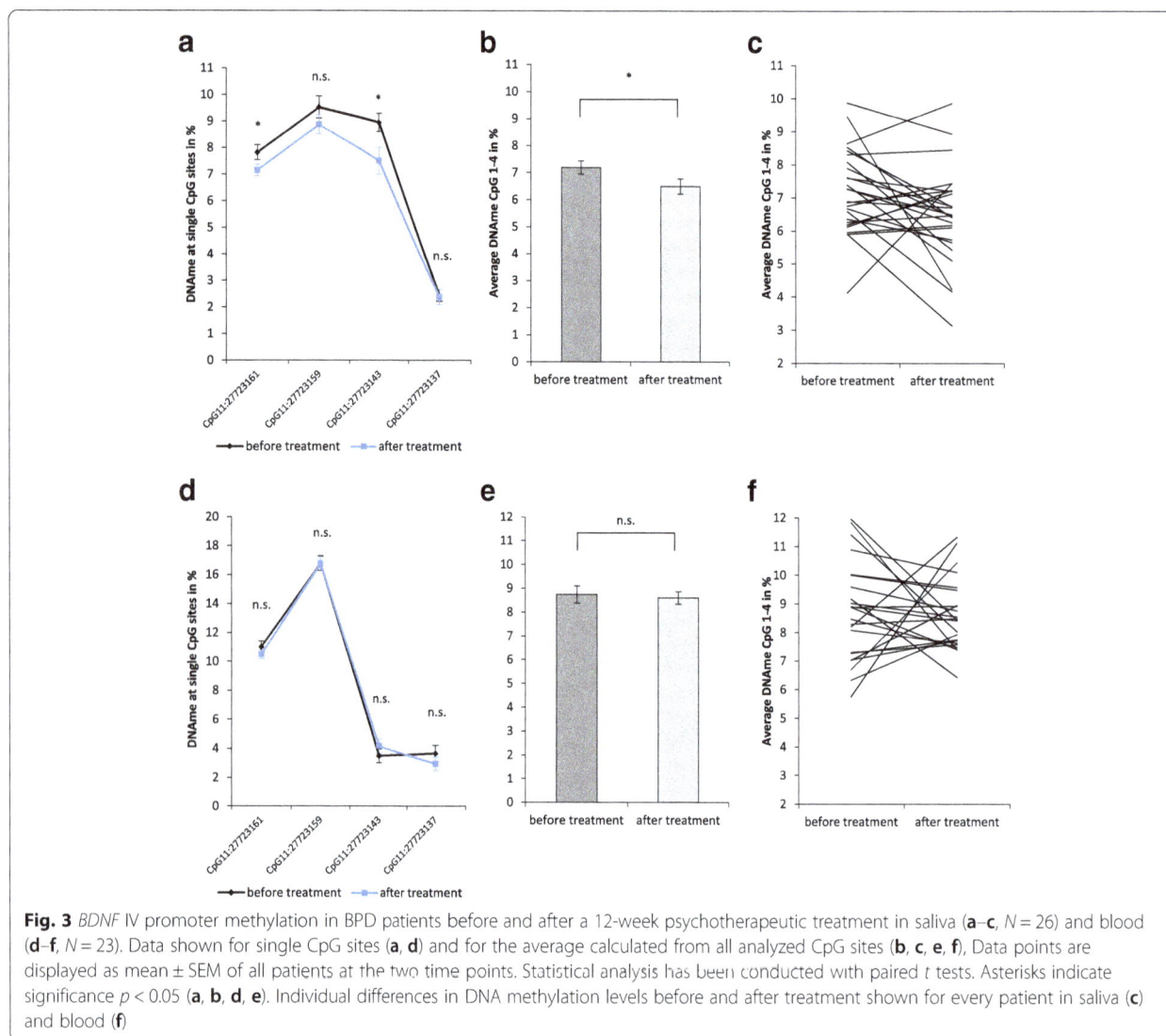

Fig. 3 *BDNF* IV promoter methylation in BPD patients before and after a 12-week psychotherapeutic treatment in saliva (**a–c**, *N* = 26) and blood (**d–f**, *N* = 23). Data shown for single CpG sites (**a**, **d**) and for the average calculated from all analyzed CpG sites (**b**, **c**, **e**, **f**), Data points are displayed as mean ± SEM of all patients at the two time points. Statistical analysis has been conducted with paired *t* tests. Asterisks indicate significance *p* < 0.05 (**a**, **b**, **d**, **e**). Individual differences in DNA methylation levels before and after treatment shown for every patient in saliva (**c**) and blood (**f**)

in our study) may have contributed to the conflicting results. With regard to the absolute levels of *BDNF,* the low levels of DNA methylation observed in our study (3-17%) were still higher than previously described for the respective CpG sites (< 5%) [20, 42]. Similarly, this discrepancy may be partially due to methodological differences (Epi-TYPER in [20]) and ethnical differences of the study cohort (Japanese cohort in [42] as compared to Caucasian cohort in the present study). Our finding of the unaltered blood DNA methylation of the *BDNF* IV promoter in BPD patients is supported by epigenome-wide studies, which also failed to provide evidence for differential *BDNF* promoter IV methylation in the blood of BPD patients [18, 19].

Table 4 Statistics for the comparison of saliva *BDNF* methylation in BPD patients before and after therapy

CpG site	Mean difference	CI lower	CI upper	*p* value	Cohen's *d*
CpG11:27723161	− 0.7	− 1.303	− 0.011	0.047	0.4
CpG11:27723159	− 0.6	− 1.562	0.282	0.165	n.a.
CpG11:27723143	− 1.4	− 2.542	− 0.324	0.013	0.5
CpG11:27723137	− 0.0	− 0.660	0.561	0.871	n.a.
Average	− 0.7	− 1.370	− 0.019	0.044	0.4

Results of paired *t* tests for salivary *BDNF* IV promoter methylation in BPD patients before (T1) and after treatment (T2) (*N* = 26). Results shown for individual CpG sites and for the average calculated from all sites
n.a. not applicable (*p* value > 0.05)

Table 5 Genomic position of analyzed CpGs within *BDNF* IV promoter

ID	Genomic position (hg19)	Differential DNAme in the context of psychiatric disorders previously analyzed in …
CpG11:27723161	chr 11: 27,723,161–27,723,162	Blood [17, 20]and saliva [68]
CpG11:27723159	chr 11: 27,723,159–27,723,160	Blood [17, 20]and saliva [68]
CpG11:27723143	chr 11: 27,723,143–27,723,144	Blood [17, 42], saliva [68], and brain [44]
CpG11:27723137	chr 11: 27,723,137–27,723,138	Blood [17, 42] and brain [44]

In contrast to the results in blood, we found significant hypermethylation of the *BDNF* IV promoter in saliva of BPD patients as compared to healthy controls. While our study is the first to analyze *BDNF* methylation in saliva samples of BPD patients, few other studies have analyzed salivary DNA methylation at the same sites within the *BDNF* IV promoter in the context of other psychiatric conditions. These studies support an association of saliva *BDNF* hypermethylation with symptoms of psychiatric diseases [21, 65, 68]. Further, the low absolute levels of saliva *BDNF* DNA methylation observed in our study (2–10%) were comparable to those previously reported in the literature, though the exact percentage of reported methylation varies between studies (1–30%). While Moser et al. report DNA methylation levels ranging from 1 to 30% in the exon IV promoter region [21], Chagnon et al. observed levels around 2–3% [65] and Januar et al. report levels between 4 and 17% [68]. Since analysis methods and study cohorts are at least partially comparable, the most likely explanation for this discrepancy is the variability in the number of CpG sites analyzed and the method of summarization of these data into reported methylation scores. However, the observed range of the saliva DNA methylation at the analyzed CpG sites in the present study is similar to the levels reported by Keller et al. [44] in human post-mortem brain tissue at the same CpG sites (5–11%). This finding further supports the significance of saliva as surrogate tissue for the brain in the study of psychiatric disorders.

Since differences in methylation between BPD patients and healthy controls were only evident in saliva, but not blood, our findings underline the importance of considering tissue-specificity of DNA methylation in biomarker studies. Salivary DNA derives from exfoliated epithelial cells and leukocytes, which migrate from the blood stream to the oral cavity [69]. Both cell types are known to express *BDNF*, though within leukocytes, all *BDNF* expression is driven by lymphocytes [70]. As there is indication for an enrichment of lymphocytes in oral samples as compared to blood [69], differential epigenetic regulation of this particular cell type may be more evident in saliva than in blood. In addition, the observed effects may also be driven by epithelial cells, as submandibular serous and ductal cells are sources of salivary BDNF protein [71] and

may therefore be dynamically regulated. Further, *BDNF* overexpression derived from salivary glands was found to influence BDNF levels in the blood and hippocampus and exert anxiolytic effects on behavior [72]. This supports a functional role for *BDNF* methylation in salivary epithelial cells. Additional studies are necessary in order to determine whether the observed alterations in salivary *BDNF* IV promoter methylation are accompanied by changes in *BDNF* expression and how these relate to psychological symptoms of BPD. However, the past years of research have shown that even small alterations in DNA methylation ($\Delta < 5\%$), as have been observed in this study, can be functionally relevant, i.e., exert influence on gene transcription [73, 74]. In fact, previous studies report similarly small changes in *BDNF* methylation associated with psychiatric symptoms ($\Delta = 0.42\%$ in [65], $\Delta = 5.4\%$ in [68]), and these findings are in accordance with the understanding of the multifactorial origin of psychiatric disorders [75]. In addition, the subtle differences in methylation in *BDNF* DNA methylation may also reflect the "tip of the iceberg," i.e., the measurable output of a complex, masked pattern of stronger, cell type-specific differential methylation. In this case, effects may be driven by buccal epithelial cells or different leukocyte subtypes contained in the saliva, as previously described in more detail. However, the detailed mechanisms underlying the differential *BDNF* IV promoter methylation in BPD patients are irrelevant to the validity of the epigenetic signal as biomarker for the disorder. With regard to that, it is important to note that despite the small absolute change, the difference in methylation between BPD patients and controls is significant and the effect size was large (Cohen's $d = 2.1$).

BDNF mRNA and protein levels were not assessed in the present study, and are difficult to assess reliably in the saliva, where protein levels are below the detection limit [76]. However, there is evidence for reduced levels of serum BDNF protein in BPD patients from previous studies [53], which is what would be expected as consequence of *BDNF* promoter hypermethylation [77]. In particular, the CpG sites analyzed in the present study are in close vicinity (– 49, – 51, – 65 and – 74 bp) to the binding site of transcription factor cAMP response element binding protein (CREB, half consensus sequence

"CGTCA" [78]). CREB controls *BDNF* transcription in a DNA methylation-dependent manner [77], indicating a plausible effect of the observed methylation difference on gene expression. Further support for the relevance of *BDNF* IV promoter hypermethylation for BPD is provided by animal experiments. These show that disruption of *BDNF* IV promoter-dependent expression results in deficits in prefrontal signaling [79–81], neurobiological changes which are also observed in BPD [82].

Lastly, we found that the level of salivary, but not blood *BDNF* IV methylation significantly decreases after patients underwent a 12-week psychotherapeutic treatment. This is particularly interesting, since the hereof predicted biological consequence, increased expression of *BDNF*, is also observed in response to antidepressant and mood-stabilizing pharmacological treatment and clinical improvement of BPD [55–59]. BPD patients did not experience any change of pharmacological treatment immediately before and during study participation. Therefore, the observed effects are unlikely to derive from psychopharmacological treatment and may present a true effect of psychotherapy. Our results are consistent with the data obtained by Perroud et al. [17], showing a decrease in *BDNF* IV methylation in BPD patients after the same psychotherapeutic intervention, though they observed the effect in the blood and not saliva. However, while Perroud et al. found the effect to be specific for treatment responders, we did not find differences in methylation change between patients with and without significant improvement of psychological symptoms after therapy. Still, the finding indicates psychotherapy-induced changes in DNA methylation. Therefore, it provides support for the conceptual premise that psychotherapeutic intervention alters biological mechanisms in a way that is comparable to pharmacological treatment [83]. Nevertheless, our results need to be interpreted with caution and the specificity of the observed effect remains to be elucidated. A major limitation of both the above-mentioned previous and the current study is the lack of appropriate control groups at the second time point of sampling, i.e., BPD patients and healthy controls without psychotherapeutic intervention. Further, potential bias may have been introduced by the cellular composition of our samples. This should be addressed in future experiments by analysis of isolated cell types, inclusion of cell counts, or application of post hoc statistical deconvolution algorithms if epigenome-wide methylation data is available [84]. One of the major confounders of cellular composition of the saliva is age [85] . However, as our sample of BPD patients and healthy control individuals was matched for age, we can exclude this as a confounder and assume that differences in cellular composition in the saliva introduced random noise rather than a systematic bias to the data. Variables that indeed differed significantly between patient

and control group and have a known influence on *BDNF* IV methylation are smoking, experience of ELS, and intake of pharmacological medication. Smoking is known to exert a broad influence on genome-wide DNA methylation with so far limited understanding of gene-specific effects [30, 31]. We found only little influence of current smoking behavior on *BDNF* DNA methylation. However, we did not assess prenatal exposure to smoking, though it is reported to have an effect on *BDNF* methylation, as well as promote vulnerability to BPD later in life [86]. Consequently, we cannot exclude the influence of prenatal exposure to smoking on the observed differences in the saliva *BDNF* methylation of BPD patients. In addition, there is evidence that ELS, such as childhood maltreatment and abuse, influences *BDNF* IV promoter methylation specifically [24–26] and may therefore have introduced systematic bias in the results. In line with this, the experience of ELS was identified as confounder in our linear model to predict DNA methylation, even though its influence was relatively small (10.2% CIE, $\beta < 0.1$). Therefore, we are not able to fully disentangle the effects of ELS and BPD on *BDNF* IV promoter methylation. Further studies will be necessary to elucidate the potential role of *BDNF* methylation in mediating vulnerability to borderline personality traits conferred by ELS [29]. With regard to intake of medication, the majority of the literature points towards a positive effect of psychopharmacological treatment on BDNF levels both in serum of patients [55, 56] as well as in cell culture experiments [58, 59, 87]. According to the DNA methylation paradigm, this increase of BDNF protein levels would correspond to a decrease in promoter methylation. Since we observed increased methylation in pharmacologically treated subjects, we therefore assume that it is more likely that medication intake has masked potential differences, rather than produced them. Further, medication did not change between T1 and T2 and is therefore unlikely to have caused the observed decrease in DNA methylation in BPD patients in response to treatment. A limitation of our study is the undefined positive predictive power of our findings, since only a limited amount of data on effect sizes for differential *BDNF* methylation in BPD was available a priori. Therefore, even though the size of our sample is in the range of, if not higher than the sample sizes reported from comparable studies (see [16, 17, 19]), the biological relevance of our finding needs to be determined in future studies and the robustness of our findings need to be confirmed by replication in independent cohorts. Further, the so far limited understanding of the dynamics of DNA methylation patterns in human peripheral tissues is increasingly investigated [88] and future studies remain to determine the stability of the observed methylation differences over time and its potential correlation or predictive value for the long-term development of psychiatric symptoms.

Conclusions

We assessed DNA methylation levels at four sites within the *BDNF* IV promoter in blood and, for the first time, saliva of BPD patients and healthy controls and found significant hypermethylation in saliva, but not blood. Further, we found that the level of salivary, but not blood *BDNF* IV methylation significantly decreases after patients underwent a 12-week psychotherapeutic treatment. As such, our study adds to a growing body of evidence for an epigenetic dysregulation of *BDNF* in BPD, even though the previously reported differential methylation in blood [17] was not evident in our study population. Further, our results highlight the importance of considering tissue-specific differences in DNA methylation and suggest the exploration of saliva-based epigenetic biomarkers in psychiatry. Our study is the first to support the validity of *BDNF* IV promoter hypermethylation as a biomarker for BPD in a tissue other than the blood and provides additional indication for the reversal of disease-associated DNA methylation patterns in response to psychotherapy.

Methods
Study population

Forty-one currently hospitalized BPD patients and 41 healthy controls without any history of psychiatric disorders were included in the study. All subjects were of Caucasian origin and both groups were matched for age and sex. BPD patients were diagnosed according to the International Personality Disorder Examination (IPDE) and met at least five diagnostic criteria of BPD as defined in the fourth edition of the Diagnostic and Statistical Manual of Mental Disorders (DSM-IV). All study participants were phenotypically characterized with the following self-report questionnaires: Symptom Checklist 90 (SCL90R) [89], Borderline Symptom List 23 (BSL23) [90], and Childhood Trauma Questionnaire (CTQ) [91]. Further questionnaires assessed demographic information along with information about nicotine and alcohol consumption (AUDIT and Fagerström-Test). GSI (global severity index = average rating given to all items) and PST scores (positive symptom total = number of symptoms/items rated higher than zero) were calculated from SCL90R. Twenty-six BPD patients completed a 12-week psychotherapeutic treatment program (dialectical behavior therapy, DBT) and for these patients, psychological symptoms were assessed a second time after completion of the program using SCL90R and BSL23. Parts of the study cohort are identical to the cohort used in [61] but only those patients with available saliva samples were included and additional patients and controls were included in the present study.

Sampling and DNA extraction

Within the first week of hospital admission (T1), saliva was collected from 41 BPD patients using the Oragene Discover DNA Collection Kit (DNA Genotek, Ottawa, Canada). Saliva from 41 control individuals was collected immediately after study inclusion using the same method. All saliva samples were stored at − 20 °C until further analysis. Venous blood was drawn from 39 of the BPD patients at T1 and from all 41 controls, collected in ethylenediaminetetraacetic acid (EDTA) tubes and stored at − 80 °C until further analysis. From the 26 patients that completed the 12-week psychotherapeutic treatment (DBT), a second saliva sample was collected during the last week of the program (T2). A second blood sample (T2) was available from 23 of these 26 patients. DNA extraction was performed using the prepIT DNA extraction Kit (DNA Genotek) for the saliva and QIAamp DNA Blood Maxi-Kit (Qiagen, Hilden, Germany) for the blood samples.

DNA methylation analysis

Five hundred nanograms genomic DNA was bisulfite converted using the EpiTect Fast Bisulfite Conversion Kit (Qiagen) and the region of interest within the *BDNF* IV promoter was amplified using the PyroMark PCR Kit (Qiagen) according to the manufacturer's instructions. PCR and sequencing primer (Metabion, Planegg, Germany) were as follows: PCR forward primer, 5′- TTT GTT GGG GTT GGA AGT GAA AAT-3′ PCR reverse primer, Biotin-5′- CCC ATC AAC TAA AAA CTC CAT TTA ATC TC-3′ (as in [92]); and sequencing primer, 5′-GTG GAT TTT TAT TTA TTT TTT TAT TTA T-3′.

Successful amplification as well as specificity of the PCR products was verified via agarose gel electrophoresis. Several PCR runs were performed as technical replicates for each sample (minimum two replications). Processing of the PCR amplicons for pyrosequencing analysis was performed according to the manufacturer's protocol and PCR products were then sequenced using the PyroMark Q24 system and the PyroMark GoldReagents (Qiagen). The level of methylation in every sample was quantified using the PyroMark Q24 software version 2.0.6 (Qiagen). The pyrosequencing assay contained six CpG sites within the *BDNF* IV promoter, but only four sites passed pyrosequencing quality control and were used for further analysis (see Table 1 and Fig. 1c for genomic position). Only samples with standard deviation of < 3% between technical replicates were included in the analysis. DNA methylation standards with 0%, 25%, 50%, 75%, and 100% methylation (Qiagen) were used to generate a standard curve and all measurements were calibrated accordingly (see Additional file 1: Figure S1). In all steps of the DNA methylation analysis (bisulfite conversion, PCR, and pyrosequencing), samples were processed in balanced design in order to avoid batch effects.

Statistical analysis

Statistical analysis was performed with SPSS (IBM, version 26). Group mean comparisons were performed with Student's t test. In addition, multiple regression analysis was performed to test the effect of group (BPD T1 vs. healthy controls) on DNA methylation, including smoking behavior (smoker vs. non-smoker) and ELS (CTQ total score) as covariates. Before and after treatment comparisons were performed using paired two-sided Student's t test. Cohen's effect size d for t test comparisons was calculated from the z-score. Differences in percentages between groups were assessed with chi-square test. Bivariate correlation analysis was performed using Pearson's correlation coefficient and 95% percentile bootstrapping was performed.

Abbreviations

BDNF: Brain-derived neurotrophic factor; BPD: Borderline personality disorder; BSL23: Borderline Symptom List 23; cAMP: Cyclic adenosine monophosphate; CIE: Change in estimate; CpG: Cytosine-phosphate-guanine; CREB: cAMP response element binding protein; CTQ: Childhood Trauma Questionnaire; DBT: Dialectical behavior therapy; DNA: Desoxyribonucleic acid; DNAme: DNA methylation; DSM-IV: Diagnostic and Statistical Manual of Mental Disorders IV; EDTA: Ethylenediaminetetraacetic acid; ELS: Early-life stress; GR/NR3C1: Glucocorticoid receptor; GSI: Global Severity Index; HTR2A: Serotonin receptor 2A; IPDE: International Personality Disorder Examination; MAOA: Monoamine oxidase A; MAOB: Monoamine oxidase B; PCR: Polymerase chain reaction; PST: Positive Symptom Total; SCL90R: Symptom Checklist-90-revised; S-COMT: Soluble catechol-O-methyltransferase

Acknowledgements

The authors thank Gisbert Farger and Danuta Altpaß for their assistance with the experimental work and Dr. Daniel Bucher and Ariane Wiegand for proofreading of the manuscript. We acknowledge support by Deutsche Forschungsgemeinschaft and Open Access Publishing Fund of University of Tübingen.

Funding

This work was funded by the NASARD Young Investigator grant (23494) from the Brain & Behavior Research Foundation to VN and by an IZKF grant (PK2015-1-11) to NK and VN. M.T. was supported with a fellowship of the German Academic Scholarship Foundation. The research group is furthermore supported by a grant from the Wilhelm-Schuler-Stiftung to VN.

Authors' contributions

AW and NK recruited study participants, performed pyrosequencing analyses, and contributed with scientific input to the design of the experiment. VN provided funding, designed, and supervised the study. KG performed pyrosequencing analysis, and FG and JBS recruited study participants. CB and MT supervised the experimental work. MT conducted the data analysis and wrote the first draft of the manuscript. VN and AW revised the manuscript critically and provided scientific input. All authors read and approved the final manuscript.

Author details

[1]Department of Psychiatry and Psychotherapy, University Hospital Tübingen, Calwerstr. 14, 72076 Tübingen, Germany. [2]Graduate Training Centre of Neuroscience, University of Tübingen, Tübingen, Germany.

References

1. American Psychiatric Association. Diagnostic and statistical manual of mental disorders. 5th ed. Washington, DC: American Psychiatric Association; 2013.
2. Grant BF, Chou SP, Goldstein RB, Huang B, Stinson FS, Saha TD, Smith SM, Dawson DA, Pulay AJ, Pickering RP, Ruan WJ. Prevalence, correlates, disability, and comorbidity of DSM-IV borderline personality disorder: results from the Wave 2 National Epidemiologic Survey on Alcohol and Related Conditions. J Clin Psychiatry. 2008;69:533–45.
3. Lenzenweger MF, Lane MC, Loranger AW, Kessler RC. DSM-IV personality disorders in the National Comorbidity Survey Replication. Biol Psychiatry. 2007;62:553–64.
4. Reichborn-Kjennerud T. The genetic epidemiology of personality disorders. Dialogues Clin Neurosci. 2010;12:103–14.
5. Gunderson JG, Zanarini MC, Choi-Kain LW, Mitchell KS, Jang KL, Hudson JI. Family study of borderline personality disorder and its sectors of psychopathology. Arch Gen Psychiatry. 2011;68:753–62.
6. Nestler EJ, Pena CJ, Kundakovic M, Mitchell A, Akbarian S. Epigenetic basis of mental illness. Neuroscientist. 2016;22(5):447-63.
7. Mostafavi Abdolmaleky H. Horizons of psychiatric genetics and epigenetics: where are we and where are we heading? Iran J Psychiatry Behav Sci. 2014;8:1–10.
8. Jones PA. Functions of DNA methylation: islands, start sites, gene bodies and beyond. Nat Rev Genet. 2012;13:484–92.
9. Yang X, Han H, De Carvalho DD, Lay FD, Jones PA, Liang G. Gene body methylation can alter gene expression and is a therapeutic target in cancer. Cancer Cell. 2014;26:577–90.
10. Shoemaker R, Deng J, Wang W, Zhang K. Allele-specific methylation is prevalent and is contributed by CpG-SNPs in the human genome. Genome Res. 2010;20:883–9.
11. Kohli RM, Zhang Y. TET enzymes, TDG and the dynamics of DNA demethylation. Nature. 2013;502:472–9.
12. Baker-Andresen D, Ratnu VS, Bredy TW. Dynamic DNA methylation: a prime candidate for genomic metaplasticity and behavioral adaptation. Trends Neurosci. 2013;36:3–13.
13. Leenen FA, Muller CP, Turner JD. DNA methylation: conducting the orchestra from exposure to phenotype? Clin Epigenetics. 2016;8:92.
14. Jones MJ, Moore SR, Kobor MS. Principles and challenges of applying epigenetic epidemiology to psychology. Annu Rev Psychol. 2018;69:459–85.
15. Edgar RD, Jones MJ, Meaney MJ, Turecki G, Kobor MS. BECon: a tool for interpreting DNA methylation findings from blood in the context of brain. Transl Psychiatry. 2017;7:e1187.
16. Dammann G, Teschler S, Haag T, Altmuller F, Tuczek F, Dammann RH. Increased DNA methylation of neuropsychiatric genes occurs in borderline personality disorder. Epigenetics. 2011;6:1454–62.
17. Perroud N, Salzmann A, Prada P, Nicastro R, Hoeppli ME, Furrer S, Ardu S, Krejci I, Karege F, Malafosse A. Response to psychotherapy in borderline personality disorder and methylation status of the BDNF gene. Transl Psychiatry. 2013;3:e207.
18. Prados J, Stenz L, Courtet P, Prada P, Nicastro R, Adouan W, Guillaume S, Olie E, Aubry JM, Dayer A, Perroud N. Borderline personality disorder and childhood maltreatment: a genome-wide methylation analysis. Genes Brain Behav. 2015;14:177–88.
19. Teschler S, Bartkuhn M, Kunzel N, Schmidt C, Kiehl S, Dammann G, Dammann R. Aberrant methylation of gene associated CpG sites occurs in borderline personality disorder. PLoS One. 2013;8:e84180.
20. Thaler L, Gauvin L, Joober R, Groleau P, de Guzman R, Ambalavanan A, Israel M, Wilson S, Steiger H. Methylation of BDNF in women with bulimic eating syndromes: associations with childhood abuse and borderline personality disorder. Prog Neuro-Psychopharmacol Biol Psychiatry. 2014;54:43–9.
21. Moser DA, Paoloni-Giacobino A, Stenz L, Adouan W, Manini A, Suardi F, Cordero MI, Vital M, Sancho Rossignol A, Rusconi-Serpa S, et al. BDNF methylation and maternal brain activity in a violence-related sample. PLoS One. 2015;10:e0143427.
22. Kim TY, Kim SJ, Chung HG, Choi JH, Kim SH, Kang JI. Epigenetic alterations of the BDNF gene in combat-related post-traumatic stress disorder. Acta Psychiatr Scand. 2017;135:170–9.
23. Peng H, Zhu Y, Strachan E, Fowler E, Bacus T, Roy-Byrne P, Goldberg J, Vaccarino V, Zhao J. Childhood trauma, DNA methylation of stress-related genes, and depression: findings from two monozygotic twin studies. Psychosom Med. 2018. Publish Ahead of Print.

24. Kundakovic M, Gudsnuk K, Herbstman JB, Tang D, Perera FP, Champagne FA. DNA methylation of BDNF as a biomarker of early-life adversity. Proc Natl Acad Sci U S A. 2015;112:6807–13.

25. Boersma GJ, Lee RS, Cordner ZA, Ewald ER, Purcell RH, Moghadam AA, Tamashiro KL. Prenatal stress decreases Bdnf expression and increases methylation of Bdnf exon IV in rats. Epigenetics. 2014;9:437–47.

26. Roth TL, Lubin FD, Funk AJ, Sweatt JD. Lasting epigenetic influence of early-life adversity on the BDNF gene. Biol Psychiatry. 2009;65:760–9.

27. Daskalakis NP, De Kloet ER, Yehuda R, Malaspina D, Kranz TM. Early life stress effects on glucocorticoid-BDNF interplay in the hippocampus. Front Mol Neurosci. 2015;8:68.

28. Jeanneteau F, Chao MV. Are BDNF and glucocorticoid activities calibrated? Neuroscience. 2013;239:173–95.

29. Pietrek C, Elbert T, Weierstall R, Muller O, Rockstroh B. Childhood adversities in relation to psychiatric disorders. Psychiatry Res. 2013;206:103–10.

30. Lee KW, Pausova Z. Cigarette smoking and DNA methylation. Front Genet. 2013;4:132.

31. Philibert RA, Beach SR, Brody GH. The DNA methylation signature of smoking: an archetype for the identification of biomarkers for behavioral illness. Neb Symp Motiv. 2014;61:109–27.

32. Toledo-Rodriguez M, Lotfipour S, Leonard G, Perron M, Richer L, Veillette S, Pausova Z, Paus T. Maternal smoking during pregnancy is associated with epigenetic modifications of the brain-derived neurotrophic factor-6 exon in adolescent offspring. Am J Med Genet B Neuropsychiatr Genet. 2010;153B:1350–4.

33. Talati A, Odgerel Z, Wickramaratne PJ, Weissman MM. Brain derived neurotrophic factor moderates associations between maternal smoking during pregnancy and offspring behavioral disorders. Psychiatry Res. 2016;245:387–91.

34. Xiao L, Kish VL, Benders KM, Wu ZX. Prenatal and early postnatal exposure to cigarette smoke decreases BDNF/TrkB signaling and increases abnormal behaviors later in life. Int J Neuropsychopharmacol. 2016;19(5):pyv117.

35. Yochum C, Doherty-Lyon S, Hoffman C, Hossain MM, Zelikoff JT, Richardson JR. Prenatal cigarette smoke exposure causes hyperactivity and aggressive behavior: role of altered catecholamines and BDNF. Exp Neurol. 2014;254:145–52.

36. Jamal M, Van der Does W, Elzinga BM, Molendijk ML, Penninx BW. Association between smoking, nicotine dependence, and BDNF Val66Met polymorphism with BDNF concentrations in serum. Nicotine Tob Res. 2015;17:323–9.

37. Colle R, Trabado S, Rotenberg S, Brailly-Tabard S, Benyamina A, Aubin HJ, Hardy P, Falissard B, Becquemont L, Verstuyft C, et al. Tobacco use is associated with increased plasma BDNF levels in depressed patients. Psychiatry Res. 2016;246:370–2.

38. Bus BA, Molendijk ML, Penninx BJ, Buitelaar JK, Kenis G, Prickaerts J, Elzinga BM, Voshaar RC. Determinants of serum brain-derived neurotrophic factor. Psychoneuroendocrinology. 2011;36:228–39.

39. D'Addario C, Dell'Osso B, Palazzo MC, Benatti B, Lietti L, Cattaneo E, Galimberti D, Fenoglio C, Cortini F, Scarpini E, et al. Selective DNA methylation of BDNF promoter in bipolar disorder: differences among patients with BDI and BDII. Neuropsychopharmacology. 2012;37:1647–55.

40. Carlberg L, Scheibelreiter J, Hassler MR, Schloegelhofer M, Schmoeger M, Ludwig B, Kasper S, Aschauer H, Egger G, Schosser A. Brain-derived neurotrophic factor (BDNF)-epigenetic regulation in unipolar and bipolar affective disorder. J Affect Disord. 2014;168:399–406.

41. Fuchikami M, Morinobu S, Segawa M, Okamoto Y, Yamawaki S, Ozaki N, Inoue T, Kusumi I, Koyama T, Tsuchiyama K, Terao T. DNA methylation profiles of the brain-derived neurotrophic factor (BDNF) gene as a potent diagnostic biomarker in major depression. PLoS One. 2011;6:e23881.

42. Ikegame T, Bundo M, Sunaga F, Asai T, Nishimura F, Yoshikawa A, Kawamura Y, Hibino H, Tochigi M, Kakiuchi C, et al. DNA methylation analysis of BDNF gene promoters in peripheral blood cells of schizophrenia patients. Neurosci Res. 2013;77:208–14.

43. Kim JM, Kang HJ, Kim SY, Kim SW, Shin IS, Kim HR, Park MH, Shin MG, Yoon JH, Yoon JS. BDNF promoter methylation associated with suicidal ideation in patients with breast cancer. Int J Psychiatry Med. 2015;49:75–94.

44. Keller S, Sarchiapone M, Zarrilli F, Videtic A, Ferraro A, Carli V, Sacchetti S, Lembo F, Angiolillo A, Jovanovic N, et al. Increased BDNF promoter methylation in the Wernicke area of suicide subjects. Arch Gen Psychiatry. 2010;67:258–67.

45. Mitchelmore C, Gede L. Brain derived neurotrophic factor: epigenetic regulation in psychiatric disorders. Brain Res. 2014;1586:162–72.

46. Zheleznyakova GY, Cao H, Schioth HB. BDNF DNA methylation changes as a biomarker of psychiatric disorders: literature review and open access database analysis. Behav Brain Funct. 2016;12:17.

47. Cunha C, Brambilla R, Thomas KL. A simple role for BDNF in learning and memory? Front Mol Neurosci. 2010;3:1.

48. Binder DK, Scharfman HE. Brain-derived neurotrophic factor. Growth Factors. 2004;22:123–31.

49. Sen S, Duman R, Sanacora G. Serum brain-derived neurotrophic factor, depression, and antidepressant medications: meta-analyses and implications. Biol Psychiatry. 2008;64:527–32.

50. Bus BA, Molendijk ML, Tendolkar I, Penninx BW, Prickaerts J, Elzinga BM, Voshaar RC. Chronic depression is associated with a pronounced decrease in serum brain-derived neurotrophic factor over time. Mol Psychiatry. 2015;20:602–8.

51. Fernandes BS, Molendijk ML, Kohler CA, Soares JC, Leite CM, Machado-Vieira R, Ribeiro TL, Silva JC, Sales PM, Quevedo J, et al. Peripheral brain-derived neurotrophic factor (BDNF) as a biomarker in bipolar disorder: a meta-analysis of 52 studies. BMC Med. 2015;13:289.

52. Green MJ, Matheson SL, Shepherd A, Weickert CS, Carr VJ. Brain-derived neurotrophic factor levels in schizophrenia: a systematic review with meta-analysis. Mol Psychiatry. 2011;16:960–72.

53. Koenigsberg HW, Yuan P, Diaz GA, Guerreri S, Dorantes C, Mayson S, Zamfirescu C, New AS, Goodman M, Manji HK, Siever LJ. Platelet protein kinase C and brain-derived neurotrophic factor levels in borderline personality disorder patients. Psychiatry Res. 2012;199:92–7.

54. Autry AE, Monteggia LM. Brain-derived neurotrophic factor and neuropsychiatric disorders. Pharmacol Rev. 2012;64:238–58.

55. Ricken R, Adli M, Lange C, Krusche E, Stamm TJ, Gaus S, Koehler S, Nase S, Bschor T, Richter C, et al. Brain-derived neurotrophic factor serum concentrations in acute depressive patients increase during lithium augmentation of antidepressants. J Clin Psychopharmacol. 2013;33:806–9.

56. Tunca Z, Ozerdem A, Ceylan D, Yalcin Y, Can G, Resmi H, Akan P, Ergor G, Aydemir O, Cengisiz C, Kerim D. Alterations in BDNF (brain derived neurotrophic factor) and GDNF (glial cell line-derived neurotrophic factor) serum levels in bipolar disorder: the role of lithium. J Affect Disord. 2014;166:193–200.

57. Molendijk ML, Bus BA, Spinhoven P, Penninx BW, Kenis G, Prickaerts J, Voshaar RC, Elzinga BM. Serum levels of brain-derived neurotrophic factor in major depressive disorder: state-trait issues, clinical features and pharmacological treatment. Mol Psychiatry. 2011;16:1088–95.

58. De-Paula VJ, Gattaz WF, Forlenza OV. Long-term lithium treatment increases intracellular and extracellular brain-derived neurotrophic factor (BDNF) in cortical and hippocampal neurons at subtherapeutic concentrations. Bipolar Disord. 2016;18:692–5.

59. Yasuda S, Liang MH, Marinova Z, Yahyavi A, Chuang DM. The mood stabilizers lithium and valproate selectively activate the promoter IV of brain-derived neurotrophic factor in neurons. Mol Psychiatry. 2009;14:51–9.

60. Yehuda R, Daskalakis NP, Desarnaud F, Makotkine I, Lehrner AL, Koch E, Flory JD, Buxbaum JD, Meaney MJ, Bierer LM. Epigenetic biomarkers as predictors and correlates of symptom improvement following psychotherapy in combat veterans with PTSD. Front Psychiatry. 2013;4:118.

61. Knoblich N, Gundel F, Bruckmann C, Becker-Sadzio J, Frischholz C, Nieratschker V. DNA methylation of APBA3 and MCF2 in borderline personality disorder: potential biomarkers for response to psychotherapy. Eur Neuropsychopharmacol. 2018;28:252–63.

62. Langie SAS, Moisse M, Declerck K, Koppen G, Godderis L, Vanden Berghe W, Drury S, De Boever P. Salivary DNA methylation profiling: aspects to consider for biomarker identification. Basic Clin Pharmacol Toxicol. 2017;121(Suppl 3):93–101.

63. Smith AK, Kilaru V, Klengel T, Mercer KB, Bradley B, Conneely KN, Ressler KJ, Binder EB. DNA extracted from saliva for methylation studies of psychiatric traits: evidence tissue specificity and relatedness to brain. Am J Med Genet B Neuropsychiatr Genet. 2015;168B:36–44.

64. Rao JS, Keleshian VL, Klein S, Rapoport SI. Epigenetic modifications in frontal cortex from Alzheimer's disease and bipolar disorder patients. Transl Psychiatry. 2012;2:e132.

65. Chagnon YC, Potvin O, Hudon C, Preville M. DNA methylation and single nucleotide variants in the brain-derived neurotrophic factor (BDNF) and oxytocin receptor (OXTR) genes are associated with anxiety/depression in older women. Front Genet. 2015;6:230.

66. Song Y, Miyaki K, Suzuki T, Sasaki Y, Tsutsumi A, Kawakami N, Shimazu A, Takahashi M, Inoue A, Kan C, et al. Altered DNA methylation status of human brain derived neurotrophis factor gene could be useful as biomarker of depression. Am J Med Genet B Neuropsychiatr Genet. 2014;165B:357–64.

67. Reddy MS, Vijay MS. Empirical reality of dialectical behavioral therapy in borderline personality. Indian J Psychol Med. 2017;39:105–8.

68. Januar V, Ancelin ML, Ritchie K, Saffery R, Ryan J. BDNF promoter methylation and genetic variation in late-life depression. Transl Psychiatry. 2015;5:e619.

69. Theda C, Hwang SH, Czajko A, Loke YJ, Leong P, Craig JM. Quantitation of the cellular content of saliva and buccal swab samples. Sci Rep. 2018;8:6944.

70. Edling AE, Nanavati T, Johnson JM, Tuohy VK. Human and murine lymphocyte neurotrophin expression is confined to B cells. J Neurosci Res. 2004;77:709–17.

71. Saruta J, Fujino K, To M, Tsukinoki K. Expression and localization of brain-derived neurotrophic factor (BDNF) mRNA and protein in human submandibular gland. Acta Histochem Cytochem. 2012;45:211–8.

72. Saruta J, To M, Sugimoto M, Yamamoto Y, Shimizu T, Nakagawa Y, Inoue H, Saito I, Tsukinoki K. Salivary gland derived BDNF overexpression in mice exerts an anxiolytic effect. Int J Mol Sci. 2017;18(9):1902.

73. Murphy SK, Adigun A, Huang Z, Overcash F, Wang F, Jirtle RL, Schildkraut JM, Murtha AP, Iversen ES, Hoyo C. Gender-specific methylation differences in relation to prenatal exposure to cigarette smoke. Gene. 2012;494:36–43.

74. Breton CV, Marsit CJ, Faustman E, Nadeau K, Goodrich JM, Dolinoy DC, Herbstman J, Holland N, LaSalle JM, Schmidt R, et al. Small-magnitude effect sizes in epigenetic end points are important in children's environmental health studies: the Children's Environmental Health and Disease Prevention Research Center's Epigenetics Working Group. Environ Health Perspect. 2017;125:511–26.

75. Sullivan PF, Daly MJ, O'Donovan M. Genetic architectures of psychiatric disorders: the emerging picture and its implications. Nat Rev Genet. 2012;13: 537–51.

76. Vrijen C, Schenk HM, Hartman CA, Oldehinkel AJ. Measuring BDNF in saliva using commercial ELISA: results from a small pilot study. Psychiatry Res. 2017;254:340–6.

77. Zheng F, Zhou X, Moon C, Wang H. Regulation of brain-derived neurotrophic factor expression in neurons. Int J Physiol Pathophysiol Pharmacol. 2012;4:188–200.

78. Zhang X, Odom DT, Koo SH, Conkright MD, Canettieri G, Best J, Chen H, Jenner R, Herbolsheimer E, Jacobsen E, et al. Genome-wide analysis of cAMP-response element binding protein occupancy, phosphorylation, and target gene activation in human tissues. Proc Natl Acad Sci U S A. 2005;102:4459–64.

79. Sakata K, Woo NH, Martinowich K, Greene JS, Schloesser RJ, Shen L, Lu B. Critical role of promoter IV-driven BDNF transcription in GABAergic transmission and synaptic plasticity in the prefrontal cortex. Proc Natl Acad Sci U S A. 2009;106:5942–7.

80. Sakata K, Jin L, Jha S. Lack of promoter IV-driven BDNF transcription results in depression-like behavior. Genes Brain Behav. 2010;9:712–21.

81. Sakata K, Duke SM. Lack of BDNF expression through promoter IV disturbs expression of monoamine genes in the frontal cortex and hippocampus. Neuroscience. 2014;260:265–75.

82. Ruocco AC, Carcone D. A neurobiological model of borderline personality disorder: systematic and integrative review. Harv Rev Psychiatry. 2016;24: 311–29.

83. Barsaglini A, Sartori G, Benetti S, Pettersson-Yeo W, Mechelli A. The effects of psychotherapy on brain function: a systematic and critical review. Prog Neurobiol. 2014;114:1–14.

84. Houseman EA, Accomando WP, Koestler DC, Christensen BC, Marsit CJ, Nelson HH, Wiencke JK, Kelsey KT. DNA methylation arrays as surrogate measures of cell mixture distribution. Bmc Bioinformatics. 2012;13

85. Eipel M, Mayer F, Arent T, Ferreira MR, Birkhofer C, Gerstenmaier U, Costa IG, Ritz-Timme S, Wagner W. Epigenetic age predictions based on buccal swabs are more precise in combination with cell type-specific DNA methylation signatures. Aging (Albany NY). 2016;8:1034–48.

86. Schwarze CE, Hellhammer DH, Frieling H, Mobascher A, Lieb K. Altered DNA methylation status (BDNF gene exon IV) associated with prenatal maternal cigarette smoking in borderline patients and healthy controls. Psychoneuroendocrinology. 2015;61:29.

87. Dwivedi T, Zhang H. Lithium-induced neuroprotection is associated with epigenetic modification of specific BDNF gene promoter and altered expression of apoptotic-regulatory proteins. Front Neurosci. 2014;8:457.

88. Forest M, O'Donnell KJ, Voisin G, Gaudreau H, MacIsaac JL, McEwen LM, Silveira PP, Steiner M, Kobor MS, Meaney MJ, Greenwood CMT. Agreement in DNA methylation levels from the Illumina 450K array across batches, tissues, and time. Epigenetics. 2018;13(1):19-32.

89. Franke GH. Symptom-Checkliste von L.R. Derogatis - Deutsche Version (SCL-90-R). Göttingen: Beltz Test; 2002.

90. Wolf M, Limberger MF, Kleindienst N, Stieglitz RD, Domsalla M, Philipsen A, Steil R, Bohus M. Short version of the borderline symptom list (BSL-23): development and psychometric evaluation. Psychother Psychosom Med Psychol. 2009;59:321–4.

91. Bernstein DP, Stein JA, Newcomb MD, Walker E, Pogge D, Ahluvalia T, Stokes J, Handelsman L, Medrano M, Desmond D, Zule W. Development and validation of a brief screening version of the Childhood Trauma Questionnaire. Child Abuse Negl. 2003;27:169–90.

92. Stenz L, Zewdie S, Laforge-Escarra T, Prados J, La Harpe R, Dayer A, Paoloni-Giacobino A, Perroud N, Aubry JM. BDNF promoter I methylation correlates between post-mortem human peripheral and brain tissues. Neurosci Res. 2015;91:1–7.

10

Triage of high-risk HPV-positive women in population-based screening by miRNA expression analysis in cervical scrapes; a feasibility study

Iris Babion[1], Barbara C. Snoek[1], Putri W. Novianti[1,2], Annelieke Jaspers[1], Nienke van Trommel[3], Daniëlle A. M. Heideman[1], Chris J. L. M. Meijer[1], Peter J. F. Snijders[1], Renske D. M. Steenbergen[1*] and Saskia M. Wilting[4]

Abstract

Background: Primary testing for high-risk HPV (hrHPV) is increasingly implemented in cervical cancer screening programs. Many hrHPV-positive women, however, harbor clinically irrelevant infections, demanding additional disease markers to prevent over-referral and over-treatment. Most promising biomarkers reflect molecular events relevant to the disease process that can be measured objectively in small amounts of clinical material, such as miRNAs. We previously identified eight miRNAs with altered expression in cervical precancer and cancer due to either methylation-mediated silencing or chromosomal alterations. In this study, we evaluated the clinical value of these eight miRNAs on cervical scrapes to triage hrHPV-positive women in cervical screening.

Results: Expression levels of the eight candidate miRNAs in cervical tissue samples ($n = 58$) and hrHPV-positive cervical scrapes from a screening population ($n = 187$) and cancer patients ($n = 38$) were verified by quantitative RT-PCR. In tissue samples, all miRNAs were significantly differentially expressed ($p < 0.05$) between normal, high-grade precancerous lesions (CIN3), and/or cancer. Expression patterns detected in cervical tissue samples were reflected in cervical scrapes, with five miRNAs showing significantly differential expression between controls and women with CIN3 and cancer. Using logistic regression analysis, a miRNA classifier was built for optimal detection of CIN3 in hrHPV-positive cervical scrapes from the screening population and its performance was evaluated using leave-one-out cross-validation. This miRNA classifier consisted of miR-15b-5p and miR-375 and detected a major subset of CIN3 as well as all carcinomas at a specificity of 70%. The CIN3 detection rate was further improved by combining the two miRNAs with HPV16/18 genotyping. Interestingly, both miRNAs affected the viability of cervical cancer cells in vitro.

Conclusions: This study shows that miRNA expression analysis in cervical scrapes is feasible and enables the early detection of cervical cancer, thus underlining the potential of miRNA expression analysis for triage of hrHPV-positive women in cervical cancer screening.

Keywords: miRNA, HPV, Cervical cancer, CIN, Scrape, Triage, Screening, qRT-PCR

* Correspondence: r.steenbergen@vumc.nl
[1]Cancer Center Amsterdam, Department of Pathology, VU University Medical Center, Amsterdam, The Netherlands
Full list of author information is available at the end of the article

Background

Cervical cancer screening by cytological examination of cervical scrapes has largely reduced the incidence and mortality rates of cervical cancer in developed countries due to early detection of well-recognizable and treatable precursor lesions (cervical intraepithelial neoplasia (CIN), graded 1–3) [1]. Persistent infection with high-risk types of the human papillomavirus (hrHPV) is a necessary cause of cervical cancer [2–4]. Testing for hrHPV DNA has been demonstrated to have a higher sensitivity for the detection of cervical high-grade CIN and cancer than the cytology-based Pap smear [5, 6]. Consequently, hrHPV testing has recently been implemented as primary screening method in The Netherlands and various other countries. As hrHPV testing also detects women with clinically irrelevant transient infections, additional triage markers are required to identify women with high-grade CIN lesions who are in need of treatment given their risk of developing cancer. Cytology is the currently recommended triage strategy for hrHPV-positive women. An ideal triage test, however, should be objective (non-morphological), available in a high-throughput format and feasible in low-resource countries. For this purpose, HPV16/18 genotyping has previously been investigated as triage test in cervical cancer screening [7–9]. Additional molecular markers reflecting the underlying carcinogenic process are highly appealing alternatives. These include DNA copy number aberrations and DNA methylation changes in the host cell genome that result in altered coding and non-coding gene expression [3].

MicroRNAs (miRNAs) belong to an abundant class of small non-coding RNAs that post-transcriptionally regulate gene expression [10]. Altered expression of miRNAs has been shown to contribute to human malignancies, including cervical cancer, by influencing expression of oncogenes and tumor suppressor genes and subsequent deregulation of important intracellular pathways (reviewed by [11]). Given their short length of approximately 22 nucleotides, miRNAs are stable biomolecules and are less prone to degradation than their longer counterparts such as mRNAs or long non-coding RNAs [10, 12, 13]. It is therefore not surprising that miRNAs have been suggested and investigated as biomarkers for cancer diagnostics and prognostics [14–16].

To identify miRNAs that are relevant to cervical carcinogenesis, we previously performed an integrative screen combining array-based miRNA expression profiles with DNA copy number aberrations and DNA methylation [17, 18]. This resulted in the identification of five miRNAs for which differential expression was associated with frequently observed chromosomal gains of chromosomes 1q and 3q (miR-9-5p, miR-15b-5p,

miR-28-5p) or losses of chromosome 11q (miR-100-5p, miR-125b-5p), and three miRNAs (miR-149-5p, miR-203a-3p, miR-375) for which gene silencing was mediated by DNA methylation of their respective promoter sequences (Table 1). Functional studies for miR-9, miR-203a, and miR-375 supported the biological relevance of these miRNA alterations, which were found to be involved in proliferation and anchorage independence of HPV-transformed cells [17–19].

In this study, we evaluated the clinical value of the eight either genetically or epigenetically deregulated miRNAs to serve as triage markers on cervical scrapes of hrHPV-positive women in cervical screening. For this purpose, we verified expression of the discovered 8 miR-NAs in 58 cervical tissues and archival cervical scrapes of 225 hrHPV-positive women, built a predictive miRNA classifier, and evaluated its performance for the detection of high-grade CIN and cancer using leave-one-out cross-validation and ROC curve analysis.

Methods

Clinical specimens

Cervical tissue samples consisted of microdissected fresh frozen specimens, of which the majority has previously been used for miRNA microarray analysis [17]. In total, 8 normal cervical epithelial samples, 18 high-grade cervical intraepithelial neoplasia (CIN2–3) lesions, 22 cervical squamous cell carcinomas (SCC), and 11 adenocarcinomas (AC) were included. All but one normal sample were hrHPV-positive. The median age per group was as follows: normal, 35 years (range 31–47); CIN2–3, 34 years (range 26–54); SCC, 48.5 years (range 25–78); and AC, 39 years (range 31–64).

Cervical scrapes of 66 hrHPV-positive women without underlying disease (Pap 1) and 121 women with CIN3 were obtained from a screening population in the Utrecht region that had been collected between January 2010 and December 2011. Original 20 ml samples were

Table 1 Candidate miRNAs

miRNA	Regulation [17]	Potential regulation mechanism [17, 18]	Class [17]
miR-9-5p	Up	Chromosomal gain (1q)	Late
miR-15b-5p	Up	Chromosomal gain (3q)	Late
miR-28-5p	Up	Chromosomal gain (3q)	Early continuous
miR-100-5p	Down	Chromosomal loss (11q)	Late
miR-125b-5p	Down	Chromosomal loss (11q)	Late
miR-149-5p	Down	DNA methylation	Early continuous
miR-203a-3p	Down	DNA methylation	Early continuous
miR-375	Down	DNA methylation	Late

concentrated and stored in 1 ml ThinPrep medium (Hologic, Vilvoorde, Belgium) at − 80 °C. For most samples, HPV genotyping was performed using the general primer GP5+/6 + –mediated PCR-enzyme immunoassay in combination with the luminex genotyping kit HPV GP at the time of sample collection [20, 21]. For samples with sufficient amounts of DNA for which no previous genotyping results were available, we used the HPV-Risk Assay (Self-screen BV, Amsterdam, The Netherlands) to complete our dataset [22]. Women without disease had a median age of 41 years (range 21–61). The median age of women with CIN3 was 35 years (range 22–60). HrHPV-positive scrapes from women with underlying cervical SCC ($n = 29$) and AC ($n = 9$, consisting of 7 AC and 2 adenosquamous carcinomas) [23, 24] were collected at the Antoni van Leeuwenhoek Hospital Amsterdam, The Netherlands, between January 2015 and March 2017. All cervical cancer samples were tested for hrHPV using the HPV-Risk Assay. Women with SCC had a median age of 51 years (range 29–86), and the median age of women with AC was 45 years (range 27–62).

RNA isolation

Total RNA was isolated using TRIzol reagent (Thermo Fisher Scientific, Landsmeer, The Netherlands) according to the manufacturer's instructions. The Qubit® microRNA Assay kit was used to quantify small RNA concentrations on a Qubit® 2.0 Fluorometer (both ThermoFisher Scientific).

Quantitative RT-PCR

Expression of hsa-miR-9-5p, hsa-miR-15b-5p, hsa-miR-28-5p, hsa-miR-100-5p, hsa-miR-125b-5p, hsa-miR-149-5p, hsa-miR-203a-3p, and hsa-miR-375 was measured using TaqMan microRNA assays (000583, 000390, 000411, 000437, 000449, 002255, 000507, 000564; Thermo Fisher Scientific). For cervical scrapes, RNU24, RNU43, U6, U75, hsa-miR-423-3p, and hsa-miR-425-5p were included as potential reference genes (001001, 001095, 001973, 001219, 002626, 001516; Thermo Fisher Scientific).

Reverse transcription (RT) of all targets was multiplexed and validated in comparison to singleplex RT reactions (data not shown). In short, a primer pool was created by combining the specific RT primers. cDNA was synthesized from 20 ng small RNA template if available, for 5 samples the maximum possible amount (< 20 ng) of RNA was used. Each 16 µl reaction contained 6 µl primer pool, 0.3 µl dNTPs (100 mM), 1.5 µl RT buffer, 0.19 µl RNase inhibitor (20 U/µl), and 3 µl Multi-Scribe Reverse Trancriptase (TaqMan microRNA Reverse Transcription kit, Thermo Fisher Scientific). Quantitative PCR reactions were performed on the ViiA™ 7 Real-Time PCR System (Thermo Fisher Scientific) in a 384-well format. Each 10 µl reaction consisted of 5 µl TaqMan® Universal Master Mix II, 0.5 µl miRNA specific TaqMan assays (Thermo Fisher Scientific), 3.5 µl H$_2$O, and 1 µl cDNA. Cycle conditions for cDNA synthesis and PCR were used according to the manufacturer's protocols.

RNU24 and miR-423-3p were selected for normalization in cervical tissue samples and scrapes using our previously published strategy (data not shown) [25]. Data were normalized to the geometric mean Ct of both reference genes applying the $2^{-\Delta C_t}$ method [26]. All samples had a reference gene geometric mean Ct ≤ 32 and were therefore considered to be suitable for miRNA expression analysis.

Statistical analysis

Statistical analysis was performed using R version 3.1.2. For logistic regression, R packages pROC and GRridge were used. The Spearman correlation coefficient (Rho) and associated p value was calculated to assess the agreement between qRT-PCR and previous microarray results. We performed an omnibus Kruskal-Wallis test to compare miRNA expression levels between normal, CIN3, SCC, and AC for each marker. Further, Wilcoxon rank test was applied with a significance level of 0.05 (two-sided) when the omnibus test showed a significant result ($p < 0.05$). p values from the post-hoc test were corrected with Benjamini-Hochberg correction method. Individual miRNA models and multi-miRNA classifiers for the detection of CIN3 were built performing univariable and multivariable logistic regression on square root transformed Ct ratios and evaluated using leave-one-out cross-validation. As a result, predicted probabilities, i.e., values between 0 and 1 representing the risk of an underlying CIN3, were calculated for each sample. For the construction of multi-miRNA classifiers, multivariable logistic regression analysis was followed by backward elimination to select relevant markers. Receiver-operated characteristic (ROC) curve analysis was carried out to evaluate the performance of the miRNA classifiers in detecting CIN3. For comparison of the obtained AUCs with a random classifier with AUC = 0.5, DeLong's test for two correlated ROC curves was used [27].

Cell culture, transfection, and cell viability assay of cervical cancer cell lines

Cervical cancer cell lines SiHa and CaSki were authenticated by STR testing using the Powerplex16 System (Promega, Leiden, The Netherlands) and cultured as described previously [28]. Cells were transiently transfected with 30 nM miRCURY LNA microRNA Power inhibitors for miR-15b-5p and negative control A (4103019, 199006; Exiqon, Vedbaek, Denmark) or 30 nM miRIDIAN microRNA mimics for miR-375 and negative control #2 (C-300682-05, CN-002000-01; GE

Dharmacon, Lafayette, CO, USA). Cells were transfected with Dharmafect 1 (GE Dharmacon) for at least 6 h according to the manufacturer's instructions. After transfection, cells were seeded in triplicate in 96-well plates (2500 cells/well). Cell viability was measured using the fluorometric CellTiter-Blue assay (Promega, Madison, WI, USA) according to the manufacturer's protocol at days 0 and 2. The average measurement of day 0 was subtracted from the measurements at day 2. Each experiment was performed at least two times.

Results

Microarray-based differential miRNA expression in cervical tissue specimens can be verified by qRT-PCR

To confirm our previously obtained microarray results, we used qRT-PCR to determine the expression levels of the eight genetically or epigenetically deregulated miRNAs in normal cervical squamous epithelium ($n = 8$), high-grade CIN lesions (CIN2–3, $n = 18$), SCC ($n = 22$), and AC ($n = 11$) tissue specimens, of which 44 had also been analyzed by microarray [17]. Except for miR-28-5p and miR-100-5p (Spearman correlation coefficient (Rho) = 0.521 and Rho = 0.645, respectively), qRT-PCR results strongly correlated with microarray results as indicated by Rho > 0.75 (Additional file 1: Figure S1). Because of the low correlations observed for miR-28-5p and miR-100-5p, both miRNAs were excluded from further analysis. Significantly differential expression between normal and CIN2-3 could be verified for 1 out of 2 upregulated miRNAs (miR-9-5p) and for 2 out of 4 downregulated miRNAs (miR-149-5p, miR-203a-3p; Additional file 2: Figure S2 and Additional file 3: Table S1). Downregulation of miR-375 in CIN2-3 compared to normal was borderline significant ($p = 0.067$). All miRNAs showed significantly differential expression between normal and SCC.

Differential miRNA expression is reflected in cervical scrapes

Next we analyzed whether altered expression of candidate miRNAs is also detectable in cervical scrapes. HrHPV-positive scrapes of women without cervical disease (normal, $n = 66$) or with underlying CIN3 ($n = 121$), SCC ($n = 29$), or AC ($n = 9$) were analyzed by qRT-PCR. All six miRNAs except for miR-9-5p could be detected in at least 99% of samples. MiR-9-5p remained undetected in about one fourth (23%, 49/212) of samples. Low expression levels of miR-9-5p were consistent with microarray and qRT-PCR results obtained in cervical tissue specimens (Fig. 1, Additional file 2: Figure S2). Because reproducibility is reduced and technical PCR noise increases when amplifying lowly abundant transcripts [29–31], we did not consider miR-9-5p a suitable biomarker and excluded it from further analysis. MiRNA

expression results obtained in hrHPV-positive cervical scrapes were generally comparable to those obtained in tissue samples (Fig. 1, Additional file 2: Figure S2 and Additional file 4: Table S2). Expression of miR-15b-5p was significantly increased in scrapes of women with CIN3 compared to controls, while miR-125b-5p and miR-375 were significantly downregulated in scrapes of women with CIN3. No significant difference between normal and CIN3 was observed for miR-149-5p and miR-203a-3p. Similar to observations in tissue samples, the largest expression change between scrapes of women with CIN3 and SCC was observed for upregulated miR-15b-5p. Expression of miR-149-5p and miR-375 was significantly decreased in scrapes of women with SCC compared to normal and CIN3. Comparison of normal controls to AC showed a significant increase in expression of all upregulated miRNAs in scrapes of AC patients. In accordance with tissue results, miR-125b-5p and miR-149-5p were significantly downregulated between normal and AC, and miR-375 did not show a significant difference between normal scrapes and those of women with AC.

Predictive miRNA classifier detects large subset of CIN3 lesions

Univariate logistic regression analysis was carried out on expression results of the five remaining markers (miR-15b-5p, miR-125b-5p, miR-149-5p, miR-203a-3p and miR-375) obtained from hrHPV-positive cervical scrapes of women without cervical disease and women with underlying CIN3, and validated by leave-one-out cross-validation. Single miRNAs achieved areas under the curve (AUC) varying from 0.523 (miR-203a-3p) to 0.605 (miR-125b-5p, Table 2, Fig. 2a).

To determine the most discriminative miRNA marker panel for CIN3, we performed multivariable logistic regression analysis followed by backward marker selection and validated results by leave-one-out cross-validation. This resulted in a 2-miRNA classifier consisting of miR-15b-5p and miR-375 with an AUC of 0.622 and optimal sensitivity and specificity of 55 and 70%, respectively (Table 2, Fig. 2b). Adding additional miRNAs to the 2-marker panel did not further improve performance.

MiRNA classifier detects all cervical carcinomas

To test how our miRNA classifiers performed in the detection of cervical carcinomas, we applied the previously determined regression models and corresponding cutoffs to our results obtained on cervical scrapes of women with underlying SCC or AC. The 2-miRNA classifier detected all SCC and all AC (Table 3). Overall, the 2-miRNA classifier achieved a CIN3+ detection rate of 65% at 70% specificity.

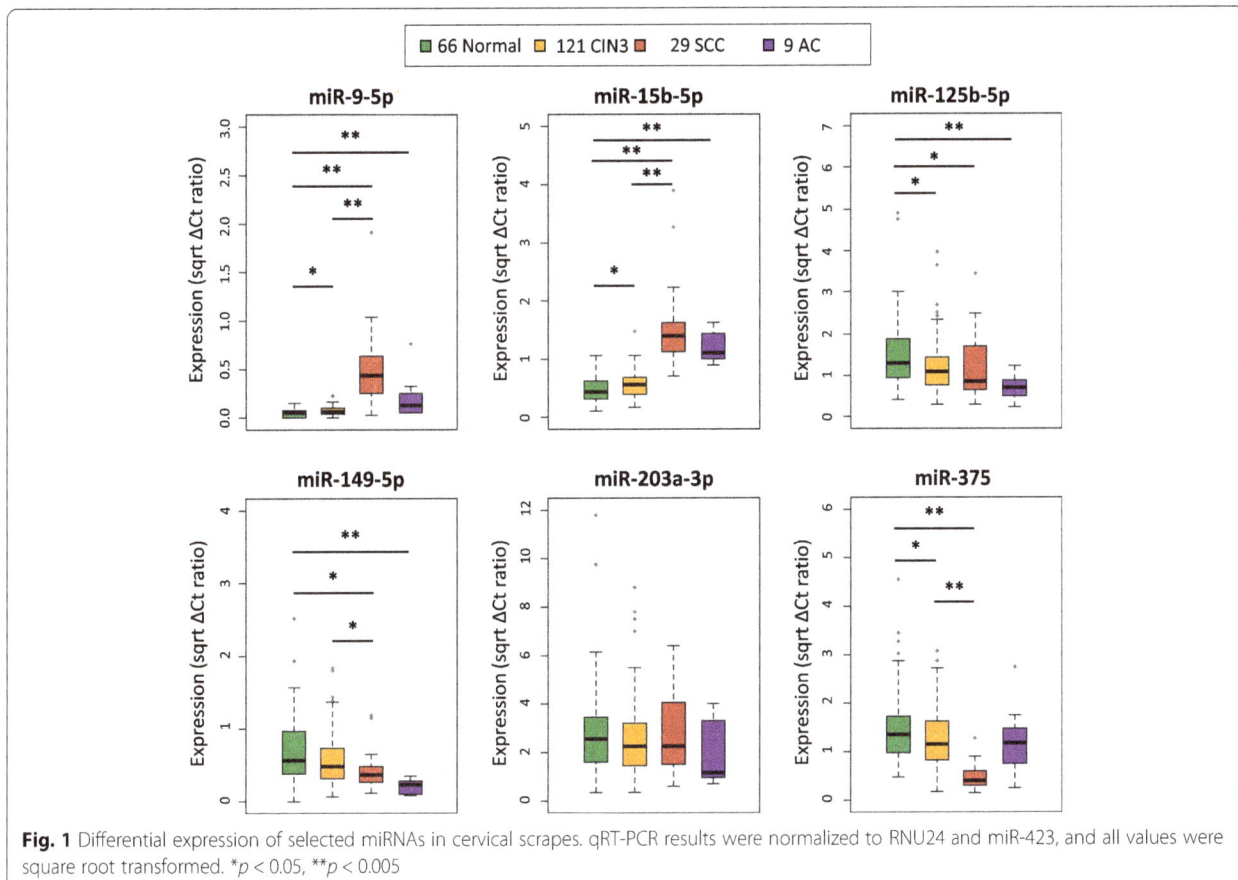

Fig. 1 Differential expression of selected miRNAs in cervical scrapes. qRT-PCR results were normalized to RNU24 and miR-423, and all values were square root transformed. *p < 0.05, **p < 0.005

HPV16/18 genotyping in conjunction with our miRNA classifier improves CIN3 detection

To compare the performance of our 2-miRNA classifier to HPV16/18 genotyping, samples were either classified as HPV16/18 positive (19 normal, 71 CIN3) or other hrHPV type positive (46 normal, 37 CIN3), for those samples for which the genotype was known ($n = 173$ out of 187). For this smaller sample set, we built (i) a new 2-miRNA classifier consisting of miR-15b and miR-375 and (ii) a logistic regression model combining the 2-miRNA classifier with HPV16/18 genotyping. Consistent with previous reports, HPV16/18 genotyping achieved 66% sensitivity and 68% specificity for CIN3 detection (Table 4) [7, 32]. The 2-miRNA classifier obtained in the smaller sample set had a comparable performance to the one obtained from the entire set of samples (Tables 3 and 4). While HPV16/18 genotyping alone was inferior to the 2-miRNA classifier ($p = 5.2$

Table 2 Comparison of optimal sensitivity and specificity between miRNA panels for the detection of CIN3 based on leave-one-out cross-validation

Panel	AUC	Cutoff	Sensitivity (%)	Specificity (%)	p value[*]
Single markers					
miR-15b-5p	0.573	0.629	62.0	56.1	0.098
miR-125b-5p	0.605	0.641	72.7	47.0	0.020
miR-149-5p	0.542	0.597	84.3	28.8	0.356
miR-203a-3p	0.523	0.654	62.0	48.5	0.619
miR-375	0.565	0.671	52.9	62.1	0.145
Two markers					
miR-15b-5p/375	0.622	0.682	54.5	69.7	0.006

[*]p value: comparison between the miRNA classifier and a random classifier with an AUC of 0.5
CIN cervical intraepithelial neoplasia, AUC area under the curve

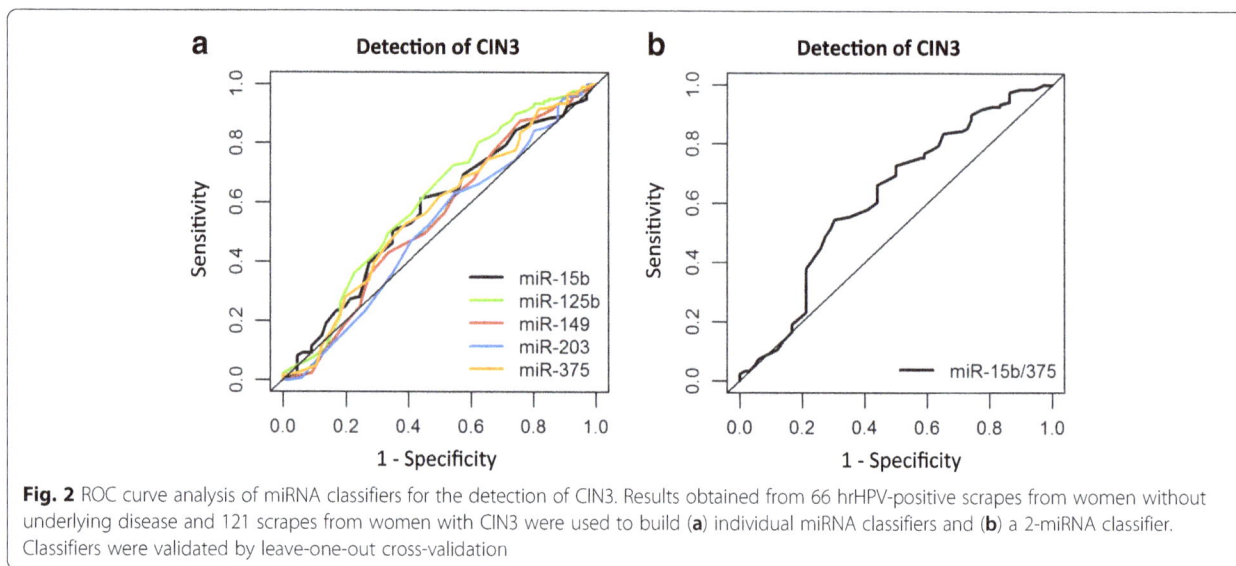

Fig. 2 ROC curve analysis of miRNA classifiers for the detection of CIN3. Results obtained from 66 hrHPV-positive scrapes from women without underlying disease and 121 scrapes from women with CIN3 were used to build (**a**) individual miRNA classifiers and (**b**) a 2-miRNA classifier. Classifiers were validated by leave-one-out cross-validation

e-16, Fig. 3), a classifier combining our two selected miRNAs with HPV16/18 genotyping had an improved performance and achieved an AUC of 0.712 (Table 4, Fig. 3). The 2-miRNA classifier adjusted by HPV16/18 type had a significantly better performance than the 2-miRNA classifier ($p = 0.011$). Including HPV16/18 genotyping in the classifier increased both sensitivity and specificity to 63 and 77%, respectively, and all SCC and AC were detected (data not shown).

Knockdown of miR-15b-5p and ectopic expression of miR-375 reduces viability in cervical cancer cells

Next, we investigated whether our miRNA markers are directly involved in cervical carcinogenesis, as is suggested by their genetic (miR-15b-5p) or epigenetic (miR-375) regulation. Transfection of cervical cancer cell lines SiHa and CaSki with miR-15b-5p inhibitors led to a reduction in cell viability, suggesting that miR-15b-5p acts as an oncomiR (Fig. 4a). Ectopic expression of

Table 3 Sensitivity of miRNA panels for the detection of SCC and AC

Panel	Sensitivity %	
	Detection of SCC	Detection of AC
Single markers		
miR-15b-5p	100	100
miR-125b-5p	69.0	100
miR-149-5p	93.1	100
miR-203a-3p	55.2	66.7
miR-375	96.6	55.6
Two markers		
miR-15b-5p/375	100	100

SCC squamous cell carcinoma, *AC* adenocarcinoma

miR-375 in SiHa and CaSki cells significantly reduced cell viability, supporting its role as tumor suppressive miRNA (Fig. 4b).

Discussion

In this study, we analyzed the triage capacity on hrHPV-positive cervical scrapes of a panel of miRNAs that exhibit either genetically or epigenetically mediated expression changes in cervical precancerous and cancerous tissue specimens and that in part have also been shown to be functionally involved in cervical carcinogenesis [17, 18]. We found that expression patterns detected in cervical tissue samples were reflected in cervical scrapes. By logistic regression analysis, a 2-miRNA classifier was built that at 70% specificity achieved 55% sensitivity for the detection of CIN3 and 100% sensitivity for the detection of SCC and AC. Upon inclusion of HPV16/18 genotyping, the sensitivity and specificity for CIN3 detection could be increased to 63 and 77%, respectively. Our data suggest that miRNA expression analysis offers a promising alternative molecular tool to triage hrHPV-positive women.

In a systematic review, Sharma et al. identified a total of 246 miRNAs that become deregulated in cervical cancer, with miR-21, miR-143, miR-145, miR-203, miR-214, and miR-218 being the most frequently described [33]. Most published studies identified deregulated miRNAs in cervical tissue samples by microarray analysis [17, 34, 35]. Studies focusing on the diagnostic or prognostic use of miRNAs detected by qRT-PCR in cervical biopsies are numerous, as are studies investigating the functional contribution of individual miRNAs to cervical cancer development. Data on the clinical applicability of miRNA expression analysis in cervical scrapes for cervical screening purposes, however, is limited. To

Table 4 Optimal sensitivity and specificity for the detection of CIN3 for hrHPV type (HPV16/18, others) and the miRNA classifier in conjunction with hrHPV type based on a smaller sample set with known hrHPV type infection and leave-one-out cross-validation

Panel	AUC	Cutoff	Sensitivity %	Specificity %	p value[*]
Single marker					
HPV type	0.445	n.a.	65.7	67.7	0.266
Multiple markers					
miR-15b-5p/375	0.622	0.656	55.6	69.2	0.008
miR-15b-5p/375/HPV	0.712	0.666	63.0	76.9	5.8 e-07

[*]p value: comparison between the miRNA classifier and a random classifier with an AUC of 0.5

CIN cervical intraepithelial neoplasia, AUC area under the curve, n.a not applicable

the best of our knowledge, only Tian et al. published on the analysis of a panel of candidate miRNA markers in HPV-positive scrapes of a gynecology outpatient clinic population to date [36]. Candidate miRNAs analyzed by Tian et al. have previously been shown to become differentially expressed during disease progression. A combination of miR-375 and miR-424 resulted in an AUC value of 0.853 for the detection of CIN3+, showing the promise of biologically relevant miRNAs as disease markers. Importantly, our study as well as the study by Tian et al. shows that the use of more than one miRNA improves detection of cervical disease. Although miR-15b-5p alone detected all carcinomas, combining miR-15b-5p with miR-375 proved beneficial for the

detection of CIN3 without a loss of sensitivity for SCC and AC. The fact that the individual miRNA performing best in the detection of CIN3 (miR-125b-5p) was not included in the 2-miRNA classifier further demonstrates that analysis of multiple complementary miRNAs can improve the detection of cervical disease. Importantly, we here show that combining miRNA profiling with HPV16/18 genotyping can further improve the detection of cervical precancer. This is especially attractive, as HPV16/18 genotyping is frequently included in clinically validated HPV tests [20, 37] and HPV16/18 genotyping and miRNA expression analysis can be performed on the same cervical scrape.

In line with Tian et al., our study shows that downregulated miRNAs can be suitable biomarkers, although the selection of downregulated markers may seem counterintuitive at first. It is important to note that the relative decrease in expression observed with cervical disease progression does not give an indication of the absolute abundance of a miRNA. Differences in performance between the study of Tian et al. and ours are most likely due to differences between study populations. While our cohort of cervical scrapes was obtained from a screening population, Tian et al. analyzed scrapes from a clinic-based referral population, which potentially contains more advanced CIN lesions. Altered expression of our candidate miRNAs is caused by either genetic or epigenetic changes which have previously been shown to be associated with cervical cancer and so-called advanced CIN3 lesions [3]. Their association with progression risk to cancer could explain why our miRNA classifiers detect only a subset of CIN3 lesions. Our 2-miRNA classifier detected all cervical cancers and 55% of CIN3 at 70% specificity, a generally accepted specificity for triage markers [38]. At present, adopted triage options for HPV-positive women include reflex cytology, HPV16/18 genotyping, repeat HPV testing, and/or repeat cytology. While triage by the current miRNA panel does not yet meet the criteria for acceptability of a triage strategy [39], we here show that triage by miRNA expression analysis is feasible and offers a promising alternative. MiRNA analysis is objective, highly reproducible,

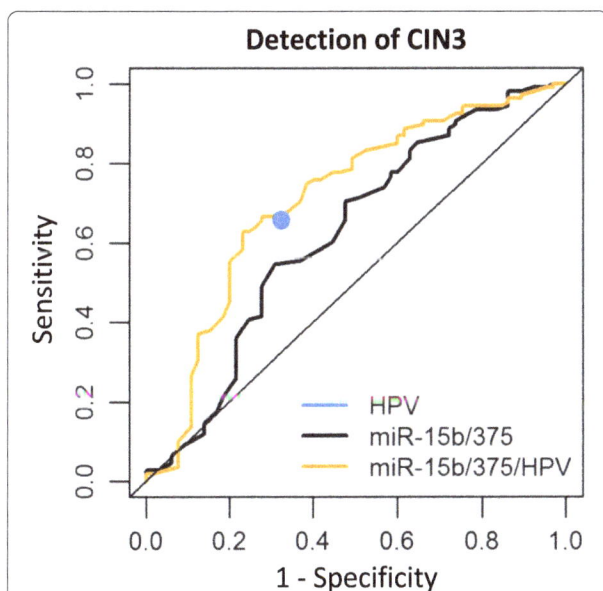

Fig. 3 ROC curve analysis of HPV16/18 genotyping and the 2-miRNA classifier for the detection of CIN3. Results obtained from scrapes with known HPV16/18 genotyping results (65 normal, 108 CIN3) were used to build classifiers for HPV16/18 genotyping (HPV), a new 2-miRNA classifier (miR-15b/375) and the 2-miRNA classifier combined with HPV16/18 genotyping (miR-15b/375/HPV). Classifiers were validated by leave-one-out cross-validation. The model miR-15b/375/HPV is significantly better than the 2-miRNA classifier (p = 0.011)

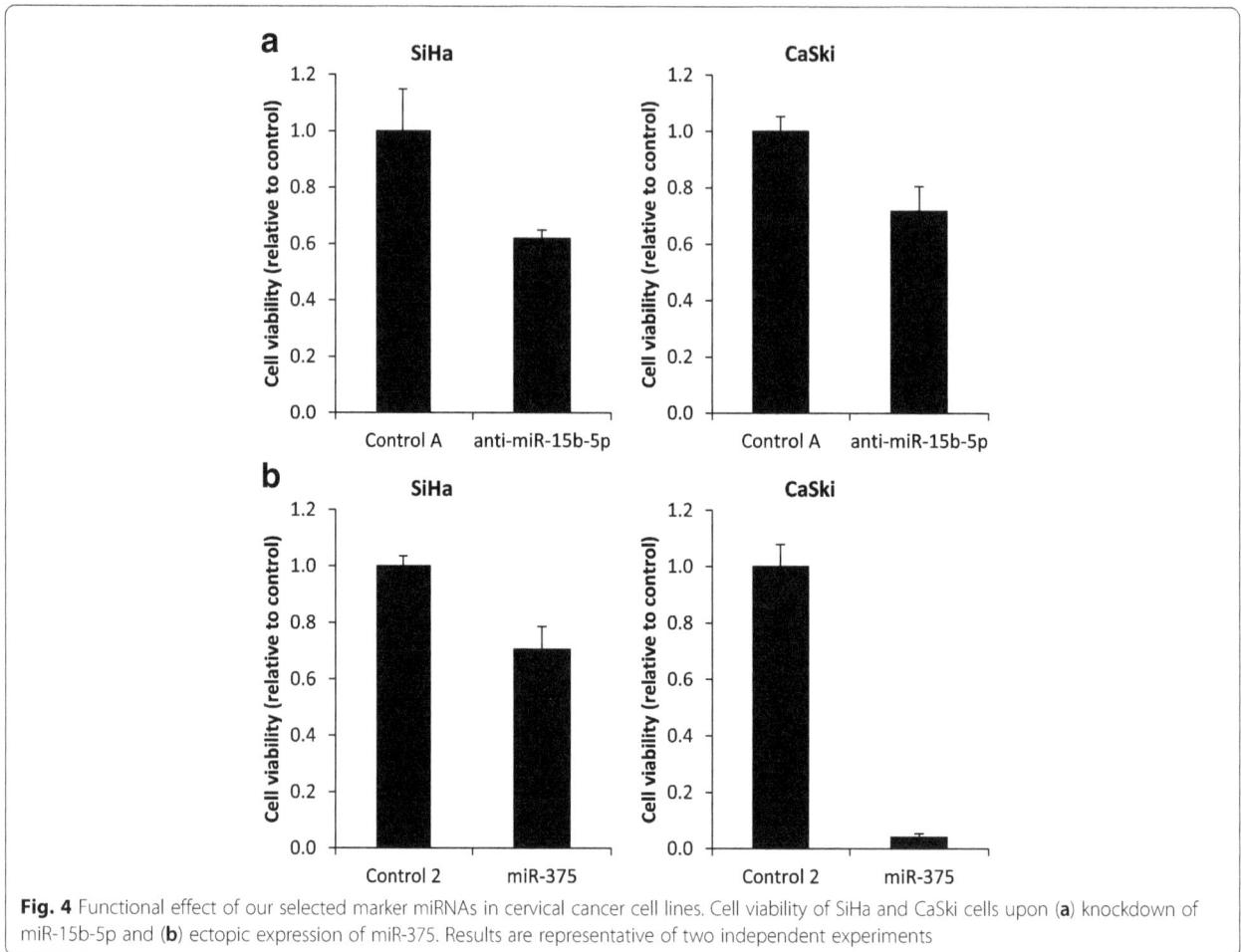

Fig. 4 Functional effect of our selected marker miRNAs in cervical cancer cell lines. Cell viability of SiHa and CaSki cells upon (**a**) knockdown of miR-15b-5p and (**b**) ectopic expression of miR-375. Results are representative of two independent experiments

and can be performed in a high-throughput manner. We do acknowledge that further panel optimization is required and expect that analysis of additional miRNAs will result in a miRNA classifier with improved performance. How an optimized miRNA panel performs in comparison to or as adjunct to cytology, HPV16/18 genotyping, DNA methylation markers, and/or other cellular markers such as p16^{INK4A}/Ki-67 will be subject of future studies.

Overexpression of miR-15b-5p has previously been associated with HPV-induced malignancies including cervical cancer, tonsillar tumors, and anal carcinomas [40, 41]. Moreover, miR-15b-5p was shown to promote cell viability, migration, and invasion in non-small cell lung cancer by targeting metastasis suppressor TIMP2 [42]. In line with this, we observed reduced cervical cancer cell viability upon knockdown of miR-15b-5p suggestive of an oncogenic role for this miRNA. Expression of miR-375 in cervical cancer, on the other hand, is downregulated by increased DNA methylation as well as by a frequently occurring focal loss of chromosome 2q35 [18, 19, 43, 44]. In line with literature, we found that ectopic expression of miR-375 in hrHPV-positive

cervical cancer cell lines reduces cell viability [19, 45]. Jung et al. previously showed that miR-375 restored major tumor suppressors p53, p21, and RB levels by deregulation of HPV16 and HPV18 viral transcripts and directly targeting E6AP [45].

One limitation of this study is that we did not include HPV-positive scrapes of women diagnosed with CIN1 and CIN2. Further validation of our 2-miRNA classifier is needed in an independent population-based screening cohort consisting of consecutive hrHPV-positive cervical scrapes including CIN1 and CIN2 lesions. In addition, the samples used in our study had been stored at room temperature for at least 1 year and at − 80 °C for another 3 to 4 years, and clinical material was limited. We showed that using as little as 20 ng of small RNA still enables the early detection of cervical cancer, but we cannot exclude that higher amounts of RNA, as also used by Tian et al., may give a better discrimination between normal and CIN3. On the other hand, our data also demonstrate that miRNAs are very stable molecules. This is of particular importance in screening settings where cervical scrape material is send to central diagnostic laboratories for molecular testing. While we analyzed a selected panel of eight miRNAs which were shown to become genetically or epigenetically deregulated during cervical carcinogenesis in cervical tissue samples, candidate miRNAs should ideally be selected directly from whole miRNome data obtained from cervical scrapes [46]. Future studies will therefore aim to identify an optimal panel of miRNAs for the detection of CIN3 and cancer.

Conclusions

In conclusion, present data show that analysis of differentially expressed miRNAs may provide an alternative molecular triage strategy in hrHPV-based cervical screening. Our data indicate that miRNAs that are genetically or epigenetically deregulated during and directly involved in disease progression are promising biomarkers for the detection of cervical cancer and a subset of CIN3 lesions. CIN3 detection was further improved by inclusion of HPV16/18 genotyping. Further optimization of the marker panel and validation in an independent cohort of hrHPV-positive cervical scrapes will reveal whether triage of hrHPV-positive women by miRNA expression analysis offers an objective and economical alternative to cytology.

Abbreviations

(hr)HPV: (High-risk) Human papillomavirus; AC: Adenocarcinoma; AUC: Area under the curve; CIN: Cervical intraepithelial neoplasia; E6AP: E6-associated protein; miRNA: MicroRNA; p21: Cyclin dependent kinase inhibitor 1A; p53: Tumor protein p53; RB: Retinoblastoma protein; ROC: Receiver-operated characteristic; SCC: Squamous cell carcinoma

Funding

This work was supported by the Dutch Cancer Society (KWF VU 2012–5708) and the European Research Council (ERC advanced 2012-AdG, proposal 322986; Mass-Care).

Authors' contributions

PJFS, CJLMM, RDMS, and SMW were involved in the conception and design of the study. Clinical material collection and data acquisition were carried out by IB, BS, AJ, NvT, DAMH, CJLMM, and SMW. IB, PWN, PJFS, CJLMM, RDMS, and SMW analyzed and interpreted the data. IB, PJFS, RDMS and SW were major contributors in writing and reviewing the manuscript. All authors read and approved the final manuscript.

Competing interests

DAMH occasionally serves on the scientific advisory board of Pfizer and Bristol-Meyer Squibb and has been on the speakers' bureau of Qiagen. PJFS, RDMS, CJLMM, and DAMH are minority stakeholders of Self-screen B.V., a spin-off company of VU University Medical Center; and since September 2017, CJLMM is director of Self-screen B.V., which holds patents related to the work. PJFS has received speakers' bureau honoraria from Roche, Qiagen, Gen-Probe, Abbott, and Seegene. He is consultant for Crucell Holland B.V. CJLMM has participated in the sponsored speaker's bureau of Merck and Qiagen and served occasionally on the scientific advisory board of Qiagen and Merck. CJLMM owns a small number of shares of Qiagen, has occasionally been consultant to Qiagen, and until April 2016 was a minority shareholder of Diassay B.V. No potential conflicts of interest were disclosed by the other authors.

Author details

[1]Cancer Center Amsterdam, Department of Pathology, VU University Medical Center, Amsterdam, The Netherlands. [2]Department of Epidemiology and Biostatistics, VU University Medical Center, Amsterdam, The Netherlands. [3]Center for Gynaecological Oncology, Antoni van Leeuwenhoek Hospital/ Netherlands Cancer Institute, Amsterdam, The Netherlands. [4]Department of Medical Oncology, Erasmus MC Cancer Institute, Erasmus University Medical Center, Rotterdam, The Netherlands.

References

1. Peto PJ, Gilham PC, Fletcher O, Matthews FE. The cervical cancer epidemic that screening has prevented in the UK. Lancet. 2004;364:249–56.
2. Walboomers JM, Jacobs MV, Manos MM, Bosch FX, Kummer JA, Shah KV, et al. Human papillomavirus is a necessary cause of invasive cervical cancer worldwide. J Pathol. 1999;189:12–9.
3. Steenbergen RDM, Snijders PJF, Heideman D a M, Meijer CJLM. Clinical implications of (epi)genetic changes in HPV-induced cervical precancerous lesions. Nat Rev Cancer. 2014;14:395–405.
4. Ferlay J, Soerjomataram I, Dikshit R, Eser S, Mathers C, Rebelo M, et al. Cancer incidence and mortality worldwide: sources, methods and major patterns in GLOBOCAN 2012. Int J Cancer. 2015;135:E359–86.
5. Arbyn M, Ronco G, Anttila A, Meijer CJLM, Poljak M, Ogilvie G, et al. Evidence regarding human papillomavirus testing in secondary prevention of cervical cancer. Vaccine. 2012;30(Suppl 5):F88–99.
6. Ronco G, Dillner J, Elfström KM, Tunesi S, Snijders PJF, Arbyn M, et al. Efficacy of HPV-based screening for prevention of invasive cervical cancer: follow-up of four European randomised controlled trials. Lancet. 2014;383:524–32.
7. Castle PE, Stoler MH, Wright TC, Sharma A, Wright TL, Behrens CM. Performance of carcinogenic human papillomavirus (HPV) testing and HPV16 or HPV18 genotyping for cervical cancer screening of women aged 25 years and older: a subanalysis of the ATHENA study. Lancet Oncol. 2011;12:880–90.
8. Cox JT, Castle PE, Behrens CM, Sharma A, Wright TC, Cuzick J, et al. Comparison of cervical cancer screening strategies incorporating different combinations of cytology, HPV testing, and genotyping for HPV 16/18: results from the ATHENA HPV study. Am J Obstet Gynecol. 2013;208:184.e1–184.e11.
9. Nakamura Y, Matsumoto K, Satoh T, Nishide K, Nozue A, Shimabukuro K, et al. HPV genotyping for triage of women with abnormal cervical cancer screening results: a multicenter prospective study. Int J Clin Oncol. 2015;20:974–81.
10. Bartel DP. MicroRNAs: Genomics, biogenesis, mechanism, and Function. Cell. 2004;116:281–97.
11. Li Y, Kowdley KV. MicroRNAs in common human diseases. Genomics Proteomics Bioinformatics. 2012;10:246–53.
12. Mraz M, Malinova K, Mayer J, Pospisilova S. MicroRNA isolation and stability in stored RNA samples. Biochem Biophys Res Commun. 2009;390:1–4.
13. Jung M, Schaefer A, Steiner I, Kempkensteffen C, Stephan C, Erbersdobler A, et al. Robust microRNA stability in degraded RNA preparations from human tissue and cell samples. Clin Chem. 2010;56:998–1006.
14. Chen X, Ba Y, Ma L, Cai X, Yin Y, Wang K, et al. Characterization of microRNAs in serum: a novel class of biomarkers for diagnosis of cancer and other diseases. Cell Res. 2008;18:997–1006.
15. Yu D-C, Li Q-G, Ding X-W, Ding Y-T. Circulating microRNAs: potential biomarkers for cancer. Int J Mol Sci. 2011;12:2055–63.
16. Cheng G. Circulating miRNAs: roles in cancer diagnosis, prognosis and therapy. Adv Drug Deliv Rev. 2015;81:75–93.
17. Wilting SM, Snijders PJF, Verlaat W, Jaspers A, M a v d W, van Wieringen WN, et al. Altered microRNA expression associated with chromosomal changes contributes to cervical carcinogenesis. Oncogene. 2013;32:106–16.
18. Wilting SM, Verlaat W, Jaspers A, Makazaji NA, Agami R, Meijer CJ, et al. Methylation-mediated transcriptional repression of microRNAs during cervical carcinogenesis. Epigenetics. 2013;8:220–8.
19. Bierkens M, Krijgsman O, Wilting SM, Bosch L, Jaspers A, Meijer GA, et al. Focal aberrations indicate EYA2 and hsa-miR-375 as oncogene and tumor suppressor in cervical carcinogenesis. Genes Chromosomes Cancer. 2013;52:56–68.
20. Hesselink AT, Berkhof J, van der Salm ML, van Splunter AP, Geelen TH, van Kemenade FJ, et al. Clinical validation of the HPV-risk assay, a novel real-time PCR assay for detection of high-risk human papillomavirus DNA by targeting the E7 region. J Clin Microbiol. 2014;52:890–6.

21. Geraets DT, Cuschieri K, de Koning MNC, van Doorn LJ, Snijders PJF, Meijer CJLM, et al. Clinical evaluation of a GP5+/6+–based luminex assay having full high-risk human papillomavirus genotyping capability and an internal control. J Clin Microbiol. 2014;52:3996–4002.

22. Polman NJ, Oštrbenk A, Xu L, Snijders PJF, Meijer CJLM, Poljak M, et al. Evaluation of the clinical performance of the HPV-risk assay using the VALGENT-3 panel. J Clin Microbiol. 2017;55:3544–51.

23. Colgan TJ, Lickrish GM. The topography and invasive potential of cervical adenocarcinoma in situ, with and without associated squamous dysplasia. Gynecol Oncol. 1990;36:246–9.

24. Bekkers RLM, Bulten J, Wiersma-van Tilburg A, Mravunac M, Schijf CPT, Massuger LFAG, et al. Coexisting high-grade glandular and squamous cervical lesions and human papillomavirus infections. Br J Cancer. 2003;89:886–90.

25. Babion I, Snoek BC, van de Wiel MA, Wilting SM, Steenbergen RDM. A strategy to find suitable reference genes for miRNA quantitative PCR analysis and its application to cervical specimens. J Mol Diagnostics. 2017; 19:625–37.

26. Livak KJ, Schmittgen TD. Analysis of relative gene expression data using real-time quantitative PCR and the 2(−Delta Delta C(T)) method. Methods. 2001;25:402–8.

27. DeLong ER, DeLong DM, Clarke-Pearson DL. Comparing the areas under two or more correlated receiver operating characteristic curves: a nonparametric approach. Biometrics. 1988;44:837–45.

28. Snellenberg S, Cillessen SAGM, Van Criekinge W, Bosch L, Meijer CJLM, Snijders PJF, et al. Methylation-mediated repression of PRDM14 contributes to apoptosis evasion in HPV-positive cancers. Carcinogenesis. 2014;35:2611–8.

29. Peccoud J, Jacob C. Theoretical uncertainty of measurements using quantitative polymerase chain reaction. Biophys J. 1996;71:101–8.

30. Bengtsson M, Hemberg M, Rorsman P, Ståhlberg A. Quantification of mRNA in single cells and modelling of RT-qPCR induced noise. BMC Mol Biol. 2008;9:63.

31. Korenková V, Scott J, Novosadová V, Jindřichová M, Langerová L, Švec D, et al. Pre-amplification in the context of high-throughput qPCR gene expression experiment. BMC Mol Biol. 2015;16:5.

32. Rijkaart DC, Berkhof J, Van Kemenade FJ, Coupe VMH, Hesselink AT, Rozendaal L, et al. Evaluation of 14 triage strategies for HPV DNA-positive women in population-based cervical screening. Int J Cancer. 2011;130:602–310.

33. Sharma G, Dua P, Agarwal SM. A comprehensive review of dysregulated miRNAs involved in cervical Cancer. Curr Genomics. 2014;15:310–23.

34. Li Y, Wang F, Xu J, Ye F, Shen Y, Zhou J, et al. Progressive miRNA expression profiles in cervical carcinogenesis and identification of HPV-related target genes for miR-29. J Pathol. 2011;224:484–95.

35. Zeng K, Zheng W, Mo X, Liu F, Li M, Liu Z, et al. Dysregulated microRNAs involved in the progression of cervical neoplasm. Arch Gynecol Obstet. 2015;292:905–13.

36. Tian Q, Li Y, Wang F, Li Y, Xu J, Shen Y, et al. MicroRNA detection in cervical exfoliated cells as a triage for human papillomavirus–positive women. J Natl Cancer Inst. 2014;106 https://doi.org/10.1093/jnci/dju241.

37. Hesselink AT, Sahli R, Berkhof J, Snijders PJF, van der Salm ML, Agard D, et al. Clinical validation of Anyplex™ II HPV HR detection according to the guidelines for HPV test requirements for cervical cancer screening. J Clin Virol. 2016;76:36–9.

38. De Strooper LMA, Meijer CJLM, Berkhof J, Hesselink AT, Snijders PJF, Steenbergen RDM, et al. Methylation analysis of the FAM19A4 gene in cervical scrapes is highly efficient in detecting cervical carcinomas and advanced CIN2/3 lesions. Cancer Prev Res. 2014;7:1251–7.

39. Dijkstra MG, van Niekerk D, Rijkaart DC, van Kemenade FJ, Heideman DAM, Snijders PJF, et al. Primary hrHPV DNA testing in cervical Cancer screening: how to manage screen-positive women? A POBASCAM trial substudy. Cancer Epidemiol Biomark Prev. 2014;23:55–63.

40. Vojtechova Z, Sabol I, Salakova M, Smahelova J, Zavadil J, Turek L, et al. Comparison of the miRNA profiles in HPV-positive and HPV-negative tonsillar tumors and a model system of human keratinocyte clones. BMC Cancer. 2016;16:382.

41. Myklebust M, Bruland O, Fluge Ø, Skarstein A. MicroRNA-15b is induced with E2F-controlled genes in HPV-related cancer. Br J Cancer. 2011;105: 1719–25.

42. Wang H, Zhan Y, Jin J, Zhang C, Li W. MicroRNA-15b promotes proliferation and invasion of non-small cell lung carcinoma cells by directly targeting TIMP2. Oncol Rep. 2017;37:3305–12.

43. Liu S, Song L, Yao H, Zhang L, Xu D, Gao F, et al. MiR-375 is epigenetically downregulated by HPV-16 E6 mediated DNMT1 upregulation and modulates EMT of cervical cancer cells by suppressing lncRNA MALAT1. PLoS One. 2016;11:e0163460.

44. Morel A, Baguet A, Perrard J, Demeret C, Jacquin E, Guenat D, et al. 5azadC treatment upregulates miR-375 level and represses HPV16 E6 expression. Oncotarget. 2017;8:46163–76.

45. Jung H, Phillips BL, Chan EK. miR-375 activates p21 and suppresses telomerase activity by coordinately regulating HPV E6/E7, E6AP, CIP2A, and 14-3-3ζ. Mol Cancer. 2014;13:80.

46. Novianti PW, Snoek BC, Wilting SM, van de Wiel MA. Better diagnostic signatures from RNAseq data through use of auxiliary co-data. Bioinformatics. 2017;33:1572–4.

47. Federa. Human Tissue and Medical Research: Code of conduct for responsible use (2011). Rotterdam: Federa; 2011. http://www.bbmri.nl/wp-content/uploads/2015/10/Federa_code_of_conduct_english.pdf. Accessed 25 Oct 2017.

11

Adipose tissue inflammation and *VDR* expression and methylation in colorectal cancer

Daniel Castellano-Castillo[1†], Sonsoles Morcillo[2†], Mercedes Clemente-Postigo[1,2*], Ana Belén Crujeiras[3,4], Jose Carlos Fernandez-García[1,2], Esperanza Torres[5], Francisco José Tinahones[1,2] and Manuel Macias-Gonzalez[1,2*]

Abstract

Background: Lack of vitamin D (VD) has been associated with colorectal cancer (CRC). VD has anti-inflammatory effects and regulates several cellular pathways by means of its receptor, including epigenetic modifications. Adipose tissue dysfunction has been related to low-grade inflammation, which is related to diseases like cancer. The aim of this study was to explore the relationship between serum 25-hydroxyvitamin D (25(OH)D), adipose tissue gene expression of VD receptor (VDR), pro-inflammatory markers, and the epigenetic factor DNA methyltransferase 3a (DNMT3A) as well as VDR promoter methylation in CRC.

Methods: Blood and visceral adipose tissue from 57 CRC and 50 healthy control subjects were collected. CRC subjects had lower serum 25(OH)D levels and higher VDR gene expression, and these were negatively correlated in the CRC group.

Results: Adipose tissue *NFκB1*, *IL6*, and *IL1B* gene expression were higher in the CRC subjects than in the control subjects. 25(OH)D correlated negatively with *NFκB1* and CRP. In turn, CRP correlated positively with *NFκB1*, *IL6*, *IL1B*, and *VDR* gene expression as well as *NFκB1* that correlated positively with *IL6* and *IL1B*. *DNMT3A* mRNA was negatively correlated with serum 25(OH)D and positively correlated with *VDR* DNA methylation. *VDR* DNA methylation at position 4 had lower levels in the CRC group. Global *NFκB1* methylation at dinucleotide 3 was lower in the CRC group.

Conclusion: Our results suggest that adipose tissue may be a key factor in CRC development. The low 25(OH)D levels and high adipose tissue *VDR* expression in CRC may, at least in part, mediate this relationship by modifying adipose tissue DNA methylation and promoting inflammation.

Keywords: Vitamin D, *VDR*, DNA methylation, Low-grade inflammation, Colorectal cancer, Adipose tissue

Background

Colorectal cancer (CRC) has become one of the most important health issues of our time due to its elevated prevalence, increasing incidence, morbidity, associated costs, and mortality rates. Several risk factors have been linked to CRC development: population aging, lack of physical activity, obesity, low fruit and vegetable intake, tobacco use, alcohol consumption, and other unknown factors [1].

Vitamin D (VD) can be incorporated from diet (vitamin D_2 or D_3) or synthetized by photoactivation of 7-dehydrocholesterol to previtamin D_3 in the skin, a process that is mediated by sunlight [2]. Then, vitamin D_2/D_3 is converted to 25-hydroxyvitamin D (25(OH)D) by CYP2R1 in the liver, which is the main form of plasma vitamin D. The conversion of 25(OH)D to the active form, the 1,25-hydroxyvitamin D (1,25(OH)D), is carried out by the enzyme CYP24A1 in the kidneys [2]. Vitamin D functions primarily through the VD receptor (VDR), which is regulated by environment, genetics, and epigenetics [2].

Several studies have related plasma 25-hydroxyvitamin D (25(OH)D) levels with CRC [3–5], finding that low circulating 25(OH)D levels have been associated with CRC [4], and

* Correspondence: mer.cp@hotmail.com; mmacias.manuel@gmail.com
†Equal contributors
[1]Unidad de Gestión Clínica de Endocrinología y Nutrición del Hospital Virgen de la Victoria, Instituto de Investigación Biomédica de Málaga (IBIMA), Universidad de Málaga, Málaga, Spain
[2]CIBER Fisiopatología de la Obesidad y Nutrición (CB06/03), Madrid, Spain
Full list of author information is available at the end of the article

high 25(OH)D levels correlate with low risk for the onset of CRC [5]. A number of studies have reported the benefits of VD in processes such as metabolic modulation, auto-immunity, cardiovascular function, and cancer [6]. In fact, it has been proposed that calcitriol has anti-tumor effects [7, 8] as well as a direct effect on tumor development by acting as a tumor repressor in many solid tumors including CRC [9]. In a clinical trial carried out with patients who suffered from colorectal adenoma, the administration of VD together with calcium was able to reduce the expression of genes implicated in CRC development [10].

A number of studies have noted the relationship between CRC and low-grade inflammation [11]. Specifically, CRC patients have dysfunctional adipose tissue that might be a key contributor to the inflammatory state, by the secretion of several detrimental molecules such as tumor necrosis factor alpha (*TNFA*), interleukin-6 (*IL6*), and nuclear factor κ-light-chain-enhancer of activated B cells 1 (*NFκB1*) [12]. Adipose tissue has traditionally only been considered as an energy storage organ. Nevertheless, the importance of this tissue in systemic physiology and especially in systemic inflammation has been pointed out in recent years [13]. Adipose tissue expresses proteins related to VD metabolism [14], and it has been proposed that it can act as VD storage tissue [15]. The active form of VD, 1,25-dihydroxyvitamin D3 ($1,25(OH)_2D_3$), is able to modify adipocyte and adipose tissue physiology via the VDR [16, 17], decreasing the expression of pro-inflammatory cytokines in adipose tissue [18]. Therefore, VD might be a key factor for the higher risk of CRC in obese subjects, since low serum 25(OH)D levels or impaired adipose tissue responsiveness to VD might lead to a higher inflammatory state, which is directly implied in cancer development. However, the precise mechanism by which VD leads to a decrease in inflammation is not completely clear.

DNA methylation is an epigenetic regulatory process in which cytosine residues are methylated normally within CpG dinucleotides, referred to as CpG, and it is usually associated with gene repression, although it has also been related to gene activation in some cases [2, 19, 20]. Epigenetic mechanisms are susceptible to environmental factors such as diet, exercise, smoking, and hormones, and could be the basis for factors associated with an increased risk of cancer development such as obesity, inflammation, diabetes, or metabolic syndrome, as well as tumor onset or development [21–26]. DNA methylation is carried out by DNA methyl-transferases *DNMT1*, *DNMT3A*, and *DNMT3B*, being *DNMT1* implied in the maintenance of DNA methylation and *DNMT3A* and *DNMT3B* in de novo DNA methylation processes. Furthermore, the relationship between vitamin D and DNA methylation has been analyzed in several studies, and 25(OH)D levels appear to control DNA methylation or demethylation [27], a mechanism in which DNA methyl-transferases could be involved [28]. Furthermore, adipose

tissue *DNMT3A* overexpression provokes a rise in adipose tissue inflammation in mice, which could be involved in adipose tissue-related diseases and CRC [29].

Therefore, we hypothesized that dysfunctional adipose tissue may play a major role in CRC development. 25(OH)D could be involved in epigenetic changes in adipose tissue triggering a change in the inflammatory profile, which could promote CRC onset and/or development. Thus, the aim of this study was to test serum levels of 25(OH)D, as well as the gene expression of the epigenetic factor *DNMT3A* and inflammatory markers in adipose tissue in CRC. We also studied *VDR* and *NFκB1* DNA methylation in adipose tissue to determine the possible role of the VD system in the epigenetic regulation of VDR and *NFκB1* gene.

Methods

Subjects

A total of 57 participants with CRC who underwent colorectal surgery and 50 control subjects who underwent hiatal hernia surgery or cholecystectomy were recruited from the Virgen de la Victoria University Hospital (Málaga, Spain) during 2012–2013.

Patients were excluded if they had cardiovascular disease, arthritis, acute inflammatory disease, infectious disease, and renal disease, and were receiving drugs that could alter the lipid or glucose profile, were undergoing treatment with calcium or vitamin D supplements, or if they consumed > 20 g ethanol per day at the time of inclusion in the study. The study was conducted in accordance with the guidelines laid down in the Declaration of Helsinki. All participants gave their written informed consent (0311/PI7), and the study was reviewed and approved by the Ethics and Research Committee of Virgen de la Victoria Hospital.

Epiploic visceral adipose (VAT) tissue was obtained during surgery, washed in physiological saline solution, and immediately frozen in liquid nitrogen. Biopsy samples were maintained at − 80 °C until analysis.

Laboratory measurements

Before surgery and after an overnight fast, blood samples were obtained from the antecubital vein and placed in vacutainer tubes (BD vacutainer™). The serum was separated by centrifugation for 15 min at 4000 rpm and immediately frozen at − 80 °C until analysis. Serum glucose, cholesterol, triglycerides, HDL cholesterol (HDL-C), and C-reactive protein (CRP) were measured in a Dimension autoanalyzer (Dade Behring Inc.) by enzymatic methods (Randox Laboratories Ltd.). LDL cholesterol (LDL-C) was calculated using the Friedewald equation. Insulin was quantified by radioimmunoassay supplied by BioSource International Inc., Camarillo, CA, USA. The homeostasis model assessment of insulin resistance (HOMA-IR) was calculated with the following equation: HOMA-IR = fasting insulin (μIU/mL) × fasting glucose (mmol/L)/22.5. Serum 25(OH)D and parathyroid hormone levels were determined by enzyme immunoassay (ELISA) kits (Immundiagnostik and DRG Diagnostics, respectively). Corrected calcium was calculated using the following equation: fasting calcium (mg/dl) + 0.8 × (4-fasting albumin (g/dl)).

Visceral adipose tissue RNA isolation and real-time quantitative PCR

Total RNA isolation from VAT was obtained using RNeasy Lipid Tissue Mini Kit (Qiagen GmbH, Hilden, Germany). The purity of the RNA was determined by the 260/280 absorbance ratio on the NanoDrop. The integrity of the total purified RNA was checked by denaturing agarose gel electrophoresis and ethidium bromide staining. For first strand cDNA synthesis, a constant amount of 1 μg of total RNA was reverse transcribed using random hexamers as primers and Transcriptor Reverse Transcriptase (Roche, Mannheim, Germany). Gene expression was assessed by real-time PCR using an Applied Biosystems 7500 Fast Real-Time PCR System (Applied Biosystems, Darmstadt, Germany) with TaqMan technology as previously described [30]. The commercially available and pre-validated TaqMan primer/probe sets used were as follows: VDR (Hs01045840_m1, RefSeq. NM_000376.2, NM_001017535.1 and NM_001017536.1), NFκB1 (Hs00765730_m1, RefSeq. NM_001165412.1 and NM_003998.3), DNMT3A (NM_001320893.1, NM_022552.4, NM_153759.3, NM_175629.2), IL6 (Hs00174131_m1; RefSeq. NM_000600.4, NM_001318095.1), IL1B (Hs00174097_m1; NM_000576.2), and PPIA (4326316E, RefSeq. NM_021130.3), used as endogenous control for the target gene in each reaction.

Protein extraction and western blot

For total protein extract preparation, adipose tissue samples were washed once in erythrocyte lysis buffer (sacarose 320 mM, Tris-HCl pH 7.5 10 mM, MgCl$_2$ 5 mM, Tritonx-100 1%) and PBS for 20 min at 4° with agitation. Samples were homogenized using T-PER tissue protein extraction reagent (Thermofisher, USA) and Ultra Turrax Homogenizer and then centrifuged to discard the pellet and the upper fatty layer. Samples were resolved by SDS-PAGE and transferred to a nitrocellulose membrane to perform the Western blotting. A mouse monoclonal anti-VDR (sc 13133, Santa Cruz Biotechnology) was used as primary antibody and a goat anti-mouse IgG-HRP (sc-2005, Santa Cruz Biotechnology) as secondary antibody. Clarity Western ECL substrate (Bio-Rad, USA) was used for detection, and the target protein was determined by using the total protein determined by ponceau staining to normalize the quantification. All experiments were performed in duplicate.

Pyrosequencing

The DNA methylation status was determined by pyrosequencing using the PyroMarkTMQ96 ID Pyrosequencing System (Qiagen). We used a premade Pyromark CpG assay for VDR (PM00051443) and NFκB1 (PM00110908). An overview of the analyzed regions for VDR and NFκB1 is depicted in Supplementary Additional files 1 and 2: Figures S1 and S2, respectively. Briefly, NFκB1 is located at chromosome 4. The region 103,423,139-103,423,177 (39 bp length) was analyzed, which contains more than 30 transcription factor binding sites (TFBS) determined by ChiP experiments by the ENCODE project [31]. Besides, the assay was located inside additional TFBS according to the Open Regulatory Annotation database (ORegAnno) [32], as SMARCA4, SPL1, STAT1, RBL2, RB1, and ETS1. VDR is located at chromosome 12. The region 48,299,419-48,299,455 (37 bp length) was analyzed, which contains several TFBS determined by ChiP experiments by the ENCODE Project [31], as POLR2A, ATF2, CTCF, EZH2, E2F6, GATA2, GATA3, CEBPB, or POL2. Additional TFBS are present according to ORegAnno [32], as SMARCA4, SPL1, STAT1, RBL2, RB1, and ETS1. DNA methylation analyses were performed using bisulfite-treated DNA followed by a highly quantitative analysis based on PCR-based pyrosequencing. The bisulfite conversion was conducted with 2-μg genomic DNA isolated from VAT using Qiazol (Qiagen) and 0.1 μM citrate ethanol solution. Then, the PCR was performed in a total volume of 25 μL, with a final primer concentration of 0.2 μM. One of the primers was biotinylated in order to purify the final PCR product using Sepharose beads. The biotinylated PCR amplification was purified using the Pyrosequencing Vacuum Prep Tool (Qiagen). Finally, 15 μL of the PCR products was pyrosequenced using the PyroMarkTMQ96 ID Pyrosequencing System, using a 0.4-μM sequencing primer.

The methylation level was expressed as the percentage of methylated cytosine over the sum of methylated and unmethylated cytosines. Non-CpG cytosine residues were used as built-in controls to verify bisulfite conversion. The values are expressed as the mean for all the sites and individually for six CpGs at the VDR gene promoter and seven CpGs at the NFκB1 promoter. We also included unmethylated and methylated DNA as controls in each run (New England Biolabs). Inter-assay precision (% CV) was < 2.5%; intra-assay (% CV) was < 1.0%.

Statistical analysis

The results are given as the mean ± SD (Table 1) and as a box plot with the minimum and maximum value (control case comparisons shown in Figs. 1, 2, and 3). Student's t test was used for comparisons of the anthropometric and biochemical characteristics as well as serum 25(OH)D levels between the CRC and control groups. Mann-Whitney U test was performed for comparisons of serum CRP and

Table 1 Anthropometric and biochemical variables of the study groups

	Control (n = 57)	CRC (n = 50)
Age (years)	64.94 ± 8.84	68.035 ± 8.43
Male/Female (%)*	68/32	45/55
BMI (kg/m²)	28.51 ± 4.21	27.61 ± 3.91
Waist (cm)	96.55 ± 11.64	97 ± 12.74
Glucose (mg/dl)	111.72 ± 28.77	125.035 ± 46.87
Insulin (µUI/ml)**	11.638 ± 6.54	6.23 ± 5.19
Triglycerides (mg/dl)*	142.3 ± 70.69	172.821 ± 87.54
Cho (mg/dl)**	220.68 ± 39.84	169.625 ± 43.57
HDL-C (mg/dl)**	53.28 ± 14.4	40.053 ± 15.12
LDL-C (mg/dl)**	136.61 ± 29.80	101.58 ± 35.67
Corrected calcium (mg/dl)**	8.99 ± 0.44	9.67 ± 0.65
Alkaline phosphatase (U/L)	72.67 ± 21.63	64.66 ± 22.81

CRC Colorectal Cancer Group, *BMI* Body Mass Index, *DM* Diabetes Mellitus, *Cho* Total Cholesterol, *HDL-C* High Density Lipoprotein Cholesterol, *LDL-C* Low density Lipoprotein Cholesterol

Results are presented as means ± S.D. $*p < 0.05$ CRC vs. Control; $**p < 0.01$ CRC vs. control according to t student's test and Chi squared test for variables expressed as percentage

PTH levels as well as for *VDR* methylation, mRNA, and protein expression levels and for *NFκB1* methylation and mRNA levels between the CRC and the control groups. Spearman's correlation analyses were performed to study the correlations between 25(OH)D and *VDR* mRNA and to study the correlations for *NFκB1* DNA methylation. Partial correlation analyses corrected by gender were used to study the correlation among the study gene expressions and plasma levels of 25(OH)D and CRP. For the analysis, non-normal distribution variables were log-transformed. The analyses were performed with SPSS (Version 15.0 for Windows; SPSS Iberica, Spain). Values were considered to be statistically significant when $p < 0.05$.

Results

Anthropometric and biochemical variables

Table 1 shows the biochemical and anthropometric characteristics of the study groups. There were no differences in age, BMI, or gender between the control and CRC groups. The CRC group had lower levels of insulin, total cholesterol, HDL-C, and LDL-C than the control group. In contrast, the CRC group presented higher levels of plasma triglycerides when compared with the control group.

Serum 25(OH)D levels and adipose tissue VDR gene and protein expression

Our results showed that 12% in the control group and 26% in the CRC group were vitamin D deficient (25(OH)D lower than 20 nmol/L) according to the Endocrine Society Clinical Practice Guideline [33], although no significant differences were found according to Fisher's test. Serum

25(OH)D levels were significantly lower in the CRC group than in the control group (Fig. 1a), while parathyroid hormone levels showed an inverse result (Fig. 1b). Contrary to serum 25(OH)D levels, adipose tissue *VDR* mRNA levels were higher in the CRC group than in the control group (Fig. 1c) which in turn correlated negatively with 25(OH)D ($r = - 0.268$; $p = 0.008$) (Fig. 1d). This correlation was maintained using a partial correlation analysis corrected by gender ($r = - 0.273$, $p = 0.01$). Accordingly, mRNA levels were translated to higher VDR protein levels in the CRC group with regard to the control group (Fig. 1e, f).

Inflammatory status and relationship with circulating vitamin D

We checked the systemic inflammatory status by measuring serum CRP, as well as the inflammatory status of adipose tissue by determining mRNA levels of *NFκB1*, *IL6*, and *IL1B* gene expression. We found higher levels of adipose tissue *NFκB1*, *IL6*, and *IL1B* mRNA levels (Fig. 2b–d) in the CRC group with regard to the control group.

25(OH)D correlated negatively with adipose tissue NFκB1 mRNA (Table 2). Concordantly, we observed that serum CRP levels were negatively correlated with serum 25(OH)D levels and positively correlated with both VDR and *NFκB1* gene expression in adipose tissue (Table 3A). In turn, there was a positive correlation between *NFκB1* mRNA and both *IL6* and *IL1B* mRNA levels (Table 3B). Furthermore, a positive correlation was found between *NFκB1* mRNA and *VDR* (Table 3B).

VDR and NFκB1 methylation and association between the epigenetic factor DNMT3A and 25(OH)D

The DNA methylation status of the *VDR* promoter was determined by pyrosequencing, but no differences between the control and CRC groups were found (Fig. 3a). When individual *VDR* CpG positions were compared, significant lower *VDR* methylation at position 4 (*VDR* P4) was found in the CRC group when compared with the control group (Fig. 3b). *NFκB1* global methylation was lower in the CRC group than in the control group. A comparative analysis at each *NFκB1* CpG analyzed showed that *NFκB1* at position 3 (*NFκB1* P3) presented a lower methylation level in CRC with regard to the control group. Moreover, a negative trend ($r = - 0.252$, $p = 0.061$) was observed between *NFκB1* mRNA levels and *NFκB1* P3 and between *VDR* mRNA and the global *NFκB1* methylation ($r = - 0.228$; $p = 0.064$). Additionally, a negative and significant correlation was found between *VDR* mRNA and *NFκB1* at position 3 (*NFκB1* P3) ($r = - 0.296$; $p = 0.015$) and at position 4 (*NFκB1* P4) ($r = - 0.327$; $p = 0.007$). Furthermore, we analyzed *DNMT3A* gene expression in adipose tissue, which was higher in the CRC group than in the control group but without getting statistic significance (Fig. 3e). We also found a negative

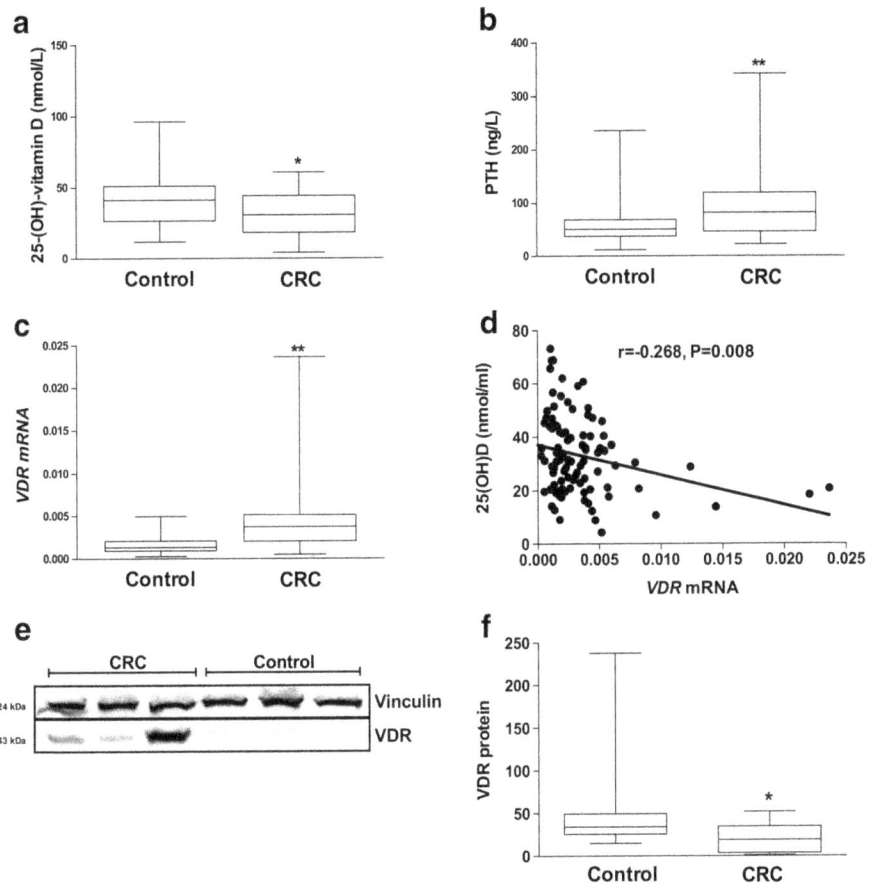

Fig. 1 Comparison of serum 25(OH)D and PTH levels and adipose tissue VDR mRNA and protein in CRC patients and controls. Comparisons were performed using Student t test (for 25(OH)D) and Mann-Whitney U test (for serum PTH and adipose tissue VDR mRNA and VRD protein). Serum levels of **a** 25(OH)D, and **b** PTH was measured by ELISA in both the control and CRC group. **c** Adipose tissue VDR mRNA expression was measured by qPCR (n = 107), and Spearman's correlation (**d**) between serum 25(OH)D and adipose tissue VDR mRNA in the whole study population was performed. Comparison of adipose tissue VDR protein (**e, f**) analyzed by Western blot (n = 18). * and ** mean $p < 0.05$ and $p < 0.01$, respectively. Parathyroid hormone (PTH), vitamin D receptor (VDR), colorectal cancer (CRC)

correlation (corrected by gender) between the gene expression of the epigenetic factor *DNMT3A* and serum 25(OH)D levels ($r = -0.264$, $p = 0.013$). There was a positive correlation between adipose tissue *DNMT3A* gene expression and adipose tissue *VDR* DNA methylation in a partial correlation corrected by gender ($r = 0.256$, $p = 0.054$). We also found a positive correlation (Spearman's correlation) between *DNMT3A* mRNA and *NFκB1* mRNA ($r = 0.279$, $p = 0.009$).

Discussion

In this study, we found lower levels of serum 25(OH)D and higher levels of CRP, which is in accordance with previous studies [34, 35]. In addition, to our knowledge, this is the first study which has aimed at analyzing the putative relationship between the VDR in adipose tissue and CRC, taking into consideration the anti-inflammatory role that has been attributed to VD [18, 36]. This is based on the hypothesis that the pro-

inflammatory profile of adipose tissue could contribute to the systemic inflammation which has been described to be related to CRC [24]. According to this hypothesis, we found that, apart from lower plasma 25(OH)D levels, CRC patients had higher adipose tissue mRNA levels of pro-inflammatory mediators. Interestingly, we also found significant differences in *VDR* gene expression between the CRC and the control group, which suggest that in fact, VD may be mediating an anti-inflammatory role in the adipose tissue of CRC patients [37]. Our study shows that adipose tissue *DNMT3A* mRNA correlates negatively with 25(OH)D and positively with adipose tissue *VDR* and *NFκB1* methylation, suggesting that VD could be involved in epigenetic modifications in both genes in adipose tissue by mechanisms involving the DNA-methyltransferase *DNMT3A*. Interestingly, the VDR CpGs analyzed were located in the promoter region of the VDR gene (Additional file 1: Figure S1) and inside several TFBS as *POLR2A, ATF2, CTCF, EZH2, E2F6,*

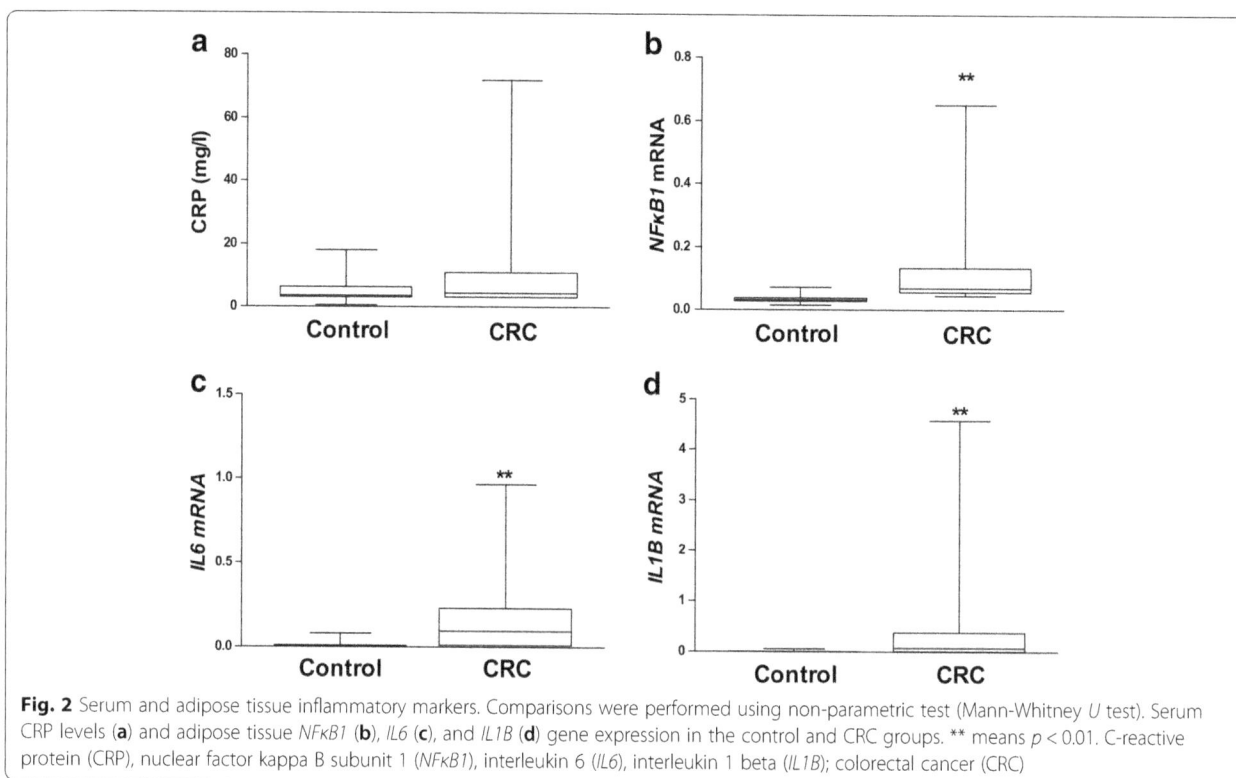

Fig. 2 Serum and adipose tissue inflammatory markers. Comparisons were performed using non-parametric test (Mann-Whitney *U* test). Serum CRP levels (**a**) and adipose tissue *NFκB1* (**b**), *IL6* (**c**), and *IL1B* (**d**) gene expression in the control and CRC groups. ** means $p < 0.01$. C-reactive protein (CRP), nuclear factor kappa B subunit 1 (*NFκB1*), interleukin 6 (*IL6*), interleukin 1 beta (*IL1B*); colorectal cancer (CRC)

GATA2, GATA3, CEBPB, or *POL2,* which some of them has been related to DNA methyltransferases recruitment [38, 39]. Changes in adipose tissue methylation status could be related to its pro-inflammatory profile, as previous studies have described a positive relationship between *DNMT3A* and inflammation in a murine model [29] as we have described in our study population.

It has been found that circulating CRP is associated with a higher risk of CRC [40], and high levels of serum CRP have been related to low levels of 25(OH)D [10], which is in agreement with our results showing a negative correlation between CRP and 25(OH)D levels. Adipose tissue dysfunction might play a crucial role in the promotion of different diseases including insulin resistance, diabetes, and cancer [41, 42]. Several mechanisms have been proposed to explain this relationship, including an altered adipokine secretion profile [24]. Some of these alterations may provoke the development of a chronic low-grade inflammatory state due to the production and secretion of pro-inflammatory cytokines by adipose tissue [41, 43, 44], which has been regarded as a favorable environment for tumor development [24]. Recently, it has been proven that cytokines secreted by adipose tissue have a direct effect on tumor aggressiveness and cancer cell migration in prostate cancer [45], and on colon cancer in mice [46]. Interestingly, it has been described that calcitriol decreases the adipose tissue chronic pro-inflammatory status by downregulating pro-

inflammatory cytokine production in a process in which *NFκB1* and *VDR* are involved [47]. Indeed, *NFκB* has been implied in cancer development [12]. Our results concur with this idea since CRC patients showed higher adipose tissue *NFκB1* gene expression in comparison with control subjects, and *NFκB1* transcription levels correlated positively to *VDR, IL6,* and *IL1B* mRNA levels, confirming the relationship between *VDR* and inflammation [47]. These facts support the idea that low circulating 25(OH)D promotes a chronic low-grade inflammatory state in adipose tissue, the effects of which could be the release of pro-inflammatory cytokines inducing or stimulating colon tumors.

Calcitriol action is mediated by its receptor, *VDR. VDR* has also been associated with CRC. Specifically, a higher tumor expression of *VDR* in CRC correlates with a better prognosis, and there is a direct relation between the tumor differentiation level and *VDR* gene expression level [48, 49]. However, to our knowledge, there are no previous studies analyzing the relationship between adipose tissue *VDR* gene expression and CRC. Here, we found that there were higher adipose tissue *VDR* mRNA and protein levels in the CRC group when compared with the control group. These high *VDR* levels in adipose tissue might be due to a compensatory mechanism in response to the low 25(OH)D levels in these subjects, and it could be a sign of VD insufficiency. Moreover, it has been

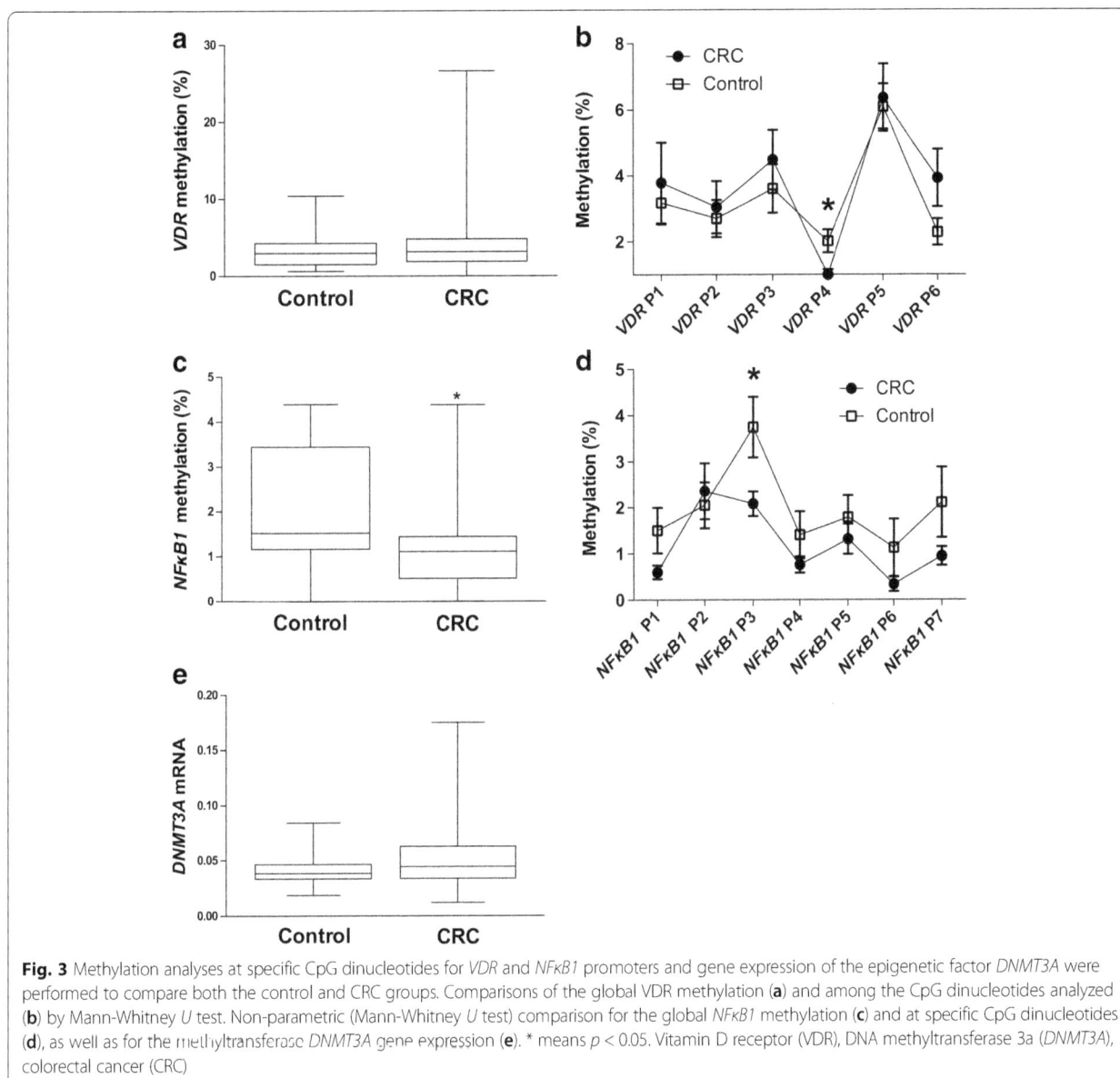

Fig. 3 Methylation analyses at specific CpG dinucleotides for *VDR* and *NFκB1* promoters and gene expression of the epigenetic factor *DNMT3A* were performed to compare both the control and CRC groups. Comparisons of the global VDR methylation (**a**) and among the CpG dinucleotides analyzed (**b**) by Mann-Whitney *U* test. Non-parametric (Mann-Whitney *U* test) comparison for the global *NFκB1* methylation (**c**) and at specific CpG dinucleotides (**d**), as well as for the methyltransferase *DNMT3A* gene expression (**e**). * means *p* < 0.05. Vitamin D receptor (VDR), DNA methyltransferase 3a (*DNMT3A*), colorectal cancer (CRC)

Table 2 Partial correlation between serum 25(OH)D and adipose tissue *NFκB1* mRNA, *IL6* mRNA and *IL1B* mRNA corrected by gender in the whole population

	25(OH)D	
	r	p
Log(*NFκB1* mRNA)	−0.232	0.041
Log(*IL6* mRNA)	−0.125	0.251
Log(*IL1B* mRNA)	−0.106	0.339

25(OH)D 25-hydroxy-vitamin D, *NFκB1* Nuclear Factor Kappa B subunit 1, *IL6* Interleukin 6, *IL1B* Interleukin 1 beta

reported that the inflammatory factor TNF can activate *VDR* gene expression [50]. So, a lack of 25(OH)D might lead to an inflammatory process which could subsequently promote *VDR* expression as we observed in our study. High *VDR* expression without its ligand, calcitriol, has been shown to have an opposite effect in gene expression regulation and could alter epigenetic marks [51, 52].

In addition, although previous studies described a relationship between methylation status and 25(OH)D [27], which agrees with our observation between *DNMT3A* and 25(OH)D levels, this phenomenon has not previously been analyzed in adipose tissue. Therefore, to our knowledge, the present study is the first one to report a negative association between 25(OH)D levels and adipose tissue *DNMT3A* gene expression. Concordantly,

Table 3 Partial correlations of C-reactive protein (A) with serum 25(OH)D, adipose tissue *VDR* mRNA, *NFκB1* mRNA, *IL6* mRNA, and *IL1B* mRNA corrected by gender. Partial correlations corrected by gender of adipose tissue *NFκB1* mRNA (B) with IL 6 mRNA, *IL1B* mRNA and *VDR* mRNA

A	Log(C-reactive protein)	
	r	p
Log(25(OH)D)	−0.270	0.011
Log(*VDR* mRNA)	0.219	0.049
Log(*NFκB1* mRNA)	0.284	0.016
Log(*IL6* mRNA)	0.245	0.029
Log(*IL1B* mRNA)	0.272	0.016
B	*NFκB1* mRNA	
	r	p
Log(*IL6* mRNA)	0.688	0.000
Log(*IL1B* mRNA)	0.778	0.000
Log(*VDR* mRNA)	0.761	0.000

25(OH)D 25-hydroxy-vitamin D, *VDR* vitamin D receptor, *NFκB1* Nuclear Factor Kappa B subunit 1, *IL6* Interleukin 6, *IL1B* Interleukin 1 beta

DNMT3A mRNA levels were positively correlated with global *VDR* promoter methylation. This could suggest an epigenetic effect in adipose tissue via VD action. Interestingly, when the methylation of key individual CpGs was analyzed, we found that methylation levels at *VDR* P4 were significantly lower in CRC than in the control subjects. However, it should also be taken into consideration that other mechanisms might be involved in the regulation of gene expressions such as histone modifications or microRNAs. Therefore, further studies will be necessary to clarify the relevance of *VDR* methylation in the regulation of its expression in adipose tissue as well as the consequences that these epigenetic changes could have in CRC. We also found a possible regulation of *NFκB1* gene expression through DNA methylation. Furthermore, we saw an association between *VDR* mRNA levels and *NFκB1* DNA methylation, which could agree with previous studies although a deeper approach would be necessary to clarify the possible relationship between *VDR* and the VD signaling with the epigenetic control in *NFκB1* gene expression.

Conclusions

Our results suggest that adipose tissue may be a key factor in CRC development. The low 25(OH)D levels in CRC and high adipose tissue *VDR* expression may, at least in part, mediate this relationship by modifying adipose tissue DNA methylation and promoting inflammation. Although more studies are needed to discover the precise mediators and mechanisms that determine this relationship, the possible mediation of adipose tissue in CRC should be borne in mind to create new treatments and preventive strategies for CRC.

Abbreviations
25(OH)D: 25-Hydroxyvitamin D; CRC: Colorectal cancer; CRP: C-reactive protein; DNMT3A: DNA methyltransferase 3a; HOMA-IR: Homeostasis model assessment of insulin resistance; IL1: Interleukin-1; IL6: Interleukin-6; NFκB1: Nuclear factor κ-light-chain-enhancer of activated B cells; TNFA: Tumor necrosis factor alpha; VAT: Visceral adipose tissue; VD: Vitamin D; VDR: Vitamin D receptor

Acknowledgements
The authors thank all the subjects for their important contribution and to Richard Carlsson for his help in the English grammar correction.

Funding
This study was supported by "Centros de Investigación En Red" (CIBER, CB06/03/0018) of the "Instituto de Salud Carlos III" (ISCIII) and grants from ISCIII (PI11/01661, PI15/0114) and co-financed by the European Regional Development Fund (FEDER). DCC was the recipient of a FPU grant from Education Ministry, Madrid, Spain (13/04211). MMG was the recipient of the Nicolas Monardes Programme from the "Servicio Andaluz de Salud, Junta de Andalucia", Spain (C-0029-2014).

Authors' contributions
The authors' responsibilities were as follows. DCC, SM, MCP, and MMG contributed to the project conception and leadership of overall research plan, writing of the first draft of the manuscript, and primary responsibility for the final content of the manuscript. DCC, SM, and MCP performed the statistical analysis. DCC, SM and ABC contributed to the bisulfite genomic sequencing and pyrosequencing assessment. DCC and MCP performed the functional and gene expression analysis. FJT, JCF, and EO contributed to the sampling and clinical data collection. MCP, JCF, EO, and FJT contributed to the interpretation of data and critical revision of the manuscript. MMG and FJT acquired funding for this study. All authors were involved in the writing of the manuscript and approving the final version of this article.

Competing interests
The authors declare that they have no competing interests.

Author details
¹1Unidad de Gestión Clínica de Endocrinología y Nutrición del Hospital Virgen de la Victoria, Instituto de Investigación Biomédica de Málaga (IBIMA), Universidad de Málaga, Málaga, Spain. ²CIBER Fisiopatología de la Obesidad y Nutrición (CB06/03), Madrid, Spain. ³Laboratory of Molecular and Cellular Endocrinology, Instituto de Investigación Sanitaria (IDIS), Complejo Hospitalario Universitario de Santiago (CHUS/SERGAS), Santiago de Compostela University (USC), Santiago de Compostela, Spain. ⁴CIBER Fisiopatología de la Obesidad y la Nutrición (CIBERobn), Madrid, Spain. ⁵Unidad de Gestión Clínica de Oncología Intercentros Hospital Universitario Virgen de la Victoria, Málaga, Spain.

References

1. Lippi G, Mattiuzzi C, Cervellin G. Meat consumption and cancer risk: a critical review of published meta-analyses. Crit Rev Oncol Hematol. 2015; https://doi.org/10.1016/j.critrevonc.2015.11.008.
2. Saccone D, Asani F, Bornman L. Regulation of the vitamin D receptor gene by environment, genetics and epigenetics. Gene. 2015;561:171–80. https://doi.org/10.1016/j.gene.2015.02.024.
3. Platz EA, Hankinson SE, Hollis BW, Colditz GA, Hunter DJ, Speizer FE, et al. Plasma 1, 25-Dihydroxy- and 25-hydroxyvitamin D and adenomatous polyps of the distal colorectum 1. Cancer Epidemiol Biomarkers Prev. 2000;9:1059–65.
4. Song M, Konijeti GG, Yuan C, Ananthakrishnan AN, Ogino S, Fuchs CS, et al. Plasma 25-hydroxyvitamin D, vitamin D binding protein, and risk of colorectal cancer in the nurses' health study. Cancer Prev Res. 2016; https://doi.org/10.1158/1940-6207.CAPR-16-0053.
5. Giovannucci E, Liu Y, Rimm EB, Hollis BW, Fuchs CS, Stampfer MJ, et al. Prospective study of predictors of vitamin D status and cancer incidence and mortality in men. J Natl Cancer Inst. 2006;98:451–9.
6. Mason RS, Sequeira VB, Gordon-Thomson C. Vitamin D: the light side of sunshine. Eur J Clin Nutr. 2011;65:986–93.
7. Peehl DM, Skowronski RJ, Leung GK, Wong ST, Stamey TA, Feldman D. Antiproliferative effects of 1,25-dihydroxyvitamin D3 on primary cultures of human prostatic cells. Cancer Res. 1994;54:805–10.
8. Flynn G, Chung I, Yu W-D, Romano M, Modzelewski RA, Johnson CS, et al. Calcitriol (1,25-dihydroxycholecalciferol) selectively inhibits proliferation of freshly isolated tumor-derived endothelial cells and induces apoptosis. Oncology. 2006;70:447–57.
9. Neska J, Swoboda P, Przybyszewska M, Kotlarz A, Bolla N, Miłoszewska J, et al. The effect of analogues of 1α,25-dihydroxyvitamin D2 on the regrowth and gene expression of human colon cancer cells refractory to 5-fluorouracil. Int J Mol Sci. 2016;17:903. https://doi.org/10.3390/ijms17060903.
10. Hopkins MH, Owen J, Ahearn T, Fedirko V, Flanders WD. Effects of supplemental vitamin D and calcium on biomarkers of inflammation in colorectal adenoma patients: a randomized, controlled clinical trial. Cancer Prev Res (Phila). 2011;4(10):1645–655.
11. Liu Z, Brooks RS, Ciappio ED, Kim SJ, Crott JW, Bennett G, et al. Diet-induced obesity elevates colonic TNF-α in mice and is accompanied by an activation of Wnt signaling: a mechanism for obesity-associated colorectal cancer. J Nutr Biochem. 2012;23:1207–13. https://doi.org/10.1016/j.jnutbio.2011.07.002.
12. Aggarwal BB. Nuclear factor-kappaB: the enemy within. Cancer Cell. 2004;6:203–8.
13. Fantuzzi G. Adipose tissue, adipokines, and inflammation. J Allergy Clin Immunol. 2005;115:911–20.
14. Wamberg L, Christiansen T, Paulsen SK, Fisker S, Rask P, Rejnmark L, et al. Expression of vitamin D-metabolizing enzymes in human adipose tissue—the effect of obesity and diet-induced weight loss. Int J Obes. 2012;37:651–7. https://doi.org/10.1038/ijo.2012.112.
15. Davis CD, Dwyer JT. The "sunshine vitamin": benefits beyond bone? J Natl Cancer Inst. 2007;99:1563–5.
16. Wood RJ. Vitamin D and adipogenesis: new molecular insights. Nutr Rev. 2008;66:40–6.
17. Ding C, Gao D, Wilding J, Trayhurn P, Bing C. Vitamin D signalling in adipose tissue. Br J Nutr. 2012;2:1–9.
18. Lira FS, Rosa JC, Cunha CA, Ribeiro EB, do Nascimento CO, Oyama LM, et al. Supplementing alpha-tocopherol (vitamin E) and vitamin D3 in high fat diet decrease IL-6 production in murine epididymal adipose tissue and 3T3-L1 adipocytes following LPS stimulation. Lipids Health Dis. 2011;10:37. https://doi.org/10.1186/1476-511X-10-37.
19. Suzuki MM, Bird A. DNA methylation landscapes provocative inside from epigenomics. Nat Rev Genet. 2008;9:465–76.
20. Rishi V, Bhattacharya P, Chatterjee R, Rozenberg J, Zhao J, Glass K, et al. CpG methylation of half-CRE sequences creates C/EBPalpha binding sites that activate some tissue-specific genes. Proc Natl Acad Sci U S A. 2010;107:20311–6. https://doi.org/10.1073/pnas.1008688107.
21. Campión J, Milagro F, Martínez JA. Epigenetics and obesity. Prog Mol Biol Transl Sci. 2010;94:291–347. https://doi.org/10.1016/B978-0-12-375003-7.00011-X.
22. Sabàtino L, Fucci A, Pancione M, Colantuoni V. PPARG epigenetic deregulation and its role in colorectal tumorigenesis. PPAR Res. 2012;2012:687492. https://doi.org/10.1155/2012/687492.
23. Sinha G. Homing in on the fat and cancer connection. J Natl Cancer Inst. 2012;104:966–7. https://doi.org/10.1093/jnci/djs306.
24. Riondino S, Roselli M, Palmirotta R, Della-Morte D, Ferroni P, Guadagni F. Obesity and colorectal cancer: role of adipokines in tumor initiation and progression. World J Gastroenterol. 2014;20:5177–90.
25. Ali O, Cerjak D, Kent JW, James R, Blangero J, Carless MA, et al. An epigenetic map of age-associated autosomal loci in northern European families at high risk for the metabolic syndrome. Clin Epigenetics. 2015;7:12. https://doi.org/10.1186/s13148-015-0048-6.
26. Uzunlulu M, Telci Caklili O, Oguz A. Association between metabolic syndrome and cancer. Ann Nutr Metab. 2016;178:173–9.
27. Zhu H, Bhagatwala J, Huang Y, Pollock NK, Parikh S, Raed A, et al. Race/ethnicity-specific association of vitamin D and global DNA methylation: cross-sectional and interventional findings. PLoS One. 2016;11:2–10.
28. Xue J, Schoenrock SA, Valdar W, Tarantino LM, Ideraabdullah FY. Maternal vitamin D depletion alters DNA methylation at imprinted loci in multiple generations. Clin Epigenetics. 2016;8:107. https://doi.org/10.1186/s13148-016-0276-4.
29. Kamei Y, Suganami T, Ehara T, Kanai S, Hayashi K, Yamamoto Y, et al. Increased expression of DNA methyltransferase 3a in obese adipose tissue: studies with transgenic mice. Obesity (Silver Spring). 2010;18:314–21. https://doi.org/10.1038/oby.2009.246.
30. Clemente-Postigo M, Muñoz-Garach A, Serrano M, Garrido-Sánchez L, Bernal-López MR, Fernández-García D, et al. Serum 25-Hydroxyvitamin D and adipose tissue vitamin D receptor gene expression: relationship with obesity and type 2 diabetes. J Clin Endocrinol Metab. 2015; https://doi.org/10.1210/jc.2014-3016.
31. Gerstein MB, Kundaje A, Hariharan M, Landt SG, Yan K, Cheng C, et al. Architecture of the human regulatory network derived from ENCODE data. Nature. 2012;488:91–100. https://doi.org/10.1038/nature11245.
32. Lesurf R, Cotto KC, Wang G, Griffith M, Kasaian K, Jones SJM, et al. ORegAnno 3.0: a community-driven resource for curated regulatory annotation. Nucleic Acids Res. 2016;44:D126–32.
33. Holick MF, Binkley NC, Bischoff-Ferrari HA, Gordon CM, Hanley DA, Heaney RP, et al. Evaluation, treatment, and prevention of vitamin D deficiency: an endocrine society clinical practice guideline. J Clin Endocrinol Metab. 2011;96:1911–30.
34. Klampfer L. Vitamin D and colon cancer. World J Gastrointest Oncol. 2014;6(11):430–37.
35. Allin KH, Bojesen SE, Nordestgaard BG. Inflammatory biomarkers and risk of cancer in 84,000 individuals from the general population. Int J Cancer. 2016;139:1493–500.
36. Krishnan AV, Feldman D. Mechanisms of the anti-cancer and anti-inflammatory actions of vitamin D. Annu Rev Pharmacol Toxicol. 2011;51:311–36. https://doi.org/10.1146/annurev-pharmtox-010510-100611.
37. Abbas MA. Physiological functions of vitamin D in adipose tissue. J Steroid Biochem Mol Biol. 2017;165:369–81. https://doi.org/10.1016/j.jsbmb.2016.08.004.
38. Velasco G, Hubé F, Rollin J, Neuillet D, Philippe C, Bouzinba-segard H. Dnmt3b recruitment through E2F6 transcriptional repressor mediates germ-line gene silencing in murine somatic tissues. 2010;107:9281–6.
39. Chou R, Yu Y, Hung M. The roles of EZH2 in cell lineage commitment. 2011;3:243–50.
40. Zhou B, Shu B, Yang J, Liu J. C-reactive protein, interleukin-6 and the risk of colorectal cancer: a meta-analysis. 2014;1397–1405.
41. Van Kruijsdijk RCM, van Der Wall E, Visseren FLJ. Obesity and cancer: the role of dysfunctional adipose tissue. Cancer Epidemiol Biomark Prev. 2009;18:2569–78.
42. Yamamoto S, Nakagawa T, Matsushita Y, Kusano S, Hayashi T, Irokawa M, et al. Visceral fat area and markers of insulin resistance in relation to colorectal neoplasia. Diabetes Care. 2010;33:184–9. https://doi.org/10.2337/dc09-1197.
43. Sikalidis AK, Varamini B. Roles of hormones and signaling molecules in describing the relationship between obesity and colon cancer. Pathol Oncol Res. 2011;17:785–90. https://doi.org/10.1007/s12253-010-9352-9.
44. Aleksandrova K, Nimptsch K, Pischon T. Influence of obesity and related metabolic alterations on colorectal cancer risk. Curr Nutr Rep. 2013;2:1–9. https://doi.org/10.1007/s13668-012-0036-9.
45. Laurent V, Guérard A, Mazerolles C, Le Gonidec S, Toulet A, Nieto L, et al. Periprostatic adipocytes act as a driving force for prostate cancer progression in obesity. Nat Commun. 2016;7:10230. https://doi.org/10.1038/ncomms10230.

46. Cao L, Liu X, Lin ED, Wang C, Choi EY, Riban V, et al. Environmental and genetic activation of a brain-adipocyte BDNF/leptin axis causes cancer remission and inhibition. Cell. 2010;142:52–64. https://doi.org/10.1016/j.cell.2010.05.029.

47. Marcotorchino J, Gouranton E, Romier B, Tourniaire F, Astier J, Malezet C, et al. Vitamin D reduces the inflammatory response and restores glucose uptake in adipocytes. Mol Nutr Food Res. 2012;56:1771–82.

48. Shabahang M, Buras RR, Davoodi F, Schumaker LM, Nauta RJ, Evans SR. 1,25-Dihydroxyvitamin D3 receptor as a marker of human colon carcinoma cell line differentiation and growth inhibition. Cancer Res. 1993;53:3712–8.

49. Evans SR, Nolla J, Hanfelt J, Shabahang M, Nauta RJ, Shchepotin IB. Vitamin D receptor expression as a predictive marker of biological behavior in human colorectal cancer. Clin Cancer Res. 1998;4:1591–5.

50. Ziv E, Koren R, Zahalka MA, Ravid A. TNF-α increases the expression and activity of vitamin D receptor in keratinocytes: role of c-Jun N-terminal kinase. Dermatoendocrinol. 2016;8:e1137399. https://doi.org/10.1080/19381980.2015.1137399.

51. Fetahu IS, Höbaus J, Kállay E. Vitamin D and the epigenome. Front Physiol. 2014;5:164. https://doi.org/10.3389/fphys.2014.00164.

52. Lee SM, Pike JW. The vitamin D receptor functions as a transcription regulator in the absence of 1,25-dihydroxyvitamin D3. J Steroid Biochem Mol Biol. 2015:4–9. https://doi.org/10.1016/j.jsbmb.2015.08.018.

12

Genetic variation affecting DNA methylation and the human imprinting disorder, Beckwith-Wiedemann syndrome

Vinod Dagar[1], Wendy Hutchison[2], Andrea Muscat[3], Anita Krishnan[4], David Hoke[5], Ashley Buckle[5], Priscillia Siswara[2], David J. Amor[1,6], Jeffrey Mann[7], Jason Pinner[8], Alison Colley[9], Meredith Wilson[10], Rani Sachdev[11], George McGillivray[6], Matthew Edwards[12], Edwin Kirk[11], Felicity Collins[10], Kristi Jones[10,13], Juliet Taylor[14], Ian Hayes[14], Elizabeth Thompson[15,16], Christopher Barnett[15], Eric Haan[15], Mary-Louise Freckmann[17], Anne Turner[11,18], Susan White[6], Ben Kamien[19], Alan Ma[10], Fiona Mackenzie[20], Gareth Baynam[20], Cathy Kiraly-Borri[20], Michael Field[19], Tracey Dudding-Byth[19,21] and Elizabeth M. Algar[1,2,22,23*] (iD)

Abstract

Background: Beckwith-Wiedemann syndrome (BWS) is an imprinting disorder with a population frequency of approximately 1 in 10,000. The most common epigenetic defect in BWS is a loss of methylation (LOM) at the 11p15.5 imprinting centre, KCNQ1OT1 TSS-DMR, and affects 50% of cases. We hypothesised that genetic factors linked to folate metabolism may play a role in BWS predisposition via effects on methylation maintenance at KCNQ1OT1 TSS-DMR.

Results: Single nucleotide variants (SNVs) in the folate pathway affecting methylenetetrahydrofolate reductase (*MTHFR*), methionine synthase reductase (*MTRR*), 5-methyltetrahydrofolate-homocysteine *S*-methyltransferase (*MTR*), cystathionine beta-synthase (*CBS*) and methionine adenosyltransferase (*MAT1A*) were examined in 55 BWS patients with KCNQ1OT1 TSS-DMR LOM and in 100 unaffected cases. *MTHFR* rs1801133: C>T was more prevalent in BWS with KCNQ1OT1 TSS-DMR LOM ($p < 0.017$); however, the relationship was not significant when the Bonferroni correction for multiple testing was applied (significance, $p = 0.0036$). None of the remaining 13 SNVs were significantly different in the two populations tested. The *DNMT1* locus was screened in 53 BWS cases, and three rare missense variants were identified in each of three patients: rs138841970: C>T, rs150331990: A>G and rs757460628: G>A encoding NP_001124295 p.Arg136Cys, p. His1118Arg and p.Arg1223His, respectively. These variants have population frequencies of less than 1 in 1000 and were absent from 100 control cases. Functional characterization using a hemimethylated DNA trapping assay revealed a reduced methyltransferase activity relative to wild-type DNMT1 for each variant ranging from 40 to 70% reduction in activity.

Conclusions: This study is the first to examine folate pathway genetics in BWS and to identify rare DNMT1 missense variants in affected individuals. Our data suggests that reduced DNMT1 activity could affect maintenance of methylation at KCNQ1OT1 TSS-DMR in some cases of BWS, possibly via a maternal effect in the early embryo. Larger cohort studies are warranted to further interrogate the relationship between impaired MTHFR enzymatic activity attributable to *MTHFR* rs1801133: C>T, dietary folate intake and BWS.

Keywords: DNA methyltransferase 1, Beckwith-Wiedemann syndrome, One-carbon pathway, Methylation

* Correspondence: elizabeth.algar@monash.edu
[1]Department of Paediatrics, University of Melbourne, Parkville 3052, Australia
[2]Pathology, Monash Health, Clayton 3168, Australia
Full list of author information is available at the end of the article

Background

The human imprinting disorder Beckwith-Wiedemann syndrome (BWS) (OMIM 130650) is characterised by overgrowth in the prenatal and postnatal period, macroglossia, umbilical hernia or exomphalos, neonatal hypoglycaemia, ear lobe creases and pits, nevi flammei, hemihyperplasia and organomegaly, particularly of the kidney, liver and pancreas. One of its more serious complications is an increased predisposition to cancer in early childhood with tumour risk segregating with distinct genetic and epigenetic subtypes (reviewed in [1–4]).

The majority of the affected children have an isolated epigenetic abnormality at the 11p15.5 imprinting centre 2 (IC2), known as KCNQ1OT1 TSS-DMR, the location of the *KCNQ1OT1/CDKN1C* locus. Fifty percent of all children with features of BWS have either mosaic or complete loss of methylation (LOM) within the *KCNQ1OT1* promoter and impaired expression of maternal *CDKN1C*, a critical regulator of growth during early development [5, 6]. For the majority of BWS cases with KCNQ1OT1 TSS-DMR imprinting disruption, the aetiology is unknown and the phenotype arises without any evidence of heritability. Rare cases have been reported with imprinting defects in KCNQ1OT1 TSS-DMR associated with inherited recessive mutations affecting *NLRP2* on 19q13.42 [7], and more recently, maternal effect missense and truncating variants in other NLRP loci, including NLRP5 and NLRP7, were reported in the mothers of offspring with multi-locus imprinting disruption (MLID) that included loss of methylation at KCNQ1OT1 TSS-DMR [8, 9]. MLID cases with methylation loss at KCNQ1OT1 TSS-DMR frequently had characteristics of BWS. Animal studies have shown that defective methylation is set in the gametes or during the first cell divisions of the embryo, and genetic modifiers and environmental factors influence this process [10]. Indeed, in BWS, the increased incidence of BWS cases with KCNQ1OT1 TSS-DMR LOM after assisted reproduction (ART) points to the involvement of environmental factors that perturb methylation at KCNQ1OT1 TSS-DMR or alternatively suggest a link between therapeutic interventions for female infertility and defective methylation [11–15].

The one-carbon pathway is the major metabolic pathway through which dietary folate is converted to methyl donor groups that subsequently methylate DNA via catalysis of the universal methyl donor S-adenosyl-methionine in the presence of DNA methyltransferase 1 (DNMT1). The key enzymes of this pathway include methylenetetrahydrofolate reductase (*MTHFR*), methionine synthase reductase (*MTRR*), 5-methyltetrahydrofolate-homocysteine S-methyltransferase (MTR), cystathionine beta-synthase (*CBS*) and methionine adenosyltransferase (*MAT1A*), and the associated effects of genetic variants with impaired enzyme activity have been documented in several studies. A common SNV (previously commonly known as c.677C>T) in *MTHFR*, rs1801133: C>T, NP_005948.3: p.Ala222Val, increases protein thermolability [16] and has been linked to vascular thrombosis, hyperhomocysteinaemia and global hypomethylation in a setting of dietary folate depletion ([17–20]. A second *MTHFR* SNV, rs1801131: A>C, NP_005948.3: p.Gln429Ala, is linked to DNA hypomethylation, independently of folate availability and acts synergistically with rs1801133 to reduce MTHFR activity [21, 22]. MTR catalyses the remethylation of homocysteine to methionine and SNV rs1805087: A>G, NP_000245.2: p.Asp919Gly alters the helix structure in the substrate binding domain leading to impaired methionine biosynthesis and reduced methyl donor availability [23–25]. *MTRR* rs1801394: A>G, NP_002445.2 p.Ile22-Met, acts synergistically with homozygous *MTHFR* rs1801133: C>T, NP_005948.3: p.Ala222Val, in the presence of low folate and/or vitamin B12 status [26].

The isoforms of Dnmt1 (Dnmt1o and Dnmt1s) play a critical role in the maintenance of DNA methylation at imprinted regions during pre-implantation mammalian development [27]. The absence of 118 N terminal amino acids allows Dnmt1o protein to accumulate to high levels in non-dividing growing oocytes [28], and expression is maintained in pre-implantation embryos in the morula and blastocyst. Howell et al. 2001 showed that *Dnmt1o*, while not essential for imprint establishment in oocytes, was required for the maintenance of methylation at imprinted loci, and heterozygous offspring of *Dnmt1o*-null mothers exhibited imprinting defects. The functions of Dnmt1o and Dnmt1 are interchangeable as Dnmt1 is itself able to maintain methylation during pre-implantation development [29, 30], and Dnmt1o can rescue *Dnmt1−/−* ES cells [31]. However, although these studies implicate DNMT1 in imprinting disorders, it has not previously been examined in the context of BWS or MLID.

In this study, we investigated the genetics of folate metabolism and maintenance of DNA methylation in cases of BWS with loss of methylation at KCNQ1OT1 TSS-DMR. This included an analysis of SNVs in *MTHFR, MTRR, MTR, MAT1A* and *CBS* predicted to alter the function and a full mutation screen of *DNMT1*. While a statistically significant association between deleterious SNVs in folate pathway genes could not be conclusively demonstrated, we identified three patients with rare missense amino acid substitutions in *DNMT1* that are represented in dbSNP at a frequency of < 0.001. Functional characterization of these variants showed a significant reduction in complex formation with hemimethylated DNA, consistent with impaired DNMT1 activity. This is the first study examining the folate pathway and the major human methyltransferase, *DNMT1*, in the most common epigenetic subtype of BWS.

Results

Analysis of *MTHFR, MTRR, MTR, MAT1A* and *CBS* in BWS cases with KCNQ1OT1 TSS-DMR LOM

The one-carbon pathway of folate metabolism is shown in Fig. 1. Coding SNVs in *MTHFR, MTRR* and *MTR* generating missense amino acid substitutions and for which previous evidence of impaired or altered enzyme function had been demonstrated in other studies were selected for investigation in the BWS study population (55 cases) and in a matched local control population (100 cases). The enzymes MAT1A and CBS were also included because rare coding SNVs were identified in genome databases with damaging polyphen scores and predicted structural effects.

All gene SNVs interrogated in the study are shown in Table 1.

Fifty-five unrelated cases with clinical features of BWS were assessed as having either complete or partial LOM at KCNQ1OT1 TSS-DMR. Ten of these 55 cases had multi-locus imprinting disruption (MLID) involving losses of methylation at additional imprinting domains including *MEST, PLAGL1, GRB10, NESPAS* and *PEG3* (Additional file 1: Table S1). A total of 11 cases had been conceived using assisted reproductive technologies (ART). Specimens were screened using HRM across selected one-carbon pathway SNVs, and those with shifted melt profiles were sequenced. Specific reaction conditions are shown in Additional file 1: Tables S2 and S3. The significance of minor allele SNV frequencies in the BWS study population for each gene was calculated using the chi-squared analysis relative to the frequencies determined in 100 control DNA specimens from the cord blood.

The MTHFR rs1801133 minor allele is more prevalent in BWS with KCNQ1OT1 TSS-DMR LOM.

Table 2 shows SNV frequencies in BWS patients with KCNQ1OT1 TSS-DMR LOM, including those with MLID, compared to controls and frequencies in dbSNP147. One SNV of 14 screened, *MTHFR* rs1801133: C>T, was significantly different when compared to the local control population with a p value of 0.0167 derived using a 2×2 contingency table. There were 43 T alleles in a total of 110 in the BWS subgroup compared to 52 T alleles in a total of 200 alleles in the control group. *MAT1A* and *CBS* minor allele frequencies were too low in both populations for meaningful statistical analysis to be done. After correcting for multiple testing of each of the 14 one-carbon pathway SNVs examined, the Bonferroni significance value was 0.0036 (0.05/14). The p value for *MTHFR* rs1801133: C>T at 0.0167 was no longer significant when this more stringent statistical test was applied to the data. Hence, although MTHFR rs1801133: C>T appears to be more prevalent in the BWS population, this finding is not statistically significant when adjustment for multiple testing is applied.

Rare variants of *DNMT1* are present in some BWS cases with KCNQ1OT1 TSS-DMR LOM

Dnmt1 and Dnmt1o proteins play a central role in the maintenance of DNA methylation during pre-implantation embryonic development, and DNMT1 is the major enzyme in the folate pathway responsible for the catalysis of *S*-adenosyl methionine, providing methyl groups for methylation of DNA. Hayward et al. [32] defined the location of human *DNMT1o* from sequence derived from EST BE537788. Primers were designed to this region (hg19 GRCh37 chr19: 10311482-10311816) and to the entire coding region of *DNMT1* (NM_001130823.1, representing the longest transcript). Variants affecting the coding regions of *DNMT1o* and *DNMT1* were screened by HRM and sequenced to

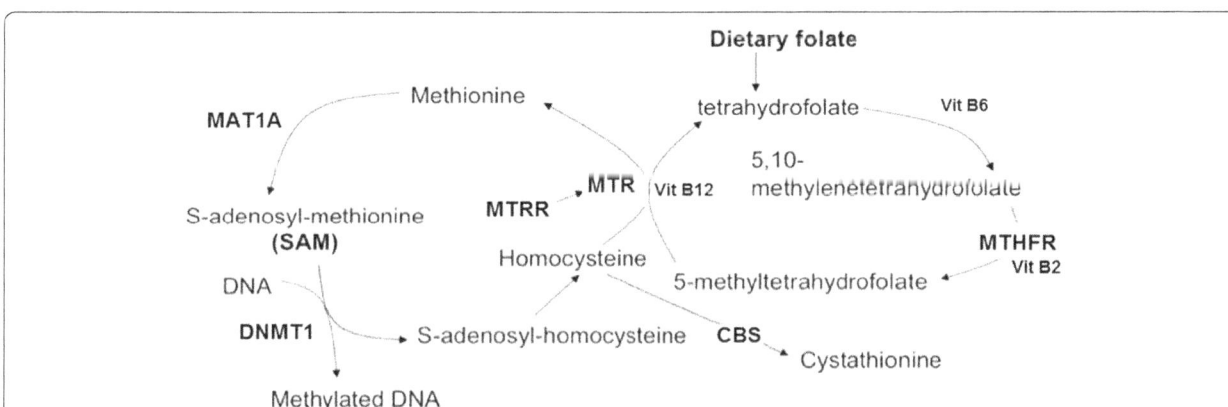

Fig. 1 The one-carbon pathway responsible for the conversion of dietary folate to methyl donor groups. The critical enzymes in the pathway examined in this study are shown in bold. MTHFR is primarily responsible for the conversion of tetrahydrofolate to methylene-tetrahydrofolate. MTRR and MTR work together to catalyse the conversion of homocysteine to methionine in the presence of the cofactor vitamin B12 and zinc, enabling the movement of the methyl group from methylene-tetrahydrofolate and recycling of tetrahydrofolate. CBS converts homocysteine in the presence of vitamin B6 to cystathione and MAT1A is responsible for converting methionine to S-adenosy-methionine (SAM), the ultimate methyl donor for DNA via catalysis by DNA methyltransferase

Table 1 SNVs interrogated in BWS patients with loss of methylation at KCNQ1OT1 TSS-DMR

Gene	SNV_1 ID	SNV_2 ID	SNV_3 ID	SNV_4 ID
MTHFR	677C>T Rs 1801133: C>T	Rs 1801131: A>C	Rs 2274976: G>A	
	NM_005957.4: c.665C>T	NM_005957.4: c.1286A>C	NM_005957.4:c.1781G>A	
	NP_005948.3 p.Ala222Val	NP_005948.3 p.Gln429Ala	NP_005948.3 p.Arg594Gln	
	A = 0.24	G = 0.24	T = 0.075	
MTRR	Rs 1801394: A>G	Rs 2287780: C>T	Rs 10380: C>T	
	NM_002454.2: c.66A>G	NM_002454.2: c.1243C>T	NM_024010.2: c.1864C>T	
	NP_002445.2 p.Ile22Met	NP_002445.2 p.Arg415Cys	NP_076915.2 p.His622Tyr	
	G = 0.36 GMAF, 0.47 ClinVar, 0.45 EXAC	T = 0.0679	T = 0.219	
MAT1A	Rs 114494303: G>A	Rs 72558181: G>A	Rs 112848063: A>G	Rs 116659053: G>A
	NM_00429.2: c.530G>A	NM_00429.2: c.791G>A	NM_00429.2: c.1061A>G	NM_00429.2: c.1066G>A
	NP_00420.1 p.Arg177Gln	NP_00420.1 p.Arg264His	NP_00420.1 p.Asp354Gly	NP_00420.1 p.Arg356Trp
	A = 0.0002	A = 0.000009		A = 0.0002
MTR	Rs 1805087: A>G			
	NM_000254.2: c.2756A>G,			
	NP_000245.2 p.Asp919Gly			
	G = 0.218			
CBS	Rs 17849313: G>C	Rs 117687681: C>T	Rs 11700812: G>A/C	
	NM_001178009.1: c.205G>C	NM_001178009.1: c.1105C>T	NM_000071.2: c.1106G>A, G>C	
	NP_000062.1 p.Ala69Pro	NP_000062.1 p.Arg369Cys	NP_001171479.1 p.Arg369His,	
		A = 0.0012	NP_001171479.1 p.Arg369Pro.	
			T/G = 0.00003	

Allele frequency data was obtained from dbSNP147 or other sources as indicated. Minor allele nucleotides on the forward genomic strand are shown. Where the alternate allele frequency is not shown, the SNV frequency is unknown. The MTHFR variant commonly referred to as c.677C>T is MTHFR: NM_005957.4 c.665C>T in HGVS format. Nucleotide numbering uses + 1 as the A of the ATG translation initiation codon

Table 2 Table showing one carbon pathway enzyme allele frequencies in 55 BWS and 100 control specimens and their significance values

Gene	SNV	BWS MAF 110 alleles	Local control MAF 200 alleles	p value BWS versus local controls	Global control MAF
MTHFR	Rs1801133: C>T	0.391	0.260	*0.0167*	0.24
	Rs1801131: A>C	0.309	0.400	0.0516	0.2494
	Rs2274976: G>A	0.045	0.060	0.6606	0.075
MTRR	Rs1801394: A>G	0.560	0.490	0.214	0.46*
	Rs2287780: C>T	0.0833	0.035	0.068	0.076
	Rs10380: C>T	0.1204	0.090	0.397	0.174
MAT1A	Rs114494303: G>A	0.01	0.00	NS	0.0002
	Rs72558181: G>A	0.01	0.00	NS	0.000009
	Rs112848063: A>G	0.00	0.00	NS	NA
	Rs116659053: G>A	0.00	0.00	NS	0.0002
MTR	Rs1805087: A>G	0.2091	0.220	0.981	0.218
CBS	Rs17849313: G>C	0.000	0.00	NS	NA
	Rs117687681: C>T	0.010	0.00	NS	NA
	Rs11700812: G>A/C	0.000	0.00	NS	NA

Global allele frequencies were derived from dbSNP147. p values were derived from chi-squared analysis with one degree of freedom

p values of significance (< 0.05) are in italics

MAF minor allele frequency, *NS* not significant, *NA* data not available

*The minor allele frequency was calculated from the mean MAF in EXAc (0.452) and Clinvar (0.47)

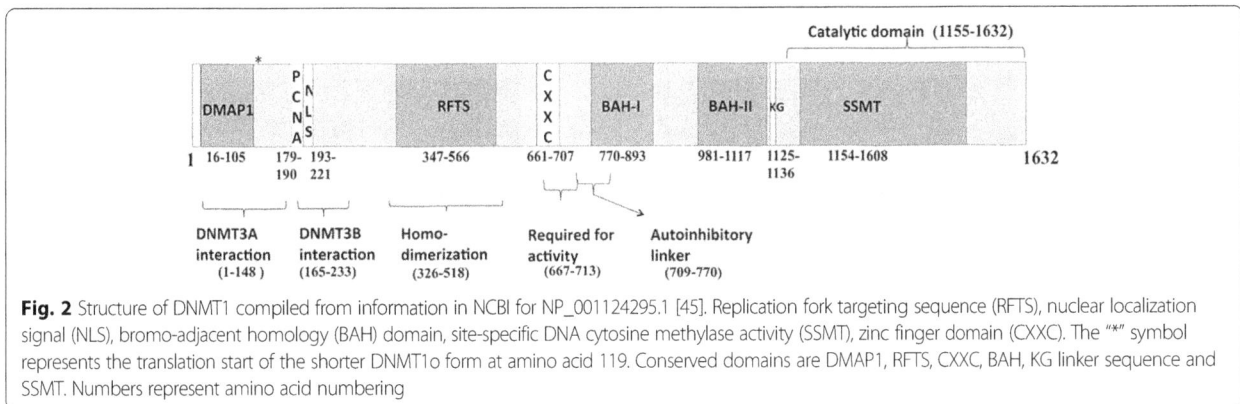

Fig. 2 Structure of DNMT1 compiled from information in NCBI for NP_001124295.1 [45]. Replication fork targeting sequence (RFTS), nuclear localization signal (NLS), bromo-adjacent homology (BAH) domain, site-specific DNA cytosine methylase activity (SSMT), zinc finger domain (CXXC). The "*" symbol represents the translation start of the shorter DNMT1o form at amino acid 119. Conserved domains are DMAP1, RFTS, CXXC, BAH, KG linker sequence and SSMT. Numbers represent amino acid numbering

confirm their identity. A schematic of DNMT1 and DNMT1o protein structure is shown in Fig. 2.

Fifty-three of the 55 BWS cases with KCNQ1OT1 TSS-DMR LOM were tested for SNVs in the coding regions of DNMT1. A total of 17 *DNMT1* SNVs were identified. No SNVs were identified in the sequence exon 1o, unique to *DNMT1* and upstream of the *DNMT1o* ATG. All of the *DNMT1* SNVs identified have been reported in dbSNP147. This database represents compiled variant data from 37 different genomic databases. Five substitutions were synonymous coding SNVs, six were located within the intronic sequence flanking exons and not predicted to affect splicing and one rare variant rs772176328: C>T, flanking exon 34 (NC_000019.10:g.10139820G>A (NM_001318731.1: c.3444-3C>T) had the potential to affect splicing but was not located within a canonical splice acceptor site. Five substitutions were missense variants with codon changes, four of which affected single patients only. Filtering of the missense *DNMT1* variants identified three with allele frequencies of less than 1 in 1000 making them potentially interesting candidates for a disorder with a population frequency of approximately 1 in 10,000 [33]. These were DNMT1 SNVs rs138841970: C>T, rs150331990: A>G and rs757460628: G>A encoding NP_001124295 p.Arg136Cys, p.His1118Arg and p.Arg1223His, respectively. Sequence traces are shown in Additional file 2: Figure S1. All

missense variants identified and their allele frequencies are described in Table 3. All were heterozygous.

All five missense variants identified, including the three rare missense variants, are predicted to have a moderate effect on protein function according to integrated analysis in Variant Effect Predictor (http://asia.ensembl.org/Tools/VEP). The variant, rs772176328: C>T, associated with a splice acceptor site, but not directly affecting a canonical base, was predicted to have a low impact on DNMT1 function. Amino acids Arg69 and Ile327 are not conserved in mouse, dog and some primates, and variants affecting these amino acid positions occur in control populations at frequencies of greater than 1 in 112 and 1 in 10, respectively, hence ruling them out as being significant in BWS. In contrast, Arg136 is conserved in all species expect dog, His1118 is conserved in all species except lamprey and Arg1223 is conserved in all species except mouse where it is leucine.

Rare variants of *DNMT1* have reduced methyltransferase activity

To directly examine the functional impact of the three rare DNMT1 missense variants, GFP-tagged DNMT1 recombinant proteins were generated and purified from Hela cells (Fig. 3 a, b).

Single nucleotide substitutions within *DNMT1* were inserted using site-directed mutagenesis (Additional file 2:

Table 3 Missense DNMT1 variants identified in BWS cases with LOM at KCNQ1OT1 TSS-DMR

SNV ID	Base change NM_001130823.1	AA change NP_001124295	Location NM_001130823.1	Ch37/Hg19 location	BWS VAF	dbSNP147 VAF	VEP
Rs 61750053	c.206G>A	p.Arg69His	Exon 3/41	Chr19:10291473	0.009	0.0089	Moderate
Rs 2228612	c.979A>G	p.Ile327Val	Exon 13/41	Chr19:10273372	0.11	0.135	Moderate
Rs 138841970	c.406C>T	p.Arg136Cys	Exon 4/41	Chr19:10291065	0.009	0.00028	Moderate
Rs 150331990	c.3353A>G	p.His1118Arg	Exon 31/41	Chr19:10251822	0.009	0.00001	Moderate
Rs 757460628	c.3668G>A	p.Arg1223His	Exon 33/41	Chr19:10250860	0.009	0.00002	Moderate

Variant allele frequencies were derived from dbSNP147. The variant effect predictor (VEP) tool was used to ascertain effects on protein function.
VAF variant allele frequency

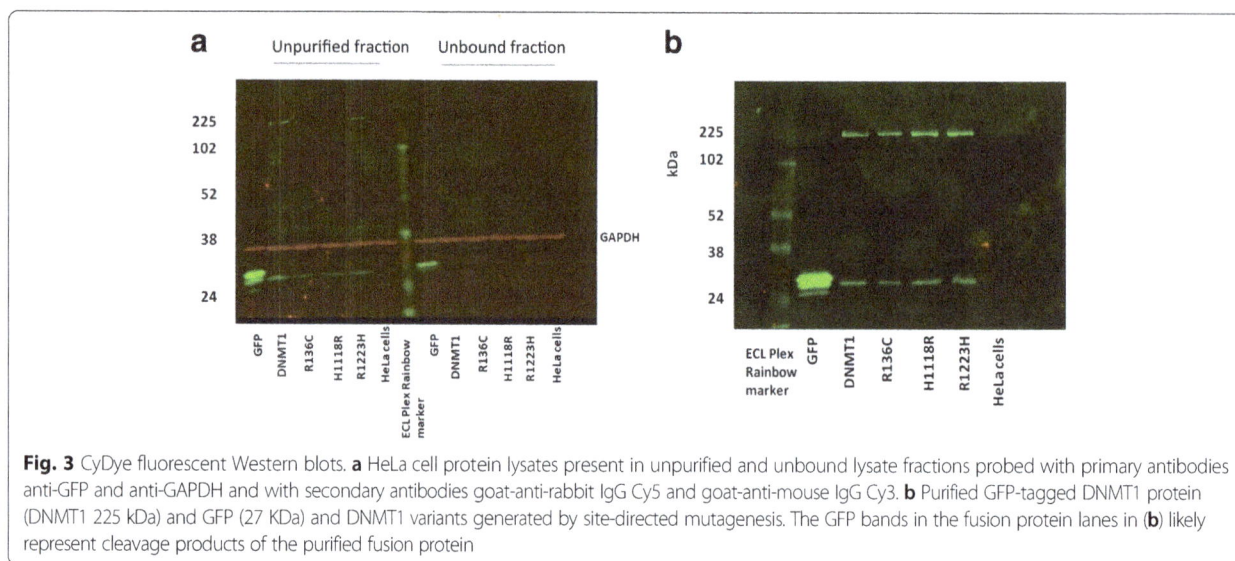

Fig. 3 CyDye fluorescent Western blots. **a** HeLa cell protein lysates present in unpurified and unbound lysate fractions probed with primary antibodies anti-GFP and anti-GAPDH and with secondary antibodies goat-anti-rabbit IgG Cy5 and goat-anti-mouse IgG Cy3. **b** Purified GFP-tagged DNMT1 protein (DNMT1 225 KDa) and GFP (27 KDa) and DNMT1 variants generated by site-directed mutagenesis. The GFP bands in the fusion protein lanes in (**b**) likely represent cleavage products of the purified fusion protein

Figure S2). Wild-type and DNMT1 mutant fusion proteins were expressed exclusively in the nucleus of Hela cells (Additional file 2: Figure S3). The functional impact of the rare missense variants on DNMT1 enzymatic activity was examined in a trapping assay previously described by Frauer and Leonhardt (2009) in which substrate is irreversibly covalently bound to DNMT1. The degree of binding is a surrogate for DNMT1 enzymatic activity as it measures the irreversible covalent enzyme-DNA complex formation as the first step of the DNA methylation reaction. Trapping activity measured relative to that of the wild-type DNMT1 protein is shown in Fig. 4.

The data in Fig. 4 shows that each missense variant exhibited reduced substrate trapping activity when compared with wild-type DNMT1 suggesting that these variants are less efficient at maintaining DNA methylation. Interestingly, each BWS case with these variants exhibited a complete LOM at KCNQ1OT1 TSS-DMR as opposed to partial or mosaic LOM the latter being a common finding in the majority of cases. The variants are predicted to affect the function of the N terminally truncated DNMT1 form, DNMT1o, in addition to DNMT1, although functional effects on DNMT1o were not examined directly. Information on these DNMT1 missense variants has been submitted to Clinvar and assigned accession numbers 3026604, 3027874 and 3028253.

It is interesting to note that *DNMT1* NM_001130823.1: c.406C>T, NP_001124295p.Arg136Cys, is located in the N-terminal domain and shows the least reduction in trapping activity whereas *DNMT1* NM_001130823.1: c.3668G>A, NP_001124295 p.Arg1223His, is located in the C-terminal catalytic domain very close to the catalytic site at p.Cys1242 and shows the maximum reduction in

trapping activity compared to wild-type DNMT1 protein. The variant, *DNMT1* NM_001130823.1: c.3353 A>G, NP_001124295 p.His1118Arg, is located adjacent to the glycine-lysine repeat region linking the BAH2 domain to the C-terminal catalytic domain and has trapping ability of approximately 50% compared to the wild-type protein.

Patient characteristics associated with variant *DNMT1*

Clinical features of patients with functionally impaired *DNMT1* variants of very low population frequency are shown in Table 4. BWS has a broad clinical presentation, and no particular feature could be ascribed to this subgroup. All cases had methylation values at KCNQ1OT1 TSS-DMR of 0.00 indicative of a complete loss of methylation in the blood. This is consistent with a defect affecting methylation establishment or maintenance very early in development either in the maternal germ cells or pre-implantation embryo. Only one of the three cases had loss of methylation at other imprinted loci consistent with MLID. Patient B96 had complete LOM at the *MEST* locus on chromosome 7q32.2 but maintained a normal methylation at *PLAGL1* (6q24), *GRB10* (7p12.1) *NESPAS* (20q13)) and *PEG3* (19q13). Interestingly, B96 had a brother who was stillborn, with an exomphalos and suspected BWS; however, this baby was born prior to the availability of molecular testing for BWS. Hence, for B96, there is a strong likelihood of an inherited predisposition. The mother of B97 was found to carry the R136C variant; however, she did not have features of BWS. Parental specimens from B96 and B66 were not available for testing. These patients also had less common variants in other folate pathway genes in varying combinations. All cases had at least two variant alleles corresponding to deleterious folate pathway polymorphisms in association with low-activity variants of DNMT1. These variants have been

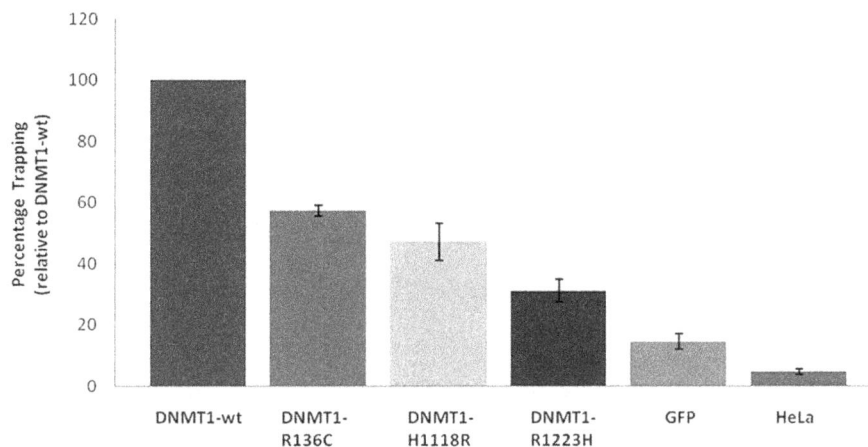

Fig. 4 DNMT1 methyltransferase trapping activity. The relative trapping ability of each DNMT1 variant is shown as a percentage relative to wild type DNMT1. Proteins from pEGFP-C1 transfected HeLa cells and non-transfected HeLa cells acted as controls. Technical replicates were performed in each assay. Four biological replicate experiments were performed for each sample and controls, except for DNMT1-R136C variant for which only three biological replicate experiments were performed. Error bars: mean ± SE

previously been shown to be associated with hypomethylation either dependent or independent of folate deficiency.

Discussion

In this paper, we have made observations that have not been previously reported. Firstly, patients with BWS and KCNQ1OT1 TSS-DMR LOM are more likely to have

Table 4 Clinical features of BWS KCNQ1OT1 TSS-DMR LOM cases with rare DNMT1 missense variants.

Clinical feature	B66 (p.Arg1223His)	B96 (p.His1118Arg)	B97 (p.Arg136Cys)
Birth weight (kg)	3.1	4.54	3.43
Neonatal hypoglycaemia	Y	N	N
Exomphalos/umbilical hernia	Y	Y	N
Macroglossia	Y	Y	Y
Macrosomia	N	Y	Y
Ear creases	Y	N	Y
Malignancy	N	N	N
Facial naevus flammeus	N	N	N
Body asymmetry	N	N	N
Genitourinary abnormality	N	N	
Hepatomegaly	Y	N	N
Nephromegaly	N	N	N
ART	Y	N	N
Family history	N	Y (sibling affected)	N
Sex	F	F	M

the low-activity *MTHFR* variant commonly known as c. 677C>T (rs1801133: C>T) although when applying a stringent statistical test for multiple testing, this association was not found to be statistically significant. BWS is a comparatively rare disorder, and examination of this relationship in larger cohorts will be required to consolidate it definitively. Secondly, we identified three rare missense variants of *DNMT1* and *DNMT1o* and characterised their capacity for maintaining DNA methylation in vitro. All variants had impaired enzymatic activity compared to wild-type *DNMT1*.

A large body of evidence has previously implicated *MTHFR* rs1801133: C>T in hyper-homocysteinaemia and DNA hypomethylation, that is potentiated by low dietary folate and homozygosity for the T allele [17–20, 22, 34–37]. *MTHFR* rs1801133: C>T causes an amino acid substitution of highly conserved alanine to valine at position 222 (p.Ala222Val) resulting in reduced enzyme activity due to increased thermolability [16]. Furthermore, BWS has been reported previously in association with homocysteinuria occurring with *CBS* enzyme deficiency [38]. Although we identified an association between the MTHFR rs1801133 T allele prevalence and BWS that was not statistically significant by a stringent statistical test, it remains to be determined whether a combination of low dietary folate and vitamin B6 and B12 deficiency, and this genotype may have a stronger association with BWS incidence. Future studies, including the prospective collection of dietary intake information, will require global collaborative efforts to examine these associations in large cohorts.

Our observations suggest that the identified low-activity *DNMT1* variants may contribute to a subgroup of BWS cases with imprinting defects through the effects on the maintenance methylation of hemimethylated DNA during DNA replication prior to implantation. Given the observation of complete loss of methylation in all three cases with variant *DNMT1*, we further propose that methylation maintenance failure at KCNQ1OT1 TSS-DMR occurs at a very early stage of embryogenesis in the cleavage embryo. Evidence from mouse models suggests a maternal effect on the maintenance of DNA methylation in the pre-implantation embryo. High levels of oocyte-derived maternal Dnmt1o are present in the cleavage embryo and protect imprinted loci from methylation loss at imprinted sites as well as in the intergenic regions. Mothers lacking Dnmt1o have abnormal imprinting in their offspring at the pre-implantation stage, including abnormal X-inactivation, in addition to placental hypomethylation [39]. Human *DNMT1o* is similarly expressed in mature oocytes and in early-stage embryonic development [32].

A direct role for DNMT1 in imprinting disorders as a result of maternal effect mutation is also suggested by the associations between the Uhrf1 protein and Dnmt1. Dnmt1 is recruited by Uhrf1 to replicating DNA [40], and intriguingly, a potentially deleterious UHRF mutation has been recently described as having a maternal effect in twins affected by MLID with loss of methylation [9]. Furthermore, another maternal effect protein, NLRP2, implicated in MLID and BWS, causes re-localization of Dnmt1 in oocytes and pre-implantation embryos [41]. Hence, there is accumulating evidence for the potential involvement of DNMT1 as a maternal effect protein associated with loss of methylation at imprinted loci.

Of the three cases with rare missense DNMT1 alleles, maternal inheritance of DNMT1 NM_001130823.1: c.406C>T, NP_001124295 p.Arg136Cys, could be demonstrated. Modes of inheritance could not be examined in the remaining two cases due to the lack of availability of parental DNA; however, case B96 had a sibling who was stillborn with exomphalos who was not tested for BWS, and the possibility of an inherited predisposition in this individual cannot be discounted. Case B66 with the variant DNMT1 NM_001130823.1: c.3668G>A, NP_001124295 p.Arg1223His, was a female conceived by intracytoplasmic sperm injection, and she also had a greater number of the clinical features of BWS when compared with the other two cases (five versus three in the other *DNMT1* variant cases). It is not known whether she had inherited the *DNMT1* variant from either of her parents; however, maternal inheritance would be consistent with recent observations in the mouse showing that oocytes deficient in *Dnmt1o* are more susceptible to imprinting defects following ART [42].

There was no reported indication of parental or familial BWS in any case. However, this might not be unexpected in a scenario where a DNMT1 mutation has a maternal effect in the pre-implantation embryo. Mothers may be mutation carriers themselves but unaffected if they had inherited a deleterious DNMT1 SNV from their fathers or had acquired one de novo. In such circumstances, only offspring arising from an oocyte expressing abnormal DNMT1 protein would be affected.

Previous studies on mouse *Dnmt1s* have identified regions required for maintenance of imprinting that are localised to the region spanning amino acids 191-394; however, none of the variants in this study are located within this domain [27]. The variant *DNMT1* NM_001130823.1: c.406C>T, NP_001124295 p.Arg136Cys, lies within an interaction site with DNMT3A suggesting the possibility of an effect on imprint establishment, given the evidence for coordination between DNMT1, DNMT3a and DNMT3b in both establishing and maintaining methylation [43, 44]. Recent studies have revealed insight into the structure of human DNMT1 protein, and conserved domains are described for DNMT1 NP_001124295.1 in the Conserved Domain Database hosted by NCBI [45–47]. None of the identified variants was located directly within the enzymatic active site at Cysteine 1242 in Ref Seq NP_001124295. Variant *DNMT1*: NP_001124295 p.His1118Arg is immediately adjacent to the second bromo-adjacent homology (BAH2) domain, and variant DNMT1: NP_001124295 p.Arg1223His lies within the catalytic domain. Histidine at 1118 is distant (> 45 Å away) from the DNA binding, SAM binding and catalytic cysteine within the catalytic domain. In the DNMT1 structures, this residue is in a short helix where it is solvent exposed and has few intra-molecular interactions (structure 3PTA in [47] and structure 4WXX in [46]). Residue Arg1223 is in the catalytic domain and distant from the DNA, SAM and Cys1242 sites (21 Å, < 15 Å, < 28 Å, respectively). This residue is leucine in mouse Dnmt1 (structure PDB ID 4DA4 [48], and both residues occupy similar structural space at the apex of a loop. In the human DNMT1 structures (PDB IDS 4WXX, 3PTA), the arginine adopts two radically side chain conformations. In both configurations, the arginine side chain does not engage in intra-molecular polar contacts and the residue is solvent exposed. The loop in which the DNMT1: NP_001124295 p.Arg1223His variant is found is added during the evolution of cytosine C5 methyltransferases. The loop is absent in the methyltransferase from Haemophilus parahaemolyticus (HhaI) [49] that has high structural similarity to the mouse and human DNMT1 catalytic domain, suggesting it is an acquired adaptation and not evolutionarily required for activity. Previous work found that *DNMT1* mutations that cause hereditary sensory neuropathy were due to protein misfolding [50]. One residue was in a hydrophobic core region while the other was in a linker region between secondary structural elements. Both mutations were found to affect the folding and stability of DNMT1 protein. In contrast, the variants reported here are in surface-exposed regions and are unlikely to be involved in the intra-molecular interactions. Therefore, they are not proposed to affect folding or stability. However, despite sharing 80% sequence identity, recent subtle differences in function between the mouse and human structures of DNMT1 protein have been recently recognised [46]. Therefore, any definitive structural effects of the identified variants are currently unclear. It may be possible that mutations exert their effects by altering conformational flexibility that is not apparent in the crystal structure. It is interesting to note however that the effect of the *DNMT1*: NP_001124295 p.Arg1223His variant on the activity was the strongest in the trapping assay and comparable to the effects described for *DNMT1* variants reported in the previous study examining hereditary neuropathies [50].

In a setting of maternal dietary folate deficiency or impaired embryonic folate metabolism, the observed decrease in DNMT1 enzymatic activity could be further exaggerated by reduced availability of the substrate *S*-adenosyl methionine (SAM) or increases in inhibitory *S*-adenosylhomocyteine (SAH). Interestingly, all cases with variant *DNMT1* had at least two variants predicted to adversely affect folate metabolism via the effects directly on *MTHFR* and methylation of tetrahydrofolate or via the effects on the conversion of homocysteine to methionine via methionine synthase reductase (MTRR) and 5-methyltetrahydrofolate-homocysteine *S*-methyltransferase (MTR) using vitamin B12 as a cofactor.

Due to their rarity in the general population, presence in a subgroup of BWS and MLID cases, and functional characterization supporting reduced methyltransferase activity, these DNMT1 variants are worthy of reporting. Ultimately, mouse models examining the effect of variant DNMT1 in the context of imprinting disruption at specific loci including KCNQ1OT1 TSS-DMR will be required for proof of association; however, larger cohort studies on families with imprinting disorders are also likely to be fruitful.

Conclusions

In conclusion, the observations from this study suggest that novel genetic factors affecting DNA methylation may cause imprinting disruption in a subgroup of BWS cases. This study paves the way for larger prospective studies in BWS and other human imprinting disorders to examine the relationship between genotypes linked to DNA methylation in concert with environmental factors, to fully elucidate the causes of abnormal genomic imprinting.

Methods

Participant recruitment

The laboratory in which this work was conducted is the primary referral laboratory for the diagnosis of BWS in Australasia. After diagnostic testing for BWS using methylation-sensitive MLPA (MS-MLPA) to interrogate imprinting defects in 11p15.5, patients with evidence of sporadic loss of methylation at KCNQ1OT1 TSS-DMR were invited to participate in this research project. Parents were asked to complete a clinical questionnaire from which data on clinical features and fertility history were collected. The project and consent forms were approved by the Human Research Ethics Committee of the Royal Children's Hospital in Melbourne (HREC 21121M), where the work was conducted. The participant recruitment extended over a period of 5 years.

Cord blood samples used as controls were obtained from the BMDI Cord Blood Bank at the Royal Children's Hospital, Melbourne, Australia. These samples were deemed unsuitable for transplantation and approved for use in this project by the local institutional ethics committee.

Molecular diagnosis of Beckwith-Wiedemann syndrome

Patients referred to the laboratory were assessed as having BWS with isolated loss of methylation at 11p15.5 KCNQ1OT1 TSS-DMR using the Salsa ME030-B1 BWS/RSS MS MLPA kit (MRC Holland). Patients with either partial or complete loss of methylation at KCNQ1OT1 TSS-DMR were included in the study. H19 methylation abnormalities and patUPD11p15 were not present in any cases included. DNA was extracted from EDTA blood using the Puregene kit (Qiagen Hilden Germany) and stored at − 20 °C prior to use.

PCR and high-resolution melting

PCR was performed in a 20-μl total volume on all samples using HotStar Taq DNA Polymerase (Qiagen). Typical cycling conditions were 95 °C for 15 min followed by 40 cycles of 95 °C for 30 s, annealing temperature for 30s, extension at 72 °C for 45 s followed by a final extension at 72 °C for 5 min. HRM reactions were performed in a total volume of 20 μL and comprised 2× HRM Sensimix (Bioline) (10 μL), 0.50 μL of forward and reverse primers at 20 μM, 1.0 μL of DNA at 10 ng/μL. Amplification reactions were 95 °C for 10 min, followed by 40 cycles of 95 °C for 15 s, annealing temperature for 10 s, 72 °C for 10 s followed by 72 °C for 5 min. Primers used in PCR, HRM and sequencing are described in the Additional file 1: Tables S2a–e, S3a–e and S4a–c.

Sanger sequencing

PCR products were treated with ExoSAP-IT (USB, Affymetrix) and sequenced with Big Dye Terminator v3.1 (BDT) mix (Applied Biosystems) according to the manufacturer's instructions. Sequences were analysed with Mutation Surveyor v 4.0 (SoftGenetics, USA).

Variant classification

Variants were examined using Polyphen (genetics.bwh.-harvard.edu/pph2/), SIFT (sift.bii.a-star.edu.sg) Variant Effect Prediction tool (https://www.ensembl.org/vep) [51], Mutation Taster (www.mutationtaster.org/) and the University of Maryland Genetic Variant Interpretation tool.

SNVs are reported relative to their cDNA reference sequences where the nucleotide numbering uses + 1 as the A of the ATG translation initiation codon. Reference sequences used are as follows: *MTHFR* NM_005957.4, *MTRR* NM_002454.2, *MAT1A* NM_00429.2, *MTR* NM_000254.2, *CBS* NM_001178009.1 and *DNMT1* NM_001130823.1. The DNMT1 genomic reference sequence used for intronic variants was NC_000019.10.

Analysis of methylation at other centres of genomic imprinting

The *PLAGL* (6q24), *GRB10* (7p12.1), *NESPAS* (20q13) and *PEG3* (19q13) loci were evaluated for methylation by pyrosequencing. Methylation at the MEST locus was evaluated by MS-MLPA.

Genomic DNA samples from 55 BWS cases with KCNQ1OT1 TSS-DMR LOM and from 13 controls were bisulphite modified using the MethylEasy DNA bisulphite modification kit (Cat No: ME-001, Human Genetic Signatures). Pyrosequencing PCR and sequencing primers were based on those described in Mackay et al. [52]. Primers for PCR are listed in Additional file 1: Table S5a, and primers used for sequencing are listed in Additional file 1: Table S5b. PCR was performed in a 40-μL total volume of 1× HotStar Master mix with 0.2 μL HotStar Taq DNA Polymerase (Cat. No: 203203, Qiagen), 0.2 μL of 20 μM forward and reverse primers, 5× Q solution (Qiagen) and 0.2 mM dNTPs. PCR cycling was at 95 °C for 15 min, followed by 45 cycles at 95 °C for 30 s, annealing temperature for 30 s and extension for 45 s at 72 °C. Pyrosequencing was performed on a PyroMark Q24 (Cat. #9001514, Qiagen) using Pyro-Mark Q24 Gold (Cat. #970802, Qiagen) according to the manufacturer's protocol. The results were analysed using PyroMark Q24 software to determine the methylation status. Thirteen control samples were used to establish the mean methylation values across the CpG sites examined. A normal range was considered to be the mean value ± two standard deviations from the mean. Patients were scored as abnormal if methylation was outside the established normal range. The *MEST* locus at 7q32.1 was examined using the SALSA MLPA kit ME032-A1 UPD7/UPD14 (MRC Holland) according to the manufacturer's instructions. Two specimens previously reported with genome-wide mosaic uniparental isodisomy

[53] were used as positive controls for loss of methylation. Loss of methylation at *MEST* was scored as positive when methylation was < 0.35.

Generation of DNMT1 plasmids

The mammalian expression vector containing the long isoform of wild-type human DNMT1 with N-terminal GFP tag in pEGFP-C1 plasmid (Clontech) was obtained from Prof. Heinrich Leonhardt (Ludwig-Maximilians-University Biocentre, Munich). The pEGFP-C1-DNMT1 construct was transfected into competent DH5-alpha cells, and construct fidelity was assessed by sequencing plasmid DNA using primers designed to *DNMT1* exons as described in the supplementary information (cDNMT1 sequencing primers).

Bacterial cultures containing pEGFP-C1-DNMT1 were grown in 2YT and kanamycin and plasmid DNA extracted with either QIAprep Spin MiniPrep kit (Cat. # 27104, Qiagen) or Plasmid Maxi kit (Cat. #12162, Qiagen) appropriate to the scale of the culture and according to the manufacturer's instructions.

Site-directed mutagenesis

DNMT1 coding variations were inserted into the wild-type *DNMT1* sequence in pEGFP-C1. Mutagenesis was performed with QuikChange II Site-Directed Mutagenesis kit (Cat. #200523, Agilent Technologies) according to the manufacturer's instructions. Mutagenic primer pairs were designed for each identified *DNMT1* sequence variant using a web-based primer design tool (www.agilent.com/genomics/qcpd) provided by Agilent Technologies. The primers are listed following. Mutated sites are underlined:

*DNMT1*406C>T, F: CCAAACCCCTTTCCAAACC T<u>T</u>GCACGCCCAGG, R: CCTGGGCGTGC<u>A</u>AGGT TTGGAAAGGGGTTTGG; *DNMT1* 3353A>G, F: GATCCTCCCAACC<u>G</u>TGCCCGTA GCCCT, R: AGGG CTACGGGCA<u>C</u>GGTTGGGAGGATC; and *DNMT1* 3668G>A F: CACCA ACTCCC<u>A</u>CGGCCAGCGGC, R: GCCGCTGGCCG<u>T</u>GGGAGTTGGTG.

Following selection in kanamycin (50 μg/mL), white colonies derived from pEGFP-C1-DNMT1 mutants were selected and sequenced to confirm the presence of the mutation. Sequence traces from mutants are shown in Additional file 2: Figure S2.

Transfection of DNMT1 into Hela cells

Wild-type *DNMT1* and *DNMT1* mutant plasmids were transfected into HeLa cells using FugeneHD (Promega) at a volumetric ratio of 3:1. Transfection efficiency was analysed by flow cytometry (BD LSR II, BD Biosciences) after 48 h. HeLa cells were transfected at a density of 1×10^5 cells per well in a 12-well plate in 1 ml of DMEM containing 10% FCS (SAFC BioSciences) and incubated at 37 °C in 5% CO_2. Nuclear GFP expression was visualised by confocal microscopy on a Leica TCS SP2. Transfection efficiencies of 60–70% were achieved.

Purification of GFP-tagged DNMT1 proteins

The GFP-Trap_A kit (Chromotek) was used to purify GFP-tagged DNMT1 proteins from HeLa cells according to the manufacturer's instructions.

Protein analysis and Western blotting

Total protein estimation using the bichoninic acid (BCA) assay (Sigma-Aldrich) was performed on 20 μL cell lysate according to the manufacturer's instructions. Western blotting with fluorescence visualization was performed as described in [54].

Purified GFP-tagged DNMT1 protein bound to beads was quantified using a DNMT1 ELISA kit (Epigentek Cat #P-3011). Standards were prepared from 7.5, 10, 12.5 and 15 ng of purified DNMT1 (supplied in the kit), and absorbance was read at 450 and 620 nm on a Multiskan EX microplate reader (Thermo Electron).

Measurement of DNA methyltransferase activity

The DNA methyltransferase activity of the generated wild-type and mutant DNMT1 proteins was measured by an irreversible covalent interaction with a hemi-methylated trapping substrate containing 5-aza-2′-deoxycytidine (5-azadC) as described in [55] and outlined below and in Additional file 2: Figure S4. This reaction is designed to irreversibly "trap" active DNMT1 in an inactive conformation by binding to the mechanism-based inhibitor 5-azadC. Capture and detection of this reaction intermediate serve as a measure of DNMT1 enzyme activity. Oligonucleotides used for the preparation of the DNA trapping substrate were synthesised by Integrated DNA Technologies. The forward oligo, MG-Upper contains a methylated cytosine (M) and the reverse 3′ end-paired Fill-in-oligo is labelled with a MAX-NHS ester fluorescent dye at its 5′ end. The Fill-in-oligo is complementary to the 3′ end of the MG-Upper oligonucleotide. Oligo sequences were as follows: MGUpper 5′ CTCAACAACTAACTACCATCMGGACCAGAA GAGTCATCATGG 3′ and Fill-in 5′MAXN-CCAT GATGACTCTTCTGGTC 3′.

Double-stranded DNA generated by oligo extension was prepared by denaturing 1 μL of each oligo at 100 μM in NEB2 buffer at 95 °C for 2 min followed by a slow cooling to 37 °C in a total final reaction volume of 15.2 μL. Hemi-methylated DNA substrate was synthesised by extension of the fill-in-oligo with the addition of 1 μL DNA Polymerase I (Large Klenow) fragment (Cat #M2201, Promega), 1 mM each of dTTP, dATP and dGTP (Cat #BIO-39025, Bioline) and 50 μM 5-aza-dCTP (Cat

#NU-1118S, Jena Bioscience) in acetylated BSA at 20 ng/μL (Cat #R3961, Promega) in a final reaction volume of 20 μL. The mix was incubated at room temperature for 10 min followed by inactivation at 75 °C for 10 min. This preparation of trapping substrate was used immediately in the in vitro DNMT1 trapping assay described below.

Fifteen nanograms of each purified pull-down GFP-tagged DNMT1 protein (bead-bound) derived from each DNMT1 protein variant was resuspended in buffer (100 mM KCl, 10 mM Tris-HCl, pH 7.6, 1 mM EDTA, 1 mM DTT) supplemented with 100 μM S-adenosyl-L--methionine (SAM) (New England Biolabs, Cat #B9003S), 4 μL end-labelled DNA trapping substrate (prepared as described above) and 160 ng/μL BSA in a total reaction volume of 200 μL. For determination of DNA methyltransferase activity, trapping was performed at 37 °C for 90 min with constant mixing. To remove unbound substrate, beads were washed twice with 1 mL of assay buffer, then resuspended in 100 μL of assay buffer and transferred to a 96-well microplate. Bound-labelled DNA trapping substrate associated with each variant and wild-type DNMT1 protein was measured by fluorescence emission on a FLUOstar Optima microplate reader (BMG Labtech). Technical duplicates were tested in each assay, and assays were performed in quadruplicate for each variant (except for DNMT1 Arg136Cys for which triplicate assays were performed) and the mean fluorescence for each DNMT1 variant was normalised to the wild-type DNMT1 fluorescence value, set to 100%. A schematic representation of the preparation of the DNA suicide substrate and the trapping assay is shown in Additional file 2: Figure S4.

Statistical analysis

Calculations of chi-squared and significance values were calculated using online analysis tools including GraphPad. Allele association was calculated using a 2 × contingency table with one degree of freedom [56]. Probability values of $p < 0.05$ were considered to be statistically significant. Pearson values for chi-squared and probability were calculated. Bonferroni correction was also applied for the analysis of folate pathway SNVs to adjust for multiple testing.

Abbreviations

BWS: Beckwith-Wiedemann syndrome; CBS: Cystathionine beta-synthase; DNMT1: DNA methyltransferase 1; MAT1A: Methionine adenosyltransferase; MLID: Multi-locus imprinting disruption; MTHFR: Methylenetetrahydrofolate reductase; MTR: 5-Methyltetrahydrofolate-homocysteine S-methyltransferase; MTRR: Methionine synthase reductase; SAH: S-adenosyl-homocysteine; SAM: S-adenosyl-methionine; SNV: Single nucleotide variant

Funding

This study was funded by the David Danks Post Graduate Scholarship (University of Melbourne) and the Children's Cancer Foundation (Murdoch Children's Research Institute). The funding bodies had no role in the design of the study, collection, analysis, interpretation of data, or in writing the manuscript.

Authors' contributions

EA and VD designed the study. VD, WH, PS and AM performed the experiments and genetic analyses. EA, VD, DA and JM analysed the data. DH and AB performed the DNMT1 protein modelling and edited the manuscript. EA wrote the manuscript. DA, JP, AC, MW, RS, GMcG, ME, EK, FC, KJ, JT, IH, ET, CB, EH, M-LF, AT, SW, BK, AMa, FM, GB, CK-B, MF and TD-B consented participants, facilitated the provision of clinical information and critically reviewed and edited the manuscript. DA and EK provided input to the statistical analysis. All authors read and approved the final manuscript.

Author details

[1]Department of Paediatrics, University of Melbourne, Parkville 3052, Australia. [2]Pathology, Monash Health, Clayton 3168, Australia. [3]School of Medicine, Deakin University, Geelong 3216, Australia. [4]Victorian Comprehensive Cancer Centre, Parkville 3052, Australia. [5]Department of Biochemistry and Molecular Biology, Monash University, Clayton 3800, Australia. [6]Murdoch Children's Research Institute, Parkville 3052, Australia. [7]Department of Anatomy and Developmental Biology, Monash University, Clayton 3800, Australia. [8]Department of Medical Genomics, Royal Prince Alfred Hospital, Camperdown 2050, Australia. [9]Clinical Genetics, Liverpool Hospital, Liverpool 2170, Australia. [10]Clinical Genetics, Children's Hospital at Westmead, Westmead 2145, Australia. [11]Centre for Clinical Genetics, Sydney Children's Hospital, Randwick 2031, Australia. [12]School of Medicine, University of Western Sydney, Penrith 2751, Australia. [13]School of Medicine, University of Sydney, Camperdown 2006, Australia. [14]Auckland District Health Board, Auckland 1023, New Zealand. [15]South Australian (SA) Clinical Genetics Service, SA Pathology, Women's and Children's Hospital, Adelaide 5000, Australia. [16]School of Medicine, University of Adelaide, Adelaide 5000, Australia. [17]Department of Clinical Genetics, Royal North Shore Hospital, St Leonards 2065, Australia. [18]School of Women's and Children's Health, University of NSW, Kensington 2052, Australia. [19]Hunter Genetics, Hunter New England Local Health District, New Lambton 2305, Australia. [20]Genetics Services of Western Australia, Crawley 6009, Australia. [21]University of Newcastle GrowUpWell Priority Research Centre, Callaghan 2308, Australia. [22]Hudson Institute of Medical Research, Clayton 3168, Australia. [23]Department of Translational Medicine, Monash University, Clayton 3168, Australia.

References

1. Weksberg R, Nishikawa J, Caluseriu O, Fei YL, Shuman C, Wei C, Steele L, Cameron J, Smith A, Ambus I, et al. Tumor development in the Beckwith-Wiedemann syndrome is associated with a variety of constitutional molecular 11p15 alterations including imprinting defects of KCNQ1OT1. Hum Mol Genet. 2001;10:2989–3000.

2. Weksberg R, Shuman C, Beckwith JB. Beckwith-Wiedemann syndrome. Eur J Hum Genet. 2010;18:8–14.

3. Mussa A, Molinatto C, Baldassarre G, Riberi E, Russo S, Larizza L, Riccio A, Ferrero GB. Cancer risk in Beckwith-Wiedemann syndrome: a systematic review and meta-analysis outlining a novel (epi)genotype specific histotype targeted screening protocol. J Pediatr. 2016;176:142–9. e141

4. Maas SM, Vansenne F, Kadouch DJ, Ibrahim A, Bliek J, Hopman S, Mannens MM, Merks JH, Maher ER, Hennekam RC. Phenotype, cancer risk, and surveillance in Beckwith-Wiedemann syndrome depending on molecular genetic subgroups. Am J Med Genet A. 2016;170:2248–60.

5. Diaz-Meyer N, Day CD, Khatod K, Maher ER, Cooper W, Reik W, Junien C, Graham G, Algar E, Der Kaloustian VM, Higgins MJ. Silencing of CDKN1C (p57KIP2) is associated with hypomethylation at KvDMR1 in Beckwith-Wiedemann syndrome. J Med Genet. 2003;40:797–801.

6. Algar E, Dagar V, Sebaj M, Pachter N. An 11p15 imprinting centre region 2 deletion in a family with Beckwith Wiedemann syndrome provides insights into imprinting control at CDKN1C. PLoS One. 2011;6:e29034.

7. Meyer E, Lim D, Pasha S, Tee LJ, Rahman F, Yates JR, Woods CG, Reik W, Maher ER. Germline mutation in NLRP2 (NALP2) in a familial imprinting disorder (Beckwith-Wiedemann syndrome). PLoS Genet. 2009;5:e1000423.

8. Docherty LE, Rezwan FI, Poole RL, Turner CL, Kivuva E, Maher ER, Smithson SF, Hamilton-Shield JP, Patalan M, Gizewska M, et al. Mutations in NLRP5 are associated with reproductive wastage and multilocus imprinting disorders in humans. Nat Commun. 2015;6:8086.

9. Begemann M, Rezwan FI, Beygo J, Docherty LE, Kolarova J, Schroeder C, Buiting K, Chokkalingam K, Degenhardt F, Wakeling EL, et al. Maternal variants in NLRP and other maternal effect proteins are associated with multilocus imprinting disturbance in offspring. J Med Genet. 2018;55(7):497–504.

10. Sato A, Otsu E, Negishi H, Utsunomiya T, Arima T. Aberrant DNA methylation of imprinted loci in superovulated oocytes. Hum Reprod. 2007;22:26–35.

11. DeBaun MR, Niemitz EL, Feinberg AP. Association of in vitro fertilization with Beckwith-Wiedemann syndrome and epigenetic alterations of LIT1 and H19. Am J Hum Genet. 2003;72:156–60.

12. Halliday J, Oke K, Breheny S, Algar E, JA D. Beckwith-Wiedemann syndrome and IVF: a case-control study. Am J Hum Genet. 2004;75:526–8.

13. Manipalviratn S, DeCherney A, Segars J. Imprinting disorders and assisted reproductive technology. Fertil Steril. 2009;91:305–15.

14. Maher ER, Afnan M, Barratt CL. Epigenetic risks related to assisted reproductive technologies: epigenetics, imprinting, ART and icebergs? Hum Reprod. 2003;18:2508–11.

15. Maher ER, Brueton LA, Bowdin SC, Luharia A, Cooper W, Cole TR, Macdonald F, Sampson JR, Barratt CL, Reik W, Hawkins MM. Beckwith-Wiedemann syndrome and assisted reproduction technology (ART). J Med Genet. 2003;40:62–4.

16. Frosst P, Blom HJ, Milos R, Goyette P, Sheppard CA, Matthews RG, Boers GJ, den Heijer M, Kluijtmans LA, van den Heuvel LP, et al. A candidate genetic risk factor for vascular disease: a common mutation in methylenetetrahydrofolate reductase. Nat Genet. 1995;10:111–3.

17. Rozen R. Molecular genetics of methylenetetrahydrofolate reductase deficiency. J Inherit Metab Dis. 1996;19:589–94.

18. Eskes TK. Open or closed? A world of difference: a history of homocysteine research. Nutr Rev. 1998;56:236–44.

19. Botto LD, Yang Q. 5,10-methylenetetrahydrofolate reductase gene variants and congenital anomalies: a HuGE review. Am J Epidemiol. 2000;151:862–77.

20. Fodinger M, Horl WH, Sunder-Plassmann G. Molecular biology of 5,10-methylenetetrahydrofolate reductase. J Nephrol. 2000;13:20–33.

21. van der Put NM, Gabreels F, Stevens EM, Smeitink JA, Trijbels FJ, Eskes TK, van den Heuvel LP, Blom HJ. A second common mutation in the methylenetetrahydrofolate reductase gene: an additional risk factor for neural-tube defects? Am J Hum Genet. 1998;62:1044–51.

22. Castro R, Rivera I, Ravasco P, Camilo ME, Jakobs C, Blom HJ, de Almeida IT. 5,10-Methylenetetrahydrofolate reductase (MTHFR) 677C-->T and 1298A-->C mutations are associated with DNA hypomethylation. J Med Genet. 2004;41:454–8.

23. Leclerc D, Campeau E, Goyette P, Adjalla CE, Christensen B, Ross M, Eydoux P, Rosenblatt DS, Rozen R, Gravel RA. Human methionine synthase: cDNA cloning and identification of mutations in patients of the cblG complementation group of folate/cobalamin disorders. Hum Mol Genet. 1996;5:1867–74.

24. Watkins D, Rosenblatt DS. Genetic heterogeneity among patients with methylcobalamin deficiency. Definition of two complementation groups, cblE and cblG. J Clin Invest. 1988;81:1690–4.

25. van der Put NM, van der Molen EF, Kluijtmans LA, Heil SG, Trijbels JM, Eskes TK, Van Oppenraaij-Emmerzaal D, Banerjee R, Blom HJ. Sequence analysis of the coding region of human methionine synthase: relevance to hyperhomocysteinaemia in neural-tube defects and vascular disease. QJM. 1997;90:511–7.

26. Vaughn JD, Bailey LB, Shelnutt KP, Dunwoody KM, Maneval DR, Davis SR, Quinlivan EP, Gregory JF 3rd, Theriaque DW, Kauwell GP. Methionine synthase reductase 66A->G polymorphism is associated with increased plasma homocysteine concentration when combined with the homozygous methylenetetrahydrofolate reductase 677C->T variant. J Nutr. 2004;134:2985–90.

27. Borowczyk E, Mohan KN, D'Aiuto L, Cirio MC, Chaillet JR. Identification of a region of the DNMT1 methyltransferase that regulates the maintenance of genomic imprints. Proc Natl Acad Sci U S A. 2009;106:20806–11.

28. Ding F, Chaillet JR. In vivo stabilization of the Dnmt1 (cytosine-5)-methyltransferase protein. Proc Natl Acad Sci U S A. 2002;99:14861–6.

29. Kurihara Y, Kawamura Y, Uchijima Y, Amamo T, Kobayashi H, Asano T, Kurihara H. Maintenance of genomic methylation patterns during preimplantation development requires the somatic form of DNA methyltransferase 1. Dev Biol. 2008;313:335–46.

30. Hirasawa R, Chiba H, Kaneda M, Tajima S, Li E, Jaenisch R, Sasaki H. Maternal and zygotic Dnmt1 are necessary and sufficient for the maintenance of DNA methylation imprints during preimplantation development. Genes Dev. 2008;22:1607–16.

31. Gaudet F, Talbot D, Leonhardt H, Jaenisch R. A short DNA methyltransferase isoform restores methylation in vivo. J Biol Chem. 1998;273:32725–9.

32. Hayward BE, De Vos M, Judson H, Hodge D, Huntriss J, Picton HM, Sheridan E, Bonthron DT. Lack of involvement of known DNA methyltransferases in familial hydatidiform mole implies the involvement of other factors in establishment of imprinting in the human female germline. BMC Genet. 2003;4:2.

33. Mussa A, Russo S, De Crescenzo A, Chiesa N, Molinatto C, Selicorni A, Richiardi L, Larizza L, Silengo MC, Riccio A, Ferrero GB. Prevalence of Beckwith-Wiedemann syndrome in north west of Italy. Am J Med Genet A. 2013;161a:2481–6.

34. Haggarty P, McCallum H, McBain H, Andrews K, Duthie S, McNeill G, Templeton A, Haites N, Campbell D, Bhattacharya S. Effect of B vitamins and genetics on success of in-vitro fertilisation: prospective cohort study. Lancet. 2006;367:1513–9.

35. Friso S, Choi SW, Girelli D, Mason JB, Dolnikowski GG, Bagley PJ, Olivieri O, Jacques PF, Rosenberg IH, Corrocher R, Selhub J. A common mutation in the 5,10-methylenetetrahydrofolate reductase gene affects genomic DNA methylation through an interaction with folate status. Proc Natl Acad Sci U S A. 2002;99:5606–11.

36. Stern LL, Mason JB, Selhub J, Choi SW. Genomic DNA hypomethylation, a characteristic of most cancers, is present in peripheral leukocytes of individuals who are homozygous for the C677T polymorphism in the methylenetetrahydrofolate reductase gene. Cancer Epidemiol Biomark Prev. 2000;9:849–53.

37. Yamada K, Chen Z, Rozen R, Matthews RG. Effects of common polymorphisms on the properties of recombinant human methylenetetrahydrofolate reductase. Proc Natl Acad Sci U S A. 2001;98:14853–8.

38. Levy HL, Vargas JE, Waisbren SE, Kurczynski TW, Roeder ER, Schwartz RS, Rosengren S, Prasad C, Greenberg CR, Gilfix BM, et al. Reproductive fitness in maternal homocystinuria due to cystathionine beta-synthase deficiency. J Inherit Metab Dis. 2002;25:299–314.

39. McGraw S, Oakes CC, Martel J, Cirio MC, de Zeeuw P, Mak W, Plass C, Bartolomei MS, Chaillet JR, Trasler JM. Loss of DNMT1o disrupts imprinted X chromosome inactivation and accentuates placental defects in females. PLoS Genet. 2013;9:e1003873.

40. Bostick M, Kim JK, Esteve PO, Clark A, Pradhan S, Jacobsen SE. UHRF1 plays a role in maintaining DNA methylation in mammalian cells. Science. 2007; 317:1760–4.

41. Mahadevan S, Sathappan V, Utama B, Lorenzo I, Kaskar K, Van den Veyver IB. Maternally expressed NLRP2 links the subcortical maternal complex (SCMC) to fertility, embryogenesis and epigenetic reprogramming. Sci Rep. 2017;7:44667.

42. Whidden LMJ, Rahimi S, Chaillet R, Chan D, Trasler JM. Compromised oocyte quality and assisted reproduction contribute to sex-specific effects on offspring outcomes and epigenetic patterning. Hum Mol Genet. 2016;25: 4649–60.

43. Kim GD, Ni J, Kelesoglu N, Roberts RJ, Pradhan S. Co-operation and communication between the human maintenance and de novo DNA (cytosine-5) methyltransferases. EMBO J. 2002;21:4183–95.

44. Li Z, Dai H, Martos SN, Xu B, Gao Y, Li T, Zhu G, Schones DE, Wang Z. Distinct roles of DNMT1-dependent and DNMT1-independent methylation patterns in the genome of mouse embryonic stem cells. Genome Biol. 2015;16:115.

45. Marchler-Bauer A, Derbyshire MK, Gonzales NR, Lu S, Chitsaz F, Geer LY, Geer RC, He J, Gwadz M, Hurwitz DI, et al. CDD: NCBI's conserved domain database. Nucleic Acids Res. 2015;43:D222–6.

46. Zhang ZM, Liu S, Lin K, Luo Y, Perry JJ, Wang Y, Song J. Crystal structure of human DNA methyltransferase 1. J Mol Biol. 2015;427:2520–31.

47. Song J, Rechkoblit O, Bestor TH, Patel DJ. Structure of DNMT1-DNA complex reveals a role for autoinhibition in maintenance DNA methylation. Science. 2011;331:1036–40.

48. Song J, Teplova M, Ishibe-Murakami S, Patel DJ. Structure-based mechanistic insights into DNMT1-mediated maintenance DNA methylation. Science. 2012;335:709–12.

49. Cheng X, Kumar S, Posfai J, Pflugrath JW, Roberts RJ. Crystal structure of the HhaI DNA methyltransferase complexed with S-adenosyl-L-methionine. Cell. 1993;74:299–307.

50. Klein CJ, Botuyan MV, Wu Y, Ward CJ, Nicholson GA, Hammans S, Hojo K, Yamanishi H, Karpf AR, Wallace DC, et al. Mutations in DNMT1 cause hereditary sensory neuropathy with dementia and hearing loss. Nat Genet. 2011;43:595–600.

51. McLaren W, Gil L, Hunt SE, Riat HS, Ritchie GRS, Thormann A, Flicek P, Cunningham F. The Ensembl variant effect predictor. Genome Biol. 2016;17:122.

52. Mackay DJ, Callaway JL, Marks SM, White HE, Acerini CL, Boonen SE, Dayanikli P, Firth HV, Goodship JA, Haemers AP, et al. Hypomethylation of multiple imprinted loci in individuals with transient neonatal diabetes is associated with mutations in ZFP57. Nat Genet. 2008;40:949–51.

53. Wilson M, Peters G, Bennetts B, McGillivray G, Wu ZH, Poon C, Algar E. The clinical phenotype of mosaicism for genome-wide paternal uniparental disomy: two new reports. Am J Med Genet A. 2008;146A: 137–48.

54. Rigby L, Muscat A, Ashley D, Algar E. Methods for the analysis of histone H3 and H4 acetylation in blood. Epigenetics. 2012;7:875–82.

55. Frauer C, Leonhardt H. A versatile non-radioactive assay for DNA methyltransferase activity and DNA binding. Nucleic Acids Res. 2009;37:e22.

56. Clarke GM, Anderson CA, Pettersson FH, Cardon LR, Morris AP, Zondervan KT. Basic statistical analysis in genetic case-control studies. Nat Protoc. 2011; 6:121–33.

13

DNA methylation and repressive H3K9 and H3K27 trimethylation in the promoter regions of PD-1, CTLA-4, TIM-3, LAG-3, TIGIT, and PD-L1 genes in human primary breast cancer

Varun Sasidharan Nair[1], Haytham El Salhat[2,3], Rowaida Z. Taha[1], Anne John[4], Bassam R. Ali[4,5] and Eyad Elkord[1,6*]

Abstract

Background: High expression of immune checkpoints in tumor microenvironment plays significant roles in inhibiting anti-tumor immunity, which is associated with poor prognosis and cancer progression. Major epigenetic modifications in both DNA and histone could be involved in upregulation of immune checkpoints in cancer.

Methods: Expressions of different immune checkpoint genes and PD-L1 were assessed using qRT-PCR, and the underlying epigenetic modifications including CpG methylation and repressive histone abundance were determined using bisulfite sequencing, and histone 3 lysine 9 trimethylation (H3K9me3) and histone 3 lysine 27 trimethylation (H3K27me3) chromatin immunoprecipitation assays (ChIP), respectively.

Results: We first assessed the expression level of six immune checkpoints/ligands and found that PD-1, CTLA-4, TIM-3, and LAG-3 were significantly upregulated in breast tumor tissues (TT), compared with breast normal tissues (NT). We investigated the epigenetic modifications beyond this upregulation in immune checkpoint genes. Interestingly, we found that CpG islands in the promoter regions of PD-1, CTLA-4, and TIM-3 were significantly hypomethylated in tumor compared with normal tissues. Additionally, CpG islands of PD-L1 promoter were completely demethylated (100%), LAG-3 were highly hypomethylated (80–90%), and TIGIT were poorly hypomethylated (20–30%), in both NT and TT. These demethylation findings are in accordance with the relative expression data that, out of all these genes, PD-L1 was highly expressed and completely demethylated and TIGIT was poorly expressed and hypermethylated in both NT and TT. Moreover, bindings of H3K9me3 and H3K27me3 were found to be reduced in the promoter loci of PD-1, CTLA-4, TIM-3, and LAG-3 in tumor tissues.

Conclusion: Our data demonstrate that both DNA and histone modifications are involved in upregulation of PD-1, CTLA-4, TIM-3, and LAG-3 in breast tumor tissue and these epigenetic modifications could be useful as diagnostic/prognostic biomarkers and/or therapeutic targets in breast cancer.

Keywords: Breast cancer, Immune checkpoints, PD-L1, DNA methylation, Histone trimethylation

* Correspondence: eelkord@hbku.edu.qa; eyad.elkord@manchester.ac.uk
[1]Cancer Research Center, Qatar Biomedical Research Institute, College of Science and Engineering, Hamad Bin Khalifa University, Qatar Foundation, Doha, Qatar
[6]Institute of Cancer Sciences, University of Manchester, Manchester, UK
Full list of author information is available at the end of the article

Background

Modifications in the epigenetic patterns of DNA are considered as an early event in the development of breast cancer [1, 2]. Aberrant DNA methylation and repressive histone modifications are associated with clinical and histopathological features of breast cancer such as tumor subtype, stage, and differentiation [3–5]. In mammalian cells, the DNA can be modified by the methylation of cytosine residues in CpG dinucleotides and the N-terminal histone modifications through methylation, acetylation, phosphorylation, and ubiquitination [6, 7]. The DNA methylation imprints can be erased through two different processes: (a) active demethylation occurs through demethylation enzymes such as ten-eleven translocation dioxygenase (TETs) and (b) passive demethylation by means of reduction in DNA methyl transferase (DNMTs) activity [8]. In addition to DNA demethylation, the global distribution of repressor histones such as H3K9me3 and H3K27me3 can also predominantly affect gene transcription [4].

Immune checkpoints are molecules contributing to the inhibitory pathways in the immune system and play pivotal roles in the immune evasion of tumor cells [9, 10]. Recent reports show that multiple immune checkpoint molecules are upregulated in the tumor microenvironment (TME) of breast cancer [11, 12], but the epigenetic modifications behind this upregulation are still not clear. Therefore, the epigenetic studies in breast TME could help to understand the molecular mechanisms behind their upregulation. Herein, for the first time, we investigated the epigenetic changes occurring in immune checkpoint molecules in breast TME. Initially, we found that immune checkpoints including PD-1, CTLA-4, TIM-3, and LAG-3 were upregulated in breast tumor tissues. In subsequent investigations, we examined the epigenetic modifications in tumor and normal tissues and found that the CpG motifs in the promoter regions of PD-1, CTLA-4, and TIM-3 genes were hypomethylated in tumor tissue, compared with normal tissue, but not significantly in LAG-3 promoter. Furthermore, the distribution of repressive histones including H3K9me3 and H3K27me3 was also reduced in the promoter regions of all four immune checkpoints in tumor compared with normal tissues. Collectively, our data reveal that upregulation of multiple immune checkpoints including PD-1, CTLA-4, and TIM-3 in breast TME depends on both DNA methylation and distribution of repressive histones, but the LAG-3 upregulation depends only on repressive histone distribution across their promoter region. Moreover, the relative expression of PD-L1 was the highest and TIGIT was the lowest in both NT and TT among all other immune checkpoint genes, and the demethylation percentage also agrees with the relative expression level; PD-L1 was totally demethylated and TIGIT was hypermethylated in both TT and NT.

Results

Upregulation of multiple immune checkpoint genes in breast tumor tissues

Various genetic and epigenetic changes that are inherent in most of the cancer cells in TME help tumor cells to develop immune resistance mechanisms, which involves multiple immune inhibitory pathways [9]. It has been reported that in the breast TME, both malignant mammary epithelial cells and tumor-infiltrating lymphocytes (TILs) express multiple immune checkpoints/ligands, including PD-1, CTLA-4, and PD-L1 to support immune evasion [13]. To investigate the expression level of various immune checkpoint molecules in the TME, we performed quantitative real-time PCR (RT-qPCR) as described in the "Methods" section. We found that PD-1, CTLA-4, TIM-3, and LAG-3 were upregulated in tumor tissue, compared with normal tissue, while there was no change in PD-L1 and TIGIT (Fig. 1a). These data show that multiple immune checkpoint genes are upregulated in breast TME, which may help the tumor cells to evade from host anti-tumor responses. Moreover, we normalized the relative expression of all immune checkpoints with TIGIT, which is poorly expressed, and found that CTLA-4 and PD-1 were highly expressed in TT compared to NT. Interestingly, PD-L1 and TIM-3 were highly expressed in both TT and NT (Fig. 1b).

DNA demethylation enzymes are upregulated in the breast tumor tissues

It has been reported that the loss of methylation imprints is one of the major epigenetic changes happening in human TME, compared with normal microenvironment [14]. The DNA methylation in the form of 5-methylcytosine (5mC) can be actively reversed to unmodified cytosine (5C) through ten-eleven translocation dioxygenase-mediated oxidation [15, 16]. Additionally, the methylation status can be dynamically regulated through the balance between TETs and DNMTs, and their occupancy in promoter sites can directly influence gene expression [17]. These reports prompt us to check the expression level of demethylation/methylation enzymes in breast TME. Interestingly, we found that TET2 and TET3 were significantly higher in the tumor tissues compared with normal tissues, but not TET1 (Fig. 1c). Our data are similar to the reports showing that out of all TET enzymes, TET2 and TET3 actively participate in DNA demethylation and not TET1 [18, 19]. Apart from the upregulation of TET2 and TET3, we also found that there is a significant downregulation of both DNMT3a and DNMT3b expression in cancer tissue compared with normal tissues (Fig. 1c). These data reveal that the epigenetic modifications such as DNA demethylation may play a predominant role in the upregulation of immune checkpoints in breast TME.

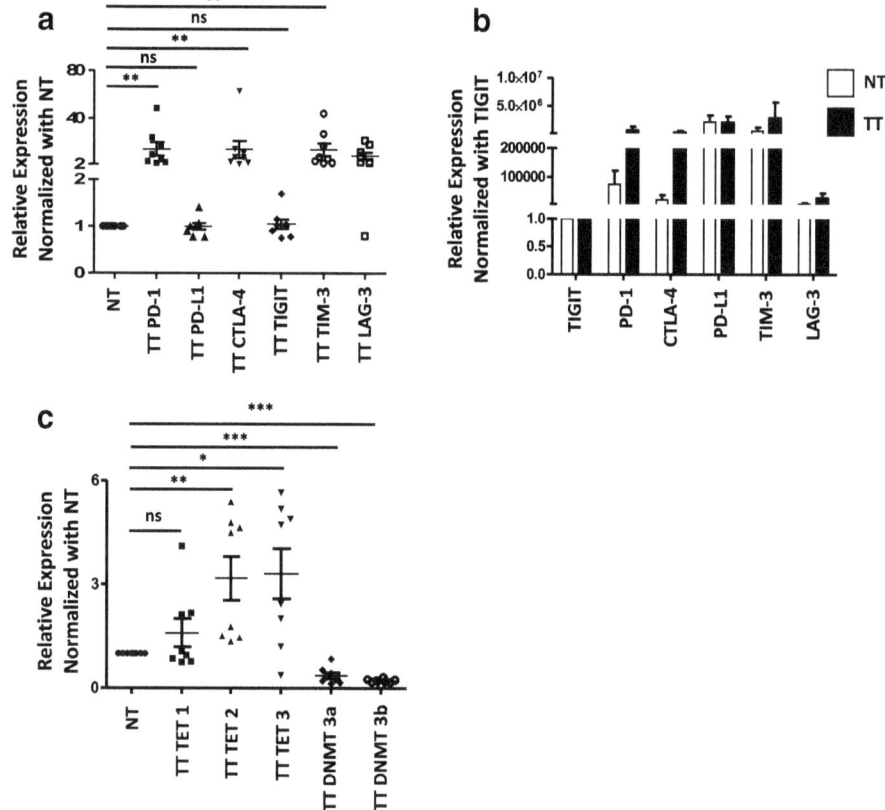

Fig. 1 Expression of immune checkpoints and PD-L1 genes and methylation/demethylation genes in breast tumor and normal tissues. RNA isolated from breast tumor and normal tissues from eight patients were reverse transcribed to cDNA. Quantitative RT-PCR was performed to assess the expression level of PD-1, PD-L1, CTLA-4, TIGIT, TIM-3, and LAG-3 (**a**); TET1, TET2, TET3, DNMT3a, and DNMT3b (**c**) from both NT and TT. The relative expression of each gene was normalized to β-actin. Absolute expression of each gene was calculated by normalizing each gene to TIGIT expression (**b**)

The promoter regions of PD-1, CTLA-4, and TIM-3 are significantly hypomethylated in tumor, compared with normal tissues

To check the DNA epigenetic modifications in immune checkpoints/ligand in the breast TME, we examined the promoter CpG methylation profile of genes including PD-1, CTLA-4, TIM-3, LAG-3, PD-L1, and TIGIT in tumor and normal tissues. It has been reported that the CpG islands (CGIs), especially those within the promoter regions, play a vital role in tumorigenesis, genome imprinting, gene silencing, and X-chromosome inactivation [20]. Due to this multifunctional importance of CGIs in transcription regulation and epigenetic modification, we intended to check the promoter CpG methylation pattern of PD-1, CTLA-4, TIM-3, LAG-3, PD-L1, and TIGIT. Herein, we selected 6 CpGs from PD-1, 4 CpGs from CTLA-4, 4 CpGs from TIM-3, 12 CpGs from LAG-3, 24 CpGs from PD-L1, and 13 CpGs from TIGIT promoters to determine the methylation profiles (Figs. 2a, c, e and g, 3a and c). Additionally, while comparing the methylation

status of tumor tissues between the eight patients, DNA demethylation percentage of CTLA-4 in TT looks more consistent than the other five genes (Figs. 2b, d, f and h, 3b and d). Interestingly, we found that the CpGs of PD-L1 promoter was completely demethylated and TIGIT was prominently methylated with no significant differences between NT and TT (Fig. 3). The average demethylation percentage of PD-1 promoter among the eight patients looks similar to CTLA-4; TT was more demethylated (90%) than NT (54%) (Fig. 4a). Furthermore, TIM-3 promoter also appears more demethylated in TT (69%) than NT (38%) (Fig. 4a). There were no significant changes in demethylation status of LAG-3 promoter in TT (91%) compared to NT (83%) (Fig. 4a). Therefore, we concluded that in breast TME, the expressions of PD-1, CTLA-4, and TIM-3 are epigenetically regulated through DNA methylation and for the LAG-3 upregulation; other epigenetic modifications might be involved. The demethylation percentage was highest in PD-L1 and lowest in TIGIT with no significant differences between

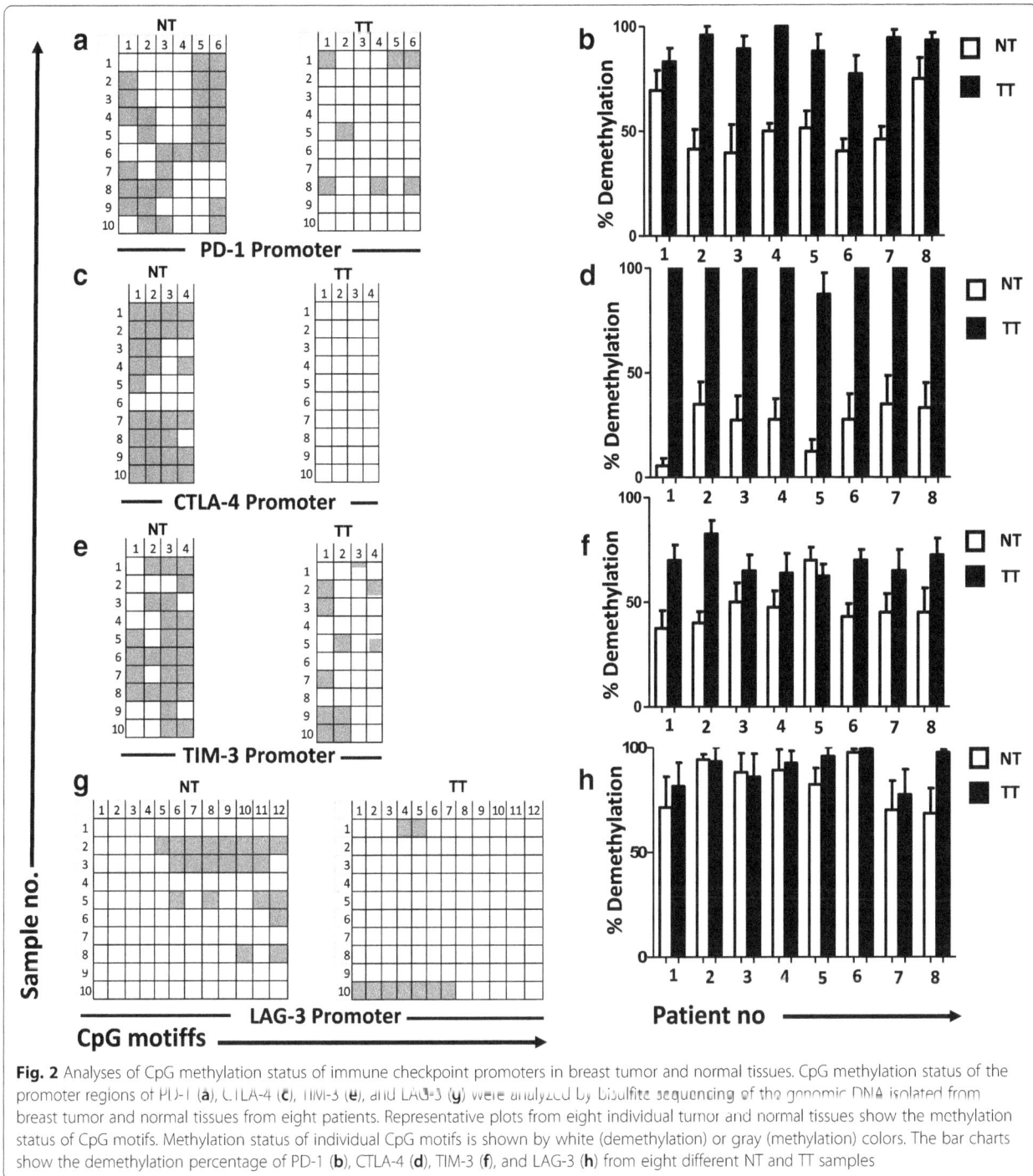

Fig. 2 Analyses of CpG methylation status of immune checkpoint promoters in breast tumor and normal tissues. CpG methylation status of the promoter regions of PD-1 (a), CTLA-4 (c), TIM-3 (e), and LAG-3 (g) were analyzed by bisulfite sequencing of the genomic DNA isolated from breast tumor and normal tissues from eight patients. Representative plots from eight individual tumor and normal tissues show the methylation status of CpG motifs. Methylation status of individual CpG motifs is shown by white (demethylation) or gray (methylation) colors. The bar charts show the demethylation percentage of PD-1 (b), CTLA-4 (d), TIM-3 (f), and LAG-3 (h) from eight different NT and TT samples

TT and NT (Fig. 4a). These data correlate with the data in Fig. 1b that there is no significant difference between the relative expression of PD-L1 and TIGIT in TT and NT. Next, we wanted to see the actual demethylation percentage in TT samples by excluding the NT demethylation percentage. In accordance with our previous results, we found that CTLA-4 is more demethylated followed by PD-1, TIM-3, LAG-3, and finally PD-L1 and TIGIT

(Fig. 4b). Additionally, we also checked the actual demethylation percentage in PD-1, CTLA-4, TIM-3, LAG-3, PD-L1, and TIGIT genes in individual patient samples and found that in TT samples, the demethylation percentage of CTLA-4 is consistently higher in all patients compared with all other five genes (Fig. 3c). Taken together, our data show that DNA demethylation plays a vital role in the upregulation of CTLA-4, PD-1, and TIM-3 in breast

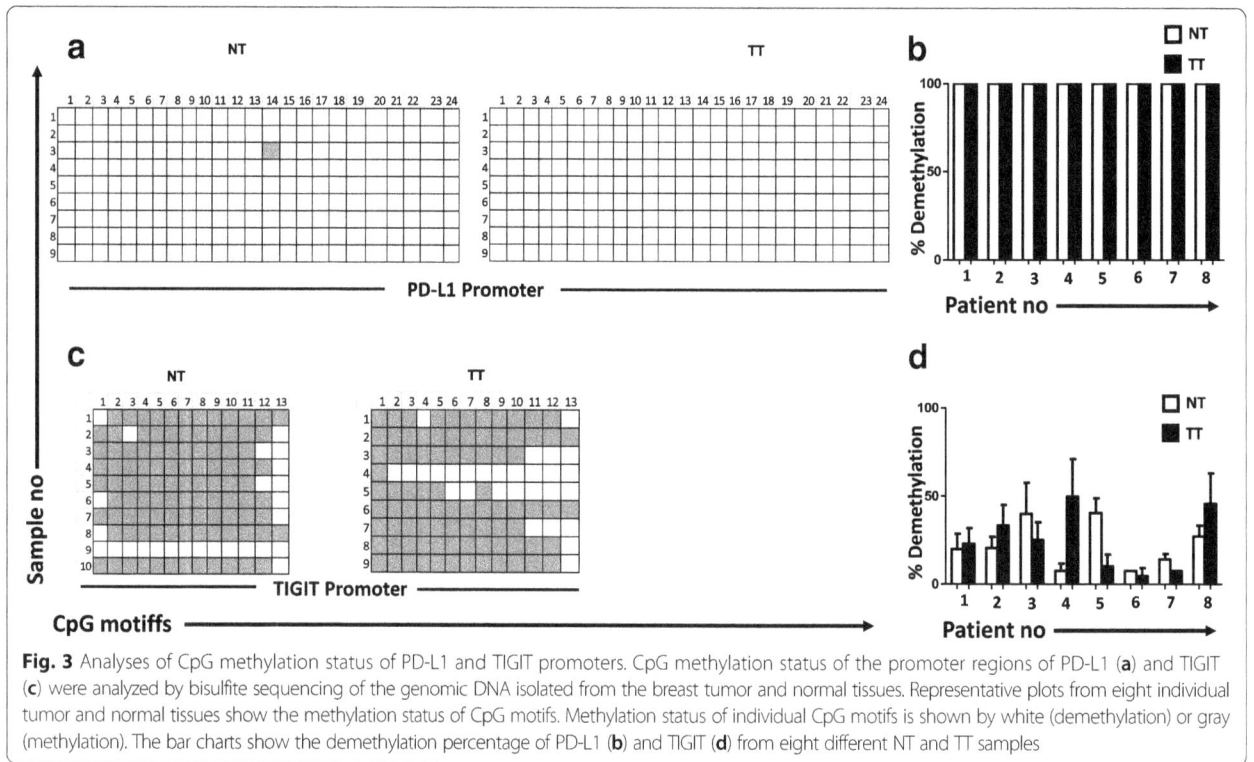

Fig. 3 Analyses of CpG methylation status of PD-L1 and TIGIT promoters. CpG methylation status of the promoter regions of PD-L1 (**a**) and TIGIT (**c**) were analyzed by bisulfite sequencing of the genomic DNA isolated from the breast tumor and normal tissues. Representative plots from eight individual tumor and normal tissues show the methylation status of CpG motifs. Methylation status of individual CpG motifs is shown by white (demethylation) or gray (methylation). The bar charts show the demethylation percentage of PD-L1 (**b**) and TIGIT (**d**) from eight different NT and TT samples

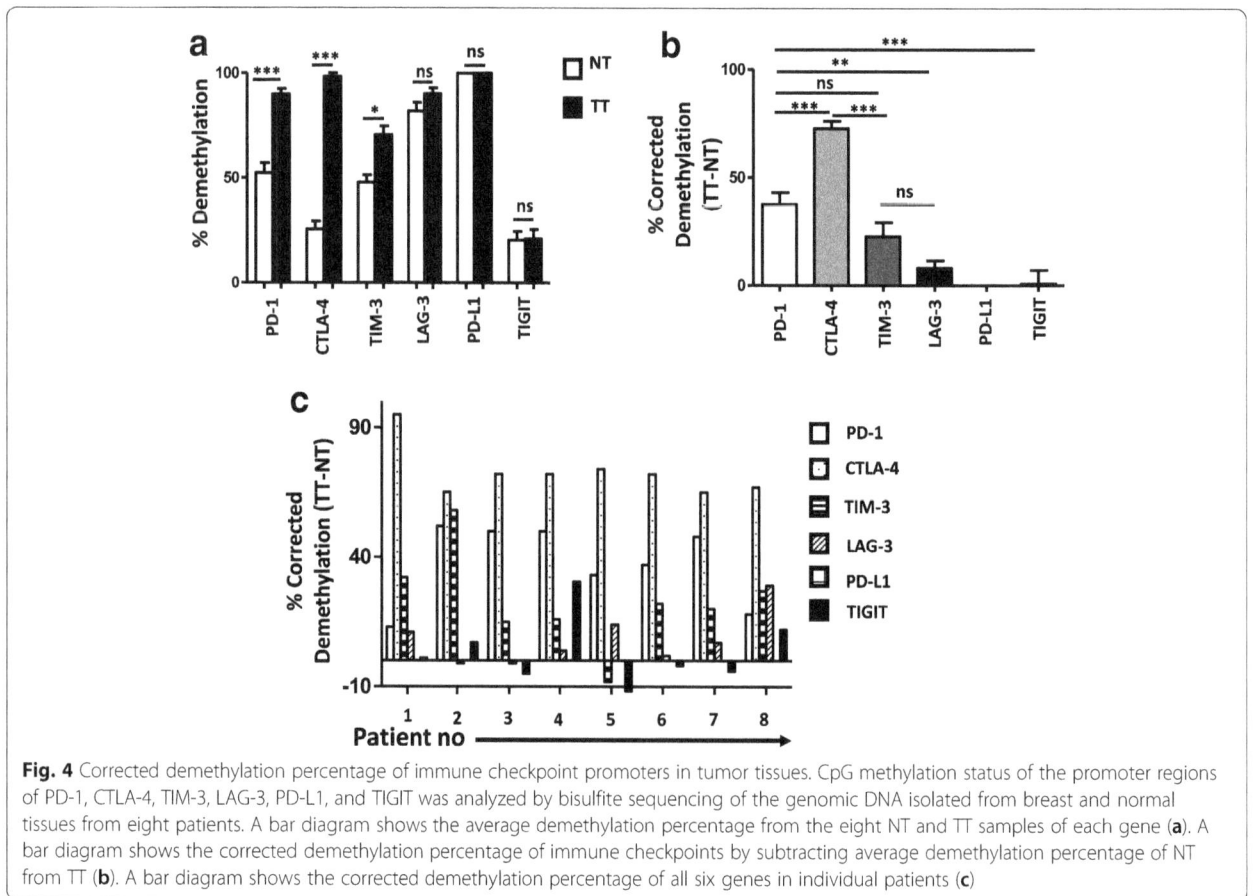

Fig. 4 Corrected demethylation percentage of immune checkpoint promoters in tumor tissues. CpG methylation status of the promoter regions of PD-1, CTLA-4, TIM-3, LAG-3, PD-L1, and TIGIT was analyzed by bisulfite sequencing of the genomic DNA isolated from breast and normal tissues from eight patients. A bar diagram shows the average demethylation percentage from the eight NT and TT samples of each gene (**a**). A bar diagram shows the corrected demethylation percentage of immune checkpoints by subtracting average demethylation percentage of NT from TT (**b**). A bar diagram shows the corrected demethylation percentage of all six genes in individual patients (**c**)

TME. Moreover, the expression of CTLA-4 could be strongly regulated by DNA methylation.

Repressive histone bindings to promotors of PD-1, CTLA-4, TIM-3, and LAG-3 are significantly reduced in breast tumor tissues

The regulation of gene expression is not limited to DNA methylation, but also depends on histone posttranslational modifications (HPTMs). It has been reported that DNA methylation can elicit the changes in chromatin structure including histone deacetylation, methylation, and local chromatin compaction [21]. H3K9me3 and H3K27me3 are two known histone marks that seem to promote chromatin compaction in promoter regions, which could be associated with hindrance of transcriptional activation [22, 23]. To quantify the binding intensity of H3K9me3 and H3K27me3 on the promoters of PD-1, CTLA-4, TIM-3, and LAG-3 in normal and breast tumor tissues, we performed a ChIP-qPCR analysis using H3K9me3 and H3K27me3 antibodies. We found that in PD-1 and CTLA-4 promoters, both repressive histones bind weakly in tumor tissues compared with normal tissues (Fig. 5a, b). Additionally, in both PD-1 and CTLA-4 promoters, H3K9me3 binds significantly weaker than H3K27me3 in tumor tissues (Fig. 5a, b). Moreover, in TIM-3 promoter, only H3K27me3 binds weakly in tumor tissues and there is no significant difference in the binding of H3K9me3 in tumor compared to normal tissues (Fig. 5c). In case of LAG-3 promoter, both repressive histones bind weakly in tumor tissues

compared to normal tissues (Fig. 5d). Collectively, our data show that the regulation of PD-1, CTLA-4, and LAG-3 were under the control of H3K9me3 and H3K27me3, but TIM-3 is regulated only by H3K27me3. In breast TME, these repressive histones fail to bind with the specific promoters of PD-1, CTLA-4, TIM-3, and LAG-3, which could lead to their upregulation of gene expression.

Discussion

Expression of immune checkpoint molecules on T cells is identified as one of the important regulatory mechanisms of immune cells to regulate responses against self-antigens [10, 24]. Reports show that individual or multiple immune checkpoints are expressed on immune cells, which can functionally synergize each other in various disease contexts [25, 26]. Even though the precise signaling pathways behind the expression of these checkpoints are poorly understood, pre-clinical studies conducting with blockade of multiple checkpoints suggest that each of these molecules follows relatively unique pathways [27, 28]. Recent advances in breast cancer research have emphasized that epigenetic modifications are correlated with cancer development and progression [5, 29, 30]. An improved understanding of these epigenetic regulations can pave the way to advance the concept of targeting immune checkpoints in cancer immunotherapy. This study critically advances our knowledge of the epigenetic modifications behind the transcriptional upregulation of PD-1, CTLA-4, TIM-3, LAG-3, TIGIT, and PD-L1 in breast tumor tissues.

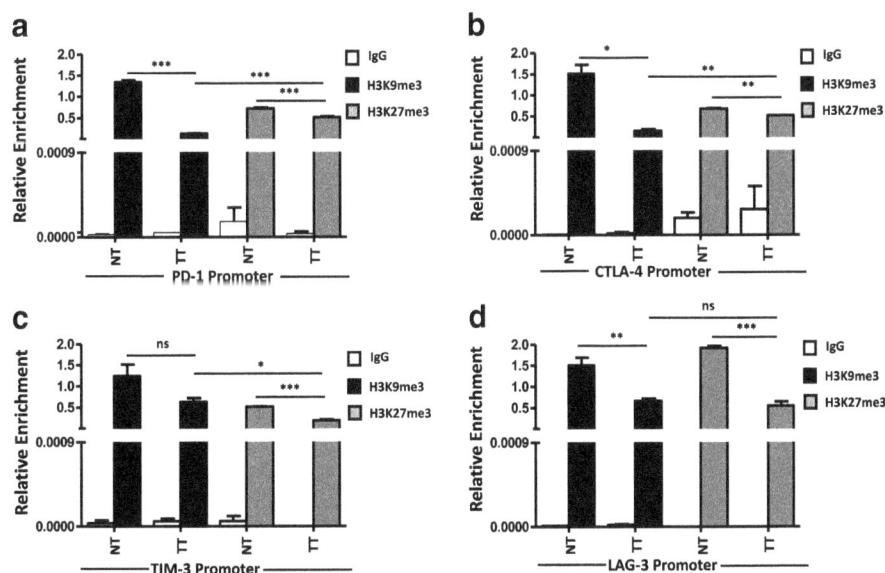

Fig. 5 Analyses of distribution of H3K9me3 and H3K27me3 across the promoters of immune checkpoints in tumor and normal tissues. Cells from two individual NT and TT samples were isolated by enzyme disaggregation. Chromatin was precipitated using H3K9me3, H3K27me3 antibodies, and control IgG as negative control. Subsequent qPCR was performed using PD-1, CTLA-4, TIM-3, and LAG-3 promoter primers and data were normalized to input. ChIP analysis of distribution of H3K9me3 and H3K27me3 at PD-1 (**a**), CTLA-4 (**b**), TIM-3 (**c**), and LAG-3 (**d**) promoter regions are shown

In breast cancer, it has been reported that multiple immune checkpoint molecules were upregulated in TILs [12, 31–33], and their expression correlates with tumor progression [13]. In our study, we checked the expression of immune checkpoints/ligand including PD-1, CTLA-4, TIGIT, TIM-3, LAG-3, and PD-L1 and found that PD-1, CTLA-4, TIM-3, and LAG-3 were upregulated in breast tumor tissues, compared with normal tissues (Fig. 1a). To investigate the molecular mechanism behind this upregulation, we checked the epigenetic modifications in these genes. Previous reports revealed that breast carcinogenesis is in fact a multistep process, which involves both genetic and epigenetic modifications [5, 29, 34], leading to genetic abnormalities in oncogenes and/or tumor suppressor genes [35–37]. These reports prompt us to check the expression of demethylation enzymes (TETs) and methylation enzymes (DNMTs) in tumor and normal tissues and found that TET2 and TET3 were upregulated, while DNMT3a and DNMT3b were downregulated in the TME (Fig. 1c). Our data are similar to previous findings that TET proteins are predominantly expressed in breast tissue [38] and play a key role in regulating hypoxia-enhanced tumor malignancy [39]. Some recent reports showed that DNMT inhibitors (DNMTi), such as 5-azacytidine and 5-decitabine, can hypomethylate the promoter region of PD-1, PD-L2, and CTLA-4 in patients with acute myeloid leukemia with myelodysplastic syndromes (AML/MDS) and upregulate their expression [40–42]. These results are in line with our findings that the downregulation of DNMT3a and 3b can significantly hypomethylate the promoter regions of PD-1, CTLA-4, and TIM-3, which in turn upregulate their expression levels in the TME (Figs. 1 and 2). Moreover, there were no changes in the methylation status of LAG-3, PD-L1, and TIGIT, indicating that genes follow different methylation patterns in the breast TME.

Various epigenetic alterations including methylation of CpG motifs in promoter regions, changes in chromatin structure, and binding of histone complexes to promoter regions can ultimately lead to the activation of oncogenes by silencing tumor suppressor genes [43]. The transcriptomic and methylation profiles of CTLA-4 and PD-1 in non-small cell lung cancer (NSCLC) patients showed that hypomethylation in the CpG islands of these genes was strongly correlated with their increased expression in the TME compared with normal tissue [44]. To reveal the underlying mechanism behind the upregulation of multiple immune checkpoints in breast tumor, we selected certain CpGs from the promoter regions of PD-1, CTLA-4, TIM-3, LAG-3, PD-L1, and TIGIT and investigated their methylation status in tumor tissues and control non-tumor tissues from all eight patients. Our results show that tumor environment alters the promoter methylation profile of PD-1, CTLA-4, and TIM-3 to extremely hypomethylated state. It has been reported that gene transcription is tightly correlated with the CpG methylation profile, where they are activated by hypomethylation and silenced by hypermethylation [45]. The promoter CpG methylation profile shows that this hypomethylation could be the reason behind the upregulation of checkpoints in breast tumor tissues (Fig. 2a, c and e). Furthermore, while comparing the six genes, CpG regions of CTLA-4 in tumor tissue were totally demethylated, which articulates that this demethylation could be a key reason behind its upregulation in breast TME. We also checked the percentage of demethylation across the eight patients and found that in PD-1 and CTLA-4, the percentage was increased consistently in tumor tissue of all patients but not in TIM-3. These data show that the consistent demethylation status of PD-1 and CTLA-4 promoters in tumor tissue could be utilized as a diagnostic marker for breast cancer. A recent study showed that PD-L1 promoter was hypomethylated in tumors with dense T cell infiltration, which correlated with adverse prognosis, and anti-PD-1 therapy could reverse this hypomethylation status [46]. Another study showed that the PD-1, CTLA-4, and PD-L1 promoter hypomethylation has a significant impact on the course of NSCLC progression [44]. These reports and our study rationalize the use of DNA methylation as a prognostic biomarker in cancer. The methylation profile analysis of PD-L1 and TIGIT showed that PD-L1 was completely demethylated and TIGIT was prominently methylated in both TT and NT (Fig. 3). This could be the reason that there were no significant changes in the relative expression between NT and TT for these two genes. Moreover, in LAG-3, we did not find a significant difference in demethylation percentage between tumor and normal tissues. This can be explained as the upregulation of LAG-3 in tumor tissue is not dependent on the DNA methylation but could be regulated by some other epigenetic modifications.

Apart from DNA methylation, post-translational histone modifications are also involved in the regulation of gene expression in breast cancer pathogenesis and its diversity [47]. It has been reported that the establishment of basic DNA methylation profile is mediated through histone modifications by recruiting DNMTs to the target CpGs [48]. To check the association of histone methyl marks in the promoter region of immune checkpoints, we selected the two known repressive histones, H3K9me3 and H3K27me3, that act to impede transcriptional elongation thereby silencing genes [49]. We found that the distribution of both trimethyl histones in the promoter region of PD-1, CTLA-4, and LAG-3 was reduced in tumor compared with normal tissues. Furthermore, only the distribution of H3K27me3 was reduced in the tumor tissue of TIM-3 promoter. These results show that the epigenetic modification behind the upregulation of

DNA methylation and repressive H3K9 and H3K27 trimethylation in the promoter regions of PD-1...

163

immune checkpoints was not limited to DNA methylation but also depends on the distribution of the methylated histones across promoters.

Immune checkpoint inhibition is considered as one of the recent successful therapeutic modalities. Despite the clinical success, one of the main limitations in immune checkpoint therapy is the low response rate among patients [50]. The dynamic and reversible nature of epigenetic modifications occurring in certain gene loci in the TME makes them a relevant target for cancer therapy [51]. Apart from DNA and histone methylation, other modifications such as histone acetylation and expression of microRNAs (miRNA) and long noncoding RNAs (lncRNAs) can also regulate immune checkpoints in the TME. Interestingly, preclinical studies showed that the histone deacetylase inhibitors (HDACi) can augment the response of PD-1 immunotherapy in lung adenocarcinoma and melanoma [52, 53]. Moreover, other reports showed that the expression of miRNAs including miR-330-5p, mir-138, and miR-424(322) regulates the expression of TIM-3, CTLA-4, and PD-1/PD-L1 in AML [52], Glioma [54], and ovarian carcinomas [55], respectively. Of note, the current scenario of epigenetic therapy is mainly focused on DNMTi and HDACi [56]. In a preclinical NSCLC study, it was shown that mocetinostat, a class I/IV HDACi, together with anti-PD-L1 antibody augmented the antitumor activity by decreasing the immune suppressive cell types and increasing CD8$^+$ T cell infiltration in the TME [57]. Some recent reports showed that in breast cancer models, HDAC inhibition together with immune checkpoint blockades can reduce tumor growth and metastasis [58, 59]. In order to improve the cancer immunotherapeutic arsenal, novel combination therapies should be established. Recent advances in research support combination of epigenetic modulators with immune checkpoint inhibitors as a more efficient approach for cancer therapy [60–62]. Our data advance the current knowledge on the importance of epigenetic modifications for the upregulation of immune checkpoints and their ligands in the breast TME.

Conclusions

In conclusion, our study shows that multiple immune checkpoints including PD-1, CTLA-4, TIM-3, and LAG-3 are upregulated in breast tumor tissues. The epigenetic modifications behind their upregulations are dependent on DNA methylation and the repressive histone distribution. Furthermore, upregulation of LAG-3 depends only upon repressive histone distribution. The overall conclusion is graphically represented in Fig. 6.

Methods
Sample collection
Tumor tissues (TT) and adjacent non-cancerous normal tissues (NT) were obtained from eight breast cancer

patients who underwent surgery at Tawam Hospital, Al Ain. All patients included in the study were treatment-naive prior to surgery. Table 1 shows the clinical and pathological characteristics of all participating subjects. The study was executed under the ethical approval by Al Ain Medical District Research Ethics committee, Al Ain, United Arab Emirates (Protocol no. 13/23-CRD 244/13). All patients provided written informed consent prior to sample collection. All experiments were performed in accordance with the relevant guidelines and regulations. After sample collection, the tissues were stored in liquid nitrogen with freezing media.

DNA and RNA isolation
DNA and RNA were isolated using RNA/DNA/Protein Purification Plus Kit (Norgen Biotek Corp, Ontario, Canada) as per manufacturer's instructions from eight TT and their corresponding NT. Briefly, frozen tissues were transferred into a mortar containing adequate amount of liquid nitrogen and grind the tissue thoroughly using a pestle followed by resuspending with lysis buffer and collection in an Eppendorf tube. The tubes were incubated at 55 °C for 10 min followed by DNA extraction using DNA extraction column. The flow-through from DNA extraction was used for RNA and protein extractions. After DNA extraction, the RNA was extracted using RNA extraction column and the flow-through was used for protein extraction. The DNA and RNA concentrations were measured using NanoDrop 2000c (Thermo scientific, Massachusetts, USA) and stored at − 80 °C.

Quantitative real-time PCR
One microgram of RNA from each sample was reverse transcribed into cDNA using QuantiTect Reverse Transcription Kit (Qiagen, Hilden, Germany). PCR reactions were performed on QuantStudio 7 Flex qPCR (Applied Biosystems, California, USA) using Fast SYBER Green Master Mix (Applied Biosystems). All data were normalized to β-actin. Non-specific amplifications were checked by the use of melting curve and agarose gel electrophoresis. The relative changes in target gene expression were analyzed by using 2$^{-\Delta\Delta CT}$ method. The absolute expression of immune checkpoints in both TT and NT was checked by comparing the relative expression values of all checkpoints normalized to the relative expression values of TIGIT. Sequences of primers are listed in Additional file 1: Table S1a. The primers were designed using Primer3 (http://www.ncbi.nlm.nih.gov/tools/primer-blast/).

CpG methylation analysis by bisulfite sequencing
The genomic DNA was extracted from tumor and normal tissues as described before and treated with bisulfite using the EZ DNA Methylation Kit (Zymo Research, Irvine, CA, United States). The bisulfite-treated DNA was then

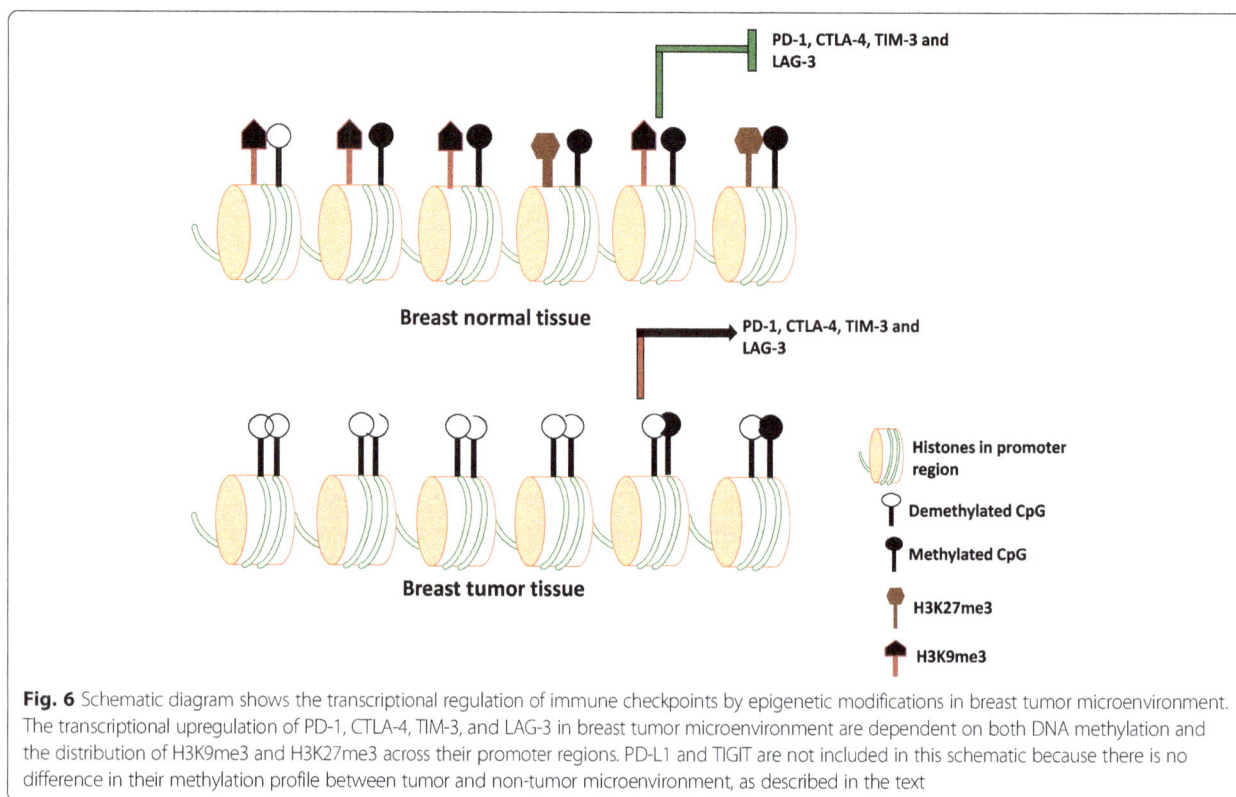

Fig. 6 Schematic diagram shows the transcriptional regulation of immune checkpoints by epigenetic modifications in breast tumor microenvironment. The transcriptional upregulation of PD-1, CTLA-4, TIM-3, and LAG-3 in breast tumor microenvironment are dependent on both DNA methylation and the distribution of H3K9me3 and H3K27me3 across their promoter regions. PD-L1 and TIGIT are not included in this schematic because there is no difference in their methylation profile between tumor and non-tumor microenvironment, as described in the text

subjected to PCR for the amplification of the promoter regions of PD-1, CTLA-4, TIM-3, and LAG-3 using Hot Start TaKaRa Taq DNA Polymerase (TaKaRa Bio, Shiga, Japan). PCR primers were designed using MethPrimer software (http://www.urogene.org/methprimer/index1.html), all are listed in Additional file 1: Table S1b. The PCR products obtained were cloned into the pGemT-easy vector (Promega, Madison, USA) using DNA Ligation Kit, Mighty Mix (TaKaRa Bio). Ten individual clones from each sample were purified using Wizard® Plus SV Minipreps DNA Purification System (Promega) and sequenced with M13-reverse/forward primers (Additional file 1: Table S1c). The promoter sequence details of immune checkpoints and PD-L1 genes are shown in Additional file 2: Figure S2 A-F.

Table 1 Characteristic features of study population

S No	Age	ER	PR	HER2	Grade	Histological grade	TNM stage
1	43	+	+	−	I	NA	IA
2	47	−	−	+	II	Moderate	IA
3	59	+	+	+	III	Poorly differentiated	IIB
4	43	−	−	+	III	Poorly differentiated	IIB
5	65	+	−	−	II	Moderate	IIB
6	41	−	−	−	III	Poorly differentiated	IIA
7	54	+	+	−	III	Poorly differentiated	IA
8	43	+	+	NA	I	Well differentiated	IA

NA not available

Enzyme disaggregation of tumor and normal tissues for cell isolation

Enzyme disaggregation (ED) of frozen tumor and normal tissues from two breast cancer patients was performed on a roller mixer at 37 °C for 60 min. Briefly, after thawing the vials, tissues were first washed with phosphate buffer saline (PBS) and mechanically cut into small fragments (2–4 mm) using a surgical scalpel. Tissues were then suspended into RPMI-1640 with 1% penicillin/streptomycin and enzyme cocktail consisting of 1 mg/ml collagenase, 100 µg/ml hyluronidase type V, and 30 IU/ml of deoxyribonuclease I (all from Sigma-Aldrich, UK). Cell suspension was then passed through a 100-µm BD Falcon cell strainer (BD Biosciences, Oxford, UK) to remove debris and aggregates. Cells were then washed with serum-free RPMI-1640 and resuspended in RPMI-1640 enriched with 10% FCS and 1% penicillin/streptomycin and used for chromatin immunoprecipitation (ChIP) experiments.

Chromatin immunoprecipitation assay

Cells isolated from NT and TT through ED were subjected to ChIP analysis using Zymo-Spin ChIP kit (Zymo Research) as per manufacturer's instructions. Briefly, after cell isolation by ED, nuclear lysate was prepared as per the protocol and sonicated using Omni Sonic Ruptor 400 Ultrasonic Homogenizer (OMNI International, GA, USA) to make small DNA fragments ranging from 100 to 1000 base pairs and then incubated with ChIP grade anti-Histone H3 (tri methyl K9) rabbit mAb (Abcam, Cambridge, United Kingdom) and anti-Histone H3 (tri methyl K27) rabbit mAb (Abcam). Isotype-matched control Ab was used as negative control. Immune complexes containing DNA fragments were precipitated using Magna A/G beads supplied with the kit. Relative enrichment of the target regions in the precipitated DNA fragments was analyzed by QuantStudio 7 Flex qPCR (Applied Biosystems) using Fast SYBER Green Master Mix (Applied Biosystems). All data were normalized to input controls. Non-specific amplification was checked by the use of melting curve and agarose gel electrophoresis. Sequences of primers are listed in Additional file 1: Table S1d.

Sanger sequencing

The purified plasmid DNA samples were subjected to sequencing using 3130X Genetic Analyzer (Applied Biosystems). Briefly, the cycle sequencing reactions of samples were performed using M-13 forward/reverse primers and BigDye Treminator V3.1 (Applied Biosystems). Thermocycler conditions were as follows: 95 °C for 5 min, 35 cycles of 95 °C for 30 s, and 60 °C for 4 min. After PCR reaction, DNA was precipitated using 125 mM EDTA and 95% ethanol by incubation at − 20 °C for 30 min. After incubation, DNA was washed twice with 70% ethanol followed by denaturation using formaldehyde. Denatured DNA was then loaded into analyzer for sequencing.

Statistical analyses

Statistical analyses were performed using GraphPad Prism 5 software (GraphPad Software, USA). We checked normality using Shapiro-Wilk normality test. Paired t test was done for the samples passed normality test, and for others, nonparametric/Wilcoxon matched-pairs signed rank test was performed. The P values are represented as follows: ***$P < 0.001$, **$P < 0.01$, and *$P < 0.05$. A P value of > 0.05 is considered statistically non-significant (NS). The data are presented as mean + standard error of the mean (SEM).

Abbreviations

ChIP: Chromatin immunoprecipitation; CpGI: CpG islands; CTLA-4: Cytotoxic T-lymphocyte associated protein 4; DNMT: DNA methyltransferase; DNMTi: DNA methyltransferase inhibitor; H3K27me3: Histone 27 lysine 9 trimethylation; H3K9me3: Histone 3 lysine 9 trimethylation; HDACi: Histone deacetylase inhibitor; LAG-3: Lymphocyte-activation gene 3; PD-1: Programmed cell death protein-1; PD-L1: Programmed death-ligand 1; RT-qPCR: Quantitative real-time PCR; TET: Ten-eleven translocation dioxygenase; TIGIT: T cell immunoreceptor with Ig and ITIM domains; TIM-3: T-cell immunoglobulin and mucin-domain containing-3

Acknowledgements

We are grateful to patients for donating samples.

Funding

This work was supported by a start-up grant [VR04] for Dr. Eyad Elkord from Qatar Biomedical research Institute, Qatar Foundation.

Authors' contributions

VSN performed the experimental work, data analysis, and wrote the manuscript. HS contributed to the sample collection and acquisition of patients' clinical data. AJ performed Sanger sequencing BA, co-supervised the project, and reviewed and corrected the manuscript. EE conceived the idea, designed the study, obtained funds, supervised the project, analyzed and interpreted the data, and wrote and revised the manuscript. All authors were involved in the final approval of the manuscript.

Competing interests

The authors declare that they have no competing interests.

Author details

[1]Cancer Research Center, Qatar Biomedical Research Institute, College of Science and Engineering, Hamad Bin Khalifa University, Qatar Foundation, Doha, Qatar. [2]Oncology Department, Al Noor Hospital, Abu Dhabi, United Arab Emirates. [3]Oncology Department, Tawam Hospital, Al Ain, United Arab Emirates. [4]Department of Pathology, College of Medicine and Health Sciences, United Arab Emirates University, Al Ain, United Arab Emirates. [5]Zayed Center for Health Sciences, United Arab Emirates University, Al Ain, United Arab Emirates. [6]Institute of Cancer Sciences, University of Manchester, Manchester, UK.

References

1. Jovanovic J, Ronneberg JA, Tost J, Kristensen V. The epigenetics of breast cancer. Mol Oncol. 2010;4:242–54.
2. van Hoesel AQ, Sato Y, Elashoff DA, Turner RR, Giuliano AE, Shamonki JM, Kuppen PJ, van de Velde CJ, Hoon DS. Assessment of DNA methylation status in early stages of breast cancer development. Br J Cancer. 2013;108:2033–8.
3. Bediaga NG, Acha-Sagredo A, Guerra I, Viguri A, Albaina C, Ruiz Diaz I, Rezola R, Alberdi MJ, Dopazo J, Montaner D, et al. DNA methylation epigenotypes in breast cancer molecular subtypes. Breast Cancer Res. 2010;12:R77.
4. Healey MA, Hu R, Beck AH, Collins LC, Schnitt SJ, Tamimi RM, Hazra A. Association of H3K9me3 and H3K27me3 repressive histone marks with breast cancer subtypes in the Nurses' Health Study. Breast Cancer Res Treat. 2014;147:639–51.
5. Karsli-Ceppioglu S, Dagdemir A, Judes G, Lebert A, Penault-Llorca F, Bignon YJ, Bernard-Gallon D. The epigenetic landscape of promoter genome-wide analysis in breast cancer. Sci Rep. 2017;7:6597.
6. Geiman TM, Robertson KD. Chromatin remodeling, histone modifications, and DNA methylation—how does it all fit together? J Cell Biochem. 2002; 87:117–25.
7. Monk M, Boubelik M, Lehnert S. Temporal and regional changes in DNA methylation in the embryonic, extraembryonic and germ cell lineages during mouse embryo development. Development. 1987;99:371–82.
8. Sadakierska-Chudy A, Kostrzewa RM, Filip M. A comprehensive view of the epigenetic landscape part I: DNA methylation, passive and active DNA demethylation pathways and histone variants. Neurotox Res. 2015;27:84–97.
9. Pardoll DM. The blockade of immune checkpoints in cancer immunotherapy. Nat Rev Cancer. 2012;12:252–64.
10. Sasidharan Nair V, Elkord E. Immune checkpoint inhibitors in cancer therapy: a focus on T-regulatory cells. Immunol Cell Biol. 2018;96:21–33.
11. Solinas C, Garaud S, De Silva P, Boisson A, Van den Eynden G, de Wind A, Risso P, Rodrigues Vitória J, Richard F, Migliori E, et al. Immune checkpoint molecules on tumor-infiltrating lymphocytes and their association with tertiary lymphoid structures in human breast cancer. Front Immunol. 2017;8:1412.
12. Syed Khaja AS, Toor SM, El Salhat H, Faour I, Ul Haq N, Ali BR, Elkord E. Preferential accumulation of regulatory T cells with highly immunosuppressive characteristics in breast tumor microenvironment. Oncotarget. 2017;8:33159–71.
13. Emens LA. Breast cancer immunobiology driving immunotherapy: vaccines and immune checkpoint blockade. Expert Rev Anticancer Ther. 2012;12:1597–611.

14. Ehrlich M. DNA hypomethylation in cancer cells. Epigenomics. 2009;1:239–59.

15. Rasmussen KD, Helin K. Role of TET enzymes in DNA methylation, development, and cancer. Genes Dev. 2016;30:733–50.

16. Tahiliani M, Koh KP, Shen Y, Pastor WA, Bandukwala H, Brudno Y, Agarwal S, Iyer LM, Liu DR, Aravind L, Rao A. Conversion of 5-methylcytosine to 5-hydroxymethylcytosine in mammalian DNA by MLL partner TET1. Science. 2009;324:930–5.

17. Nair VS, Song MH, Ko M, Oh KI. DNA demethylation of the Foxp3 enhancer is maintained through modulation of ten-eleven-translocation and DNA methyltransferases. Mol Cells. 2016;39:888–97.

18. Sasidharan Nair V, Song MH, Oh KI. Vitamin C facilitates demethylation of the Foxp3 enhancer in a Tet-dependent manner. J Immunol. 2016;196:2119–31.

19. Wu X, Zhang Y. TET-mediated active DNA demethylation: mechanism, function and beyond. Nat Rev Genet. 2017;18:517–34.

20. Takai D, Jones PA. Comprehensive analysis of CpG islands in human chromosomes 21 and 22. Proc Natl Acad Sci U S A. 2002;99:3740–5.

21. Miller JL, Grant PA. The role of DNA methylation and histone modifications in transcriptional regulation in humans. Subcell Biochem. 2013;61:289–317.

22. Liu F, Wang L, Perna F, Nimer SD. Beyond transcription factors: how oncogenic signalling reshapes the epigenetic landscape. Nat Rev Cancer. 2016;16:359–72.

23. Zhang T, Cooper S, Brockdorff N. The interplay of histone modifications—writers that read. EMBO Rep. 2015;16:1467–81.

24. Chaudhary B, Elkord E. Regulatory T cells in the tumor microenvironment and cancer progression: role and therapeutic targeting. Vaccines (Basel). 2016;4 https://doi.org/10.3390/vaccines4030028.

25. Liu J, Yuan Y, Chen W, Putra J, Suriawinata AA, Schenk AD, Miller HE, Guleria I, Barth RJ, Huang YH, Wang L. Immune-checkpoint proteins VISTA and PD-1 nonredundantly regulate murine T-cell responses. Proc Natl Acad Sci U S A. 2015;112:6682–7.

26. Nirschl CJ, Drake CG. Molecular pathways: coexpression of immune checkpoint molecules: signaling pathways and implications for cancer immunotherapy. Clin Cancer Res. 2013;19:4917–24.

27. Karachaliou N, Gonzalez-Cao M, Sosa A, Berenguer J, Bracht JWP, Ito M, Rosell R. The combination of checkpoint immunotherapy and targeted therapy in cancer. Ann Transl Med. 2017;5:388.

28. Swart M, Verbrugge I, Beltman JB. Combination approaches with immune-checkpoint blockade in cancer therapy. Front Oncol. 2016;6:233.

29. Fleischer T, Tekpli X, Mathelier A, Wang S, Nebdal D, Dhakal HP, Sahlberg KK, Schlichting E, Oslo Breast Cancer Research C, Borresen-Dale AL, et al. DNA methylation at enhancers identifies distinct breast cancer lineages. Nat Commun 2017; 8:1379.

30. Terry MB, McDonald JA, Wu HC, Eng S, Santella RM. Epigenetic biomarkers of breast cancer risk: across the breast cancer prevention continuum. Adv Exp Med Biol. 2016;882:33–68.

31. Burugu S, Gao D, Leung S, Chia SK, Nielsen TO. LAG-3+ tumor infiltrating lymphocytes in breast cancer: clinical correlates and association with PD-1/PD-L1+ tumors. Ann Oncol. 2017;28(12):2977–84.

32. Mao H, Zhang L, Yang Y, Zuo W, Bi Y, Gao W, Deng B, Sun J, Shao Q, Qu X. New insights of CTLA-4 into its biological function in breast cancer. Curr Cancer Drug Targets. 2010;10:728–36.

33. Zhu S, Lin J, Qiao G, Wang X, Xu Y. Tim-3 identifies exhausted follicular helper T cells in breast cancer patients. Immunobiology. 2016;221:986–93.

34. Troester MA, Hoadley KA, D'Arcy M, Cherniack AD, Stewart C, Koboldt DC, Robertson AG, Mahurkar S, Shen H, Wilkerson MD, et al. DNA defects, epigenetics, and gene expression in cancer-adjacent breast: a study from The Cancer Genome Atlas. NPJ Breast Cancer. 2016;2:16007.

35. Antoniou AC, Easton DF. Models of genetic susceptibility to breast cancer. Oncogene. 2006;25:5898–905.

36. Michailidou K, Lindstrom S, Dennis J, Beesley J, Hui S, Kar S, Lemacon A, Soucy P, Glubb D, Rostamianfar A, et al. Association analysis identifies 65 new breast cancer risk loci. Nature. 2017;551:92–4.

37. Nielsen FC, van Overeem Hansen T, Sorensen CS. Hereditary breast and ovarian cancer: new genes in confined pathways. Nat Rev Cancer. 2016;16: 599–612.

38. Wu MJ, Kim MR, Chen YS, Yang JY, Chang CJ. Retinoic acid directs breast cancer cell state changes through regulation of TET2-PKCzeta pathway. Oncogene. 2017;36:3193–206.

39. Wu MZ, Chen SF, Nieh S, Benner C, Ger LP, Jan CI, Ma L, Chen CH, Hishida T, Chang HT, et al. Hypoxia drives breast tumor malignancy through a TET-TNFalpha-p38-MAPK signaling axis. Cancer Res. 2015;75:3912–24.

40. Daver N, Boddu P, Garcia-Manero G, Yadav SS, Sharma P, Allison J, Kantarjian H. Hypomethylating agents in combination with immune checkpoint inhibitors in acute myeloid leukemia and myelodysplastic syndromes. Leukemia. 2018;32:1094–105.

41. Orskov AD, Treppendahl MB, Skovbo A, Holm MS, Friis LS, Hokland M, Gronbaek K. Hypomethylation and up-regulation of PD-1 in T cells by azacytidine in MDS/AML patients: a rationale for combined targeting of PD-1 and DNA methylation. Oncotarget. 2015;6:9612–26.

42. Yang H, Bueso-Ramos C, DiNardo C, Estecio MR, Davanlou M, Geng QR, Fang Z, Nguyen M, Pierce S, Wei Y, et al. Expression of PD-L1, PD-L2, PD-1 and CTLA4 in myelodysplastic syndromes is enhanced by treatment with hypomethylating agents. Leukemia. 2014;28:1280–8.

43. Dworkin AM, Huang TH, Toland AE. Epigenetic alterations in the breast: implications for breast cancer detection, prognosis and treatment. Semin Cancer Biol. 2009;19:165–71.

44. Marwitz S, Scheufele S, Perner S, Reck M, Ammerpohl O, Goldmann T. Epigenetic modifications of the immune-checkpoint genes CTLA4 and PDCD1 in non-small cell lung cancer results in increased expression. Clin Epigenetics. 2017;9:51.

45. Deaton AM, Bird A. CpG islands and the regulation of transcription. Genes Dev. 2011;25:1010–22.

46. Zhang Y, Xiang C, Wang Y, Duan Y, Liu C, Zhang Y. PD-L1 promoter methylation mediates the resistance response to anti-PD-1 therapy in NSCLC patients with EGFR-TKI resistance. Oncotarget. 2017;8:101535–44.

47. Judes G, Dagdemir A, Karsli-Ceppioglu S, Lebert A, Echegut M, Ngollo M, Bignon YJ, Penault-Llorca F, Bernard-Gallon D. H3K4 acetylation, H3K9 acetylation and H3K27 methylation in breast tumor molecular subtypes. Epigenomics. 2016;8:909–24.

48. Ooi SK, Qiu C, Bernstein E, Li K, Jia D, Yang Z, Erdjument-Bromage H, Tempst P, Lin SP, Allis CD, et al. DNMT3L connects unmethylated lysine 4 of histone H3 to de novo methylation of DNA. Nature. 2007;448:714–7.

49. Cedar H, Bergman Y. Linking DNA methylation and histone modification: patterns and paradigms. Nat Rev Genet. 2009;10:295–304.

50. Ribas A, Hamid O, Daud A, Hodi FS, Wolchok JD, Kefford R, Joshua AM, Patnaik A, Hwu WJ, Weber JS, et al. Association of pembrolizumab with tumor response and survival among patients with advanced melanoma. JAMA. 2016;315:1600–9.

51. Kanwal R, Gupta S. Epigenetic modifications in cancer. Clin Genet. 2012;81: 303–11.

52. Woods DM, Sodre AL, Villagra A, Sarnaik A, Sotomayor EM, Weber J. HDAC inhibition upregulates PD-1 ligands in melanoma and augments immunotherapy with PD-1 blockade. Cancer Immunol Res. 2015;3:1375–85.

53. Zheng H, Zhao W, Yan C, Watson CC, Massengill M, Xie M, Massengill C, Noyes DR, Martinez GV, Afzal R, et al. HDAC inhibitors enhance T-cell chemokine expression and augment response to PD-1 immunotherapy in lung adenocarcinoma. Clin Cancer Res. 2016;22:4119–32.

54. Wei J, Nduom EK, Kong LY, Hashimoto Y, Xu S, Gabrusiewicz K, Ling X, Huang N, Qiao W, Zhou S, et al. MiR-138 exerts anti-glioma efficacy by targeting immune checkpoints. Neuro-Oncology. 2016;18:639–48.

55. Xu S, Tao Z, Hai B, Liang H, Shi Y, Wang T, Song W, Chen Y, OuYang J, Chen J, et al. miR-424(322) reverses chemoresistance via T-cell immune response activation by blocking the PD-L1 immune checkpoint. Nat Commun. 2016;7: 11406.

56. Sigalotti L, Fratta E, Coral S, Maio M. Epigenetic drugs as immunomodulators for combination therapies in solid tumors. Pharmacol Ther. 2014;142:339–50.

57. Briere D, Sudhakar N, Woods DM, Hallin J, Engstrom LD, Aranda R, Chiang H, Sodre AL, Olson P, Weber JS, Christensen JG. The class I/IV HDAC inhibitor mocetinostat increases tumor antigen presentation, decreases immune suppressive cell types and augments checkpoint inhibitor therapy. Cancer Immunol Immunother. 2018;67:381–92.

58. Guerriero JL, Sotayo A, Ponichtera HE, Castrillon JA, Pourzia AL, Schad S, Johnson SF, Carrasco RD, Lazo S, Bronson RT, et al. Class IIa HDAC inhibition reduces breast tumours and metastases through anti-tumour macrophages. Nature. 2017;543:428–32.

59. Terranova-Barberio M, Thomas S, Ali N, Pawlowska N, Park J, Krings G, Rosenblum MD, Budillon A, Munster PN. HDAC inhibition potentiates immunotherapy in triple negative breast cancer. Oncotarget. 2017;8: 114156–72.

14

An epigenetic classifier for early stage lung cancer

Yun Su[1*], Hong Bin Fang[2] and Feng Jiang[3]

Abstract

Background: Methylated genes detected in sputum are promise biomarkers for lung cancer. Yet the current PCR technologies for quantification of DNA methylation and diagnostic value of the sputum biomarkers are not sufficient to be used for lung cancer early detection. The emerging droplet digital PCR (ddPCR) is a straightforward means for precise, direct, and absolute quantification of nucleic acids. Here, we investigate whether ddPCR can sensitively and robustly quantify DNA methylation in sputum for more precise diagnosis of lung cancer.

Results: First, the analytic performance of methylation-specific ddPCR (ddMSP) and quantitative methylation-specific PCR (qMSP) is determined in methylated and unmethylated DNA samples. Second, 29 genes, previously proposed as potential sputum biomarkers for lung cancer, are analyzed by using ddMSP in a training set of 127 lung cancer patients and 159 controls. ddMSP has higher sensitivity, precision, and reproducibility for quantification of methylation compared with qMSP (all $p < 0.05$). A classifier comprising four sputum methylation biomarkers for lung cancer is developed by using ddMSP, producing 86.6% sensitivity and 90.6% specificity, independent of stage and histology of lung cancer (all $p > 0.05$). The classifier has higher accuracy compared with sputum cytology (88.8 vs. 70.6%, $p < 0.01$). The diagnostic performance is confirmed in a testing set of 89 cases and 107 controls.

Conclusions: ddMSP is a robust tool for reliable quantification of DNA methylation in sputum, and the epigenetic classifier could help diagnose lung cancer at the early stage.

Keywords: ddPCR, DNA methylation, Sputum, Diagnosis, Lung cancer

Background

Lung cancer is the leading cause of cancer death among men and women [1]. More than 85% lung tumors are non-small cell lung cancers (NSCLCs), which consist of adenocarcinoma (AC), squamous cell carcinoma (SCC), and large cell carcinoma (LC). Cigarette smoking is the foremost cause of NSCLC [2]. People who smoke cigarettes are nearly 30 times more likely to get lung cancer or die from lung cancer than people who do not smoke. Even smoking a few cigarettes a day or smoking occasionally increases the risk of lung cancer. Individuals who quit smoking have a lower risk of lung cancer than if they had continued to smoke, but their risk is higher than the risk for people who never smoked. The National Lung Screening Trial (NLST) results show that using low-dose CT (LDCT) for the early detection of

lung cancer in smokers can reduce the mortality by 20% as compared to chest X-rays [1]. Therefore, LDCT is recently recommended to be used for lung cancer early detection among smokers [3, 4]. However, LDCT is associated with over-diagnosis, excessive cost, and radiation exposure, limiting its clinical applications [3–5]. The development of noninvasive approaches that can accurately and cost-effectively diagnose early stage lung cancer among smokers remains clinically important [6].

Lung cancer develops from a field defect characterized by an accumulation of molecular abnormalities resulted from repeated exposure of the airway of the smokers to the tobacco-related carcinogens [7–9]. Regardless of the anatomic location relative to the tumors, the molecular alterations observed in the large bronchial airway might reflect the altered changes existed in lung tumors [9–11]. Sputum is defined as secretions from the airways and contains bronchial epithelial cells exfoliated from the airways or lungs [12]. Therefore, the analysis of exfoliated bronchial

* Correspondence: yunsu326@yahoo.com
[1]Department of Surgery, Jiangsu Province Hospital of Nanjing University of Chinese Medicine, 138 Xianlin Road, Nanjing 210023, China
Full list of author information is available at the end of the article

epitheliums in sputum for the molecular changes may provide a useful tool for noninvasively and cost-effectively diagnosing lung cancer.

DNA methylations of tumor suppressor genes (TSGs) are early molecular events in lung carcinogenesis and thus show great promise as biomarkers for early stage lung cancer [6, 11, 13–34]. Conventional qPCR-based platforms, particularly, methylation-specific PCR (qMSP), have been used for detecting DNA methylation of TSGs in sputum [13]. However, qMSP has some weaknesses, limiting its use in the clinical settings. For example, qMSP is an indirect approach, which requires internal controls for data normalization [35]. Furthermore, qMSP's sensitivity for analyzing low copy number of genes is poor. This is particularly challenging for quantification of DNA methylation in bronchial epitheliums, as the large excess of non-epithelial cells in sputum could obscure detection of the relative scarcity of methylated DNA from the exfoliated bronchial epitheliums. A more sensitive, precise, and reproducibility method for quantification of methylated DNA in sputum would provide a useful means for noninvasive diagnosis of lung cancer.

Droplet digital PCR (ddPCR) is a direct method for quantitatively measuring nucleic acids [36–45], since it depends on limiting partition of the PCR volume, where a positive result of a large number of microreactions indicates the presence of a single molecule in a given reaction. The number of positive reactions, together with Poisson's distribution, can be used to produce a straight and high-confidence measurement of the original target concentration [43]. Furthermore, ddPCR does not require the reliance on rate-based measurements, endogenous controls, and the use of calibration curves. In addition, previous studies including our own research have demonstrated that ddPCR can quantify low-abundance nucleic acids and has higher sensitivity and precision than does conventional PCR [36, 37, 46]. The objective of this study is to investigate whether methylation-specific ddPCR (ddMSP) could sensitively and robustly quantify DNA methylations in sputum and hence develop a biomarker-based classifier for early stage lung cancer.

Methods
Study population
The study protocol was approved by the local Institutional Review Board. The participants in this study were recruited from the hospital at the point of their referral for suspected lung cancer between the ages of 55–80. Written informed consent was obtained from all enrolled subjects. Exclusion criteria included pregnancy, current pulmonary infection, surgery within 6 months, radiotherapy within 1 year, and life expectancy of < 1 year. Clinical diagnosis of lung cancer was made using histopathologic examinations of specimens obtained by CT-guided transthoracic needle biopsy, transbronchial biopsy, videotape-assisted thoracoscopic surgery, or surgical resection. The surgical pathologic staging was determined according to the TNM classification of the International Union Against Cancer with the 8th American Joint Committee on Cancer and the International Staging System for Lung Cancer. Histopathological classification was determined according to the World Health Organization classification. A total of 482 subjects including 216 lung cancer patients and 266 cancer-free smokers were recruited. The 216 lung cancer patients were diagnosed with NSCLC consisting of 55 stage I cases, 55 stage II cases, 50 stage III cases, and 56 stage IV cases. One hundred and twelve cases were AC, 91 were SCC, and 13 were LC. The 266 cancer-free patients who were smokers and served as control subjects had granulomatous inflammation ($n = 117$), nonspecific inflammatory changes ($n = 105$) or lung infections ($n = 44$). The cancer-free smokers had been followed for at least 2 years, and none had any evidence of cancer. No difference of age, gender, and smoking status was observed in the lung cancer cases vs. controls (All $p > 0.05$). To refine the biomarkers whose changes specific to NSCLC, the cases were matched to the controls on gender, age, race, and smoking status as a nested case-control study. The cases and controls were then randomly split into a training set and a testing set by using a random number generator. The training set consisted of 127 lung cancer patients and 159 cancer-free controls. The testing set comprised 89 lung cancer patients and 107 cancer-free controls. The demographic and clinical characteristics of the two cohorts are presented in Tables 1 and 2.

Sample collection and sputum cytology
Sputum was collected from the participants as described in previous reports [47–54]. Briefly, to reduce the percentage of oral epithelial cells in the sputum, subjects were asked to blow their nose, rinse their mouth, and swallow water to minimize contamination of squamous cells from postnasal drip and saliva. Sputum samples were then coughed in a sterile container and processed within 2 h. To further minimize oral squamous cell contamination, opaque or dense portions that looked different from saliva under the inverted microscope were selected using blunt forceps from expectorate. The samples were processed on ice in 4 volumes of 0.1% dithiothreitol (Sigma-Aldrich, St. Louis, Mo) followed by 4 volumes of phosphate-buffered saline (PBS) (Sigma-Aldrich). The cell suspension was filtered through 45-μm nylon gauzes (BNSH Thompson, Scarborough, ON, Canada). Absolute cell numbers and cell viability were quantitated by using a hemacytometer with trypan blue. Two cytocentrifuge slides

Table 1 Characteristics of NSCLC patients and cancer-free smokers in a training set

	NSCLC cases (n = 127)	Controls (n = 159)	p value
Age	65.48 (SD 12.32)	65.63 (SD 11.56)	0.32
Sex			0.35
Female	45	56	
Male	82	103	
Smoking pack-years (median)	35.23	33.79	0.34
Stage			
Stage I	33		
Stage II	32		
Stage III	29		
Stage IV	33		
Histological type			
Adenocarcinoma	63		
Squamous cell carcinoma	57		
Large cell carcinoma	7		

Abbreviations: NSCLC non-small cell lung cancer

were prepared from aliquots of cell suspension by using a cytospin machine (Shandon, Pittsburgh, PA) and were then stained with the Papanicolaou staining technique [12]. A sputum sample was considered adequate if lung macrophages or Curschmann spirals were present on the slides [11, 12]. Cytologic diagnosis was performed on the cytospin slides using the classification of Saccomanno et al. [12]. The remaining cells are stored at − 80 °C until used.

Table 2 Characteristics of NSCLC patients and cancer-free smokers in a testing set

	NSCLC cases (n = 89)	Controls (n = 107)	p value
Age	65.25 (SD 11.28)	65.36 (SD 11.48)	0.30
Sex			0.36
Female	31	37	
Male	58	70	
Smoking pack-years (median)	35.76	33.29	0.32
Stage			
Stage I	22		
Stage II	23		
Stage III	21		
Stage IV	23		
Histological type			
Adenocarcinoma	49		
Squamous cell carcinoma	34		
Large cell carcinoma	6		

Abbreviations: NSCLC non-small cell lung cancer

DNA isolation and bisulfite conversion

We extracted DNA from the specimens using DNeasy kit (Qiagen, Valencia, CA) as previously described [14]. We eluted DNA with 50 μL of elution buffer (10 mmol/L Tris-Cl, pH 8.5) (Sigma-Aldrich Corporation). DNA was quantified by using the Quantifiler Human DNA Quantification kit (Applied Biosystems, Foster City, CA). Bisulfite conversion was carried out on DNA by using the Zymo EZ DNA Methylation Kit (Zymo Research, Irvine, CA) according to the manufacturer's protocol.

Serially diluted methylated/unmethylated DNA specimens

We purchased 100% methylated and 100% unmethylated control human DNA samples (Zymo Research). We isolated DNA from sputum of a healthy nonsmoker whose sputum DNA did not harbor DNA methylation of TSGs, including *RASSF1A*, *3OST2*, and *PRDM14* [14]. To determine limit of quantification (LOQ) of an assay, we diluted methylated DNA into the sputum DNA sample in the following concentrations: 100, 25, 6.25, 1.56, 0.39, 0.1, 0.04, and 0% methylated DNA. To determine limits of detection (LOD) of an assay, we prepared serially diluted samples containing 5000, 2500, 1250, 625, 313, 156, and 0 pg methylated DNA in H2O.

Quantification of DNA methylation in sputum by ddMSP

We added bisulfite-treated DNA (2 μL) to ddPCR mixture (18 μL) containing 2 × ddPCR Supermix for probes (no-dUTP), 750 nmol/L of each primer and 250 nmol/L of the corresponding probe in a final volume of 20 μL. Twenty-nine genes were selected for DNA methylation analysis, since the genes were previously reported as potential sputum methylation biomarkers for lung cancer [6, 13–34]. The 29 genes are *3OST2, APC, CDH1, CDO1, CXCL, CYGB, DAL-1, DAPK, DCR2, FAM19A4, FHIT, GATA, H-cadherin, HOXA9, JPH3, KIFLA, MAGE, p16, PAX5, PCDH20, PHACTR3, PRDM14, RARβ, RASSF1A, SOX17, SULF2, TAC1, TCF2L,* and *ZFP42* (Additional file 1: Table S1). Primers and probes of the targeted genes were designed in the studies [6, 13–34]. A thermocycling protocol (95 °C × 10 min; 40 cycles of [94 °C × 30s, 60 °C × 60s], 98 °C × 10 min) was undertaken in a Bio-Rad C1000 (Bio-Rad, Pleasanton, CA). The PCR plate was transferred to the QX100 Droplet Reader (Bio-Rad) for automatic reading of samples in all wells. We used QuantaSoft 1.7.4 analysis software (Bio-Rad) and Poisson statistics to compute droplet concentrations (copies/μL; PCR scale). Only tests that had at least 10,000 droplets were used for the ddMSP analysis [36, 37]. All assays were done in triplicates, and one no-template control and two interplate controls were carried along in each experiment.

Quantification of DNA methylation in sputum by qMSP

qMSP was done as previously described [13, 14]. The cycle threshold (Ct) values for each gene were determined. Ct values above 35 were censored according to previous recommendations [13, 14, 55–58]. To determine methylation level of target genes in a given sample, we normalized Ct values of the target genes in relation to that the of *myoblast determination protein one* (*MYOD1*) [13, 32]. The percentage of methylated reference (PMR) was defined as target gene/*MYOD1* ratio of the sample divided by target gene/*MYOD1* ratio of the calibrator DNA (methylated control DNA) and multiplying by 100 [14].

Comparison of tolerance of ddMSP and qMSP to PCR inhibitors

To determine tolerance of ddMSP and qMSP to inhibitory substances of PCR, we directly introduced inhibitors, sodium dodecyl sulfate (SDS), and heparin (Sigma-Aldrich Corporation), into the PCR reactions [59, 60]. Differences in the resulting inhibition curves and the half-maximal inhibitory concentrations (IC50) were assessed and compared as described previously [59, 60].

Statistical analysis

We used t test to determine significant differences of values of each gene between cases and controls. We used log transformation of the molecular results and applied Pearson's correlation analysis to assess relationship between DNA methylation and demographic characteristics of subjects. We calculated coefficient of variations (CV) to determine the variation between different measurements. We performed the linear regression between different measurements of the assays and the amount of input DNA. We used the receiver-operator characteristic (ROC) curve and area under the curve (AUC) to determine accuracy, sensitivity, and specificity of each gene or the tests. We employed logistic regression models with constrained parameters as in least absolute shrinkage and selection operator (LASSO) based on ROC criterion to eliminate the irrelevant genes and optimize a composite biomarker panel (classifier). The optimal panel of biomarkers was blindly applied to the testing data set to confirm the diagnostic value by comparing the AUC with the goodness-of-fit statistics [61].

Results

ddMSP has higher sensitivity, precision, and reproducibility for quantification of DNA methylation compared with qMSP

In methylated DNA serially diluted in sputum DNA of a healthy nonsmoker, ddMSP generated at least 10,000 droplets passing through a fluorescence detector. The results suggested that the specimens were successfully "read" by ddPCR. ddMSP detected methylated genes (*RASSF1A*, *3OST2*, and *PRDM14*) at a concentration of 0.04% (LOQ = 0.04%)(R^2 = 0.966) (Fig. 1a), whereas qMSP detected the methylation at a concentration of 0.10% (LOQ = 0.10%)(R^2 = 0.935) (p = 0.008) (Fig. 1b). There was excellent linearity between the methylated DNA input and values measured by both qMSP and ddMSP (all $R^2 \geq 0.93$). Furthermore, the dispersion of values of the four analyses of the specimen was lower with ddMSP than with qMSP. The repeated measurements by ddMSP had a lower CV value compared with those determined by qMSP (p = 0.03) (Additional file 1: Table S2). Therefore, ddMSP had a higher precision for quantification of methylation compared to qMSP (p = 0.03) (Additional file 1: Table S2).

To determine the absolute LOD of the two platforms, 100% methylated DNA serially diluted into water and then tested by ddMSP and qMSP. The smallest amount of methylated DNA that can be reliably measured by ddMSP was 156 pg/μL (Fig. 1c), suggesting that ddMSP had a LOD of 156 pg/μL. qMSP produced more than 35 Ct values for the samples that had less than 313 pg methylated DNA per microliter, yielding a LOD of 313 pg/μL (Fig. 1d). Therefore, ddMSP had higher sensitivity as demonstrated by lower LOQ and LOD than did qMSP in the serial dilutions of DNA control samples (all p < 0.001).

To determine reproducibility of ddMSP and qMSP, the diluted samples were independently analyzed. The CVs of repeated measures by ddMSP on different days were more than twofold lower compared with those determined by qMSP (Additional file 1: Table S3). Furthermore, the CVs of repeated measures by different research staff using ddMSP were at least twofold lower than did those generated by qMSP (Additional file 1: Table S4). Therefore, ddMSP had a higher reproducibility than did qMSP for quantification of DNA methylation.

To evaluate analytic performance of ddMSP and qMSP in clinical sputum samples, sputum of 20 lung cancer patients and 20 cancer-free controls was tested for *RASSF1A*, whose aberrant methylation level was shown to be elevated in sputum of lung cancer patients [13, 14, 55–58]. Each well of the samples contained at least 10,000 droplets (Fig. 2a). Therefore, ddMSP analysis of DNA methylation could successfully be performed in clinical sputum specimens. *RASSF1A* analyzed by both the techniques displayed a high methylation level in lung cancer patients vs. controls (all p < 0.05). In the ddMSP assay, a specimen with ≥ one copy of DNA methylation of *RASSF1A* per microliter was considered to be positive. When the criteria was used, of 20 sputum specimens of lung cancer patients, 11 (55%) had positive methylation of the gene detected by ddMSP. In the qMSP assay, a PMR ≥ 1% was classified as positive for *RASSF1A* in a given sample [62].

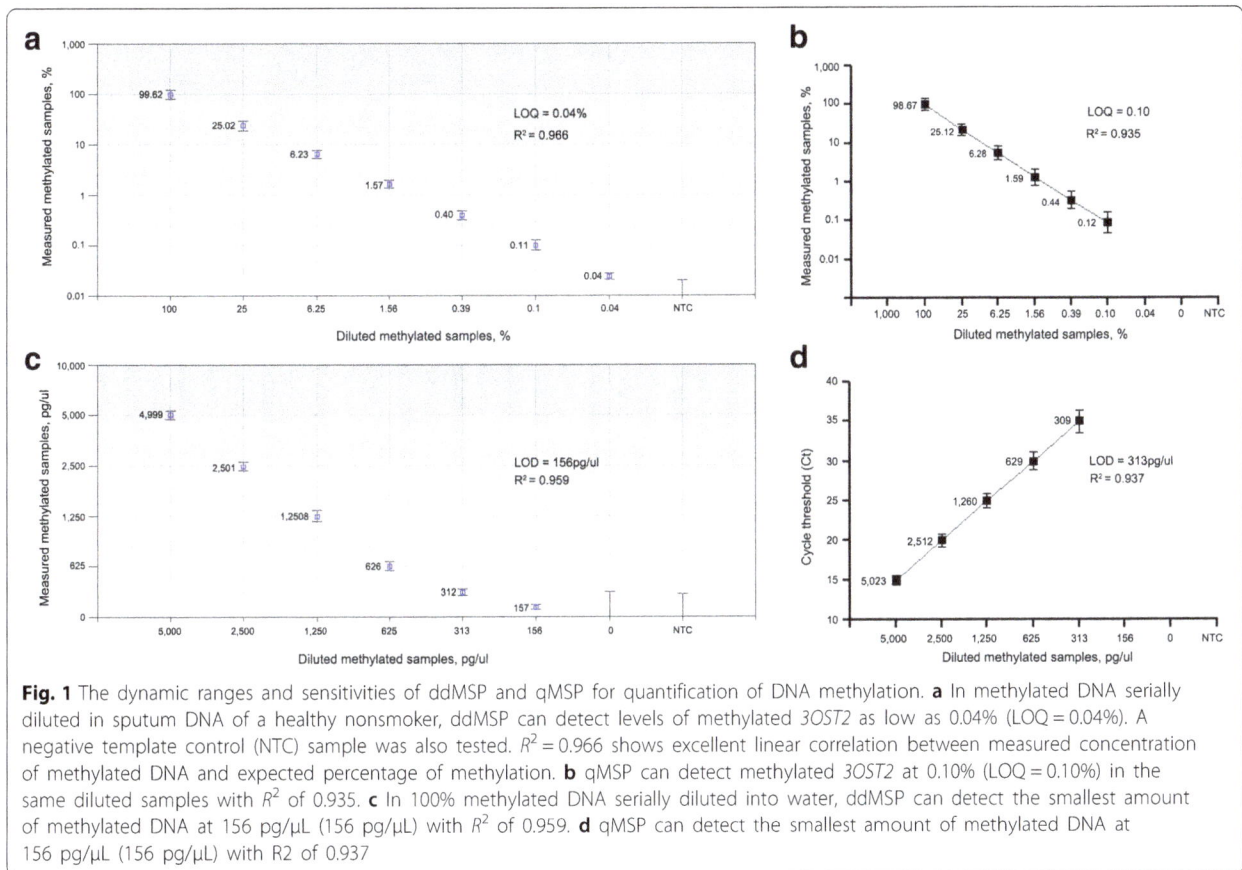

Fig. 1 The dynamic ranges and sensitivities of ddMSP and qMSP for quantification of DNA methylation. **a** In methylated DNA serially diluted in sputum DNA of a healthy nonsmoker, ddMSP can detect levels of methylated *3OST2* as low as 0.04% (LOQ = 0.04%). A negative template control (NTC) sample was also tested. $R^2 = 0.966$ shows excellent linear correlation between measured concentration of methylated DNA and expected percentage of methylation. **b** qMSP can detect methylated *3OST2* at 0.10% (LOQ = 0.10%) in the same diluted samples with R^2 of 0.935. **c** In 100% methylated DNA serially diluted into water, ddMSP can detect the smallest amount of methylated DNA at 156 pg/µL (156 pg/µL) with R^2 of 0.959. **d** qMSP can detect the smallest amount of methylated DNA at 156 pg/µL (156 pg/µL) with R2 of 0.937

When the criteria was used, 9 (45%) were positive for *RASSF1A* by qMSP. The same 4 sputum specimens of control subjects had positive methylation of the gene detected by both ddMSP and qMSP. Therefore, ddMSP analysis of DNA methylation of *RASSF1A* in sputum had a higher sensitivity (55%) than did qMSP (45%) ($p = 0.01$) for distinguishing lung cancer patients from control subjects, while maintaining the same specificity (80%) (Additional file 1: Figure S1). Furthermore, the CVs of repeated measures by ddMSP on different days by different researchers were approximately twofold lower compared with those generated by qMSP. Altogether, in clinical sputum specimens, ddMSP also exhibited higher sensitivity, accuracy, and reproducibility than did qMSP for quantification of DNA methylation.

To compare the tolerance of ddMSP and qMSP to PCR inhibitors, we added SDS and heparin directly into the PCR reactions and then calculated log IC50 values from the resulting inhibition curves. We found greater than a half log increase in IC50 of ddMSP over qMSP for both SDS and heparin (all $p < 0.05$), implying that ddMSP tolerated the presence of the inhibitors better than qMSP.

Diagnostic performance of ddMSP quantified-sputum methylation biomarkers for lung cancer

We first evaluated DNA methylation of 29 genes in the training cohort of 127 NSCLC patients and 159 controls. All the 29 genes displayed a higher level of methylation in patients vs. controls (all $p < 0.05$). ROC curve and AUC analysis showed that the genes had 29–88% sensitivities and 26–92% specificities in differentiating lung cancer patients from healthy controls (Additional file 1: Table S1). Since methylation levels of genes did not follow a normal distribution, we used the log transformation of ddPCR results. We then applied multivariate logistic regression models with stepwise regression based on ROC curve to develop a prediction classifier. Four genes (*HOXA9*, *RASSF1A*, *SOX17*, and *TAC1*) were identified as the best biomarkers (all $p < 0.001$) and incorporated into a logistic classifier: Probability of lung cancer = $e^x/(1 + e^x)$, where $x = 1.69 + 1.48 \times \log (HOXA9) - 1.25 \times \log (RASSF1A) + 0.27 \times \log (SOX17) + 0.16 \times \log (TAC1)$. The logistic classifier produced 0.92 AUC for lung cancer detection (Fig. 2b). Furthermore, Pearson correlation among methylation levels of the four genes was low ($p > 0.05$), implying that their diagnostic values were complementary to each other. Using Youden's index, we set up

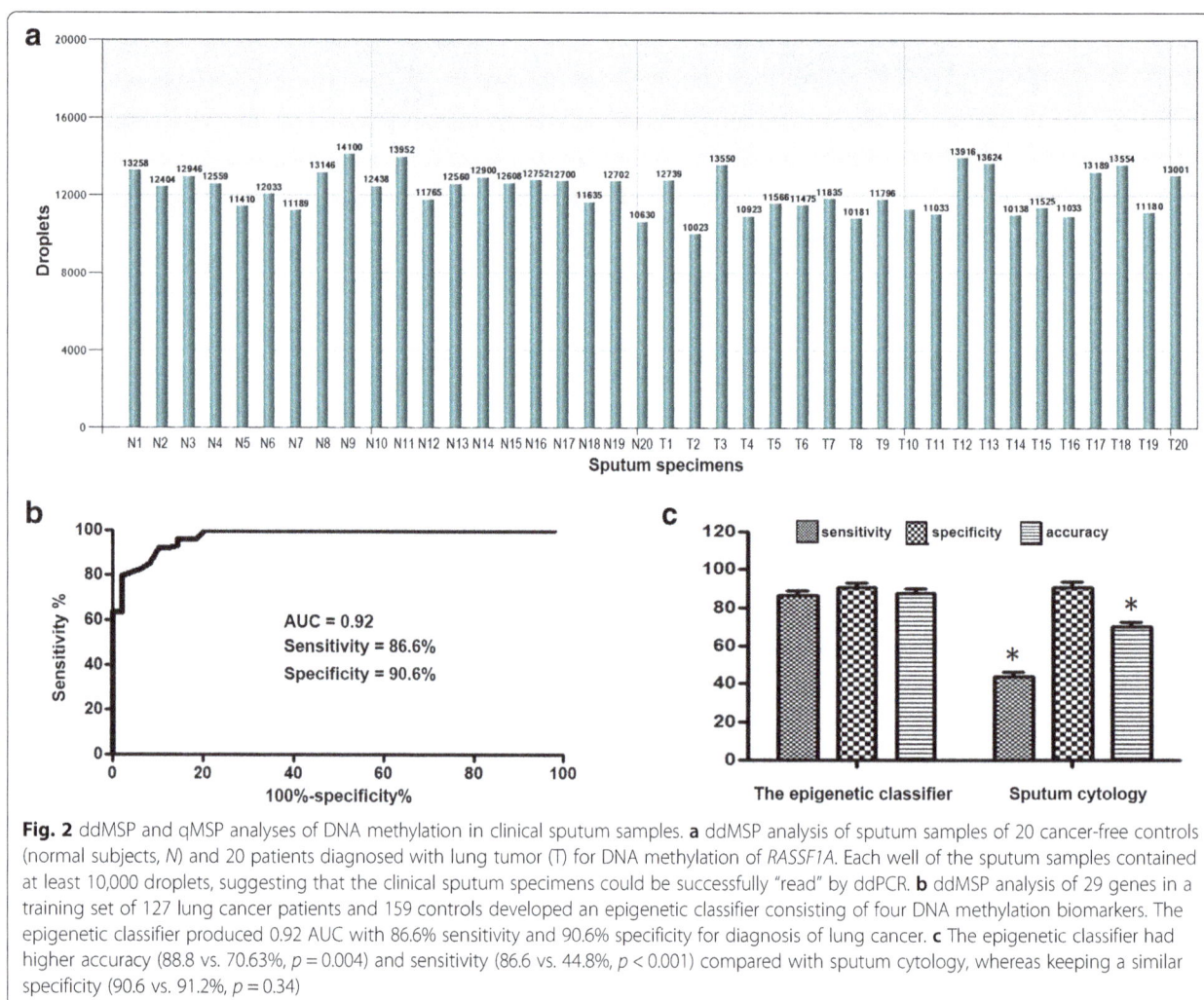

Fig. 2 ddMSP and qMSP analyses of DNA methylation in clinical sputum samples. **a** ddMSP analysis of sputum samples of 20 cancer-free controls (normal subjects, N) and 20 patients diagnosed with lung tumor (T) for DNA methylation of *RASSF1A*. Each well of the sputum samples contained at least 10,000 droplets, suggesting that the clinical sputum specimens could be successfully "read" by ddPCR. **b** ddMSP analysis of 29 genes in a training set of 127 lung cancer patients and 159 controls developed an epigenetic classifier consisting of four DNA methylation biomarkers. The epigenetic classifier produced 0.92 AUC with 86.6% sensitivity and 90.6% specificity for diagnosis of lung cancer. **c** The epigenetic classifier had higher accuracy (88.8 vs. 70.63%, $p = 0.004$) and sensitivity (86.6 vs. 44.8%, $p < 0.001$) compared with sputum cytology, whereas keeping a similar specificity (90.6 vs. 91.2%, $p = 0.34$)

optimal cutoff at 1.28 for the prediction classifier. Subsequently, combined use of the four genes by simply calculating the equation produced 86.6% sensitivity and 90.6% specificity. In addition, including other genes in the prediction classifier did not improve the accuracy for lung cancer diagnosis. The prevalence of the DNA methylation of the four genes was related with pack-years of smoking ($p = 0.03$). Since the cases and controls were matched 1:1 by age, gender, and smoking status as a nested case-control study, we adjusted the parameters during model building. The logistic classifier did not show special association with stage and histological type of lung cancer, and patients' age, gender, and smoking status (all $p > 0.05$).

Moreover, the logistic classifier had higher accuracy (88.8 vs. 70.63%, $p = 0.004$) and sensitivity (86.6 vs. 44.8%, $p < 0.001$) than did sputum cytology, while maintaining a similar specificity (90.6 vs. 91.2%, $p = 0.34$) (Fig. 2c). The integrated use of the biomarkers and sputum cytology did not significantly increase the diagnostic value.

Validating the panel of ddMSP-quantified methylation biomarkers in a testing cohort

In the testing cohort, the panel of the four genes had 85.4% sensitivity and 91.6% specificity in differentiating lung cancer patients from controls (Table 3). In line with findings in the training set, the logistic classifier was not

Table 3 The diagnostic performance of the epigenetic classifier and sputum cytology in a testing set

	Accuracy (%) (95% CI)*	Sensitivity (%) (95% CI)*	Specificity (%) (95% CI)
The epigenetic classifier	88.78 (83.50 to 92.83)	85.39 (76.32 to 91.99)	91.59 (84.63 to 96.08)
Sputum cytology	71.43 (64.56 to 77.64)	46.07 (35.44 to 56.96)	92.52 (85.80 to 96.72)

Abbreviations: NSCLC non-small cell lung cancer, *CI* confidence interval
*$p < 0.05$

associated with patient's age, gender, and smoking status, as well as histological type and stage of NSCLC (all $p > 0.05$). Moreover, the logistic classifier yielded higher accuracy (88.8 vs. 71.4%, $p = 0.002$) and sensitivity (85.4 vs. 46.1%, $p < 0.001$), while keeping a similar specificity (91.6 vs. 92.5%, $p = 0.45$), as compared with sputum cytology (Table 3). Taken together, the validation data confirmed the potential of the ddMSP-quantified sputum biomarkers as a sensitive classifier for the early detection of lung cancer.

Discussion

This current study presents the earliest assessment of ddPCR, an emerging technique, for quantitative detection of DNA methylation in sputum. We find that ddMSP can absolutely and robustly quantify DNA methylation in sputum without requiring external references. Therefore, determination of DNA methylation in sputum by ddMSP is highly efficient, and data handling is forthright. Furthermore, our head-to-head comparison of ddMSP and qMSP reveals that ddMSP displays higher precision and reproducibility in measuring copy number of DNA methylation in both control DNA samples and clinical sputum specimens. The sensitivity of conventional qMSP for analyzing low-abundance methylated DNA is poor. This is particularly challenging for the determination of DNA methylation in bronchial epitheliums, since the large excess of normal cells in sputum could obscure detection of the relative scarcity of methylated DNA. We find that ddMSP has a higher sensitivity to quantify cancer-specific methylation and thus could overcome the obstacle of qMSP. In addition, the total time required for ddMSP is about twofold shorter than did qMSP and might be further reduced when an automated system is used [63, 64]. Moreover, ddMSP is not expensive and tolerates the PCR inhibitors better compared with conventional qMSP. Altogether, ddMSP is a straightforward and robust approach for accurate quantification of DNA methylation in sputum.

Importantly, using ddMSP, we develop and validate a DNA methylation-based classifier that has higher accuracy and sensitivity compared with sputum cytology, the clinical gold standard. Furthermore, ddMSP analysis of the four genes by simply calculating the equation would be a convenient tool to be used in the clinics. In addition, the diagnostic performance of the logistic classifier is independent of stage and histological type of the NSCLC, as well as age, gender, and smoking status of subjects. Therefore, the classifier has an important characteristic if it is employed for more precisely and easily identifying early stage lung cancer among smokers.

However, some limitations do exist in this present study: (i) we evaluate ddMSP for quantification of DNA methylation using a retrospective cases and controls, which may produce selection bias and overfitting. Furthermore, the cases and controls are hospital-based patients, and not representative of the smokers in a screening setting for lung cancer early detection. We will perform a large trial to prospectively validate if the logistic classifier could help identify lung cancer at the early stage in a screening setting among smokers. (ii) the overall sensitivity and specificity of the DNA methylation-based classifier are 86.6 and 90.6%, which are not high enough for clinical diagnosis of NSCLC. The integration of the methylation biomarkers with other classes of biomarkers, such as microRNAs [36, 47–52, 65–67] or DNA mutations [33], is one path to improve the early detection of lung cancer [14]. (iii) since there is no sample left from the patients of the training and cohorts, we are not able to test the classification performance of qMSP in all the samples of the training and testing cohorts. We are consenting new cases and controls and collecting specimens and will then compare performance of qMSP and ddMSP in the same samples. (iv) like qMSP, ddMSP has the same limitations as do other PCR-based platforms. For instance, large experiments can become quite labor intensive to perform, when multiple genes are targeted. In this present study, we use 96-well PCR plates. Given the four genes to be analyzed with duplication, we only test 12 clinical samples at one time. In the future, we will use 484-well PCR plates, in which, we could simultaneously test 60 samples.

Conclusion

ddMSP could be a sensitive and robust tool for reliable quantitation of sputum methylation biomarkers. The ddMSP-quantified methylation classifier may provide a potential diagnostic test for the early detection of lung cancer and thus reduce the deaths and costs associated with the disease. Nevertheless, the continued development of this new technology, and further exploring its value for routine use for the early detection of lung cancer would be required.

Acknowledgements
This study was supported in part by a grant for cancer research from Jiangsu Province Hospital of Nanjing University of Chinese Medicine (Y, S).

Authors' contributions
YS, HF, and FJ conducted the experiments and participated in study design, coordination, and data interpretation, and preparing the manuscript. All authors read and approved the final manuscript.

Competing interests
The authors declare that they have no competing interests.

Author details
[1]Department of Surgery, Jiangsu Province Hospital of Nanjing University of Chinese Medicine, 138 Xianlin Road, Nanjing 210023, China. [2]Department of Biostatistics, Bioinformatics and Biomathematics, Georgetown University Medical Center, 4000 Reservoir Road, N.W, Washington D.C. 20057, USA. [3]Department of Pathology, University of Maryland School of Medicine, Baltimore, MD, USA.

References

1. Aberle DR, Adams AM, Berg CD, Black WC, Clapp JD, Fagerstrom RM. Reduced lung-cancer mortality with low-dose computed tomographic screening. N Engl J Med. 2011;365:395–409.

2. Blumer G. Cigarette smoking and cancer of the lung. Ill Med J. 1951;100:98–9.

3. Patz EF Jr, Pinsky P, Gatsonis C, Sicks JD, Kramer BS, Tammemagi MC. Overdiagnosis in low-dose computed tomography screening for lung cancer. JAMA Intern Med. 2014;174:269–74.

4. Aberle DR, Berg CD, Black WC, Church TR, Fagerstrom RM, Galen B. The national lung screening trial: overview and study design. Radiology. 2011; 258:243–53.

5. Sant M, Allemani C, Santaquilani M, Knijn A, Marchesi F, Capocaccia R. EUROCARE-4. Survival of cancer patients diagnosed in 1995-1999. Results and commentary. Eur J Cancer. 2009;45:931–91.

6. Hubers AJ, Prinsen CF, Sozzi G, Witte BI, Thunnissen E. Molecular sputum analysis for the diagnosis of lung cancer. Br J Cancer. 2013;109:530–7.

7. Belinsky SA. Gene-promoter hypermethylation as a biomarker in lung cancer. Nat Rev Cancer. 2004;4:707–17.

8. Grossman DC, Curry SJ, Owens DK, Barry MJ, Davidson KW, Doubeni CA. Screening for adolescent idiopathic scoliosis: US preventive services task force recommendation statement. JAMA. 2018;319:165–72.

9. Brody JS, Spira A. State of the art. Chronic obstructive pulmonary disease, inflammation, and lung cancer. Proc Am Thorac Soc. 2006;3:535–7.

10. Kadara H, Wistuba II. Field cancerization in non-small cell lung cancer: implications in disease pathogenesis. Proc Am Thorac Soc. 2012;9:38–42.

11. Belinsky SA, Liechty KC, Gentry FD, Wolf HJ, Rogers J, Vu K. Promoter hypermethylation of multiple genes in sputum precedes lung cancer incidence in a high-risk cohort. Cancer Res. 2006;66:3338–44.

12. Saccomanno G, Saunders RP, Archer VE, Auerbach O, Kuschner M, Beckler PA. Cancer of the lung: the cytology of sputum prior to the development of carcinoma. Acta Cytol. 1965;9:413–23.

13. Hubers AJ, Heideman DA, Burgers SA, Herder GJ, Sterk PJ, Rhodius RJ. DNA hypermethylation analysis in sputum for the diagnosis of lung cancer: training validation set approach. Br J Cancer. 2015;112:1105–13.

14. Su Y, Fang H, Jiang F. Integrating DNA methylation and microRNA biomarkers in sputum for lung cancer detection. Clin Epigenetics. 2016;8:109.

15. Liu D, Peng H, Sun Q, Zhao Z, Yu X, Ge S. The indirect efficacy comparison of DNA methylation in sputum for early screening and auxiliary detection of lung cancer: a meta-analysis. Int J Environ Res Public Health. 2017; 23:14–9.

16. Hsu HS, Chen TP, Wen CK, Hung CH, Chen CY, Chen JT. Multiple genetic and epigenetic biomarkers for lung cancer detection in cytologically negative sputum and a nested case-control study for risk assessment. J Pathol. 2007;213:412–9.

17. Guzman L, Depix MS, Salinas AM, Roldan R, Aguayo F, Silva A. Analysis of aberrant methylation on promoter sequences of tumor suppressor genes and total DNA in sputum samples: a promising tool for early detection of COPD and lung cancer in smokers. Diagn Pathol. 2012;7:87.

18. Herman JG, Graff JR, Myohanen S, Nelkin BD, Baylin SB. Methylation-specific PCR: a novel PCR assay for methylation status of CpG islands. Proc Natl Acad Sci U S A. 1996;93:9821–6.

19. Wang X, Cao A, Peng M, Hu C, Liu D, Gu T. The value of chest CT scan and tumor markers detection in sputum for early diagnosis of peripheral lung cancer. Zhongguo Fei Ai Za Zhi. 2004;7:58–63.

20. Leng S, Wu G, Klinge DM, Thomas CL, Casas E, Picchi MA. Gene methylation biomarkers in sputum as a classifier for lung cancer risk. Oncotarget. 2017;8: 63978–85.

21. Belinsky SA, Leng S, Wu G, Thomas CL, Picchi MA, Lee SJ. Gene methylation biomarkers in sputum and plasma as predictors for lung cancer recurrence. Cancer Prev Res (Phila). 2017;10:635–40.

22. Miyake M, Gomes Giacoia E, Aguilar Palacios D, Rosser CJ. Lung cancer risk assessment for smokers: gene promoter methylation signature in sputum. Biomark Med. 2012;6:512.

23. Leng S, Do K, Yingling CM, Picchi MA, Wolf HJ, Kennedy TC. Defining a gene promoter methylation signature in sputum for lung cancer risk assessment. Clin Cancer Res. 2012;18:3387–95.

24. Hwang SH, Kim KU, Kim JE, Kim HH, Lee MK, Lee CH. Detection of HOXA9 gene methylation in tumor tissues and induced sputum samples from primary lung cancer patients. Clin Chem Lab Med. 2011;49:699–704.

25. Liu Y, Lan Q, Shen M, Jin J, Mumford J, Ren D. Aberrant gene promoter methylation in sputum from individuals exposed to smoky coal emissions. Anticancer Res. 2008;28:2061–6.

26. Belinsky SA, Grimes MJ, Casas E, Stidley CA, Franklin WA, Bocklage TJ. Predicting gene promoter methylation in non-small-cell lung cancer by evaluating sputum and serum. Br J Cancer. 2007;96:1278–83.

27. Su SB, Yang LJ, Zhang W, Jin YL, Nie JH, Tong J. p16 and MGMT gene methylation in sputum cells of uranium workers. Zhonghua Lao Dong Wei Sheng Zhi Ye Bing Za Zhi. 2006;24:92–5.

28. Belinsky SA, Klinge DM, Dekker JD, Smith MW, Bocklage TJ, Gilliland FD. Gene promoter methylation in plasma and sputum increases with lung cancer risk. Clin Cancer Res. 2005;11:6505–11.

29. Olaussen KA, Soria JC, Park YW, Kim HJ, Kim SH, Ro JY. Assessing abnormal gene promoter methylation in paraffin-embedded sputum from patients with NSCLC. Eur J Cancer. 2005;41:2112–9.

30. Hubers AJ, Heideman DA, Duin S, Witte BI, de Koning HJ, Groen HJ. DNA hypermethylation analysis in sputum of asymptomatic subjects at risk for lung cancer participating in the NELSON trial: argument for maximum screening interval of 2 years. J Clin Pathol. 2017;7:250–4.

31. Hubers AJ, Brinkman P, Boksem RJ, Rhodius RJ, Witte BI, Zwinderman AH. Combined sputum hypermethylation and eNose analysis for lung cancer diagnosis. J Clin Pathol. 2014;67:707–11.

32. Hubers AJ, van der Drift MA, Prinsen CF, Witte BI, Wang Y, Shivapurkar N. Methylation analysis in spontaneous sputum for lung cancer diagnosis. Lung Cancer. 2014;84:127–33.

33. Hubers AJ, Heideman DA, Yatabe Y, Wood MD, Tull J, Taron M, et al. EGFR mutation analysis in sputum of lung cancer patients: a multitechnique study. Lung Cancer. 2013;82(1):38–43.

34. Hubers AJ, Heideman DA, Herder GJ, Burgers SA, Sterk PJ, Kunst PW. Prolonged sampling of spontaneous sputum improves sensitivity of hypermethylation analysis for lung cancer. J Clin Pathol. 2012;65:541–5.

35. Hindson CM, Chevillet JR, Briggs HA, Gallichotte EN, Ruf IK, Hindson BJ. Absolute quantification by droplet digital PCR versus analog real-time PCR. Nat Methods. 2013;10:1003–5.

36. Li N, Ma J, Guarnera MA, Fang H, Cai L, Jiang F. Digital PCR quantification of miRNAs in sputum for diagnosis of lung cancer. J Cancer Res Clin Oncol. 2014;140:145–50.

37. Ma J, Li N, Guarnera M, Jiang F. Quantification of plasma miRNAs by digital PCR for cancer diagnosis. Biomark Insights. 2013;8:127–36.

38. Bhat S, Herrmann J, Armishaw P, Corbisier P, Emslie KR. Single molecule detection in nanofluidic digital array enables accurate measurement of DNA copy number. Anal Bioanal Chem. 2009;394:457–67.

39. Kiss MM, Ortoleva-Donnelly L, Beer NR, Warner J, Bailey CG, Colston BW. High-throughput quantitative polymerase chain reaction in picoliter droplets. Anal Chem. 2008;80:8975 81.

40. Kreutz JE, Munson T, Huynh T, Shen F, Du W, Ismagilov RF. Theoretical design and analysis of multivolume digital assays with wide dynamic range validated experimentally with microfluidic digital PCR. Anal Chem. 2011;83: 8158–68.

41. Pinheiro LB, Coleman VA, Hindson CM, Herrmann J, Hindson BJ, Bhat S. Evaluation of a droplet digital polymerase chain reaction format for DNA copy number quantification. Anal Chem. 2012;84:1003–11.

42. Pohl G, Shih IM. Principle and applications of digital PCR. Expert Rev Mol Diagn. 2004;4:41–7.

43. Vogelstein B, Kinzler KW. Digital PCR. Proc Natl Acad Sci U S A. 1999;96: 9236–41.

44. Hayden RT, Gu Z, Ingersoll J, Abdul-Ali D, Shi L, Pounds S, et al. Comparison of droplet digital PCR to real-time PCR for quantitative detection of cytomegalovirus. J Clin Microbiol. 2013;51(2):540–6.

45. Day E, Dear PH, McCaughan F. Digital PCR strategies in the development and analysis of molecular biomarkers for personalized medicine. Methods. 2013;59:101–7.

46. Li H, Jiang Z, Leng Q, Bai F, Wang J, Ding X. A prediction model for distinguishing lung squamous cell carcinoma from adenocarcinoma. Oncotarget. 2017;8:50704–14.

47. Yu L, Todd NW, Xing L, Xie Y, Zhang H, Liu Z. Early detection of lung adenocarcinoma in sputum by a panel of microRNA markers. Int J Cancer. 2010;127:2870–8.

48. Xing L, Todd NW, Yu L, Fang H, Jiang F. Early detection of squamous cell lung cancer in sputum by a panel of microRNA markers. Mod Pathol. 2010; 23:1157–64.

49. Xie Y, Todd NW, Liu Z, Zhan M, Fang H, Peng H. Altered miRNA expression in sputum for diagnosis of non-small cell lung cancer. Lung Cancer. 2010; 67:170–6.

50. Anjuman N, Li N, Guarnera M, Stass SA, Jiang F. Evaluation of lung flute in sputum samples for molecular analysis of lung cancer. Clin Transl Med. 2013;2:15.

51. Jiang F, Todd NW, Li R, Zhang H, Fang H, Stass SA. A panel of sputum-based genomic marker for early detection of lung cancer. Cancer Prev Res (Phila). 2010;3:1571–8.

52. Jiang F, Todd NW, Qiu Q, Liu Z, Katz RL, Stass SA. Combined genetic analysis of sputum and computed tomography for noninvasive diagnosis of non-small-cell lung cancer. Lung Cancer. 2009;66:58–63.

53. Qiu Q, Todd NW, Li R, Peng H, Liu Z, Yfantis HG. Magnetic enrichment of bronchial epithelial cells from sputum for lung cancer diagnosis. Cancer. 2008;114:275–83.

54. Li R, Todd NW, Qiu Q, Fan T, Zhao RY, Rodgers WH. Genetic deletions in sputum as diagnostic markers for early detection of stage I non-small cell lung cancer. Clin Cancer Res. 2007;13:482–7.

55. Li W, Deng J, Jiang P, Zeng X, Hu S, Tang J. Methylation of the RASSF1A and RARbeta genes as a candidate biomarker for lung cancer. Exp Ther Med. 2012;3:1067–71.

56. Lee SM, Lee WK, Kim DS, Park JY. Quantitative promoter hypermethylation analysis of RASSF1A in lung cancer: comparison with methylation-specific PCR technique and clinical significance. Mol Med Rep. 2012;5:239–44.

57. Fischer JR, Ohnmacht U, Rieger N, Zemaitis M, Stoffregen C, Manegold C. Prognostic significance of RASSF1A promoter methylation on survival of non-small cell lung cancer patients treated with gemcitabine. Lung Cancer. 2007;56:115–23.

58. Chen H, Suzuki M, Nakamura Y, Ohira M, Ando S, Iida T. Aberrant methylation of RASGRF2 and RASSF1A in human non-small cell lung cancer. Oncol Rep. 2006;15:1281–5.

59. Dingle TC, Sedlak RH, Cook L, Jerome KR. Tolerance of droplet-digital PCR vs real-time quantitative PCR to inhibitory substances. Clin Chem. 2013;59: 1670–2.

60. Wilson IG. Inhibition and facilitation of nucleic acid amplification. Appl Environ Microbiol. 1997;63:3741–51.

61. Lemeshow S, Hosmer DW Jr. A review of goodness of fit statistics for use in the development of logistic regression models. Am J Epidemiol. 1982;115: 92–106.

62. Grote HJ, Schmiemann V, Geddert H, Bocking A, Kappes R, Gabbert HE. Methylation of RAS association domain family protein 1A as a biomarker of lung cancer. Cancer. 2006;108:129–34.

63. Kurimoto K, Hayashi M, Guerrero-Preston R, Koike M, Kanda M, Hirabayashi S. PAX5 gene as a novel methylation marker that predicts both clinical outcome and cisplatin sensitivity in esophageal squamous cell carcinoma. Epigenetics. 2017;12: 865–74.

64. Campomenosi P, Gini E, Noonan DM, Poli A, D'Antona P, Rotolo N. A comparison between quantitative PCR and droplet digital PCR technologies for circulating microRNA quantification in human lung cancer. BMC Biotechnol. 2016;16:60.

65. Shen J, Liao J, Guarnera MA, Fang H, Cai L, Stass SA. Analysis of MicroRNAs in sputum to improve computed tomography for lung cancer diagnosis. J Thorac Oncol. 2014;9:33–40.

66. Su J, Liao J, Gao L, Shen J, Guarnera MA, Zhan M. Analysis of small nucleolar RNAs in sputum for lung cancer diagnosis. Oncotarget. 2016;7:5131–42.

67. Xing L, Su J, Guarnera MA, Zhang H, Cai L, Zhou R. Sputum microRNA biomarkers for identifying lung cancer in indeterminate solitary pulmonary nodules. Clin Cancer Res. 2015;21:484–9.

Increased epigenetic age in normal breast tissue from luminal breast cancer patients

Erin W. Hofstatter[1][*][†] , Steve Horvath[2,3][†], Disha Dalela[4], Piyush Gupta[5], Anees B. Chagpar[6], Vikram B. Wali[1], Veerle Bossuyt[7], Anna Maria Storniolo[8], Christos Hatzis[1], Gauri Patwardhan[1], Marie-Kristin Von Wahlde[1,9], Meghan Butler[4], Lianne Epstein[1], Karen Stavris[4], Tracy Sturrock[4], Alexander Au[4,10], Stephanie Kwei[4] and Lajos Pusztai[1]

Abstract

Background: Age is one of the most important risk factors for developing breast cancer. However, age-related changes in normal breast tissue that potentially lead to breast cancer are incompletely understood. Quantifying tissue-level DNA methylation can contribute to understanding these processes. We hypothesized that occurrence of breast cancer should be associated with an acceleration of epigenetic aging in normal breast tissue.

Results: Ninety-six normal breast tissue samples were obtained from 88 subjects (breast cancer = 35 subjects/40 samples, unaffected = 53 subjects/53 samples). Normal tissue samples from breast cancer patients were obtained from distant non-tumor sites of primary mastectomy specimens, while samples from unaffected women were obtained from the Komen Tissue Bank ($n = 25$) and from non-cancer-related breast surgery specimens ($n = 28$). Patients were further stratified into four cohorts: age < 50 years with and without breast cancer and age ≥ 50 with and without breast cancer. The Illumina HumanMethylation450k BeadChip microarray was used to generate methylation profiles from extracted DNA samples. Data was analyzed using the "Epigenetic Clock," a published biomarker of aging based on a defined set of 353 CpGs in the human genome. The resulting age estimate, DNA methylation age, was related to chronological age and to breast cancer status.
The DNAmAge of normal breast tissue was strongly correlated with chronological age ($r = 0.712$, $p < 0.001$). Compared to unaffected peers, breast cancer patients exhibited significant age acceleration in their normal breast tissue ($p = 0.002$). Multivariate analysis revealed that epigenetic age acceleration in the normal breast tissue of subjects with cancer remained significant after adjusting for clinical and demographic variables. Additionally, smoking was found to be positively correlated with epigenetic aging in normal breast tissue ($p = 0.012$).

Conclusions: Women with luminal breast cancer exhibit significant epigenetic age acceleration in normal adjacent breast tissue, which is consistent with an analogous finding in malignant breast tissue. Smoking is also associated with epigenetic age acceleration in normal breast tissue. Further studies are needed to determine whether epigenetic age acceleration in normal breast tissue is predictive of incident breast cancer and whether this mediates the risk of chronological age on breast cancer risk.

Keywords: Humans, DNA methylation, Genome, Multivariate analysis, Epigenetics, Breast, Epigenomics, Breast neoplasms, Biomarkers, Smoking

* Correspondence: erin.hofstatter@yale.edu
†Erin W. Hofstatter and Steve Horvath contributed equally to this work.
[1]Department of Internal Medicine, Section of Medical Oncology, Yale School of Medicine, 300 George Street, Suite 120, New Haven, CT 06511, USA
Full list of author information is available at the end of the article

Background

Breast cancer represents 15% of all new cancer cases in the US, and with 252,710 estimated new cases in 2017, it has the highest cancer-related incidence in women in the country [1]. Age is one of the strongest risk factors for developing breast cancer and is most frequently diagnosed among women aged 55 to 64. However, the factors that mediate the effect of chronological age on breast cancer are not fully known. Since epigenetic changes are one of the hallmarks of aging, it is plausible that age-related epigenetic changes may play a role in conferring breast cancer risk.

Historically, studies of the effect of age on breast cancer have been limited by the lack of suitable molecular biomarkers of tissue age. Several studies have explored whether telomere shortening is associated with increased risk and earlier occurrence of familial breast cancer, but the reported effect sizes are relatively weak and require additional validation [2, 3].

It has recently been recognized that DNA methylation levels lend themselves for defining a highly accurate biomarker of tissue age ("epigenetic clock") that applies to all human tissues and cell types [4]. This epigenetic biomarker is based on the weighted average DNA methylation level of 353 cytosine-phosphate-guanines (CpGs). The age estimate (in unit of years) is referred to as "DNA methylation age" (DNAmAge) or "epigenetic age." By contrasting DNAmAge with an individual's chronological age, one can define a measure of epigenetic age acceleration. For instance, a woman whose blood tissue has a higher DNAmAge than expected based upon her chronological age is said to exhibit positive age acceleration in blood. Recent studies support the idea that these measures are at least passive biomarkers of biological age. To elaborate, the epigenetic age of blood has been found to be predictive of all-cause mortality [2, 3], lung cancer [5], frailty [6], and cognitive and physical functioning [7]. Further, the utility of the epigenetic clock method using various tissues and organs has been demonstrated in several applications including Alzheimer's disease [8], centenarian status [8, 9], obesity [10], menopause [11], and osteoarthritis [12].

An increasing body of literature suggests that epigenetic age acceleration in blood is predictive of various cancers [5, 13] including breast cancer [14]. Cancer greatly disrupts the epigenetic age of the affected (malignant) tissue [4, 15]. While some cancer types are associated with positive age acceleration, others are associated with negative age acceleration [4, 15]. We have recently shown that *malignant* breast cancer samples from luminal breast cancer exhibit strong positive age acceleration, which contrasts sharply with the negative age acceleration in basal breast cancers [4, 15]. However, it is unknown whether these age acceleration effects can also be observed in a *normal* adjacent tissue. Here, we address

this question by correlating epigenetic age acceleration in normal breast tissue samples with breast cancer disease status. We find that normal breast tissue samples from breast cancer cases exhibit positive age acceleration compared to normal breast tissue samples from controls. These age acceleration effects are independent of various confounders such as chronological age, ethnicity, age at menarche, number of live births, and menstrual status. In a secondary analysis, we found that smoking is associated with positive epigenetic age acceleration in normal breast tissue.

Methods

Study specimens

This was a multicenter cross-sectional study performed on fresh frozen samples of normal breast tissue that were collected from four cohorts of women, namely age < 50 years with and without breast cancer and age ≥ 50 with and without breast cancer. Normal breast tissue in patients with breast cancer was defined as histologically benign tissue at least 3 cm away from the primary tumor margin. These samples were obtained prospectively from patients undergoing primary total mastectomy for stage 0–III breast cancer at the Yale Breast Center. Eligible patients were those who had not received chemotherapy, radiation, or endocrine therapy prior to surgery. Normal breast tissue from non-cancer patients was obtained from the Susan G. Komen Tissue Bank at IU Simon Cancer Center and prospectively from women presenting for reduction mammoplasty at Yale New Haven Hospital. Clinical data collected for each subject included age, height, weight, ethnicity, medical history, reproductive history, tobacco and alcohol use, family history of breast cancer, and tumor characteristics. The study was approved by the institutional review board, and written informed consent was obtained from all patients in compliance with the protocol.

The Susan G. Komen Tissue Bank (KTB) is a unique resource that has helped in the understanding of normal breast biology. All participant samples from the KTB group are unaffected tissue donors without a cancer history, and study samples were anonymized in accordance to the protocol. The study population from the hospital prospective cohort included women from all age groups that consented for the study, and patients that had received neoadjuvant treatment were excluded. The tissue samples were further categorized based on tumor molecular subtypes.

Tissue processing

The breast tissue was sampled as six individual core pieces that were histologically benign, and within 5 min of procurement, each piece was embedded in a cassette that was subsequently placed in a 10% buffered formalin solution and stored at room temperature. The cores were then flash frozen with liquid nitrogen at − 166.2 °C. The cryo-vials with at least 50 mg of breast tissue per sample were shipped to the lab where the DNA was extracted using the Qiagen All Prep Universal kit. Samples were processed as whole tissue, and DNA was re-extracted from samples that had low DNA yield because of increased fatty tissue. The extracted DNA was then used for bisulfite sequencing experiments.

DNA extraction and methylation studies
Zymo EZ DNA methylation KIT (Zymo Research, Orange, CA, USA) was used to obtain bisulfite conversion and subsequent hybridization, and scanning was performed with the HumanMethylation450k BeadChip (Illumina, San Diego, CA) and iScan (Illumina) according to the manufacturers' protocol with standard settings. DNA methylation levels (β) were quantified using the "noob" normalization method [16]. Specifically, the β value was calculated as a ratio of the intensity of fluorescent signals from the methylated and the unmethylated sites:

$\beta = \max(M,0)/[\max(M,0) + \max(U,0) + 100]$.

M = methylated signals.

U = unmethylated signal.

Thus, β values ranged from 0 to 1 (completely unmethylated to completely methylated).

DNAmAge was then calculated, which has been described in detail elsewhere [4]. Briefly, the epigenetic clock is defined as a prediction method of age based on the DNA methylation levels of 353 CpGs. Predicted age, referred to as DNAmAge, correlates with chronological age in multiple different cell types (CD4+ T cells, monocytes, B cells, neurons), tissues, and organs, including whole blood, brain, breast, kidney, liver, and lung [4].

Internal validation cohort
Five sets of duplicate samples were analyzed from the cancer cohort in order to examine for concordance.

Statistical methods
Patient variables
Baseline patient characteristics were compared in the cancer and control arm to identify any differences in the study cohort. The continuous variables were analyzed using the unpaired student t test and presented as mean values with 95% confidence intervals. The categorical variables were analyzed using the chi-square test and presented as frequency percentages. A multivariate logistic regression analysis was then performed to identify significant co-variates for the breast cancer status.

Epigenetic variables
Despite high correlations, DNAmAge estimates can deviate substantially from chronological age at the individual level; by adjusting for chronological age, we can arrive at a measure of epigenetic age acceleration. DNA methylation age was regressed on chronological age (at the time of breast sample collection) using linear regression. Age acceleration was then defined as raw residuals resulting from the model. Thus, a positive or negative value indicates that a given breast sample is older or younger than expected based on chronological age, respectively. This measure of age acceleration is not correlated with chronological age ($r = 0$) and has a mean value of zero. All measures were calculated using a previously published online version of the DNAmAge calculator. We further calculated the mean methylation levels in the two groups. Pearson correlation statistic of methylation levels against age was calculated for cancer and control groups. Non-parametric tests were performed to test for mean differences in all the epigenetic variables within the two cohorts.

Regression models (univariate, multivariate, and IPWRA)
A linear regression model was plotted to define the collinearity of the DNAmAge with the age variable. The residuals from the plot were utilized to define the age acceleration residuals as mentioned before. A univariate and multivariate linear regression analysis was then performed to identify predictors of DNAmAge and age acceleration residuals. The p value < 0.05 was considered statistically significant. A regression adjustment model with inverse probability weighting (IPWRA) was created to address for the potential confounding variables. This treatment effects model was further bootstrapped for 500 repetitions to identify the 95% confidence intervals of the average treatment effect in population and the potential-outcome means. Average treatment effect in this model can be defined as the additional DNAmAge years of the tissue sample in breast cancer patients compared to controls in a matched population.

Predictive function of epigenetic variables—ROC curves
Receiver operating characteristic (ROC) were plotted for breast cancer status as the reference variable and age, DNAmAge, mean methylation by sample, age acceleration difference, and age acceleration residuals as classification variables. DeLong method was used to calculate the standard errors, and binomial confidence intervals were calculated. The ROC curves were plotted based on the binomial fit models, and the AUC was calculated. The sensitivity and specificity of the

most predictive epigenetic variable was then calculated based on the ROC curve.

All the tables, graphs and statistical analysis was performed using STATA version 15.1 (StataCorp LLC, TX, USA). Original datasets used for statistical analysis are included as Additional files 1 and 2.

Results

Sample characteristics

Ninety-six normal breast tissue samples were obtained from 88 subjects (breast cancer = 35 subjects/40 samples, unaffected = 53 subjects/53 samples). Normal tissue samples from breast cancer patients were obtained from distant non-tumor sites of primary mastectomy specimens, while samples from unaffected women were obtained from the Komen Tissue Bank ($n = 25$) and from non-cancer related breast surgery specimens ($n = 28$). Three patients that received neoadjuvant chemotherapy in the cancer arm were excluded from analysis. Five additional samples were taken from specimens with breast cancer to serve as internal controls for studying any variations within the breast tissue. Samples from the breast cancer patients were classified as the "cancer arm," and those from unaffected patients were classified as the "control arm."

Patient demographics

The baseline characteristics for the cancer arm and control arm have been summarized in Table 1. The mean age of patients was 49.7 years versus 45.9 years in the cancer arm and the control arm, respectively ($p = 0.126$). Most of the patients in our study cohort were Caucasian (86%) and non-Hispanic (91.4%). The average body mass index of the cancer group was 27 kg/m^2. Forty percent of patients were ever-smokers, and 62% are current alcohol users. There was significantly higher alcohol consumption in the control group than the cancer group (72% vs 47%, $p = 0.019$). The patients were mostly premenopausal (60%), and 74% were ever-pregnant. The median live birth count was 2, and 41% patients had a history of breastfeeding. The mean age at menarche and mean age at first live birth were not significant between the two cohorts. Within the cancer cohort, patients were randomly distributed in terms of the pathological stage (0–III). Forty-five percent had a positive family history of breast cancer, and 95% of patients had ER+/PR+ tumors. Her2neu was positive in 7.5% of tumor samples, while 15% of patients were not typed for Her2neu. One patient in the control group was BRCA-positive, who had undergone a risk-reduction mastectomy. This patient was excluded

from univariate and multivariate analyses. Further multivariate logistic regression analysis revealed that alcohol consumption and post-menopausal status was significantly different in the two cohorts. The details of the analysis have been summarized in Table 2.

CpG methylation levels and the "epigenetic clock" analysis

The estimated DNAmAge (derived from the epigenetic clock) based on tissue CpG mean methylation levels highly correlated with the chronological age of the patients at the time of breast tissue collection ($r = 0.712$, $p < 0.001$, Spearman's correlation test) (Fig. 1), (Table 3). This further confirmed the findings we had published previously that tissue-level methylation can serve as a predictor for the aging process in an individual [17]. Despite an increasing trend, it can be noted that the tissue epigenetic age varies widely for each individual. The cancer cohort showed a higher mean of DNAmAge than the control cohort on univariate analysis ($p = 0.021$, Student's t test) and remained statistically significant even after matching for age and smoking status ($p = 0.009$). (Table 3) To eliminate the effect of age, we regressed the DNAmAge values over the age variable to calculate the age acceleration residuals. The cancer cohort exhibited a significant positive age acceleration (positive residual coefficient) correlation compared to the control samples ($p < 0.001$, Student's t test) (Fig. 2d). All samples but one in the cancer cohort were ER+ and/or PR+ (luminal subtype). The single basal subtype did not show a positive age acceleration; however, no conclusion could be drawn from a single value. Three patients from the luminal subtypes were Her2+. Though these three patients had a positive age acceleration with respect to the controls, it was not significantly different from the Her2-negative cancer cohort (RR – 0.001, SE – 0.006, $p = 0.237$).

Predictors of DNAmAge and age acceleration residuals—univariate and multivariate analyses and inverse probability weighted regression adjustment (IPWRA) analysis

A univariate analysis revealed that age ($p < 0.001$), breast cancer status ($p = 0.021$), smoking (pack years) ($p = 0.013$), more than one live birth ($p < 0.01$), and post-menopausal status ($p < 0.001$) were significantly associated with DNAmAge. However, on the multivariate analysis only age ($p < 0.001$), breast cancer status ($p = 0.009$), and smoking pack years ($p = 0.022$) remained significant. Since DNAmAge has a very strong correlation with age of the individual ($r = 0.713$), it can be hypothesized that the effect of breast cancer status or any other covariate will be diminished. To adjust for this, we calculated an age-adjusted measure of DNAmAge as age acceleration residual, which is independent of the age of the patient

Table 1 Demographic variables of the cancer and control arms

Variables	Breast cancer N (%)/mean (95% CI)	Controls N (%)/mean (95% CI)	p value
Total cohort samples	40	53	
Age (years)	49.7 (46.32–53.02)	45.9 (40.29–51.55)	0.126
Age category			0.742
< 50 years	24 (60%)	30 (57%)	
≥ 50 years	16 (40%)	23 (43%)	
Ethnicity			0.076
White	31 (78%)	49 (92%)	
African Americans	4 (10%)	3 (6%)	
Others	5 (13%)	1 (2%)	
Ashkenazi Jew	6 (15%)	3 (6%)	0.162
Height (in.)	64.02 (63.10–64.94)	63.96 (63.19–64.73)	0.45
Weight (lbs)	157.22 (146.54–167.90)	157.50 (148.59–166.41)	0.483
BMI (kg/m^2)			0.446
< 18.5	0 (0%)	1 (2%)	
18.5–24.9	21 (53%)	22 (42%)	
25.0–29.9	8 (20%)	17 (32%)	
> 30	11 (28%)	13 (25%)	
Tobacco use			0.696
No	25 (63%)	31 (58%)	
Yes	15 (38%)	22 (42%)	
Smoking (pack years)	3.73 (1.06–6.41)	3.86 (1.06–6.59)	0.475
Current alcohol use			0.019
No	20 (52%)	15 (28%)	
Yes	18 (47%)	38 (72%)	
Positive family history of breast cancer	18 (45%)	11 (21%)	0.012
Age at menarche (years)	12.37 (11.72–13.03)	12.54 (12.20–12.87)	0.671
Menopausal status			0.212
Pre-menopausal	27 (68%)	29 (55%)	
Post-menopausal	13 (33%)	24 (45%)	
Ever pregnant			0.266
No	8 (20%)	16 (30%)	
Yes	32 (80%)	37 (70%)	
No. of times pregnant	2.6 (1.94–3.25)	1.94 (1.48–2.39)	0.049
Age at first childbirth	25.73 (23.24–28.99)	25.61 (24.21–27.01)	0.465

Table 1 Demographic variables of the cancer and control arms (*Continued*)

Variables	Breast cancer N (%)/mean (95% CI)	Controls N (%)/mean (95% CI)	p value
(years)			
Number of live births	1.97 (1.54–2.40)	1.57 (1.23–1.92)	0.073
Breastfeeding			0.567
No	25 (63%)	30 (57%)	
Yes	15 (38%)	23 (43%)	
ER/PR status			NA
ER+/PR+	38 (95%)	–	
ER+/PR-	1 (2.5%)	–	
ER-/PR+	0 (0)		
ER-/PR-	1 (2.5%)	–	
Her2 status			NA
Not typed	6 (15%)	–	
Her-	31 (78%)	–	
Her+	3 (7.5%)	–	

(vide supra). This can be seen in Fig. 2 where age acceleration residual ($p < 0.001$) (Fig. 2d) has a stronger correlation than DNAmAge ($p = 0.007$). A multivariate analysis on age acceleration residuals revealed that only breast cancer status ($p = 0.009$) and smoking pack years ($p = 0.022$) were significant predictors of this epigenetic variable (Table 3). Further, breast cancer status is a much stronger predictor (coefficient = 4.489) of increased age acceleration residual than the smoking pack years (coefficient = 0.178) (Table 2).

In a secondary analysis, we examined the correlation of smoking pack years with the DNAmAge of the sampled breast tissue. Age acceleration residual was correlated with tobacco variables ($r = 0.21$, $p = 0.047$ for total years of smoking, $r = 0.26$, $p = 0.014$ cigarettes per day, and $r = 0.26$, $p = 0.015$ smoking pack years) in the complete cohort. Similar trends were also noted in the control group (Fig. 3a–f). Though a positive correlation was also noted in the cancer group, it did not reach statistical significance (Fig. 3g–i). These results need to be interpreted with caution as the study was not designed initially to identify smoking as a potential driver of tissue-level epigenetic changes.

Our study population had a selection bias in the age of presentation of the cancer and control population. This can be identified in Fig. 1, where most of the patients in the cancer cohort were in the age group 45 to 65 years whereas the control group were either below or above this age group. To adjust for

Table 2 Multivariate logistic regression predicting breast cancer

Logistic regression					Number of obs	57
					LR chi2(9)	25.9
					Prob > χ^2	0.0021
Log likelihood			− 25.488985		Pseudo R^2	0.3369
Breast cancer status	Odds ratio	Std. err.	z	$p > z$	[95% conf.	Interval]
Age	1.11	0.07	1.79	0.07	0.99	1.25
Age of first live birth	1.04	0.08	0.50	0.62	0.89	1.22
Age of menarche	1.33	0.38	0.99	0.32	0.76	2.34
Current alcohol intake	0.21	0.16	− 2.06	0.04	0.05	0.93
BMI	0.95	0.07	− 0.78	0.44	0.82	1.09
Ever breast fed	0.61	0.50	− 0.60	0.55	0.12	3.06
Family history	2.37	1.91	1.07	0.28	0.49	11.51
Post- vs pre-menopausal	0.01	0.02	− 2.60	0.01	0.00	0.32
Smoking (py)	0.89	0.08	− 1.29	0.20	0.74	1.06

this, we created an IPWRA model based on predictors of DNAmAge (linear-dependent outcome variable) and breast cancer status (logistic-dependent treatment variable), accounting for age and smoking as independent outcome variables and current alcohol use and menstrual status as independent treatment variables, to identify the average treatment effect. The iterations were further bootstrapped to 500 reps to calculate the 95% CI. The analysis revealed that breast cancer status was significantly associated with a higher DNAmAge score with an average treatment effect of 3.98 years ($p = 0.003$) (Table 4).

Predictive function of the epigenetic variables

The receiver operating characteristic (ROC) were plotted to identify the accuracy of the epigenetic variables in predicting breast cancer (Fig. 4). Age is considered a strong risk factor for breast cancer; thus, its ROC curve was considered as the baseline for comparison (AUC = 0.527). Like age, DNAmAge (AUC = 0.578) was not a good predictor for breast cancer status, and the curve closely resembled the age binomial fit model. This can be attributed to age being a stronger predictor for DNAmAge than breast cancer. Age difference calculated as the difference of the epigenetic age from the chronological age did not reach desired predictive accuracy as well.

Both mean methylation by sample and age acceleration residuals lead to ROC curves that lie above the reference line (AUC = 0.687 and AUC = 0.689, respectively) (Fig. 4). The mean age acceleration for the control cohort was − 1.67 which corresponded to a sensitivity of 82.5% and specificity of 49.06% with a positive likelihood ratio 1.62 and negative likelihood ratio 0.35. The mean age acceleration residual for cancer cohort was 2.21 which corresponded to a sensitivity of 47.50% and specificity of 75.47% with a positive likelihood ratio 1.94 and negative likelihood ratio 0.69. The tradeoff was achieved at − 0.920 with 80% sensitivity and 57% specificity.

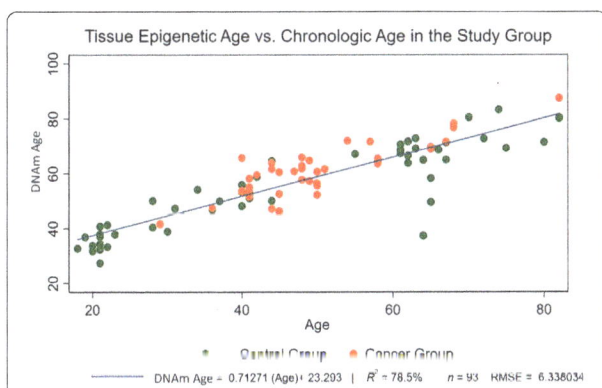

Fig. 1 Tissue epigenetic age versus chronological age. DNA methylation age estimate based on 353 CpGs (y-axis) versus chronological age. All samples are normal breast tissue samples; normal tissue samples from cancer patients were obtained from mastectomy specimens > 3 cm from tumor margin. Samples (points) are colored by disease status of the donor: red = breast cancer and green = control. A linear regression line has been added. Age acceleration is defined as raw residual resulting from the regression model, i.e., the (signed) vertical distance to the line. Points above and below the line exhibit positive and negative epigenetic age acceleration, respectively. The high Pearson correlation coefficient $r = 0.712$, ($p < 0.001$) reflects the strong linear relationship between DNAmAge and chronological age at the time of breast sample collection

Discussion

To our knowledge, this is the first study that has analyzed the epigenetic age variables of the adjacent

Table 3 Univariate and multivariate analyses of factors affecting DNAmAge and age acceleration residuals

	Univariate analysis			Multivariate analysis		
	Coef.	Std. err.	p > t	Coef.	Std. err.	p > t
DNAmAge						
Age	*0.712*	*0.039*	*< 0.001*	*0.807*	*0.095*	*< 0.001*
Breast cancer vs controls	*6.551*	*2.78*	*0.021*	*4.489*	*1.663*	*0.009*
BMI	0.148	0.238	0.534	0.164	0.143	0.256
Current alcohol use	− 2.833	2.904	0.332	–	–	–
Smoking (py)	*0.407*	*0.16*	*0.013*	*0.177*	*0.075*	*0.022*
Age at menarche	0.322	0.959	0.738	0.948	0.49	0.057
Age at first live birth	0.03	0.251	0.905	–	–	–
Count of live births						
1	2.292	5.494	0.678	− 4.92	3.268	0.137
1+	14.395	2.887	< 0.001	− 1.536	2.138	0.475
Breast fed	5.286	2.83	0.065	–	–	–
Post- vs pre-menopausal	18.645	2.138	< 0.001	− 3.982	3.006	0.19
Hispanic	− 5.924	5.018	0.241	− 3.921	3.223	0.228
Race						
White	− 0.059	5.815	0.992	0.709	3.088	0.819
African Americans	− 2.142	7.643	0.78	0.196	4.219	0.963
Age Acc. Residuals						
Age	0.000	0.039	1	0.095	0.095	0.324
Breast cancer vs controls	*3.878*	*1.264*	*0.003*	*4.489*	*1.664*	*0.009*
BMI	0.117	0.11	0.288	0.164	0.143	0.256
Current alcohol use	− 2.484	1.349	0.068	–	–	–
Smoking (py)	*0.174*	*0.074*	*0.022*	*0.178*	*0.076*	*0.022*
Age at menarche	0.358	0.454	0.433	0.949	0.491	0.057
Age at first live birth	− 0.169	0.153	0.274	–	–	–
Count of live births						
1	− 1.598	2.9	0.583	− 4.92	3.268	0.137
1+	0.041	1.52	0.979	− 1.536	2.138	0.475
Breast fed	− 2.28	1.315	0.086	–	–	–
Post vs pre-menopausal	− 1.351	1.335	0.314	− 3.982	3.006	0.19
Hispanic	0.636	2.342	0.786	− 3.921	3.223	0.228
Race						
White	− 1.063	2.685	0.693	0.709	3.088	0.819
African Americans	1.082	3.529	0.76	0.196	4.219	0.963

Variables in italics are those which reached statistical significance

"normal" breast tissue in patients with breast cancer. Our cross-sectional analysis suggests that both epigenetic age acceleration and mean methylation in adjacent breast tissue are predictive of breast cancer status, but these findings require validation in prospective cohort studies. Age, along with breast cancer status and smoking, are independent predictors of epigenetic age of breast tissue.

It is unknown what age-related genetic changes come in effect to increase the incidence of breast cancer in the age group 45–65 years and whether the changes are limited to the site of tumor origin or are present in the entire breast tissue. The concept of field cancerization is well-known in other regions of the body where it has been attributed to exposure to exogenous factors; however, the role of endogenous factors like chronic cell cycling or age-related epigenetic silencing of various genetic pathways in making a tissue more vulnerable to oncogenic transformation is not fully identified. Certain aging processes can accelerate or hinder tumorigenesis in a tissue-specific manner which has been discussed elsewhere [18]. Its specific role in the breast cancer is yet to be elucidated.

Our study highlights the treatment effects analysis which suggests that the normal tissue in the breast cancer patients was at least half a decade older in terms of cumulative epigenetic damage in an age-matched comparison. While this finding may initially seem to have little clinical significance, it is interesting to note that the age acceleration residuals were in complete contrast within the two cohorts. Unaffected individuals had a negative mean age acceleration residual, suggesting that the rate of increase of breast tissue age was slowing down in terms of chronological age, compared to the patients with breast cancer who had positive age acceleration residual, suggesting that the breast tissue was aging at a faster rate than the individual herself. The ROC curves further suggest that higher age acceleration in the breast cancer cohort was specific for breast cancer occurrence. Although our cross-sectional model does not lend itself for dissecting cause and effect relationships, the significant age acceleration observed in patients with luminal breast cancers supports the hypothesis that DNAmAge of normal breast tissue in women with breast cancer increases at a higher rate than in an unaffected individual. As such, our findings suggest that a breast tissue biomarker of accelerated aging may exist that could potentially be associated with the future development of breast cancer.

Future studies will need to test the hypothesis that breast tissue is more predictive of incident breast cancer than blood tissue, which has previously been

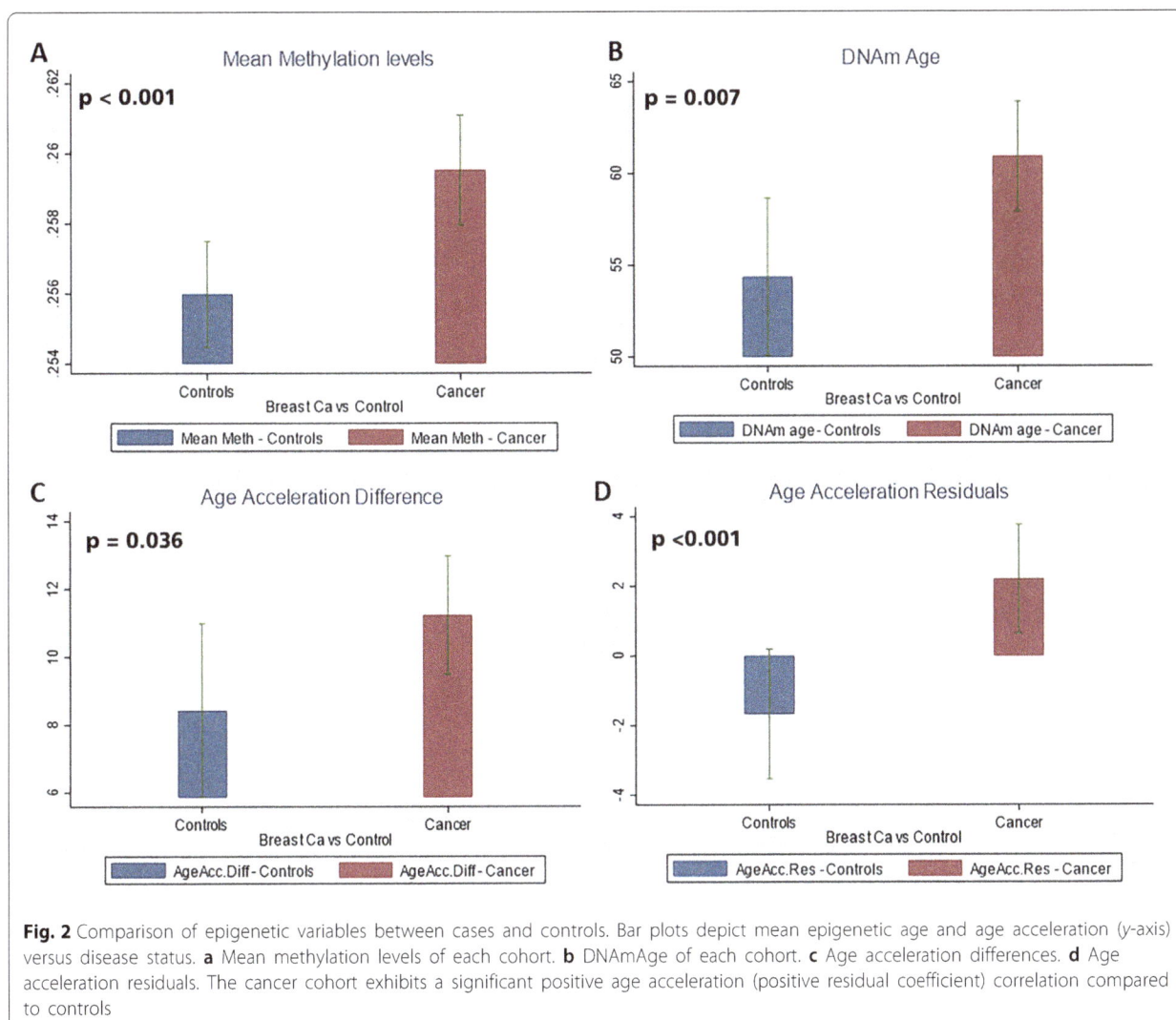

Fig. 2 Comparison of epigenetic variables between cases and controls. Bar plots depict mean epigenetic age and age acceleration (y-axis) versus disease status. **a** Mean methylation levels of each cohort. **b** DNAmAge of each cohort. **c** Age acceleration differences. **d** Age acceleration residuals. The cancer cohort exhibits a significant positive age acceleration (positive residual coefficient) correlation compared to controls

shown to have a positive, but relatively weak, predictive association [14]. This hypothesis is indirectly supported by the finding that DNA methylation levels in breast tissue are more predictive of the endogenous hormonal milieu in unaffected women compared to blood [19]. Thus, it will be interesting to study whether DNA methylation changes precede actual occurrence of the breast cancer in patients with hormone-responsive breast cancers.

The positive association of smoking with the DNA-mAge as well as age acceleration residual is an interesting and unexpected finding in our study. Previous studies failed to detect such an effect in blood [20], liver, or adipose tissue [10]. Taken together, these findings corroborate the hypothesis that many stress factors affect epigenetic age acceleration in a tissue-specific manner. Ever-smokers have been found to have a modest increase in the incidence of breast cancer, particularly in females who started

smoking in their adolescence. Although our study does not include data on the exact time interval since smoking initiation and/or smoking cessation and acquisition of data, the association of an overall impact of smoking on DNA methylation is intriguing and merits further study.

We recently published our findings that breast tissue ages faster than blood in unaffected women, as measured by DNA methylation [17]. From the current study, we further extend our understanding of the normal breast tissue, where we identify that patients with hormone-responsive breast cancer have higher epigenetic age acceleration compared to age-matched controls. Given that breast tissue age could be considered a function of multiple variables orchestrating in sync in response to endogenous and exogenous factors during an individual's lifetime (such as age of menarche, use of hormone replacement therapy, alcohol use, and others), epigenetic

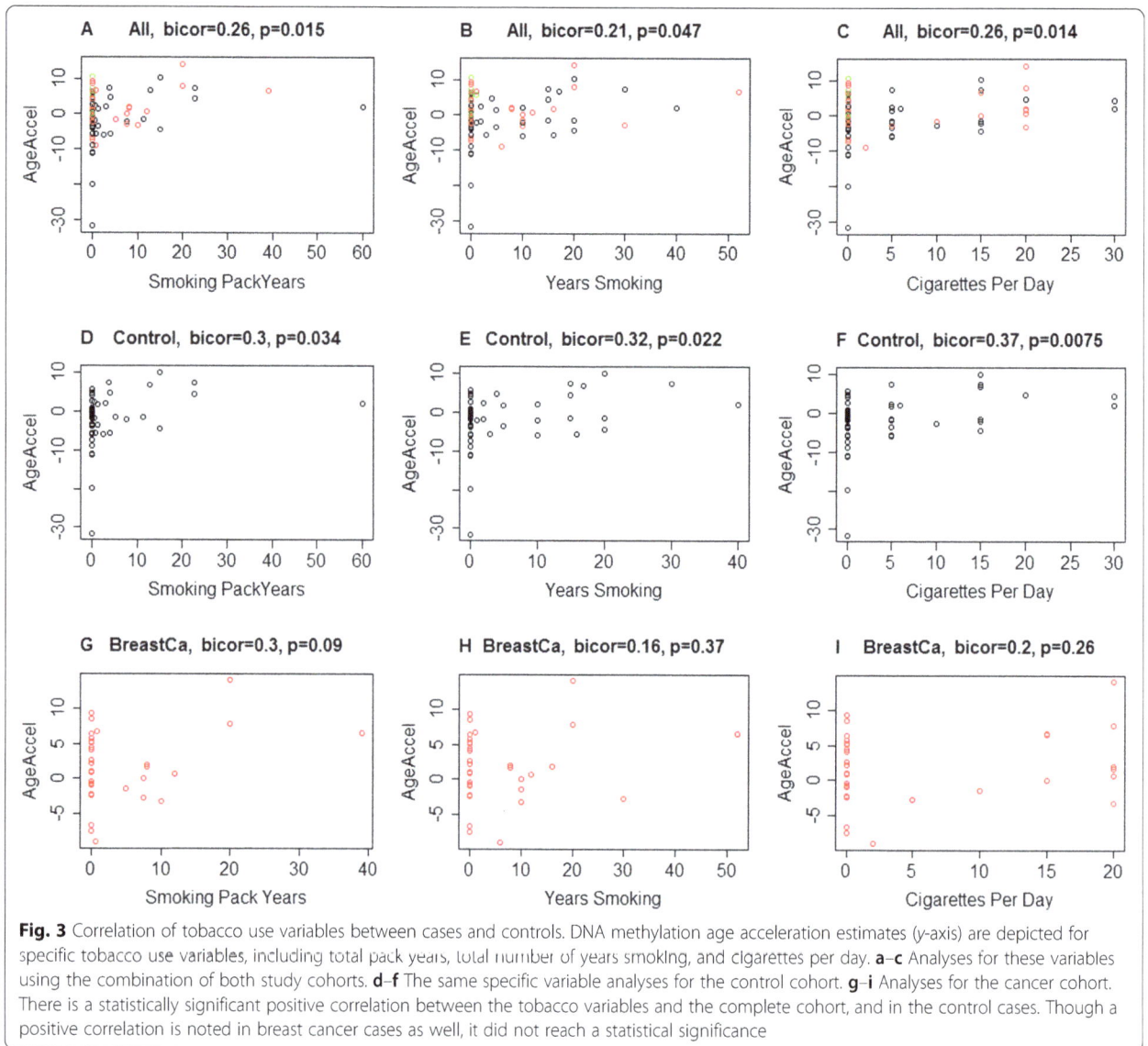

Fig. 3 Correlation of tobacco use variables between cases and controls. DNA methylation age acceleration estimates (y-axis) are depicted for specific tobacco use variables, including total pack years, total number of years smoking, and cigarettes per day. **a–c** Analyses for these variables using the combination of both study cohorts. **d–f** The same specific variable analyses for the control cohort. **g–i** Analyses for the cancer cohort. There is a statistically significant positive correlation between the tobacco variables and the complete cohort, and in the control cases. Though a positive correlation is noted in breast cancer cases as well, it did not reach a statistical significance

aging may serve as a useful surrogate marker of this changing internal milieu, and offer insight into future breast cancer risk.

We acknowledge the limitations of our study, including the aforementioned small sample size and inability to extrapolate findings to all breast cancer subtypes. Our study involved mainly luminal breast cancer samples. We had one ER-negative/PR-negative sample

(which exhibited negative age acceleration) and one ER+/PR-negative sample, and thus, no definite conclusions could be drawn from them. We were also not able to evaluate the effect of BRCA mutations on epigenetic age acceleration since our study involved only a single BRCA mutation carrier who had not (yet) developed breast cancer at the time of sample collection. Further, no significant correlation could be drawn based on the

Table 4 Regression adjustment model with inverse showing average treatment effects (ATE) and potential-outcome mean (POmean)

DNAmAge	Groups	Coef.	Bootstrap Std. err.	z	p > z	[95% conf. interval]	
ATE	Cancer vs control group	3.98337	1.333459	2.99	0.003	1.369837	6.596902
POmean	Control	55.60416	1.642661	33.85	0	52.38461	58.82372

Treatment-effects estimation: Number of obs = 85; Estimator: IPW regression adjustment; Outcome model: linear; Treatment model: logit; Bootstrap Iterations: 500

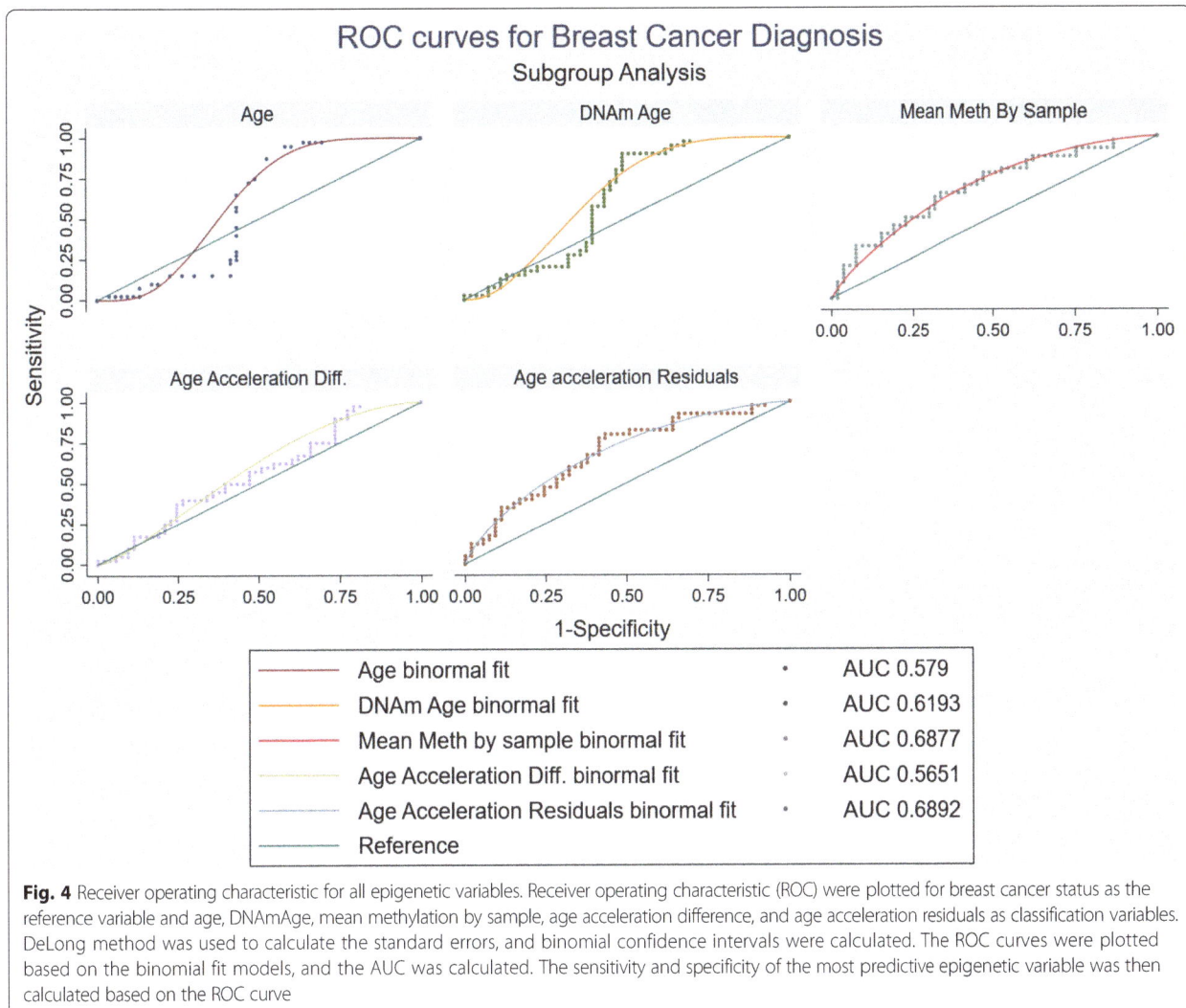

Fig. 4 Receiver operating characteristic for all epigenetic variables. Receiver operating characteristic (ROC) were plotted for breast cancer status as the reference variable and age, DNAmAge, mean methylation by sample, age acceleration difference, and age acceleration residuals as classification variables. DeLong method was used to calculate the standard errors, and binomial confidence intervals were calculated. The ROC curves were plotted based on the binomial fit models, and the AUC was calculated. The sensitivity and specificity of the most predictive epigenetic variable was then calculated based on the ROC curve

pathologic stage of the tumor as the sample size was not powered for such an analysis. An additional limitation of our study was the difference in age distribution of the cancer cohort as compared to the unaffected cohort, though statistical measures were taken to account for this difference. Future studies with closely age-matched cohorts would be helpful to corroborate our findings. Finally, and of note, we did not isolate any specific cell type within the whole breast sample for the epigenetic age analysis. Thus, we cannot account for the specific cell type, if any, that is primarily responsible for the DNAmAge acceleration in the normal breast. Future studies should be considered to determine the epigenetic ages of individual cell types, as compared to whole tissue epigenetic age analysis.

Conclusions

In summary, our study demonstrates that epigenetic age acceleration of the "normal" breast tissue in patients with luminal breast cancer was significantly higher than that of unaffected women. We also observed that the difference was maintained when adjusted for potential clinical confounders. Further larger prospective studies will be required to identify the temporal trend of the observed epigenetic aging and its possible use as a predictive biomarker.

Abbreviations
AUC: Area under the curve; CI: Confidence interval; CpGs: Cytosine-phosphate-guanines; DNAmAge: DNA methylation age; ER: Estrogen receptor; IPWRA: Inverse probability weighted regression adjustment; KTB: Komen Tissue Bank; PR: Progesterone receptor; ROC: Receiver operating characteristic

Acknowledgements
The authors wish to acknowledge Jill Henry and Theresa Mathieson of the Komen Tissue Bank for their assistance in sample acquisition, and Jaime

Miller and Guilin Wang of the Yale Center for Genome Analysis for their assistance in DNA methylation tissue analysis.

Funding
This work was supported by the Terri Brodeur Breast Cancer Research Foundation (Hofstatter), the Lion Heart Foundation (Hofstatter), and the NCI P30 Cancer Clinical Investigator Team Leadership Award (Hofstatter). Additional support came from NIH/NIA 5R01AG042511-02 (Horvath) and NIH/NIA U34AG051425-01 (Horvath). The funding bodies played no role in the design and conduct of the study; the collection, management, analysis, and interpretation of the data; preparation, review, or approval of the manuscript; and decision to submit the manuscript for publication. EH received philanthropic funding from Chute for the Cure.

Authors' contributions
EH and LP contributed to the conception and design. EH, AC, VW, VB, AS, GP, MVW, MB, LE, KS, TS, AA, and SK contributed to the acquisition of data. EH, SH, DD, PG, CH, and LP contributed to the analysis and interpretation of data. EH, SH, DD, PG, AC, VW, and LP contributed to the manuscript writing/revision. All authors read and approved the final manuscript.

Competing interests
The employer of SH, the Regents of the University of California, hold a patent on the epigenetic clock method which names SH as inventor. The other authors declare that they have no competing interests.

Author details
[1]Department of Internal Medicine, Section of Medical Oncology, Yale School of Medicine, 300 George Street, Suite 120, New Haven, CT 06511, USA. [2]Department of Human Genetics, David Geffen School of Medicine, University of California Los Angeles, Los Angeles, CA 90095, USA. [3]Department of Biostatistics, Fielding School of Public Health, University of California Los Angeles, Los Angeles, CA 90095, USA. [4]Department of Pharmacology, Yale School of Medicine, 333 Cedar Street, New Haven, CT 06511, USA. [5]Department of Surgery, Memorial Sloan Kettering Cancer Center, New York 10065, USA. [6]Department of Surgery, Yale School of Medicine, 330 Cedar Street, New Haven, CT 06511, USA. [7]Department of Pathology, Yale School of Medicine, 330 Cedar Street, New Haven, CT 06511, USA. [8]Department of Internal Medicine, Indiana University Melvin and Bren Simon Cancer Center, Indianapolis, IN 46202, USA. [9]Department of Obstetrics and Gynecology, Münster University Hospital, Münster, Germany. [10]Department of Clinical Surgery, Perelman School of Medicine, University of Pennsylvania, Philadelphia, PA 19104, USA.

References
1. Howlader N, Noone AM, Krapcho M, Miller D, Bishop K, Kosary CL, Yu M, Ruhl J, Tatalovich Z, Mariotto A, Lewis DR, Chen HS, Feuer EJ, Cronin KA (eds). SEER Cancer Statistics Review, 1975-2014, National Cancer Institute. Bethesda, MD, http://seer.cancer.gov/csr/1975_2014/, based on November 2016 SEER data submission, posted to the SEER web site, April 2017.
2. Pellatt AJ, Wolff RK, Torres-Mejia G, John EM, Herrick JS, Lundgreen A, Baumgartner KB, Giuliano AR, Hines LM, Fejerman L, et al. Telomere length, telomere-related genes, and breast cancer risk: the breast cancer health disparities study. Genes Chromosomes Cancer. 2013;52(7):595–609.
3. Martinez-Delgado B, Yanowsky K, Inglada-Perez L, Domingo S, Urioste M, Osorio A, Benitez J. Genetic anticipation is associated with telomere shortening in hereditary breast cancer. PLoS Genet. 2011;7(7):e1002182.
4. Horvath S. DNA methylation age of human tissues and cell types. Genome Biol. 2013;14:R115.
5. Levine ME, Hosgood HD, Chen B, Absher D, Assimes T, Horvath S. DNA methylation age of blood predicts future onset of lung cancer in the women's health initiative. Aging (Albany NY). 2015;7(9):690–700.
6. Breitling LPH, Saum KU, Perna L, Schöttker B, Holleczek B, Brenner H. Frailty is associated with the epigenetic clock but not with telomere length in a German cohort. Clin Epigenetics. 2016;8:21. https://doi.org/10.1186/s13148-016-0186-5.
7. Marioni RE, Shah S, McRae AF, Ritchie SJ, Muniz-Terrera G, Harris SE. The epigenetic clock is correlated with physical and cognitive fitness in the Lothian Birth Cohort 1936. Int J Epidemiol. 2015;44(4):1388–96. https://doi.org/10.1093/ije/dyu277.
8. Levine ME, Lu AT, Bennett DA, Horvath S. Epigenetic age of the pre-frontal cortex is associated with neuritic plaques, amyloid load, and Alzheimer's disease related cognitive functioning. Aging (Albany NY). 2015;7(12):1198–211.
9. Horvath S, Mah V, Lu AT, Woo JS, Choi OW, Jasinska AJ, Riancho JA, Tung S, Coles NS, Braun J, et al. The cerebellum ages slowly according to the epigenetic clock. Aging (Albany NY). 2015;7(5):294–306.
10. Horvath S, Erhart W, Brosch M, Ammerpohl O, von Schonfels W, Ahrens M, Heits N, Bell JT, Tsai PC, Spector TD, et al. Obesity accelerates epigenetic aging of human liver. Proc Natl Acad Sci U S A. 2014;111(43):15538–43.
11. Levine ME, Lu AT, Chen BH, Hernandez DG, Singleton AB, Ferrucci L, Bandinelli S, Salfati E, Manson JE, Quach A, et al. Menopause accelerates biological aging. Proc Natl Acad Sci U S A. 2016;113(33):9327–32.
12. Vidal L, Lopez-Golan Y, Rego-Perez I, Horvath S, Blanco FJ, Riancho JA, Gomez-Reino JJ, Gonzalez A. Specific increase of methylation age in osteoarthritis cartilage. Osteoarthr Cartil. 2016;24:S63.
13. Zheng Y, Joyce BT, Colicino E, Liu L, Zhang W, Dai Q, Shrubsole MJ, Kibbe WA, Gao T, Zhang Z, et al. Blood epigenetic age may predict cancer incidence and mortality. EBioMedicine. 2016;5:68–73.
14. Ambatipudi S, Horvath S, Perrier F, Cuenin C, Hernandez-Vargas H, Le Calvez-Kelm F, Durand G, Byrnes G, Ferrari P, Bouaoun L, et al. DNA methylome analysis identifies accelerated epigenetic ageing associated with postmenopausal breast cancer susceptibility. Eur J Cancer. 2017;75:299–307.
15. Horvath S. Erratum to: DNA methylation age of human tissues and cell types. Genome Biol. 2015;16:96.
16. Triche TJ, Weisenberger DJ, Van Den Berg D, Laird PW, Siegmund KD. Low-level processing of Illumina Infinium DNA methylation BeadArrays. Nucleic Acids Res. 2013;41(7):e90.
17. Sehl ME, Henry JE, Storniolo AM, Ganz PA, Horvath S. DNA methylation age is elevated in breast tissue of non-cancer affected women. Breast Cancer Res Treat. 2017;164(1):209–19.
18. de Magalhaes JP. How ageing processes influence cancer. Nat Rev Cancer. 2013;13(5):357–65.
19. Johnson KC, Houseman EA, King JE, Christensen BC. Normal breast tissue DNA methylation differences at regulatory elements are associated with the cancer risk factor age. Breast Cancer Res. 2017;19(1):81.
20. Quach A, Levine ME, Tanaka T, Lu AT, Chen BH, Ferrucci L, Ritz B, Bandinelli S, Neuhouser ML, Beasley JM, Snetselaar L, Wallace RB, Tsao PS, Absher D, Assimes TL, Stewart JD, Li Y, Hou L, Baccarelli AA, Whitsel EA, Horvath S. Epigenetic clock analysis of diet, exercise, education, and lifestyle factors. Aging (Albany NY). 2017;9(2):419-46. https://doi.org/10.18632/aging.101168.

16

Characteristic profiles of DNA epigenetic modifications in colon cancer and its predisposing conditions—benign adenomas and inflammatory bowel disease

Tomasz Dziaman[1,7]* ⓘ, Daniel Gackowski[1], Jolanta Guz[1], Kinga Linowiecka[1], Magdalena Bodnar[2,6], Marta Starczak[1], Ewelina Zarakowska[1], Martyna Modrzejewska[1], Anna Szpila[1], Justyna Szpotan[1], Maciej Gawronski[1], Anna Labejszo[1], Ariel Liebert[4], Zbigniew Banaszkiewicz[3], Maria Klopocka[4], Marek Foksinski[1], Andrzej Marszalek[2,5] and Ryszard Olinski[1,7]*

Abstract

Background: Active demethylation of 5-methyl-2′-deoxycytidine (5-mdC) in DNA occurs by oxidation to 5-(hydroxymethyl)-2′-deoxycytidine (5-hmdC) and further oxidation to 5-formyl-2′-deoxycytidine (5-fdC) and 5-carboxy-2′-deoxycytidine (5-cadC), and is carried out by enzymes of the ten-eleven translocation family (TETs 1, 2, 3). Decreased level of epigenetic DNA modifications in cancer tissue may be a consequence of reduced activity/expression of TET proteins. To determine the role of epigenetic DNA modifications in colon cancer development, we analyzed their levels in normal colon and various colonic pathologies. Moreover, we determined the expressions of TETs at mRNA and protein level.

The study included material from patients with inflammatory bowel disease (IBD), benign polyps (AD), and colorectal cancer (CRC). The levels of epigenetic DNA modifications and 8-oxo-7,8-dihydro-2′-deoxyguanosine (8-oxodG) in examined tissues were determined by means of isotope-dilution automated online two-dimensional ultraperformance liquid chromatography with tandem mass spectrometry (2D-UPLC-MS/MS). The expressions of *TET* mRNA were measured with RT-qPCR, and the expressions of TET proteins were determined immunohistochemically.

Results: IBD was characterized by the highest level of 8-oxodG among all analyzed tissues, as well as by a decrease in 5-hmdC and 5-mdC levels (at a midrange between normal colon and CRC). AD had the lowest levels of 5-hmdC and 5-mdC of all examined tissues and showed an increase in 8-oxodG and 5-(hydroxymethyl)-2′-deoxyuridine (5-hmdU) levels. CRC was characterized by lower levels of 5-hmdC and 5-mdC, the lowest level of 5-fdC among all analyzed tissues, and relatively high content of 5-cadC. The expression of *TET1* mRNA in CRC and AD was significantly weaker than in IBD and normal colon. Furthermore, CRC and AD showed significantly lower levels of *TET2* and *AID* mRNA than normal colonic tissue.

(Continued on next page)

* Correspondence: tomekd@cm.umk.pl; ryszardo@cm.umk.pl
[1]Department of Clinical Biochemistry, Faculty of Pharmacy, Collegium Medicum in Bydgoszcz, Nicolaus Copernicus University in Torun, Torun, Poland
Full list of author information is available at the end of the article

(Continued from previous page)

Conclusions: Our findings suggest that a complex relationship between aberrant pattern of DNA epigenetic modification and cancer development does not depend solely on the transcriptional status of TET proteins, but also on the characteristics of premalignant/malignant cells. This study showed for the first time that the examined colonic pathologies had their unique epigenetic marks, distinguishing them from each other, as well as from normal colonic tissue. A decrease in 5-fdC level may be a characteristic feature of largely undifferentiated cancer cells.

Keywords: DNA epigenetic modification, Ten-eleven translocation protein, Colon cancer, Inflammatory bowel disease, Adenoma, Demethylation,

Background

During the last decade, one of the hot topics in oncogenesis was the so-called cancer epigenome, having implications for cancer promotion and progression. This, in turn, is linked with a plethora of abnormalities based on somatic heritable modifications that are not caused by alterations in primary sequence of DNA.

Methylation of cytosine, usually in CpG dinucleotides, is a key epigenetic modification exerting a profound impact on gene repression, cellular identity, and organismal fate [1]. However, equally important is an opposite reaction, DNA demethylation, resulting in activation of previously silenced genes. Although a large body of evidence suggests that active demethylation may occur in mammalian cells, its molecular background is still unclear (for review, see [2]). The most plausible mechanism behind the active demethylation of 5-methyl-2′-deoxycytidine (5-mdC) moiety in DNA involves ten-eleven translocation (TET) proteins, which catalyze oxidation of 5-mdC to form 5-(hydroxy-methyl)-2′-deoxycytidine (5-hmdC) and further oxidation reactions that generate 5-formyl-2′-deoxycytidine (5-fdC) and 5-carboxy-2′-deoxycytidine (5-cadC) [2, 3]. Evidence from experimental studies supports the hypothesis that TET enzymes may be also involved in the synthesis of 5-(hydroxymethyl)-2′-deoxyuridine (5-hmdU), a molecule with epigenetic function [4].

Several recent studies showed that the level of 5-hmdC in many various types of human malignancies, including CRC, is profoundly reduced [5–7] and the degree of the reduction is proportional to tumor stage [8].

Either the mechanism or the reason behind the decrease in 5-hmdC level in cancer tissues is still not fully understood. Perhaps, this phenomenon reflects a decrease in the activity/expression of TET proteins [9]. However, it also cannot be excluded that the regulatory mechanisms of active DNA demethylation are determined by external conditions (e.g., chronic inflammation, oxidative stress, nutritional status), which results in a release of different products.

Chronic inflammation being a direct consequence of inflammatory bowel disease (IBD) is considered the most important etiological factor of sporadic colorectal malignancies [10]. Epigenetic modification of DNA is a dynamic molecular process, being a form of response to inflammation-related environmental/metabolic changes.

The downstream steps of active demethylation process may be, at least partially, responsible for the loss of 5-mdC. Furthermore, 5-fdC and 5-cadC were shown to be recognized by a larger number of proteins than 5-hmdC, despite markedly higher level of the latter [11, 12].

In the vast majority of previous studies, 5-hmdC, 5-fdC, and 5-cadC were determined semi-quantitatively, by means of immunohistochemistry; consequently, the results of these might be biased due to ultra-low content of these modifications in genomic DNA of the tumor [7]. It should be also stressed that the accuracy of immunohistochemical studies depends largely on the sensitivity/specificity of antibodies against a given modification.

In our present study, instead of using a semiquantitive method with anti-5-hmdC antibodies, we determined 5-mdC, 5-hmdC, 5-fdC, 5-cadC, and 5-hmU with a highly specific and highly sensitive method developed recently in our laboratory: isotope-dilution automated online two-dimensional ultra-performance liquid chromatography with tandem mass spectrometry (2D-UPLC-MS/MS) [13].

To provide a better insight in the relationship between epigenetic DNA modifications and factors which may influence formation thereof and to determine their role in CRC development, we analyzed their levels in normal colon and various colonic pathologies, which predispose to CRC development. Moreover, we determined the expressions of TETs and AID at mRNA and protein level.

The study included samples from patients with CRC ($n = 97$, both from the tumor and from normal colonic tissue), colon adenomas (AD, $n = 39$), and IBD ($n = 49$). Since both CRC and chronic inflammation are associated with oxidative stress, aside from the epigenetic DNA modifications, we also determined an established marker of oxidatively modified DNA, 8-oxodG. The rationale of the study was to fill the gap in existing knowledge, explaining how conditions which predispose to CRC development can influence the synthesis of TET-mediated DNA modifications and oxidatively modified DNA.

Methods
Study group
The study material originated from three groups of patients with (1) IBD ($n = 49$, median age 35 years, 53% of women), (2) AD, i.e., histologically confirmed adenoma tubulare (90%) or adenoma tubulovillosum (10%) ($n = 39$, median age 65 years, 46% of women), and (3) CRC, i.e., histologically confirmed stage A (8%), stage B (45%), stage C (29%), or stage D (9%) adenocarcinoma, or malignant polyps (9%) ($n = 97$, median age 65 years, 46% of women). None of the study subjects were related with one another, and all of them were Caucasians. All participants of the study were recruited in a hospital setting (Collegium Medicum, Nicolaus Copernicus University, Bydgoszcz, Poland) and subjected to colonoscopy. At the enrollment, all subjects completed a questionnaire containing information about their demographics, smoking, diet, and medical history. The study groups were matched for eating habits, age, body weight, and smoking status. No significant intergroup differences were found in terms of body weight and body stature of male and female subjects. To make the study groups even more homogenous, the subjects who reported overeating or use of dietary supplements during a month preceding the study were not included in the analysis. The questionnaire survey was conducted by the team physician (Dr. Banaszkiewicz, Dr. Klopocka).

Preparation of tissue microarrays (TMA) for immunochemical analysis
Immunohistochemical studies were performed using archived formaldehyde-fixed paraffin-embedded (FFPE) tissue sections derived in the Department of Clinical Pathomorphology, Collegium Medicum in Bydgoszcz, Nicolaus Copernicus University in Torun.

Hematoxylin and eosin (H&E)-stained microscopic slides of archived FFPE tissue sections (donor blocks) were used to identify representative tumor areas with at least 80% tumor cells. Then, two such regions, each 2 mm in diameter, were transferred from the donor blocks to a recipient TMA block using an automated tissue arrayer (TMA Master3D HISTECH, Budapest, Hungary). The same procedure was repeated for normal tissue located at least 2 cm from the tumor resection margin. Then, another set of H&E-stained slides was prepared to verify the accuracy of the TMA blocks. TMA blocks were verified and double-checked by two independent pathologists.

Immunohistochemistry
Immunohistochemical staining was carried out as described elsewhere [14–16], and the results were standardized against a series of positive and negative controls. Positive control staining was performed on a model tissue section selected according to The Human Protein Atlas (http://www.proteinatlas.org) [17] and antibody specification (Additional file 1: Table S1) and the antibody datasheet. Negative controls were prepared from the examined tissues treated with 1% solution of bovine serum albumin (BSA) in phosphate buffered saline (PBS), instead of the primary antibody. Paraffin TMA blocks and archived FFPE tissue sections were cut with a manual rotary microtome (AccuCut, Sakura, Torrance, USA) to obtain 4-μm slices, which were then processed routinely and mounted on extra adhesive slides (SuperFrostPlus, MenzelGlasser, Braunschweig, Germany).

The deparaffinization, rehydration, and antigen retrieval were carried out in PT-Link system (Dako, Agilent Technologies, USA). The slides were heated for 20 min in Epitope Retrieval Solution high-pH (95–98 °C; Dako, Agilent Technologies). Then, the activity of endogenous peroxidase was blocked by a 15-min incubation with 3% H_2O_2 solution, and non-specific binding was eliminated by a 15-min incubation with 5% BSA solution; both reactions were carried out at room temperature. Subsequently, the slides were incubated with primary antibodies against TET1, TET2, and TET3 (specified in Additional file 1: Table S1). The antibody complexes were detected with En-Vision Flex Anti-Mouse/Rabbit HRP-Labeled Polymer (Dako, Agilent Technologies) and localized using 3–3′diaminobenzidine (DAB) as a chromogen. Finally, the slides were counterstained with hematoxylin, subsequently dehydrated, cleared in series of xylenes, and coverslipped using mounting medium (Dako, Agilent Technologies).

Evaluation of protein expression based on immunohistochemical staining
Each slide was examined under ECLIPSE E400 light microscope (Nikon Instruments Europe, Amsterdam, Netherlands) with the low-power (20×) objective. The result of immunohistochemical staining was expressed according to Immunoreactive Remmele-Stegner (IRS) score [18], described in detail in our previous papers [14–16, 19]. Total IRS score (from 0 to 12) was obtained by multiplying the staining intensity score (0—negative, 1—weak staining, 2—moderate staining, 3—strong staining) by the relative proportion of immunolabeled specimen area (0—none; 1—less than 10%; 2—10 to 50%; 3—50 to 80%; 4—at least 80%).

Extraction of DNA from tissues and its hydrolysis to deoxynucleosides
DNA from examined fresh frozen tissues was isolated as described elsewhere [20], with some modifications. Isolated DNA was dissolved in 100 mM ammonium acetate (Sigma-Aldrich) containing 0.1 mM $ZnCl_2$ (pH 4.3). The dissolved DNA samples (50 μl) were mixed with 1 U of

nuclease P1 (Sigma-Aldrich) and tetrahydrouridine (Calbiochem) (as cytidine deaminase inhibitor, 10 µg per sample) and incubated at 37 °C for 1 h. Subsequently, 12 µl 5% (v/v) NH₄OH (JT Baker) and 1.3 U of alkaline phosphatase (Sigma-Aldrich) were added to each sample following 1-h incubation at 37 °C. Finally, all DNA hydrolysates were acidified with CH₃COOH (Sigma-Aldrich) (to final v/v concentration of 2%) and ultrafiltered prior to injection.

Isolation of DNA and determination of epigenetic modifications and 8-oxodG in DNA isolates

The methodology used to determine 5-methyl-2′-deoxycytidine (5-mdC), 5-hydroxymethyl-2′-deoxycytidine (5-hmdC), 5-formyl-2′-deoxycytidine (5-fdC), 5-carboxy-2′deoxycytidine (5-cadC), 5-(hydroxymethyl)-2′-deoxyuridine (5-hmdU), and 8-oxodG levels by means of 2D-UPLC-MS/MS has been described elsewhere [13]. Transition patterns and specific detector settings for all analyzed compounds are presented in the Additional file 2: Table S2.

Gene expression analysis

Isolated leukocytes were stored at − 80 °C until the analysis. RNA was isolated with MagNA Pure 2.0 (Roche) following the standard procedures. Concentration and purity of RNA aliquots were verified spectrophotometrically with NanoDrop 2000 (Thermo Scientific). A_{260}/A_{280} ratio was used as an indicator of protein contamination and A_{260}/A_{230} ratio as a measure of contamination with polysaccharides, phenol, and/or chaotropic salts. Quality and integrity of total RNA were assessed by visualization of 28S/18S/5.8S rRNA band pattern in a 1.2% agarose gel. Non-denaturing electrophoresis was carried out at 95 V for 20 min in TBE buffer (Tris – Boric Acid – EDTA). The gel was stained with ethidium bromide or SimplySafe and visualized using GBox EF Gel Documentation System (SynGene). Purified RNA was stored at − 80 °C. The samples with RNA concentrations greater than 50 ng/µl were qualified for further analysis. 0.5 microgram of total RNA from each sample (in 20-µl volume) was used for cDNA synthesis by reverse transcription with High-Capacity cDNA Reverse Transcription Kit (Applied Biosystems, catalog no. 43-688-14), according to the manufacturer's instruction. The reaction was carried out with Mastercycler Nexus Gradient thermocycler (Eppendorf). To exclude contamination with genomic DNA, reverse transcriptase reaction included also a negative control. cDNA was either used for qPCR setup immediately after obtaining or stored at − 20 °C. The RT-qPCR complies with the Minimum Information for Publication of Quantitative Real-time PCR Experiments (MIQE) guidelines. Three gene transcripts, TET1, TET2, and TET3, were analyzed

by relative quantitative RT-PCR (RT-qPCR) with relevant primers and short hydrolysis probes substituted with Locked Nucleic Acids from the Universal Probe Library (UPL, Roche) (see: Additional file 3: Table S3). The probes were labeled with fluorescein (FAM) at the 5′-end and with a dark quencher dye at the 3′-end. Expressions of target genes were normalized for two selected reference genes, HMBS (GeneID: 3145) and TBP (GeneID: 6908), using UPL Ready Assay #100092149 and #100092158, respectively. Real-time PCR mixes (in 20 µl volumes) were prepared from cDNA following the standard procedures for LightCycler480 Probes Master (Roche), provided with the reagent set. The reactions were carried out on 96-well plates. Aside from the proper samples, each plate included also no-template control and no-RT control. Quantitative real-time PCR was carried out with LightCycler 480 II, using the following cycling parameters: 10 s at 95 °C, followed by 45 repeats 10 s each at 95 °C; 30 s at 58 °C; and finally, 1 s at 72 °C with acquisition mode (parameters of wavelength excitation and detection equal 465 and 510 nm, respectively). The reaction for each gene was standardized against a standard curve, to estimate amplification efficiency. Standardization procedure included preparation of 10-fold serial dilutions with controlled relative amount of targeted template. The efficiency of amplification was assessed based on a slope of the standard curve. Standard dilutions were amplified in separate wells, but within the same run. Then, the samples were subjected to qPCR with measurement of C_t, and amplification efficiencies were automatically calculated and displayed on the analysis window of LightCycler 480 software, version 1.5.1.62 (Roche). The same software was also used for sample setup, real-time PCR analysis, and calculation of relative C_t values referred to as "ratios."

Statistical methods

The results are presented as medians, interquartile ranges, and non-outlier ranges. Normal distribution of the study variables was verified with Kolmogorov-Smirnov test with Lilliefors correction and based on visual inspection of plotted histograms. Variables with non-normal distributions (5-hmdC, 5-fdC, 5-cadC, 5-hmdU, 8-oxodG concentration and TETs, AID mRNA expression) were subjected to Box-Cox transformation prior to statistical analyses with parametric tests. Normalized data were subjected to one-way analysis of variance (ANOVA) followed by LSD and Tukey post hoc tests. Associations between pairs of variables were assessed based on Pearson correlation coefficients for raw or normalized data, where applicable. All statistical transformations and analyses were carried out with STATISTICA 13.1 PL [Dell Inc. (2016). Dell Statistica (data analysis software system), version 13.

software.dell.com.]. The results were considered statistically significant at P values lower than 0.05.

Results

Levels of epigenetic modifications and 8-oxodGuo in DNA from tissue specimens

The highest levels of 5-mdC and 5-hmdC were found in normal colonic tissue, followed by IBD, AD, and CRC specimens (Fig. 1a, b); the level of 5-mdC in AD turned out to be significantly lower than in other tissues. In turn, CRC specimens were characterized by significantly lower levels of 5-fdC than other samples (Fig. 1c). The level of 5-cadC in AD was significantly (2- to 2.5-fold) lower than in other tissues; in turn, the highest level of this modification was found in normal colonic tissue (Fig. 1d). We also analyzed

possible association between level of the epigenetic modifications and tumor progression reflected in tumor stage from A to D. Significant decrease of 5-mdC, 5-hmdC, and 5-fdC was characteristic for early stage of CRC development (stage A), and no further changes were observed along the disease progression.

The highest levels of 5-hmdU and 8-oxodG were observed in IBD and AD and the lowest in CRC and normal colonic tissue; also, these intergroup differences were statistically significant (Fig. 1e, f).

Furthermore, significant correlations were found in the levels of 5-mdC, 5-cadC, 8-oxodG, and 5-hmdU between CRC and normal colon (Fig. 2).

We have analyzed relationship/correlation between age and 5-hmCyt (and other modifications). However in

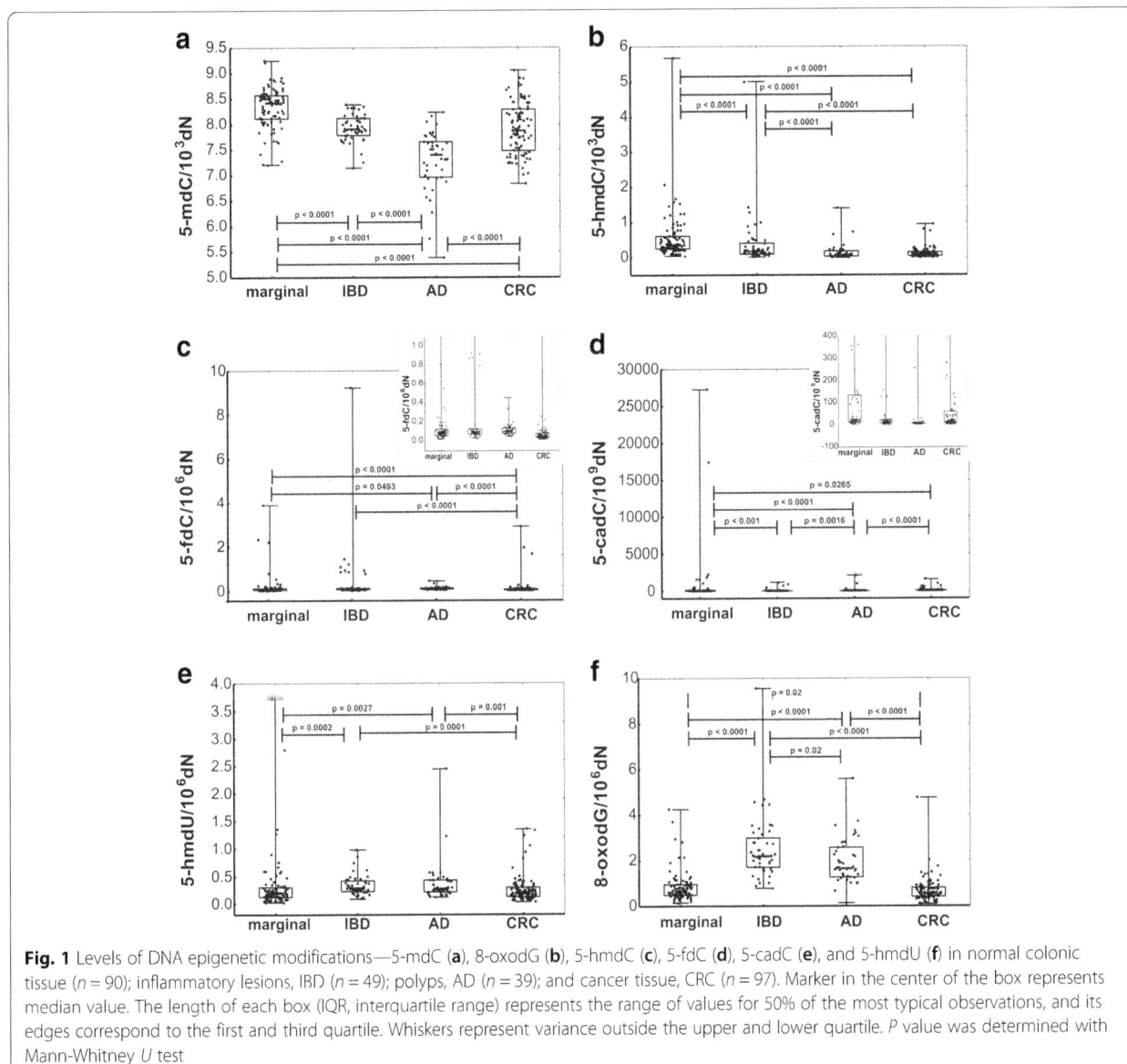

Fig. 1 Levels of DNA epigenetic modifications—5-mdC (**a**), 8-oxodG (**b**), 5-hmdC (**c**), 5-fdC (**d**), 5-cadC (**e**), and 5-hmdU (**f**) in normal colonic tissue ($n = 90$); inflammatory lesions, IBD ($n = 49$); polyps, AD ($n = 39$); and cancer tissue, CRC ($n = 97$). Marker in the center of the box represents median value. The length of each box (IQR, interquartile range) represents the range of values for 50% of the most typical observations, and its edges correspond to the first and third quartile. Whiskers represent variance outside the upper and lower quartile. P value was determined with Mann-Whitney U test

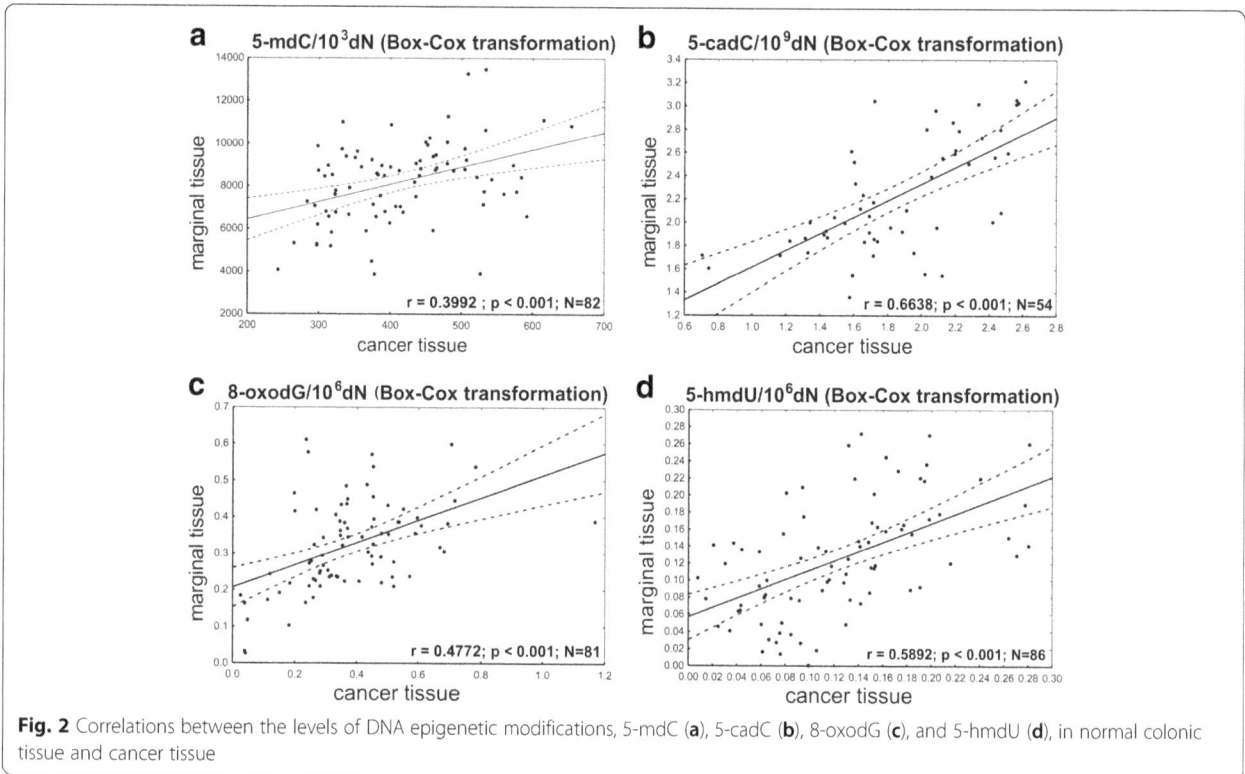

Fig. 2 Correlations between the levels of DNA epigenetic modifications, 5-mdC (**a**), 5-cadC (**b**), 8-oxodG (**c**), and 5-hmdU (**d**), in normal colonic tissue and cancer tissue

CRC patients as well as in other groups, no such correlation was found.

Expression of TET and AID mRNA

The expression of *TET1* in AD and CRC was significantly weaker than in normal colonic tissue and IBD (Fig. 3a). The expression of *TET2* in normal colonic tissue was significantly weaker than in AD and CRC; moreover, a significant difference was found in *TET2* expressions in IBD and AD (Fig. 3b). The examined tissues did not differ significantly in terms of *TET3* expressions (Fig. 3c). Irrespective of the examined tissue, the levels of *AID* mRNA were very low or below the detection threshold. Nevertheless, the levels of *AID* mRNA in CRC turned out to be significantly lower than in other tissues (Fig. 3d). No statistically significant correlations were found between TETs expression and epigenetic DNA modifications (data not shown).

Immunohistochemical analysis of protein expression

Immunoreactivity to anti-TET1 antibodies in CRC turned out to be significantly lower than in normal colonic tissue (Fig. 4). In the case of TET2, immunohistochemical analysis was on the borderline of statistical significance with $p = 0.06$.

Discussion

Although a molecular link between adenomas, chronic inflammation, and carcinogenesis is still not completely understood, a major contributor to CRC development seems to be aberrant methylation of DNA and oxidatively damaged DNA. A growing body of evidence suggests that decreased levels of 5-mdC (for review, see: [21]) and 5-hmdC [22] may be found not only in human malignancies but also in their precursor lesions, such as adenomas. This implies that the level of this modification may decrease gradually throughout carcinogenesis. However, it is still unclear if hypomethylation is a late or early event in cancer development, and whether this process is directly involved in carcinogenesis (for review, see: [21]). Therefore, the aim of this study was to verify if CRC and its precursor lesions differ from normal colonic tissue in the levels of DNA epigenetic modifications.

Similar to previous studies, we demonstrated that 5-hmdC level in CRC was several times lower than in normal colonic tissue. However, the level of this modification in cancer precursor lesions still raises some controversies. In some studies, the levels of 5-hmdC in benign lesions were shown to be lower than in normal tissues [7, 22]. However, in a recent study, the results of which were published in *Cell* [6], melanocytes forming benign nevi showed relatively high levels of 5-hmdC, whereas a significant decrease or complete loss of this epigenetic mark was observed in melanoma cells. It should be stressed that in all these studies, 5-hmdC was determined with a less accurate semiquantitative

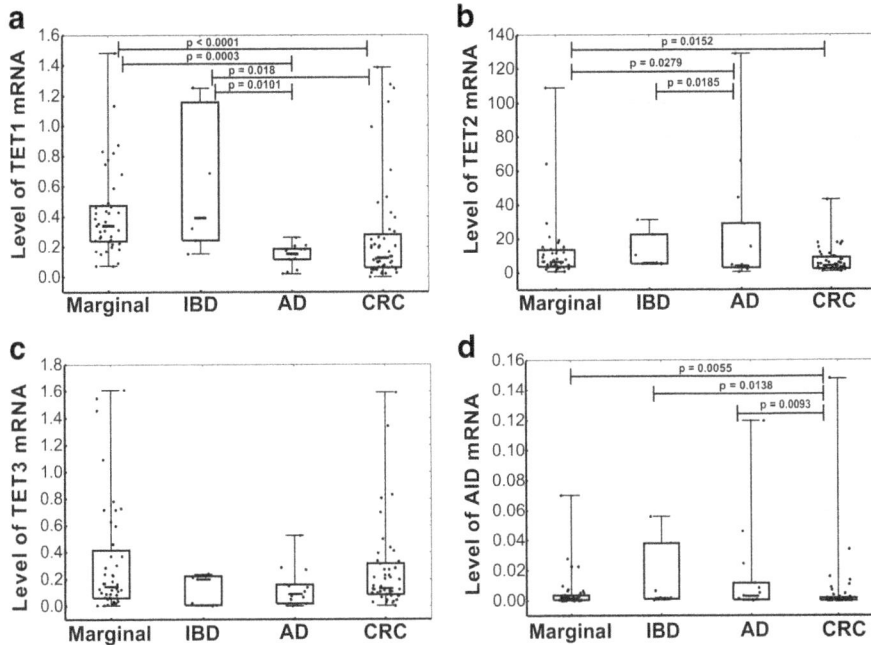

Fig. 3 Expressions of *TET1* (**a**), *TET2* (**b**), *TET3* (**c**), and *AID* (**d**) mRNA in normal colonic tissue, cancer tissue (CRC, $n = 49$), inflammatory lesions (IBD, $n = 7$), and polyps (AD, $n = 14$). Marker in the center of the box represents median value. The length of each box (IQR, interquartile range) represents the range of values for 50% of the most typical observations, and its edges correspond to the first and third quartile. Whiskers represent variance outside the upper and lower quartile. *P* value was determined with Mann-Whitney *U* test

method. Our present study, involving highly accurate quantitative technique for 5-hmdC determination, demonstrated that the level of this modification in AD and CRC was essentially the same, approximately four times lower than in normal colonic tissue. These findings are consistent with the results published by Uribe-Lewis et al. [22], who also showed that 5-hmdC levels in CRC and adenoma were substantially lower than in normal colon. However, to the best of our knowledge, our present study was the first one to show that the level of 5-hmdC in IBD was significantly lower than in normal colonic tissue, at a midrange between the values found in this material and in CRC (Fig. 1b).

Interestingly, a significant decrease in 5-fdC content was observed solely in CRC, and the level of this modification in both types of precursor lesions, IBD and AD, was essentially the same as in normal colonic tissue (Fig. 1c). Furthermore, both IBD and AD were characterized by significantly higher levels of 8-oxodG (the marker of oxidative stress) than CRC and normal colon (Fig. 1f). It should be remembered that the induction of oxidative stress in a cell culture was previously shown to contribute to a decrease in 5-hmdC level [23].

The level of another higher-order oxidative modification of 5-mdC, i.e., 5-cadC, was significantly higher in CRC than in AD or IBD (Fig. 1a, d). Furthermore, we found a significant correlation between the levels of this modification in CRC and normal colonic tissue (Fig. 2).

Previous semiquantitative studies with specific antibodies demonstrated elevated levels of 5-cadC in human breast cancer and gliomas [24].

Recent evidence suggests that oncogenic transcription factors, Myc and Max, and perhaps also an array of regulatory proteins, can specifically recognize 5-cadC, having lesser affinity for 5-fdC and showing only a trace of affinity towards 5-mdC and 5-hmdC. It should be remembered that dysregulation of MYC-MAX transcriptional network is a common mechanism driving progression of human malignancies [25]. This may at least partially explain higher levels of 5-cadC found in cancer tissue. Moreover, Xiong et al. [26] showed recently that Sall4, an oncogenic protein being overexpressed in colon cancer [27], may cooperate with TET2, catalyzing oxidation of 5-hmdC and contributing to formation of 5-cadC. Another study demonstrated that TET3 may specifically bind to 5-cadC, initiating BER pathway and thus activating the process of demethylation [28].

Intriguingly, the analyses of associations between overall survival and the levels of epigenetic modifications in CRC patients demonstrated that the only correlation of longer survival was low level of 5-cadC in marginal tissue (Fig. 5). Hence, an important question arises why this parameter is a meaningful predictor of longer survival in cancer patients? Although histopathological examination did not demonstrate presence of cancer cells in marginal/normal tissue, the molecular assays

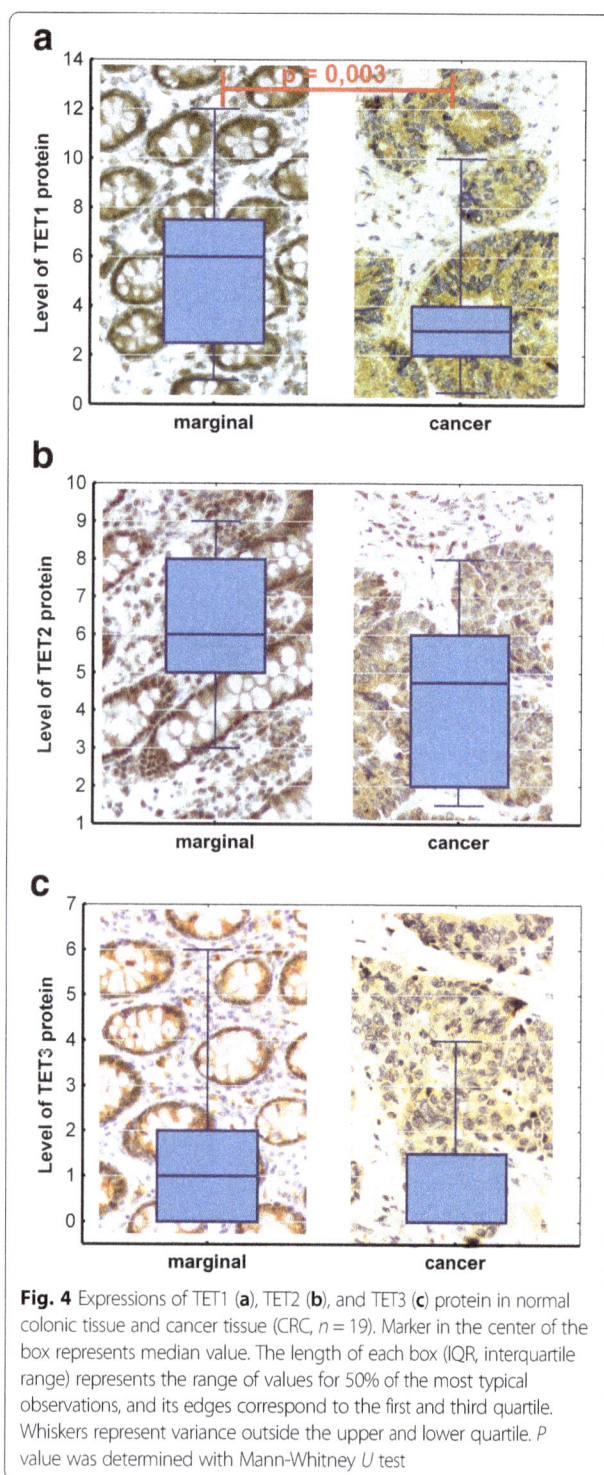

Fig. 4 Expressions of TET1 (**a**), TET2 (**b**), and TET3 (**c**) protein in normal colonic tissue and cancer tissue (CRC, $n = 19$). Marker in the center of the box represents median value. The length of each box (IQR, interquartile range) represents the range of values for 50% of the most typical observations, and its edges correspond to the first and third quartile. Whiskers represent variance outside the upper and lower quartile. P value was determined with Mann-Whitney U test

in CRC and normal colonic tissue and a relatively high content of this modification in CRC, one can expect that marginal tissue with lower level of 5-cadC is less likely to contain cancer cells.

Both CRC and its precursor lesions, especially AD, showed significantly lower levels of 5-mdC than normal colonic tissue (Fig. 1). A dramatic decrease in 5-mdC and 5-hmdC levels in AD may contribute to genomic instability and thus represent a decisive step in CRC development. Interestingly, a substantial decrease in the levels of these modifications in AD (observed also in IBD specimens) co-existed with an increase in 5-hmU, 8-oxodG, and 5-fdC content. This suggests that the decrease in 5-mdC level observed in cancer precursor lesions may be associated with the recently proposed phenomenon of processive DNA demethylation. Plausibly, 5-fdC, 5-hmd, and perhaps also 8-oxodG initiate processive demethylation of DNA, as proposed by Franchini et al. [31, 32]. In line with this hypothesis, an alternative pathway, the so-called processive DNA demethylation, exists aside from the active process involved in local and specific demethylation of DNA. According to the authors of this hypothesis, a single initiating event (such as a certain mismatch, e.g., 5-hmUra-G) may trigger processive demethylation of numerous 5-mdCs (and perhaps also 5-hmdCs) on the same locus via long-path BER, DNA mismatch repair (MMR), or nucleotide excision repair (NER) pathway. Recent experiments with cell-free extracts and circular heteroduplex DNA substrate demonstrated that 5-hmU may trigger the removal of distant epigenetic modifications (5-mdC and 5-hmdC) on MMR- and long-path BER-dependent pathway [33].

Our present study showed that the expression of *TET1* mRNA in CRC and AD was significantly weaker than in IBD and normal colon (Fig. 3). Furthermore, CRC and AD showed significantly lower levels of *TET2* and *AID* mRNA than normal colonic tissue. However, at a protein level, the only significant difference between the examined tissues was found in the case of *TET1*, significantly more abundant in normal colon than in CRC.

A main factor contributing to a decrease in the activity of TET proteins are mutations in catalytic domains of these enzymes [34]. Another reason behind the reduced activity of TETs may be an inhibitory effect of accumulated onco-metabolites, such as 2-OH-glutarate [35, 36], resulting primarily from the presence of IDH1/2 mutations. However, these mutations were observed mainly in hematopoietic malignances and are rare or completely absent in solid tumors, such as CRC [37–39]. This implies that a decrease in 5-hmdC level may be caused by other factors than TET/IDH mutations, for example oxidative stress. Indeed, recent evidence suggests that oxidative stress may contribute to post-translational

detected the cells being clonally related to the tumor (field cancerization) [29]. Moreover, in the case of CRC colon marginal tissue, field cancerization may involve up to 10-cm patches [30]. Therefore, the relatively large specimen of marginal tissue used for DNA isolation likely corresponded to the area of field cancerization. Considering a strong correlation between 5-cadC levels

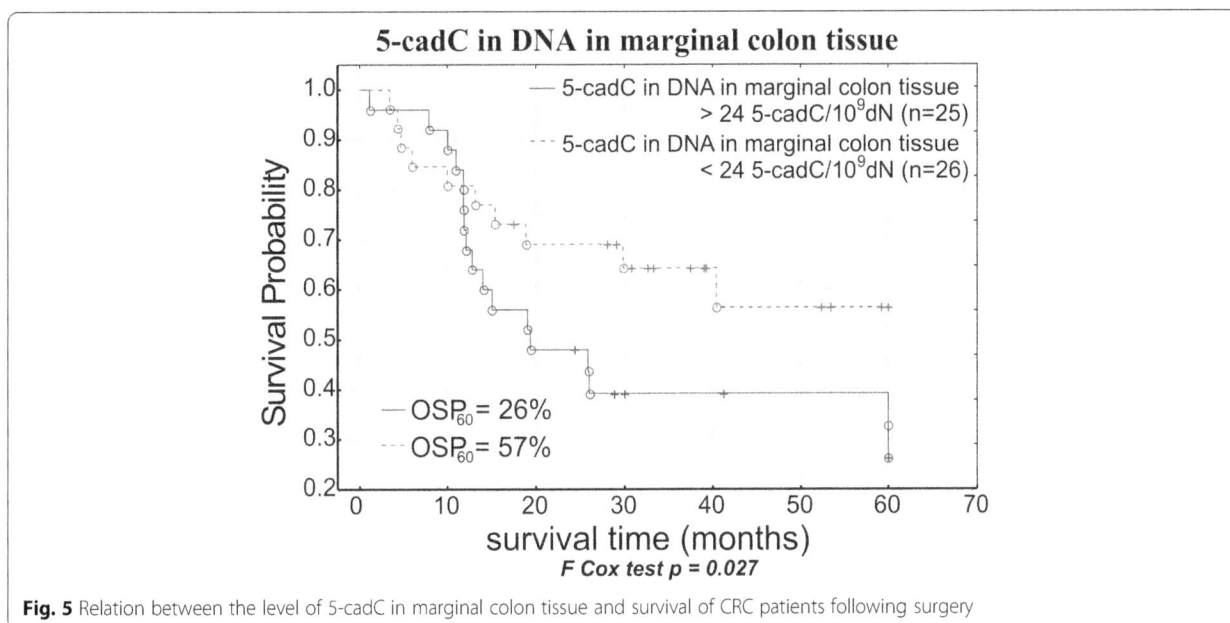

5-cadC in DNA in marginal colon tissue

Fig. 5 Relation between the level of 5-cadC in marginal colon tissue and survival of CRC patients following surgery

modulation of TET2 [40]. Recently, it was demonstrated that the inhibition of TET proteins may be a direct consequence of hypoxia [41]. Hypoxia is a common phenomenon in solid tumors, which may at least partially explain a decrease in 5-hmdC and 5-fdC levels observed in CRC. Interestingly, hypoxia increases overall oxidative stress and can change redox status of the cell [42].

Since the shape of TET co-substrates (2-ketoglutarate, Fe^{+2}) depends on the redox state of the cell, the change in the activity of these enzymes may reflect the severity of oxidative stress. Furthermore, it cannot be excluded that also superoxide (O^{-2}), an anion radical of dioxygen and the precursor of free radicals, plays an important role in TET-mediated active DNA demethylation [43, 44]. Thus, changes in the activity of TET proteins may result from a persistent increase in the severity of oxidative stress, which promotes aberrant generation of DNA epigenetic modifications during iterative oxidation of 5-mdC. In this study, we found elevated levels of 8-oxodG in IBD and AD. Of note, level of 8-oxodG in DNA may directly inform about oxidative stress in nuclei of cells, where epigenetic processes take place. Recently, it was also demonstrated that 8-oxodG may serve as a demethylation signal [45]: binding to 8-oxodG; OGG1 glycosylase may recruit TET1 which in turn may be involved in specific DNA demethylation in response to oxidative stress/oxidatively damaged DNA. This may at least partially explain a decrease in 5-mdC level observed in AD and IBD, i.e., in precursor lesions characterized by elevated levels of 8-oxodG.

Conclusion

Our hereby presented findings suggest that a complex relationship between aberrant pattern of DNA epigenetic modification and cancer development does not depend solely on the transcriptional status of TET proteins, but also on the characteristics of premalignant/malignant cells. This in turn implies that epigenetic modification of DNA is linked to oxidative stress. However, the exact character of this complex relationship is still poorly understood.

Our findings are consistent with the results of previous studies, showing that aberrant methylation of DNA occurs at very early stages of CRC development. Moreover, the hereby presented data add to existing evidence, showing that a decrease in the level of epigenetic marks is characteristic for early stages of CRC development, and further progression of the tumor is not associated with any additional changes in these parameters. To the best of our knowledge, this study was the first one to show that CRC, AD, and IBD had their unique epigenetic marks, distinguishing them from each other as well as from normal colonic tissue: (i) IBD was characterized by the highest level of 8-oxodG among all analyzed tissues, as well as by a decrease in 5-hmdC and 5-mdC levels (at a midrange between normal colon and CRC); (ii) AD had the lowest levels of 5-hmdC and 5-mdC of all examined tissues and showed an increase in 8-oxodG and 5-hmdU levels; (iii) CRC was characterized by lower levels of 5-hmdC and 5-mdC, the lowest level of 5-fdC among all analyzed tissues, and relatively high content of 5-cadC. This implies that a decrease in 5-hmdC level is not a unique feature of CRC (as previously reported) and can be also found in its precursor lesions, in particular in AD. The mechanism behind a substantial decrease in 5-fdC generation at advanced stages of carcinogenesis is still unclear, and the same refers to the consequences of this phenomenon. A recent observation that 5-fdC is rich in active enhancers involved in tissue development/differentiation [46] sheds a new light on these relationships, implying that reduced level of this modification may be a characteristic feature of largely undifferentiated cancer cells.

It cannot be excluded that the analysis of a larger spectrum of DNA epigenetic modifications, rather than solely 5-hmdC, supported by a transcriptional information, might provide a better insight in carcinogenesis, risk factors of CRC, and perhaps also therapy of this malignancy.

Abbreviations
2D-UPLC-MS/MS: Two-dimensional ultra-performance liquid chromatography with tandem mass spectrometry; 5-cadC: 5-Carboxy-2'deoxycytidine; 5-fdC: 5-Formyl-2'-deoxycytidine; 5-hmdC: 5-Hydroxymethyl-2'-deoxycytidine; 5-hmdU: 5-(Hydroxymethyl)-2'-deoxyuridine; 5-mdC: 5-Methyl-2'-deoxycytidine; 8-oxodG: 8-Oxo-2'-deoxyguanosine; AD: Adenoma; AID: Activation-induced cytidine deaminase protein; CRC: Colorectal cancer; FFPE: Formaldehyde-fixed paraffin-embedded; IBD: Inflammatory bowel disease; TET: Ten-eleven translocation protein; TMA: Tissue microarrays

Funding
This work was supported by the Polish National Science Center [grant no. 2013/09/B/NZ5/00767].

Authors' contributions
RO, AM, MF, ZB, MK, DG, and TD designed the research. ZB, MK, and ALi recruited the participants of the study. AM and MB performed the immunochemical analysis. TD, MS, EZ, MM, AS, JS, MG, KL, and ALa performed the isolation of DNA and its hydrolysis to deoxynucleosides. DG and MS performed determination of the epigenetic modifications in DNA. TD, JG, and KL performed isolation of RNA and gene expression analysis. TD, DG, and MF performed statistical analysis. TD, MF, and RO supervised the research. TD and RO wrote the manuscript. RO, AM, MF, ZB, MK, DG, and TD revised and edited the manuscript. All authors read and approved the final manuscript.

Competing interests
The authors declare that they have no competing interests.

Author details
[1]Department of Clinical Biochemistry, Faculty of Pharmacy, Collegium Medicum in Bydgoszcz, Nicolaus Copernicus University in Torun, Torun, Poland. [2]Department of Clinical Pathomorphology, Faculty of Medicine, Collegium Medicum in Bydgoszcz, Nicolaus Copernicus University in Torun, Torun, Poland. [3]Department of Surgery, Faculty of Medicine, Collegium Medicum in Bydgoszcz, Nicolaus Copernicus University in Torun, Torun, Poland. [4]Department of Vascular Diseases and Internal Medicine, Faculty of Health Sciences, Collegium Medicum in Bydgoszcz, Nicolaus Copernicus University in Torun, Torun, Poland. [5]Department of Oncologic Pathology and Prophylaxis, Poznan University of Medical Sciences and Greater Poland Cancer Center, Poznan, Poland. [6]Department of Otolaryngology and Laryngeal Oncology, K. Marcinkowski University of Medical Sciences, Poznan, Poland. [7]Department of Clinical Biochemistry, Collegium Medicum in Bydgoszcz, Nicolaus Copernicus University, Karlowicza 24, 85-095 Bydgoszcz, Poland.

References
1. Feng S, Jacobsen SE, Reik W. Epigenetic reprogramming in plant and animal development. Science. 2010;330:622–7.
2. Bhutani N, Burns DM, Blau HM. DNA demethylation dynamics. Cell. 2011; 146:866–72.
3. Tahiliani M, Koh KP, Shen Y, Pastor WA, Bandukwala H, Brudno Y, Agarwal S, Iyer LM, Liu DR, Aravind L, Rao A. Conversion of 5-methylcytosine to 5-hydroxymethylcytosine in mammalian DNA by MLL partner TET1. Science. 2009;324:930–5.
4. Pfaffeneder T, Spada F, Wagner M, Brandmayr C, Laube SK, Eisen D, Truss M, Steinbacher J, Hackner B, Kotljarova O, Schuermann D, Michalakis S, Kosmatchev O, Schiesser S, Steigenberger B, Raddaoui N, Kashiwazaki G, Muller U, Spruijt CG, Vermeulen M, Leonhardt H, Schar P, Muller M, Carell T. Tet oxidizes thymine to 5-hydroxymethyluracil in mouse embryonic stem cell DNA. NatChemBiol. 2014;10:574–81.
5. Jin SG, Jiang Y, Qiu R, Rauch TA, Wang Y, Schackert G, Krex D, Lu Q, Pfeifer GP. 5-Hydroxymethylcytosine is strongly depleted in human cancers but its levels do not correlate with IDH1 mutations. Cancer Res. 2011;71:7360–5.
6. Lian CG, Xu Y, Ceol C, Wu F, Larson A, Dresser K, Xu W, Tan L, Hu Y, Zhan Q, Lee CW, Hu D, Lian BQ, Kleffel S, Yang Y, Neiswender J, Khorasani AJ, Fang R, Lezcano C, Duncan LM, Scolyer RA, Thompson JF, Kakavand H, Houvras Y, Zon LI, Mihm MC Jr, Kaiser UB, Schatton T, Woda BA, Murphy GF, Shi YG. Loss of 5-hydroxymethylcytosine is an epigenetic hallmark of melanoma. Cell. 2012;150:1135–46.
7. Yang H, Liu Y, Bai F, Zhang JY, Ma SH, Liu J, Xu ZD, Zhu HG, Ling ZQ, Ye D, Guan KL, Xiong Y. Tumor development is associated with decrease of TET gene expression and 5-methylcytosine hydroxylation. Oncogene. 2013;32: 663–9.
8. Chen ML, Shen F, Huang W, Qi JH, Wang Y, Feng YQ, Liu SM, Yuan BF. Quantification of 5-methylcytosine and 5-hydroxymethylcytosine in genomic DNA from hepatocellular carcinoma tissues by capillary hydrophilic-interaction liquid chromatography/quadrupole TOF mass spectrometry. Clin Chem. 2013;59:824–32.
9. Cimmino L, Abdel-Wahab O, Levine RL, Aifantis I. TET family proteins and their role in stem cell differentiation and transformation. Cell Stem Cell. 2011;9:193–204.
10. Kraus S, Arber N. Inflammation and colorectal cancer. CurrOpinPharmacol. 2009;9:405–10.
11. Iurlaro M, Ficz G, Oxley D, Raiber EA, Bachman M, Booth MJ, Andrews S, Balasubramanian S, Reik W. A screen for hydroxymethylcytosine and formylcytosine binding proteins suggests functions in transcription and chromatin regulation. Genome Biol. 2013;14:R119.
12. Spruijt CG, Gnerlich F, Smits AH, Pfaffeneder T, Jansen PW, Bauer C, Munzel M, Wagner M, Muller M, Khan F, Eberl HC, Mensinga A, Brinkman AB, Lephikov K, Muller U, Walter J, Boelens R, van IH, Leonhardt H, Carell T, Vermeulen M. Dynamic readers for 5-(hydroxy)methylcytosine and its oxidized derivatives. Cell. 2013;152: 1146–59.
13. Gackowski D, Starczak M, Zarakowska E, Modrzejewska M, Szpila A, Banaszkiewicz Z, Olinski R. Accurate, direct, and high-throughput analyses of a broad spectrum of endogenously generated DNA base modifications with isotope-dilution two-dimensional ultraperformance liquid chromatography with tandem mass spectrometry: possible clinical implication. AnalChem. 2016;88:12128–36.
14. Bodnar M, Szylberg L, Kazmierczak W, Marszalek A. Tumor progression driven by pathways activating matrix metalloproteinases and their inhibitors. JOral PatholMed. 2015;44:437–43.
15. Bodnar M, Luczak M, Bednarek K, Szylberg L, Marszalek A, Grenman R, Szyfter K, Jarmuz-Szymczak M, Giefing M. Proteomic profiling identifies the inorganic pyrophosphatase (PPA1) protein as a potential biomarker of metastasis in laryngeal squamous cell carcinoma. AminoAcids. 2016;48: 1469–76.
16. Bodnar M, Burduk P, Antosik P, Jarmuz-Szymczak M, Wierzbicka M, Marszalek A. Assessment of BRAF V600E (VE1) protein expression and BRAF gene mutation status in codon 600 in benign and malignant salivary gland neoplasms. JOral PatholMed. 2017;46:340–5.
17. Uhlen M, Oksvold P, Fagerberg L, Lundberg E, Jonasson K, Forsberg M, Zwahlen M, Kampf C, Wester K, Hober S, Wernerus H, Bjorling L, Ponten F. Towards a knowledge-based human protein atlas. NatBiotechnol. 2010;28: 1248–50.

18. Remmele W, Stegner HE. Recommendation for uniform definition of an immunoreactive score (IRS) for immunohistochemical estrogen receptor detection (ER-ICA) in breast cancer tissue. Pathologe. 1987;8:138–40.

19. Burduk PK, Bodnar M, Sawicki P, Szylberg L, Wisniewska E, Kazmierczak W, Martynska M, Marszalek A. Expression of metalloproteinases 2 and 9 and tissue inhibitors 1 and 2 as predictors of lymph node metastases in oropharyngeal squamous cell carcinoma. Head Neck. 2015;37:418–22.

20. Guz J, Foksinski M, Siomek A, Gackowski D, Rozalski R, Dziaman T, Szpila A, Olinski R. The relationship between 8-oxo-7,8-dihydro-2'-deoxyguanosine level and extent of cytosine methylation in leukocytes DNA of healthy subjects and in patients with colon adenomas and carcinomas. MutatRes. 2008;640:170–3.

21. Herceg Z, Vaissiere T. Epigenetic mechanisms and cancer: an interface between the environment and the genome. Epigenetics. 2011;6:804–19.

22. Uribe-Lewis S, Stark R, Carroll T, Dunning MJ, Bachman M, Ito Y, Stojic L, Halim S, Vowler SL, Lynch AG, Delatte B, de Bony EJ, Colin L, Defrance M, Krueger F, Silva AL, Ten HR, Ibrahim AE, Fuks F, Murrell A. 5-hydroxymethylcytosine marks promoters in colon that resist DNA hypermethylation in cancer. Genome Biol. 2015;16:69.

23. Delatte B, Jeschke J, Defrance M, Bachman M, Creppe C, Calonne E, Bizet M, Deplus R, Marroqui L, Libin M, Ravichandran M, Mascart F, Eizirik DL, Murrell A, Jurkowski TP, Fuks F. Genome-wide hydroxymethylcytosine pattern changes in response to oxidative stress. SciRep. 2015;5:12714.

24. Eleftheriou M, Pascual AJ, Wheldon LM, Perry C, Abakir A, Arora A, Johnson AD, Auer DT, Ellis IO, Madhusudan S, Ruzov A. 5-Carboxylcytosine levels are elevated in human breast cancers and gliomas. ClinEpigenetics. 2015;7:88.

25. Wang D, Hashimoto H, Zhang X, Barwick BG, Lonial S, Boise LH, Vertino PM, Cheng X. MAX is an epigenetic sensor of 5-carboxylcytosine and is altered in multiple myeloma. Nucleic Acids Res. 2017;45:2396–407.

26. Xiong J, Zhang Z, Chen J, Huang H, Xu Y, Ding X, Zheng Y, Nishinakamura R, Xu GL, Wang H, Chen S, Gao S, Zhu B. Cooperative action between SALL4A and TET proteins in stepwise oxidation of 5-methylcytosine. Mol Cell. 2016;64:913–25.

27. Cheng J, Deng R, Zhang P, Wu C, Wu K, Shi L, Liu X, Bai J, Deng M, Shuai X, Gao J, Wang G, Tao K. miR-219-5p plays a tumor suppressive role in colon cancer by targeting oncogene Sall4. Oncol Rep. 2015;34:1923–32.

28. Jin SG, Zhang ZM, Dunwell TL, Harter MR, Wu X, Johnson J, Li Z, Liu J, Szabo PE, Lu Q, Xu GL, Song J, Pfeifer GP. Tet3 reads 5-carboxylcytosine through its CXXC domain and is a potential guardian against neurodegeneration. Cell Rep. 2016;14:493–505.

29. Braakhuis BJ, Tabor MP, Kummer JA, Leemans CR, Brakenhoff RH. A genetic explanation of Slaughter's concept of field cancerization: evidence and clinical implications. Cancer Res. 2003;63:1727–30.

30. Hawthorn L, Lan L, Mojica W. Evidence for field effect cancerization in colorectal cancer. Genomics. 2014;103:211–21.

31. Franchini DM, Chan CF, Morgan H, Incorvaia E, Rangam G, Dean W, Santos F, Reik W, Petersen-Mahrt SK. Processive DNA demethylation via DNA deaminase-induced lesion resolution. PLoSOne. 2014;9:e97754

32. Olinski R, Starczak M, Gackowski D. Enigmatic 5-hydroxymethyluracil: oxidatively modified base, epigenetic mark or both? MutatResRevMutatRes. 2016;767:59–66.

33. Grin I, Ishchenko AA. An interplay of the base excision repair and mismatch repair pathways in active DNA demethylation. Nucleic Acids Res. 2016;44:3713–27.

34. Kohli RM, Zhang Y. TET enzymes, TDG and the dynamics of DNA demethylation. Nature. 2013;502:472–9.

35. Xu W, Yang H, Liu Y, Yang Y, Wang P, Kim SH, Ito S, Yang C, Wang P, Xiao MT, Liu LX, Jiang WQ, Liu J, Zhang JY, Wang B, Frye S, Zhang Y, Xu YH, Lei QY, Guan KL, Zhao SM, Xiong Y. Oncometabolite 2-hydroxyglutarate is a competitive inhibitor of alpha-ketoglutarate-dependent dioxygenases. Cancer Cell. 2011;19:17–30.

36. Figueroa ME, Bdel-Wahab O, Lu C, Ward PS, Patel J, Shih A, Li Y, Bhagwat N, Vasanthakumar A, Fernandez HF, Tallman MS, Sun Z, Wolniak K, Peeters JK, Liu W, Choe SE, Fantin VR, Paietta E, Lowenberg B, Licht JD, Godley LA, Delwel R, Valk PJ, Thompson CB, Levine RL, Melnick A. Leukemic IDH1 and IDH2 mutations result in a hypermethylation phenotype, disrupt TET2 function, and impair hematopoietic differentiation. Cancer Cell. 2010;18:553–67.

37. Wu X, Zhang Y. TET-mediated active DNA demethylation: mechanism, function and beyond. NatRevGenet. 2017;18:517–34.

38. Kan Z, Jaiswal BS, Stinson J, Janakiraman V, Bhatt D, Stern HM, Yue P, Haverty PM, Bourgon R, Zheng J, Moorhead M, Chaudhuri S, Tomsho LP, Peters BA, Pujara K, Cordes S, Davis DP, Carlton VE, Yuan W, Li L, Wang W, Eigenbrot C, Kaminker JS, Eberhard DA, Waring P, Schuster SC, Modrusan Z, Zhang Z, Stokoe D, de Sauvage FJ, Faham M, Seshagiri S. Diverse somatic mutation patterns and pathway alterations in human cancers. Nature. 2010; 466:869–73.

39. Seshagiri S, Stawiski EW, Durinck S, Modrusan Z, Storm EE, Conboy CB, Chaudhuri S, Guan Y, Janakiraman V, Jaiswal BS, Guillory J, Ha C, Dijkgraaf GJ, Stinson J, Gnad F, Huntley MA, Degenhardt JD, Haverty PM, Bourgon R, Wang W, Koeppen H, Gentleman R, Starr TK, Zhang Z, Largaespada DA, Wu TD, de Sauvage FJ. Recurrent R-spondin fusions in colon cancer. Nature. 2012;488:660–4.

40. Zhang YW, Wang Z, Xie W, Cai Y, Xia L, Easwaran H, Luo J, Yen RC, Li Y, Baylin SB. Acetylation enhances TET2 function in protecting against abnormal DNA methylation during oxidative stress. MolCell. 2017;65:323–35.

41. Thienpont B, Steinbacher J, Zhao H, D'Anna F, Kuchnio A, Ploumakis A, Ghesquiere B, Van DL, Boeckx B, Schoonjans L, Hermans E, Amant F, Kristensen VN, Koh KP, Mazzone M, Coleman ML, Carell T, Carmeliet P, Lambrechts D. Tumour hypoxia causes DNA hypermethylation by reducing TET activity. Nature. 2016;537:63–8.

42. Debevec T, Millet GP, Pialoux V. Hypoxia-induced oxidative stress modulation with physical activity. Front Physiol. 2017;8:84.

43. Afanas'ev I. Mechanisms of superoxide signaling in epigenetic processes: relation to aging and cancer. Aging Dis. 2015;6:216–27.

44. Cyr AR, Domann FE. The redox basis of epigenetic modifications: from mechanisms to functional consequences. AntioxidRedoxSignal. 2011;15:551–89.

45. Zhou X, Zhuang Z, Wang W, He L, Wu H, Cao Y, Pan F, Zhao J, Hu Z, Sekhar C, Guo Z. OGG1 is essential in oxidative stress induced DNA demethylation. Cell Signal. 2016;28:1163–71.

46. Iurlaro M, McInroy GR, Burgess HE, Dean W, Raiber EA, Bachman M, Beraldi D, Balasubramanian S, Reik W. In vivo genome-wide profiling reveals a tissue-specific role for 5-formylcytosine. Genome Biol. 2016;17:141.

17

Inverse association between estrogen receptor-α DNA methylation and breast composition in adolescent Chilean girls

Alexandra M Binder[1†], Leah T Stiemsma[1†], Kristen Keller[2], Sanne D van Otterdijk[3], Verónica Mericq[4], Ana Pereira[4], José L Santos[5], John Shepherd[6] and Karin B Michels[1*]

Abstract

Background: Estrogen receptor-α (ER-α) is a transcriptional regulator, which mediates estrogen-dependent breast development, as well as breast tumorigenesis. The influence of epigenetic regulation of ER-α on adolescent breast composition has not been previously studied and could serve as a marker of pubertal health and susceptibility to breast cancer. We investigated the association between ER-α DNA methylation in leukocytes and breast composition in adolescent Chilean girls enrolled in the Growth and Obesity Cohort Study (GOCS) in Santiago, Chile. Breast composition (total breast volume (BV; cm^3), fibroglandular volume (FGV; cm^3), and percent fibroglandular volume (%FGV)) was measured at breast Tanner stage 4 (B4). ER-α promoter DNA methylation was assessed by pyrosequencing in blood samples collected at breast Tanner stages 2 (B2; $n = 256$) and B4 ($n = 338$).

Results: After adjusting for fat percentage at breast density measurement, ER-α methylation at B2, and cellular heterogeneity, we observed an inverse association between B4 average ER-α DNA methylation and BV and FGV. Geometric mean BV was 15% lower (95% CI: − 28%, − 1%) among girls in the highest quartile of B4 ER-α methylation (6.96–23.60%) relative to the lowest (0.78–3.37%). Similarly, FGV was 19% lower (95% CI: − 33%, − 2%) among girls in the highest quartile of B4 ER-α methylation relative to the lowest. The association between ER-α methylation and breast composition was not significantly modified by body fat percentage and was not influenced by pubertal timing.

Conclusions: These findings suggest that the methylation profile of ER-α may modulate adolescent response to estrogen and breast composition, which may influence breast cancer risk in adulthood.

Keywords: Estrogen receptor-α, DNA methylation, Epigenetics, Breast density, Fibroglandular volume

Background

Estrogen receptor-α (ER-α) is a ligand-activated transcriptional regulator, which mediates the action of estrogen and contributes to normal breast development and breast tumorigenesis [1]. Collectively, estrogen and its receptors (ER-α and β) regulate breast epithelial cell proliferation, differentiation, and apoptosis [1]. A majority of literature concerning ER-α is focused on its role in breast cancer; notably, two thirds of all breast cancer cases are associated with overexpression of ER-α [2, 3]. These ER+ tumors respond well to selective estrogen receptor modulators (e.g., tamoxifen), which competitively bind to estrogen receptors to prevent estrogen-dependent cancer growth [4]. DNA methylation of the ER-α promoter blocks the expression of ER-α [5–8]. Consequently, the DNA methylation profile of ER-α is currently being explored as a predictor of breast cancer incidence and prognosis (i.e., lower ER-α DNA methylation may be indicative of increased breast cancer risk). Due to its vital role in mediating the mammary tissue response to estrogen, ER-α methylation could also be considered as a potential marker of pubertal health, particularly in relation to mammary gland development.

* Correspondence: k.michels@ucla.edu

Alexandra M Binder and Leah T Stiemsma are co-first authors.

[†]Alexandra M Binder and Leah T Stiemsma contributed equally to this work.

[1]Department of Epidemiology, Fielding School of Public Health, University of California, Los Angeles 90095, USA

Full list of author information is available at the end of the article

ER-α plays a crucial role in mediating the action of estrogen in normal breast tissue and in regulating mammary gland development [9, 10]. ER-α knockout mice display decreased mammary epithelial cell proliferation and limited ductal growth [11, 12]. ER-α is also a major contributor to normal reproductive development [13, 14]. Knockout ER-α mice and mice with mutated ER- α are infertile and display a decreased response to estrogen [13, 14], suggesting normal ER-α expression is necessary to regulate the response to estrogen and guide normal pubertal development.

There have been no studies to date exploring the epigenetic regulation of ER-α in relation to adolescent breast development in humans. Variants in the ER-α gene (ESR1) have been associated with the increased percent fibroglandular volume (%FGV) in pre- and post-menopausal women [15–17], supporting a role of ER-α in regulating breast tissue composition in humans. The objective of this study was to analyze ER-α promoter DNA methylation in leukocytes during the pubertal time period (at breast Tanner stages 2 (B2) and 4 (B4)), in relation to total breast volume (BV), fibroglandular (FGV), and %FGV measured at B4 in a prospective cohort of girls enrolled in the Growth and Obesity Cohort Study (GOCS) in Santiago, Chile. Given the potential influence of the peripheral conversion of estrogen on ER-α regulation, the majority of which occurs in adipose tissue, we also evaluate potential effect modification of this relation by adolescent adiposity (body fat percentage) [18]. Further, we analyze effect modification by exposure to endocrine-disrupting chemicals (EDCs; phthalates and phenols), which mimic or antagonize the effects of endogenous hormones [19–21]. The methylation profile of ER-α in adolescence may represent an additional marker of pubertal health and a potential marker of breast cancer risk in adulthood.

Results
Demographics of Chilean girls enrolled in the Growth and Obesity Cohort Study
This study includes 429 Chilean girls enrolled in the Growth and Obesity Cohort Study (GOCS) and assessed for breast development at B4 ($n = 345$) and ER-α promoter DNA methylation at B2 ($n = 256$) and B4 ($n = 338$). The median age at methylation assessment was 10.1 years at B2 and 11.1 years at B4. It should be noted that the B2 assessment may not accurately represent age at thelarche, of which the median age was 9.3 years. The median age at menarche was 11.9 years. Body fat percentage was measured at B4, concurrent with breast composition measurements (median fat percentage = 26 %). The remaining demographics for this cohort are summarized in Table 1.

Table 1 Demographic characteristics of 429 Chilean girls participating in GOCS and included in this analysis

Covariate	Breast Tanner stage	Demographics	
Age at visit, years	B2	n	256
		Median	10.1
		25th–75th percentiles	9.4–10.8
	B4	n	358
		Median	11.1
		25th–75th percentiles	10.6–11.8
Fibroglandular volume (% DV/BV)	FGV	n	345
		Median	76.8
		25th–75th percentiles	58.7–98.4
	BV	n	345
		Median	200.5
		25th–75th percentiles	144.7–278.7
	%FGV	n	345
		Median	37.9
		25th–75th percentiles	27.2–53.4
Age at menarche, years		n	379
		Median	11.9
		25th–75th percentiles	11.2–12.4
Fat percentage at Tanner 4		n	357
		Median	26.0
		25th–75th percentiles	22.5–29.8
Maternal education	Completed secondary	n	328
		%	76.5
	Completed post-secondary	n	101
		%	23.5
ER-α methylation	B2	n	256
		Median	6.0
		25th–75th percentiles	4.0–8.8
	B4	n	338
		Median	7.0
		25th–75th percentiles	4.3–9.4

ER-α methylation is moderately correlated between B2 and B4
ER-α methylation at B2 and B4 was assessed across 10 CpG sites (located within the 5′ untranslated region

(5'UTR) of the *ESR1* gene) in blood samples from adolescent Chilean girls. Due to the high correlation in percent methylation across the interrogated CpG loci (Spearman rho = 0.65–98; Additional file 1: Figure S1), we summarized the methylation level of the ER-α promoter by the mean across all sites. Average ER-α methylation was moderately correlated between B2 and B4 (Spearman rho = 0.244, *p* = 0.002); the intra-individual correlation in methylation across Tanner stage was not improved after correction for cellular heterogeneity (Spearman rho = 0.215; *p* = 0.009). We also compared the level of methylation between B2 and B4 (paired *t* test) and found no statistically significant differences between these time points.

ER-α methylation at B4 is inversely associated with B4 breast composition

We first investigated the influence of ER-α methylation at B2 and B4 on adolescent (B4) breast composition, including total breast volume (BV; cm³), fibroglandular volume (FGV; cm³), and percent fibroglandular volume (%FGV). Average B2 ER-α methylation was not associated with any of these measures of breast composition in either unadjusted or adjusted models (Tables 2, 3, and 4). In contrast, we detected an inverse association between average B4 ER-α methylation and total BV, as well as FGV, after adjusting for B2 ER-α methylation, fat percentage at density measurement, and cellular heterogeneity (Fig. 1; Tables 2 and 3). Among girls in the same quartile of B2 ER-α methylation, those in the highest quartile (Q4) of B4 methylation (6.96–23.60%) had 15% lower (0.85; 95% confidence interval (CI): 0.72–0.99) geometric mean BV than girls in the lowest quartile (Q1) of B4 methylation (0.78–3.37%), adjusting for fat percentage and cellular heterogeneity. Similarly, geometric mean FGV was 19% lower (0.81; 95% CI: 0.67–0.98) among girls in the highest B4 methylation quartile relative to the lowest, adjusting for B2 ER-α methylation, fat percentage, and cellular heterogeneity. These associations were consistent after further adjustment for age at breast density measurement and maternal education (Tables 2 and 3). We observed a similar relation between B4 ER-α methylation and BV in models that were not adjusted for B2 ER-α methylation. However, these associations did not reach statistical significance (*p* > 0.05). Given the similar influence of B4 ER-α methylation on total BV and FGV, there was no association between ER-α methylation and %FGV. The impact of ER-α methylation on FGV and total BV at B4 did not related to age at menarche. Neither B2 nor B4 methylation was significantly associated with the timing of menarche, before or after adjustment for potential confounding variables (Table 5).

Table 2 ER-α methylation at B4 is inversely associated with B4 total BV in Chilean girls enrolled in GOCS

Stage label	Relative change in geometric mean BV (95% CI)		
	Model 1[a]	Model 2[b]	Model 3[c]
Tanner 2			
Quartiles[d]			
Q2	0.91 (0.79–1.05)	0.89 (0.76–1.03)	0.89 (0.77–1.04)
Q3	1.04 (0.90–1.21)	1.05 (0.90–1.22)	1.05 (0.90–1.22)
Q4	1.03 (0.89–1.19)	1.02 (0.88–1.19)	1.03 (0.89–1.20)
Linear model[e]			
	1.03 (0.96–1.09)	1.01 (0.95–1.08)	1.02 (0.95–1.09)
Tanner 4			
Quartiles[d]			
Q2	0.91 (0.82–1.00)	0.95 (0.86–1.06)	0.95 (0.86–1.06)
Q3	1.03 (0.93–1.14)	0.99 (0.89–1.10)	0.99 (0.89–1.10)
Q4	0.94 (0.85–1.04)	0.92 (0.83–1.02)	0.92 (0.83–1.02)
Linear model[e]			
	0.98 (0.94–1.03)	0.96 (0.91–1.00)	0.96 (0.91–1.00)
Tanner 2 (2 and 4)[f]			
Quartiles[d]			
Q2	0.89 (0.77–1.03)	0.90 (0.77–1.05)	0.90 (0.77–1.05)
Q3	1.07 (0.92–1.24)	1.08 (0.92–1.27)	1.08 (0.92–1.27)
Q4	1.00 (0.86–1.17)	1.02 (0.87–1.19)	1.01 (0.86–1.19)
Linear model[e]			
	1.02 (0.95–1.09)	1.00 (0.94–1.08)	1.00 (0.93–1.08)
Tanner 4 (2 and 4)[g]			
Quartiles[d]			
Q2	0.93 (0.81–1.07)	0.95 (0.82–1.10)	0.95 (0.82–1.10)
Q3	1.10 (0.94–1.28)	1.03 (0.88–1.21)	1.03 (0.88–1.21)
Q4	0.89 (0.77–1.04)	*0.85 (0.72–0.99)**	*0.85 (0.72–0.99)**
Linear model[e]			
	0.98 (0.91–1.04)	*0.93 (0.86–1.00)**	*0.93 (0.86–1.00)**

[a]Association with mean ER-α methylation adjusting for fat percentage at breast density measurement
[b]Association with cell composition corrected mean ER-α methylation adjusting for fat percentage at breast density measurement
[c]Model 2 additionally adjusted for age at breast density measurement and maternal education
[d]Quartiles for Tanner 2 methylation: Q1 [1.17, 4.05], Q2 (4.05, 6.04], Q3 (6.04, 8.85], Q4 (8.85, 29.30]; quartiles for Tanner 2 methylation after correction for cellular heterogeneity: Q1 [0.98, 3.49], Q2 (3.49, 5.03], Q3 (5.03, 7.34], Q4 (7.34, 24.8]. Quartiles for Tanner 4 methylation: Q1 [1.10, 4.27], Q2 (4.27, 7.05], Q3 (7.05, 9.37], Q4 (9.37, 32.00]; quartiles for Tanner 4 methylation after correction for cellular heterogeneity: Q1 [0.78, 3.37], Q2 (3.37, 5.28], Q3 (5.28, 6.96], Q4 (6.96, 23.60]
[e]Reporting relative change in geometric mean BV per doubling of percent methylation
[f]Modeling B2 and B4 ER-α methylation simultaneously, reporting association with B2 ER-α methylation
[g]Modeling B2 and B4 ER-α methylation simultaneously, reporting association with B4 ER-α methylation
**p*<0.05, Wald test

Table 3 ER-α methylation at B4 is inversely associated with B4 FGV in Chilean girls enrolled in GOCS

Stage label	Relative change in geometric mean FGV (95% CI)		
	Model 1[a]	Model 2[b]	Model 3[c]
Tanner 2			
Quartiles[d]			
Q2	0.95 (0.80–1.12)	0.92 (0.77–1.10)	0.93 (0.77–1.11)
Q3	1.10 (0.92–1.31)	1.13 (0.94–1.37)	1.14 (0.95–1.37)
Q4	1.04 (0.88–1.25)	1.04 (0.87–1.24)	1.05 (0.88–1.27)
Linear model[e]			
	1.02 (0.95–1.10)	1.01 (0.93–1.09)	1.01 (0.94–1.09)
Tanner 4			
Quartiles[d]			
Q2	0.91 (0.80–1.03)	0.94 (0.83–1.07)	0.94 (0.83–1.08)
Q3	0.99 (0.87–1.12)	0.98 (0.86–1.11)	0.99 (0.87–1.13)
Q4	0.94 (0.83–1.07)	0.92 (0.81–1.04)	0.92 (0.81–1.05)
Linear model[e]			
	0.97 (0.92–1.03)	0.95 (0.90–1.01)	0.96 (0.90–1.01)
Tanner 2 (2 and 4)[f]			
Quartiles[d]			
Q2	0.93 (0.78–1.11)	0.92 (0.76–1.10)	0.92 (0.76–1.11)
Q3	1.14 (0.95–1.37)	1.20 (0.99–1.44)	1.20 (0.99–1.45)
Q4	1.02 (0.85–1.23)	1.05 (0.87–1.27)	1.05 (0.87–1.27)
Linear model[e]			
	1.02 (0.94–1.10)	1.01 (0.93–1.10)	1.02 (0.93–1.11)
Tanner 4 (2 and 4)[g]			
Quartiles[d]			
Q2	0.90 (0.76–1.06)	0.90 (0.76–1.07)	0.90 (0.76–1.07)
Q3	1.07 (0.89–1.28)	1.05 (0.87–1.26)	1.05 (0.87–1.27)
Q4	0.91 (0.76–1.09)	*0.81 (0.67–0.98)**	*0.81 (0.67–0.98)**
Linear model[e]			
	0.97 (0.90–1.05)	*0.91 (0.83–0.99)**	*0.91 (0.83–0.99)**

[a]Association with mean ER-α methylation adjusting for fat percentage at breast density measurement
[b]Association with cell composition corrected mean ER-α methylation adjusting for fat percentage at breast density measurement
[c]Model 2 additionally adjusted for age at breast density measurement and maternal education
[d]Quartiles for Tanner 2 methylation: Q1 [1.17, 4.05], Q2 (4.05, 6.04], Q3 (6.04, 8.85], Q4 (8.85, 29.30]; quartiles for Tanner 2 methylation after correction for cellular heterogeneity: Q1 [0.98, 3.49], Q2 (3.49, 5.03], Q3 (5.03, 7.34], Q4 (7.34, 24.8]. Quartiles for Tanner 4 methylation: Q1 [1.10, 4.27], Q2 (4.27, 7.05], Q3 (7.05, 9.37], Q4 (9.37, 32.00]; quartiles for Tanner 4 methylation after correction for cellular heterogeneity: Q1 [0.78, 3.37], Q2 (3.37, 5.28], Q3 (5.28, 6.96], Q4 (6.96, 23.60]
[e]Reporting relative change in geometric mean FGV per doubling of percent methylation
[f]Modeling B2 and B4 ER-α methylation simultaneously, reporting association with B2 ER-α methylation
[g]Modeling B2 and B4 ER-α methylation simultaneously, reporting association with B4 ER-α methylation
*p<0.05, Wald test

Table 4 ER-α methylation is not associated with B4 %FGV in Chilean girls enrolled in GOCS

Stage label	Relative change in geometric mean %FGV (95% CI)		
	Model 1[a]	Model 2[b]	Model 3[c]
Tanner 2			
Quartiles[d]			
Q2	1.04 (0.94–1.14)	1.03 (0.93–1.15)	1.04 (0.94–1.15)
Q3	1.05 (0.95–1.17)	1.08 (0.97–1.20)	1.08 (0.97–1.21)
Q4	1.01 (0.92–1.12)	1.01 (0.91–1.13)	1.02 (0.92–1.13)
Linear model[e]			
	1.00 (0.96–1.04)	1.00 (0.95–1.04)	1.00 (0.95–1.04)
Tanner 4			
Quartiles[d]			
Q2	1.01 (0.93–1.09)	0.99 (0.91–1.07)	0.99 (0.92–1.07)
Q3	0.96 (0.89–1.04)	0.99 (0.91–1.07)	1.00 (0.92–1.08)
Q4	1.01 (0.93–1.09)	1.00 (0.93–1.08)	1.01 (0.93–1.09)
Linear model[e]			
	0.99 (0.96–1.02)	1.00 (0.96–1.03)	1.00 (0.97–1.04)
Tanner 2 (2 and 4)[f]			
Quartiles[d]			
Q2	1.04 (0.93–1.15)	1.02 (0.91–1.14)	1.02 (0.91–1.14)
Q3	1.07 (0.95–1.19)	1.10 (0.99–1.23)	1.10 (0.98–1.23)
Q4	1.01 (0.91–1.13)	1.03 (0.92–1.15)	1.04 (0.93–1.16)
Linear model[e]			
	1.00 (0.95–1.05)	1.01 (0.96–1.06)	1.01 (0.96–1.06)
Tanner 4 (2 and 4)[g]			
Quartiles[d]			
Q2	0.97 (0.88–1.07)	0.95 (0.86–1.05)	0.96 (0.86–1.06)
Q3	0.98 (0.88–1.09)	1.02 (0.91–1.14)	1.02 (0.92–1.14)
Q4	1.02 (0.92–1.14)	0.96 (0.86–1.08)	0.96 (0.86–1.08)
Linear model[e]			
	1.00 (0.96 1.05)	0.99 (0.94–1.04)	0.99 (0.94–1.04)

[a]Association with mean ER-α methylation adjusting for fat percentage at breast density measurement
[b]Association with cell composition corrected mean ER-α methylation adjusting for fat percentage at breast density measurement
[c]Model 2 additionally adjusted for age at breast density measurement and maternal education
[d]Quartiles for Tanner 2 methylation: Q1 [1.17, 4.05], Q2 (4.05, 6.04], Q3 (6.04, 8.85], Q4 (8.85, 29.30]; quartiles for Tanner 2 methylation after correction for cellular heterogeneity: Q1 [0.98, 3.49], Q2 (3.49, 5.03], Q3 (5.03, 7.34], Q4 (7.34, 24.8]. Quartiles for Tanner 4 methylation: Q1 [1.10, 4.27], Q2 (4.27, 7.05], Q3 (7.05, 9.37], Q4 (9.37, 32.00]; quartiles for Tanner 4 methylation after correction for cellular heterogeneity: Q1 [0.78, 3.37], Q2 (3.37, 5.28], Q3 (5.28, 6.96], Q4 (6.96, 23.60]
[e]Reporting relative change in geometric mean %FGV per doubling of percent methylation
[f]Modeling B2 and B4 ER-α methylation simultaneously, reporting association with B2 ER-α methylation
[g]Modeling B2 and B4 ER-α methylation simultaneously, reporting association with B4 ER-α methylation

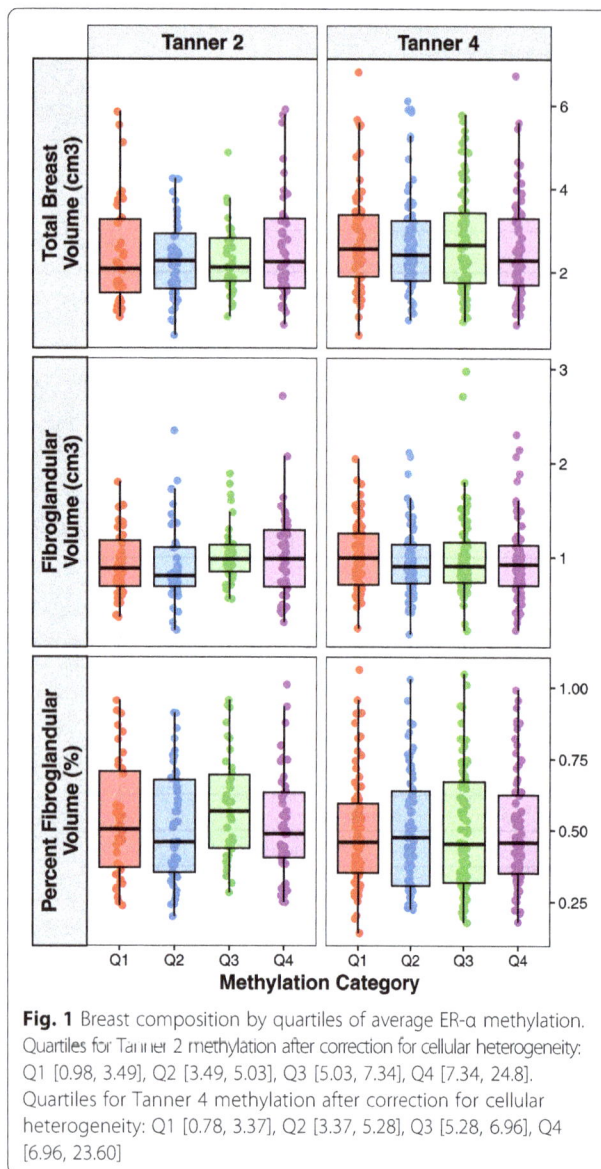

Fig. 1 Breast composition by quartiles of average ER-α methylation. Quartiles for Tanner 2 methylation after correction for cellular heterogeneity: Q1 [0.98, 3.49], Q2 [3.49, 5.03], Q3 [5.03, 7.34], Q4 [7.34, 24.8]. Quartiles for Tanner 4 methylation after correction for cellular heterogeneity: Q1 [0.78, 3.37], Q2 [3.37, 5.28], Q3 [5.28, 6.96], Q4 [6.96, 23.60]

Table 5 ER-α methylation is not associated with age at menarche in Chilean girls enrolled in GOCS

Stage label	Relative time to menarche (95% CI)		
	Model 1[a]	Model 2[b]	Model 3[c]
Tanner 2			
Quartiles[d]			
Q2	0.98 (0.96–1.00)	0.99 (0.97–1.02)	1.00 (0.97–1.03)
Q3	0.99 (0.97–1.01)	0.98 (0.95–1.00)	0.98 (0.95–1.00)
Q4	0.98 (0.96–1.00)	0.98 (0.96–1.01)	0.99 (0.96–1.02)
Linear model[e]			
	0.99 (0.98–1.00)	0.99 (0.98–1.00)	0.99 (0.98–1.01)
Tanner 4			
Quartiles[d]			
Q2	1.00 (0.98–1.02)	1.01 (0.98–1.03)	1.01 (0.98–1.03)
Q3	0.99 (0.97–1.02)	0.99 (0.97–1.01)	0.99 (0.97–1.01)
Q4	1.00 (0.97–1.02)	1.01 (0.98–1.03)	1.01 (0.98–1.03)
Linear model[e]			
	1.00 (0.99–1.01)	1.00 (0.99–1.01)	1.00 (0.99–1.01)
Tanner 2 (2 and 4)[f]			
Quartiles[d]			
Q2	0.98 (0.95–1.01)	0.99 (0.96–1.03)	1.00 (0.97–1.03)
Q3	0.99 (0.96–1.02)	0.98 (0.94–1.00)	0.97 (0.94–1.01)
Q4	0.98 (0.95–1.01)	0.98 (0.95–1.01)	0.98 (0.95–1.01)
Linear model[e]			
	0.99 (0.98–1.01)	0.99 (0.98–1.00)	0.99 (0.98–1.00)
Tanner 4 (2 and 4)[g]			
Quartiles[d]			
Q2	1.00 (0.97–1.03)	1.01 (0.98–1.04)	1.01 (0.98–1.04)
Q3	1.01 (0.98–1.04)	1.00 (0.97–1.03)	1.00 (0.97–1.03)
Q4	0.99 (0.96–1.03)	1.01 (0.98–1.05)	1.01 (0.98–1.05)
Linear model[e]			
	1.00 (0.99–1.02)	1.01 (0.99–1.02)	1.01 (0.99–1.02)

[a]Relative time to menarche associated with mean ER-α methylation estimated via accelerated failure time model
[b]Association with cell composition corrected mean ER-α methylation
[c]Model 2 additionally adjusted for fat percentage at breast density measurement and maternal education
[d]Quartiles for Tanner 2 methylation: Q1 [1.17, 4.05], Q2 [4.05, 6.04], Q3 [6.04, 8.85], Q4 [8.85, 29.30]; Quartiles for Tanner 2 methylation after correction for cellular heterogeneity: Q1 [0.98, 3.49], Q2 [3.49, 5.03], Q3 [5.03, 7.34], Q4 [7.34, 24.8]. Quartiles for Tanner 4 methylation: Q1 [1.10, 4.27], Q2 [4.27, 7.05], Q3 [7.05, 9.37], Q4 [9.37, 32.00]; Quartiles for Tanner 4 methylation after correction for cellular heterogeneity: Q1 [0.78, 3.37], Q2 [3.37, 5.28], Q3 [5.28, 6.96], Q4 [6.96, 23.60]
[e]Reporting relative time to menarche per doubling of percent methylation
[f]Modeling B2 and B4 ER-α methylation simultaneously, reporting association with B2 ER-α methylation
[g]Modeling B2 and B4 ER-α methylation simultaneously, reporting association with B4 ER-α methylation

Associations between ER-α methylation and breast composition are not modified by body fat percentage

We next evaluated whether the association between ER-α methylation and breast composition was modified by body fat percentage at B4. Percent body fat did not significantly modify the association between either B2 or B4 ER-α methylation and breast composition (results not shown). Likewise, percent body fat did not significantly interact with log-transformed ER-α methylation (%) to influence menarcheal age.

Exposure to EDCs may modify the association between B2 ER-α methylation and B4 breast composition

Similarly, we postulated exposure to exogenous chemicals that mimic or antagonize the body's endogenous hormones may modify the relation between ER-α methylation and breast composition. Urinary biomarkers of 26 phenols and phthalates were measured among 200 girls at B1 and B4; of these girls, DNA methylation results were available for 149 girls at B2 and 186 at B4. We previously observed no statistically significant difference in the influence of B1 and B4 phenol and phthalate concentrations on adolescent breast density in this population [publication accepted - in process]. Biomarker concentrations of monocarboxyisononyl phthalate (MCNP) significantly modified the influence of log-transformed B2 ER-α methylation on BV (likelihood ratio test (LRT), $p = 0.036$) and FGV (LRT, $p = 0.014$). The association between B2 ER-α methylation and FGV was also modified by average levels of both benzophenone-3 (LRT, $p = 0.023$) and methyl paraben urinary concentration (LRT, $p = 0.041$). In each of these cases, the impact of B2 ER-α methylation on either BV or FGV appeared to be in opposite directions for girls

with low biomarker concentrations compared to those with high biomarker concentrations (Fig. 2; Table 6). However, none of these associations, stratified by dichotomized EDC category, reached statistical significance (Table 6; $p > 0.05$). The influence of B4 ER-α methylation on the breast measurements was not significantly modified by any of the measured EDCs. While we did detect a significant interaction between propyl paraben and log-transformed B2 ER-α methylation on the timing of menarche, the interaction was no longer statistically significant after the exclusion of one influential observation. We note that these associations should be interpreted with caution given the limited power to account for the role of type-I error inflation.

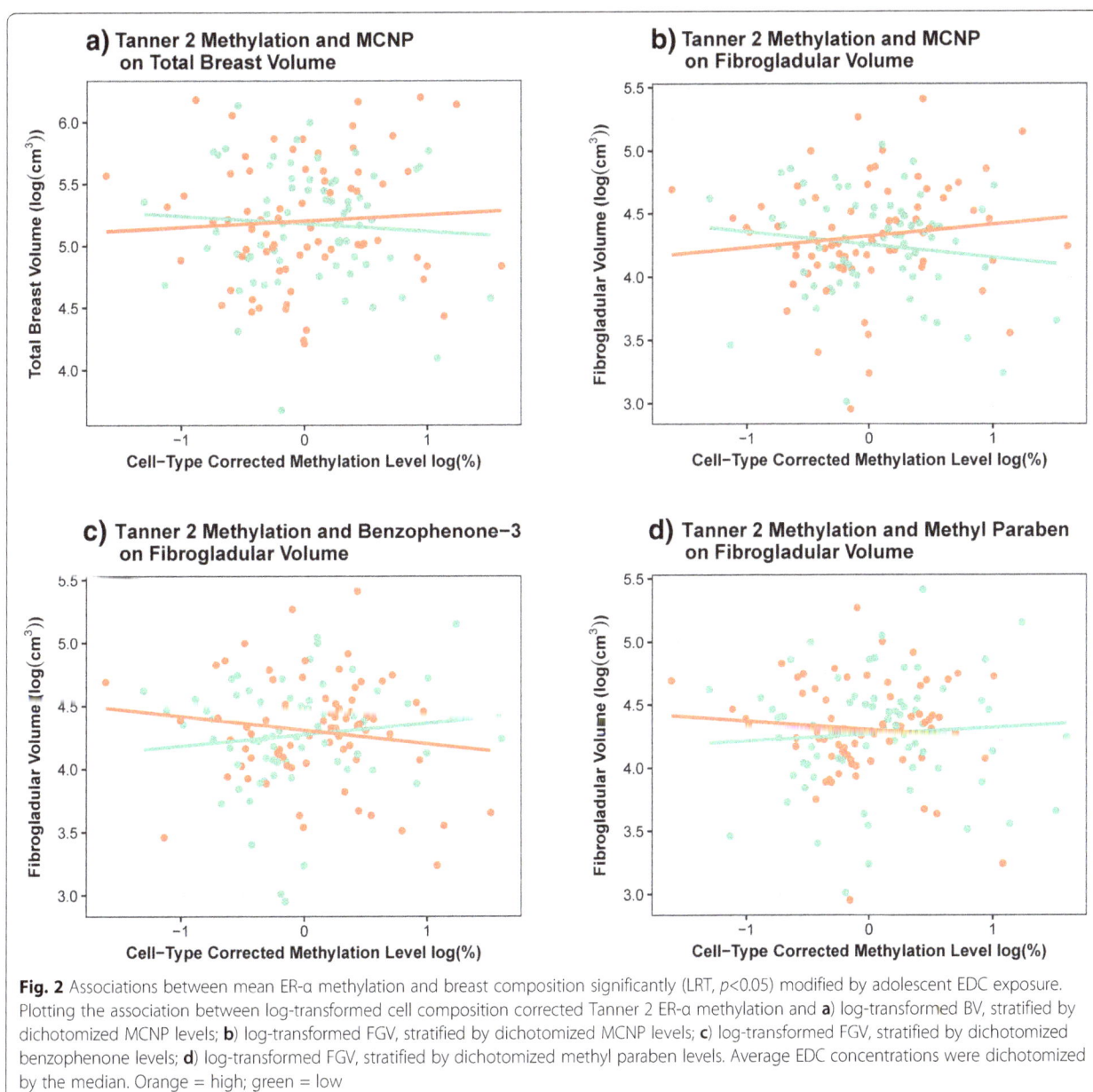

Fig. 2 Associations between mean ER-α methylation and breast composition significantly (LRT, $p<0.05$) modified by adolescent EDC exposure. Plotting the association between log-transformed cell composition corrected Tanner 2 ER-α methylation and **a)** log-transformed BV, stratified by dichotomized MCNP levels; **b)** log-transformed FGV, stratified by dichotomized MCNP levels; **c)** log-transformed FGV, stratified by dichotomized benzophenone levels; **d)** log-transformed FGV, stratified by dichotomized methyl paraben levels. Average EDC concentrations were dichotomized by the median. Orange = high; green = low

Table 6 Relative change in geometric mean B4 breast composition (95% CI) associated with a doubling of cell composition corrected mean Tanner 2 ER-α methylation that is significantly (LRT, p<0.05) modified by specific EDC biomarker concentrations

Outcome		EDC category[b]	
EDC	LRT p value[a]	High	Low
Total breast volume (cm³)			
MCNP	0.036	1.03 (0.93–1.14)	0.97 (0.87–1.09)
Fibroglandular volume (cm³)			
MCNP	0.014	1.06 (0.95–1.19)	0.93 (0.82–1.07)
Benzophenone-3	0.023	0.93 (0.82–1.05)	1.07 (0.94–1.21)
Methyl paraben	0.041	0.95 (0.83–1.09)	1.04 (0.93–1.17)

[a]Likelihood ratio test (LRT) p-value comparing a model for log transformed breast composition that includes log-transformed cell composition corrected mean ER-α methylation, log-transformed EDC biomarker concentration, fat percentage and age at breast density measurement, and maternal education, to a model that additionally includes an interaction between log-transformed methylation level and log transformed EDC biomarker concentration. Restricting to models for which the statistical interaction term significantly (p<0.05) improved model fit
[b]Relative change in geometric mean breast composition associated with a doubling of percent methylation, stratifying by dichotomized (by the median) EDC metabolite concentrations, adjusting for fat percentage and age at breast density measurement, and maternal education

Discussion

In this prospective cohort of Chilean girls, average B4 ER-α promoter DNA methylation was inversely associated with total BV and FGV measured at B4, adjusting for B2 ER-α methylation, cellular heterogeneity, and fat percentage at breast density measurement. Among individuals that were in the same quartile of B2 ER-α methylation, those in the lowest quartile of B4 ER-α methylation had greater BV and FGV than those in the highest quartile at B4. In other words, we observed a relative change in breast composition between groups that had the greatest divergence in ER-α methylation after B2. Due to similar associations with both total BV and FGV, epigenetic regulation of ER-α was not associated with %FGV in adolescence. Although ER-α has been reported to regulate reproductive development [13, 14], we did not observe it to be associated with menarcheal age. This could be attributed to the fact that endometrium growth is modulated by both ER-α and β [22, 23]. These findings were also not modified by adolescent body fat percentage, which suggests peripheral conversion of estrogen did not modulate the association between epigenetic regulation of its receptor and breast development at this stage. Lastly, we provide cursory evidence to support effect modification by exposure to specific EDCs on the relation between B2 ER-α methylation and B4 breast composition.

Promoter methylation of ER-α is highly correlated with its expression pattern [7, 8, 24, 25]. Accordingly, the observed inverse association between ER-α methylation and FGV and BV may reflect diminished sensitivity to estrogen-stimulated mammary epithelial cell proliferation and ductal growth [11, 12]. The association with ER-α methylation varied by developmental stage (B2 versus B4); only B4 ER-α methylation was associated with adolescent breast composition. Given B4 ER-α methylation and breast composition were measured concurrently, it is possible that decreased B4 ER-α methylation was a consequence of breast composition. However, mouse knockouts of *ERS1* suggest ER-α is a requisite for normal mammary gland and reproductive development [10, 26, 27]. Direct action of estrogen on its receptors initiates mammary epithelial cell proliferation by inducing expression of proliferative markers (e.g., Ki67). Subsequently, ER-α expression is reduced, while the proliferative markers remain expressed [10, 28], allowing for continued ductal growth. The inverse association at B4 is potentially due to continued downregulation of the *ESR1* gene. *ESR1* downregulation also correlates with the upregulation of inhibitory markers (e.g., TGF-β), which induce cell cycle arrest and may reduce epithelial proliferation in mammary tissue in the later stages of breast maturation [28–30]. Shepherd et al. report that the peak total FGV occurs at B4; hence, in this cohort, breast composition measurements were performed only at B4 [31]. Consequently, we cannot report on the association between B2 ER-α methylation and initiation of breast budding, beginning at B2. Perhaps we did not see an inverse association between B2 epigenetic regulation of ER-α and B4 breast composition due to the necessity for estrogen-stimulated mammary epithelial cell proliferation at the onset of ductal development. As breast maturation advances toward B4, however, there is a progressive reduction in ER-α expression associated with diminished mammary cell proliferation and enhanced ductal differentiation [28, 32]. Further, the B2 methylation assessment does not truly represent thelarche in this cohort and it is possible this may affect our analysis at B2.

We can only provide cursory evidence of the role of adolescent exposure to EDCs on breast development. However, exposure to high levels of EDCs appears to have differential effects on the relation between B2 ER-α methylation and BV and FGV. Among girls with high EDC exposure, we observed an inverse association between B2 methylation and FGV, suggesting that EDC exposure may decrease expression of ER-α and subsequently, FGV. The positive association between B2 ER-α methylation and BV among girls exposed to high levels of EDCs may be attributed to increased peripheral conversion of estrogen and subsequent increases in adiposity and BV.

Modulation of adolescent breast development by ER-α regulation could have future implications for breast cancer risk. Increased proportion of dense breast tissue (breast density, percent fibroglandular volume) in adults is one of the strongest and most consistent risk factors for breast cancer [33–35]. Peak breast density is postulated to be established during adolescence [36, 37], at which time the susceptibility of the developing mammary tissue to carcinogens is strongly enhanced. Correspondingly, Boyd and colleagues have speculated that women at high risk of breast cancer could be identified at an early age based on a breast density measurement [37]. The importance of pubertal development in breast cancer etiology is further highlighted by the inverse association between both age at breast bud development (thelarche) and age at menarche and breast cancer incidence [38–40]. In this study, epigenetic regulation of ER-α was not associated with age at menarche. This is perhaps due to our analysis of ER-α in blood, as pubertal timing is largely regulated by neuronal ER-α [41, 42]. The hypothalamic-pituitary-gonadal axis is also coordinated by many hormones (gonadotropic releasing hormone, testosterone, etc.) and endogenous and exogenous factors beyond estrogen [43], which may explain the lack of association between epigenetic regulation of ER-α and pubertal timing. Finally, it is possible this epigenetic signature is transient, instigating changes in pubertal breast development during a key developmental window of susceptibility for breast cancer. However, it is vital that ER-α methylation be assessed at additional time points throughout the life course to determine whether this methylation signature remains stable through post-pubertal mammary gland development.

In addition to addressing a major gap in our understanding of how ER-α regulation modifies adolescent breast development in humans, our study has a number of strengths. This investigation was conducted in a large, well-characterized longitudinal pediatric cohort. Assessment of ER-α methylation at two pubertal time points facilitated the identification of time-varying associations between epigenetic regulation of ER-α and breast composition. Measurement of body fat and urinary EDC biomarkers enabled examination of endogenous and exogenous modifiers of hormone regulation and potential impact on breast development. However, despite our relatively large sample size, after adjusting for multiple testing, we had limited power to identify significant interactions between EDC biomarker concentrations and ER-α methylation on breast composition. Another limitation of this study was the assessment of ER-α methylation in blood rather than breast tissue; however, in a pediatric cohort, biopsies of the target tissue (breast) are not feasible. Gene-specific methylation profiles are mildly correlated among whole blood and breast tumor samples; however, blood-derived DNA typically displays a lower methylation frequency for particular genes when compared to breast or tumor tissues [44, 45]. This limits the potential for ER-α blood DNA promoter methylation to serve as a surrogate marker of adolescent breast tissue methylation. However, as blood DNA methylation is currently being explored as a marker of breast cancer risk and breast tumor development [46], the blood epigenetic profile of ER-α may serve as a marker of adolescent breast composition. Additionally, due to our restriction to a Chilean cohort, we also note that the observed associations may not be generalizable to all populations as race/ethnicity may be associated with differential methylation profiles [47] and/or varied timing of breast maturation [48]. Finally, we do not yet know which of these girls may develop breast cancer in their lifetime, and thus, we cannot conclude that adolescent breast composition or the regulation of ER-α is predictive of breast cancer development in adulthood.

Conclusion

Our study outlines the potential influence of ER-α epigenetic regulation on breast development in humans. Specifically, we identified an inverse association between increased ER-α DNA promoter methylation and total BV and FGV at B4 in Chilean girls. Future work in this research area should consider other endogenous and exogenous factors (e.g., dietary patterns) influencing adolescent ER-α methylation and implications for breast composition. To better characterize the role of ER-α in initiating breast development, researchers should also consider the analysis of the ER-α methylation profile and expression pattern at B1, prior to the onset of mammary gland development. Further, as breast cancer typically develops later in life, researchers should consider assessing ER-α methylation at later stages of development and during periods of significant hormonal shifts (B5, during pregnancy, and prior to menopause). Finally, it is important to note that follow-up proof-of-concept studies in humans and animal models are needed to verify our findings. For example, in vitro and/or in vivo experimental analyses should be applied to elucidate the feedback relation between estrogen levels and epigenetic regulation of ER-α during this critical window of breast development in adolescence. In addition, it will be important for future studies to assess the role of other biological pathways and genetic components, which may be modified by environmental factors and associated with pubertal development. In conclusion, this study greatly expands upon the current literature surrounding the role of ER-α in breast development by providing evidence in humans to support ER-α as a key modifier of pubertal breast composition and a potential risk marker for breast cancer in adulthood.

Methods

Study population

This study includes a subcohort of 429 Chilean girls enrolled in the Growth and Obesity Cohort Study (GOCS) with blood samples collected at B2 and/or at B4. Details of GOCS have been previously described [49]. Briefly, 1190 singleton children born at term (37–42 weeks) were enrolled in the study in 2006 when they were 2.6–4.0 years of age. All participants had a birth weight between 2500 and 4500 g. Children with any physical, medical, or endocrine diseases that might impact growth or puberty were excluded from the study. Children were physically assessed annually from 2006 to 2010 at the Institute of Nutrition and Food Technology Health Clinic in Santiago, Chile. From 2011 onward, the participants were physically assessed every 6 months. GOCS children were recruited from public nursery schools and are thus representative of low- to middle-income Chilean children from the southeast area of Santiago. The study protocol was approved by the Ethics Committee of the Institute of Nutrition and Food Technology, University of Chile. All parents and/or legal guardians gave signed informed consent prior to the data collection and children gave their assent.

Dense breast tissue assessment

Assessment of breast density at B4 in GOCS has been previously described [36]. Briefly, breast development was assessed visually and by palpation by a single female trained dietitian (kappa with pediatric endocrinologist = 0.9) at clinical visits approximately every 6 months, beginning in 2009, using Tanner's rating scale [50, 51]. At the first B4 visit, breast fibroglandular volume (FGV; cm^3), total breast volume (BV; cm^3), and percentage of fibroglandular volume (%FGV = FGV/BV × 100) were measured via dual-energy X-ray absorptiometry (DXA) in the left and right breasts. DXA has been previously validated and correlates strongly with mammography [31, 52, 53]. The dosage of radiation exhibited by this assessment is extremely low, lower than that received during a transcontinental flight, limiting any significant health risks associated with this X-ray method [54]. Each breast was scanned using GE iDXA system software (version 13.6, GE Healthcare, Madison, WI, USA). Breast composition was derived from a two-compartment model of adipose and fibroglandular tissues using the software developed by Dr. Shepherd and colleagues, Department of Radiology and Biomedical Imaging, University of California, San Francisco (version 5). A quality control phantom that contained reference breast density materials was scanned throughout the study to ensure stable calibration. Values from the left and right breasts are averaged for all analyses.

Biospecimen collection

Fasting blood samples were collected at B2 and B4 for ER-α methylation analysis. DNA was extracted from the blood leukocytes using the QIAamp DNA Blood Mini Kit (Qiagen). Fasting spot urine samples were collected

between 10 AM and 12 PM in polypropylene sterile cups and were immediately vortexed and aliquoted. They were collected at breast Tanner stages 1 (B1) and B4 for analysis of exposure to EDCs.

ER-α methylation analysis
Polymerase chain reaction (PCR)

Genomic DNA was treated with bisulphite salt using the EZ DNA Methylation-Gold kit (Zymo Research, Cat. No. D5007) according to the manufacturer's protocol. DNA was amplified in 20-μl PCR reactions, containing 10 μl of Hot StarTaq Master Mix Kit (Qiagen, Cat. No 203446), 150 ng of each primer, and ~ 20 ng modified DNA. PCR was performed with one cycle of 95 °C for 15 min, 40 cycles of 95 °C for 30 s, 57–63 °C for 30 s, and 72 °C for 30 s, followed by one cycle of 72 °C for 10 min. The reverse primer included a 5′-biotin label to allow subsequent analysis by pyrosequencing. Primer sequences can be found in (Additional file 1: Table S1). PCRs were performed in duplicate using 96-well plates. Each PCR plate contained the participants' DNA samples, as well as three dH_2O samples as non-template controls and three samples with known methylation status as positive controls.

Pyrosequencing

Pyrosequencing was performed on a PyroMark Q24 MD pyrosequencer (Qiagen, Cat. No 9001514) according to the manufacturer's recommendations. The primers were designed using the primer design program "PSQ assay" (Biotage), using the ER-α gene sequence that was obtained from the GenBank entry on NCBI (Additional file 1: Table S1).

Assay validation was carried out on samples of known methylation status, using the EpiTect Control DNA and Control DNA Set (Qiagen, Cat. No. 59568). All pyrosequencing analyses were performed in duplicate. If the duplicates of the individual samples showed a difference < 5% of methylation, the average methylation of the two measurements was used for further analyses. When the difference was > 5%, a third measurement was performed. Due to the high correlation in percent methylation across the 10 interrogated CpG loci, ER-α methylation was summarized by average methylation across pyrosequenced loci 1–8. Loci 9 and 10 were not included in this average due to low resolution at the end of the sequencing reads in approximately 50% of the samples. Average ER-α methylation independent of blood composition was estimated by regressing log-transformed ER-α methylation on the proportion of monocytes, basophils, eosinophils, neutrophils, and lymphocytes, stratified by breast Tanner stage at ER-α methylation measurement. The exponentiated residuals were used in subsequent models that we note were corrected for cellular heterogeneity.

Endocrine-disrupting chemicals

Urinary biomarker concentrations of 26 phenols and phthalates were measured among a subset of 200 GOCS girls at breast B1 and B4. EDC assays were performed at the Centers for Disease Control and Prevention (CDC) National Center for Environmental Health Laboratory using previously described analytical methods [55, 56]. The analysis of blinded specimens by the CDC laboratory was determined not to constitute engagement in human subjects' research. Concentrations below the limit of detection (LOD) were given an imputed value equal to LOD/sqrt(2). EDC biomarker concentrations (ng/ml) were corrected for specific gravity. Dilution adjustment was performed using the formula $P_c = P[(1.015 - 1)/(SG - 1)]$, where P_c is the specific gravity-corrected biomarker concentration, P is the observed biomarker concentration, SG is the specific gravity of the urine sample, and 1.015 is the median SG of the study population [55–58]. The analysis was restricted to the subset of 21 EDCs for which biomarker concentrations were above the LOD in at least 75% of the samples. For this study, EDC measurements were averaged across B1 and B4.

Age at menarche

Prior to the onset of B4, girls were asked to report their first menstrual bleeding at each 6-month visit. After achieving B4, girls were contacted by study dietitians every 3 months to survey whether the girl had reached menarche. During this phone interview, a questionnaire was used to differentiate menarche from other potential causes of vaginal bleeding, such as vaginal infection, urinary infection, or trauma. Longitudinal follow-up of participants enabled the confirmation of menarche onset.

Covariates

Additional covariates included in this analysis were age at methylation assessment (B2 and B4), body fat percentage, and maternal education. All additional covariates were measured at B4. Maternal education status was self-reported by mothers at an in-clinic study visit and categorized as secondary or post-secondary for this study. Compared with BMI, body fat percentage is a more precise measurement of adolescent fat distribution. Fat percentage was estimated at each visit using Tanita-BC-418 MA bioelectrical impedance measurements (Tanita-Corporation, Tokyo, Japan), according to the manufacturer's guidelines and at a measurement frequency of 50 kHz (accuracy 0.1 kg) [59].

Statistical analyses

All breast measurements were log-transformed prior to analysis. Linear models were used to estimate the association between ER-α methylation and breast composition, adjusting for fat percentage at breast density measurement. We considered models additionally adjusted for cellular heterogeneity and further adjusted for age at breast density measurement and maternal education. We independently modeled the association between B2 average ER-α methylation and breast composition ($N = 177$; $N = 164$ correcting for cellular heterogeneity), as well as the association between average B4 ER-α methylation and breast composition ($N = 329$; $N = 303$ correcting for cellular heterogeneity). To identify time-dependent associations between ER-α methylation and breast composition, we also simultaneously modeled the influence of both B2 ER-α methylation and B4 ER-α methylation on these breast measurements ($N = 161$; $N = 142$ correcting for cellular heterogeneity). ER-α methylation was modeled both as quartiles and continuously as log-transformed percent methylation. Estimated associations and 95% confidence intervals (CI) between ER-α methylation and breast measurements were exponentiated to provide the percent change in geometric mean breast density measurement. When modeling methylation continuously, we report the percent change in geometric mean breast density measurement given a doubling in percent methylation. Accelerated failure time models were used to assess the influence of ER-α methylation on time to menarche, assuming a Weibull distribution. For incident cases, survival time was the age at menarche, estimated based on the time between the self-reported date of first menses and date of birth. Survival time for right-censored individuals was the age at last clinic visit, based on the time between the date of last visit and date of birth. Similar to the breast measurement models, time to menarche was modeled as a function of B2 ER-α methylation and B4 ER-α methylation both separately and together, adjusting for cellular heterogeneity. To assess whether B4 fat percentage significantly modified the association between log-transformed B2 ER-α methylation and breast measurement, we compared the fit of a model with and without an interaction term between these two dependent variables (likelihood ratio test (LRT)), adjusting for cellular heterogeneity. We similarly evaluated whether there was a statistically significant interaction between log-transformed average EDC biomarker concentration and log-transformed B2 ER-α methylation on breast measurement, adjusting for cellular heterogeneity and fat percentage. Each biomarker was modeled separately. Analogously, we analyzed effect modification by both fat percentage and EDC exposure on the association between B4 ER-α methylation and breast measurement, as well as on the impact of B2 ER-α methylation and B4 ER-α methylation on time to menarche, respectively. Among models significantly modified by EDC biomarker concentration (LRT, $p < 0.05$), the association between log-transformed ER-α methylation and breast measurement is reported stratified by dichotomized EDC level (high vs low relative to the median). All analyses were performed using R version 3.4.1 and visualized using ggplot2.

Abbreviations

%FGV: Percent fibroglandular volume; B1–B4: Breast Tanner stages 1–4; BMI: Body mass index; BV: Breast volume; CDC: Center for Disease Control; DXA: Dual-energy X-ray absorptiometry; EDC: Endocrine-disrupting chemical; ER-α: Estrogen receptor-alpha; FGV: Fibroglandular volume; GOCS: Growth and Obesity Cohort Study; LOD: Limit of detection; LRT: Likelihood ratio test; UTR: Untranslated region

Funding

This work was supported by the Public Health Service grant R01CA158313 from the National Cancer Institute, National Institutes of Health, US Department of Health and Human Services (to KBM). This publication was also partially made possible by the Breast Cancer and the Environment Research Program (BCERP) award number U01ES026130 from the National Institute of Environmental Health Sciences (NIEHS) and the National Cancer Institute (NCI), NIH, DHHS (to KBM). During preparation and submission of this manuscript, LTS was supported by a T-32 training grant 5T32CA009142-37 from the National Cancer Institute, National Institutes of Health.

Authors' contributions

AMB, JS, and KBM designed the research plan; AMB and KK conducted the statistical analyses; AMB and LTS interpreted the results and co-wrote the manuscript; SDV conducted DNA methylation assays; AP, and VM acquired the clinical data analyzed in this study; JLS organized and processed the biospecimens; JS oversaw the breast composition measurements and interpretation; AMB, LTS, SDV, VM, AP, JLS, JS, CC, and KBM provided critical revision of the manuscript for important intellectual content; AMB, LTS, and KBM had primary responsibility for final content. All authors read and approved the final manuscript.

Author details

[1]Department of Epidemiology, Fielding School of Public Health, University of California, Los Angeles 90095, USA. [2]Department of Biostatistics, Fielding School of Public Health, University of California, Los Angeles 90095, USA. [3]Institute for Prevention and Cancer Epidemiology, Faculty of Medicine and Medical Center, University of Freiburg, Freiburg im Breisgau, Germany. [4]Institute of Nutrition and Food Technology, University of Chile, Santiago, Chile. [5]Department of Nutrition, Diabetes and Metabolism, School of Medicine, Pontificia Universidad Católica de Chile, Santiago, Chile. [6]Population Sciences in the Pacific Program, University of Hawaii Cancer Center, Honolulu, HI 96813, USA.

References

1. Anderson E. The role of oestrogen and progesterone receptors in human mammary development and tumorigenesis. Breast Cancer Res. 2002;4(5): 197–201.
2. Hagrass HA, Pasha HF, Ali AM. Estrogen receptor alpha (ERalpha) promoter methylation status in tumor and serum DNA in Egyptian breast cancer patients. Gene. 2014;552(1):81–6.
3. Williams KE, Anderton DL, Lee MP, Pentecost BT, Arcaro KF. High-density array analysis of DNA methylation in tamoxifen-resistant breast cancer cell lines. Epigenetics. 2014;9(2):297–307.
4. Early Breast Cancer Trialists' Collaborative G, Davies C, Godwin J, Gray R, Clarke M, Cutter D, Darby S, McGale P, Pan HC, Taylor C, et al. Relevance of breast cancer hormone receptors and other factors to the efficacy of adjuvant tamoxifen: patient-level meta-analysis of randomised trials. Lancet. 2011;378(9793):771–84.
5. Mao X, Qiao Z, Fan C, Guo A, Yu X, Jin F. Expression pattern and methylation of estrogen receptor alpha in breast intraductal proliferative lesions. Oncol Rep. 2016;36(4):1868–74.
6. Ung M, Ma X, Johnson KC, Christensen BC, Cheng C. Effect of estrogen receptor alpha binding on functional DNA methylation in breast cancer. Epigenetics. 2014;9(4):523–32.
7. Lapidus RG, Ferguson AT, Ottaviano YL, Parl FF, Smith HS, Weitzman SA, Baylin SB, Issa JP, Davidson NE. Methylation of estrogen and progesterone receptor gene 5′ CpG islands correlates with lack of estrogen and progesterone receptor gene expression in breast tumors. Clin Cancer Res. 1996;2(5):805–10.
8. Ottaviano YL, Issa JP, Parl FF, Smith HS, Baylin SB, Davidson NE. Methylation of the estrogen receptor gene CpG island marks loss of estrogen receptor expression in human breast cancer cells. Cancer Res. 1994;54(10):2552–5.
9. Saji S, Jensen EV, Nilsson S, Rylander T, Warner M, Gustafsson JA. Estrogen receptors alpha and beta in the rodent mammary gland. Proc Natl Acad Sci U S A. 2000;97(1):337–42.
10. Cheng G, Weihua Z, Warner M, Gustafsson JA. Estrogen receptors ER alpha and ER beta in proliferation in the rodent mammary gland. Proc Natl Acad Sci U S A. 2004;101(11):3739–46.
11. Mueller SO, Clark JA, Myers PH, Korach KS. Mammary gland development in adult mice requires epithelial and stromal estrogen receptor alpha. Endocrinology. 2002;143(6):2357–65.
12. Haslam SZ, Woodward TL. Host microenvironment in breast cancer development: epithelial-cell-stromal-cell interactions and steroid hormone action in normal and cancerous mammary gland. Breast Cancer Res. 2003;5(4):208–15.
13. Sinkevicius KW, Woloszyn K, Laine M, Jackson KS, Greene GL, Woodruff TK, Burdette JE. Characterization of the ovarian and reproductive abnormalities in prepubertal and adult estrogen non-responsive estrogen receptor alpha knock-in (ENERKI) mice. Steroids. 2009;74(12):913–9.
14. Gieske MC, Kim HJ, Legan SJ, Koo Y, Krust A, Chambon P, Ko C. Pituitary gonadotroph estrogen receptor-alpha is necessary for fertility in females. Endocrinology. 2008;149(1):20–7.
15. Gomes-Rochette NF, Souza LS, Tommasi BO, Pedrosa DF, Eis SR, Fin IDF, Vieira FLH, Graceli JB, Rangel LBA, Silva IV. Association of PvuII and XbaI polymorphisms on estrogen receptor alpha (ESR1) gene to changes into serum lipid profile of postmenopausal women: effects of aging, body mass index and breast cancer incidence. PLoS One. 2017;12(2). https://doi.org/10.1371/journal.pone.0169266.
16. Souza MA, Fonseca Ade M, Bagnoli VR, Barros N, Neves EM, Moraes SD, Hortense VH, Soares JM, Baracat EC. The expression of the estrogen receptor in obese patients with high breast density (HBD). Gynecol Endocrinol. 2014;30(1):78–80.
17. Tchatchou S, Jung A, Hemminki K, Sutter C, Wappenschmidt B, Bugert P, Weber BH, Niederacher D, Arnold N, Varon-Mateeva R, et al. A variant affecting a putative miRNA target site in estrogen receptor (ESR) 1 is associated with breast cancer risk in premenopausal women. Carcinogenesis. 2009;30(1):59–64.
18. Siiteri PK. Adipose tissue as a source of hormones. Am J Clin Nutr. 1987;45(1 Suppl):277–82.
19. Markey CM, Luque EH, Munoz De Toro M, Sonnenschein C, Soto AM. In utero exposure to bisphenol A alters the development and tissue organization of the mouse mammary gland. Biol Reprod. 2001;65(4):1215–23.
20. Rudel R. Predicting health effects of exposures to compounds with estrogenic activity: methodological issues. Environ Health Perspect. 1997; 105(Suppl 3):655–63.
21. Kuiper GG, Lemmen JG, Carlsson B, Corton JC, Safe SH, van der Saag PT, van der Burg B, Gustafsson JA. Interaction of estrogenic chemicals and phytoestrogens with estrogen receptor beta. Endocrinology. 1998; 139(10):4252–63.
22. Valladares F, Frias I, Baez D, Garcia C, Lopez FJ, Fraser JD, Rodriguez Y, Reyes R, Diaz-Flores L, Bello AR. Characterization of estrogen receptors alpha and beta in uterine leiomyoma cells. Fertil Steril. 2006;86(6):1736–43.

23. Collins F, MacPherson S, Brown P, Bombail V, Williams AR, Anderson RA, Jabbour HN, Saunders PT. Expression of oestrogen receptors, ERalpha, ERbeta, and ERbeta variants, in endometrial cancers and evidence that prostaglandin F may play a role in regulating expression of ERalpha. BMC Cancer. 2009;9:330.

24. Tsuboi K, Nagatomo T, Gohno T, Higuchi T, Sasaki S, Fujiki N, Kurosumi M, Takei H, Yamaguchi Y, Niwa T, et al. Single CpG site methylation controls estrogen receptor gene transcription and correlates with hormone therapy resistance. J Steroid Biochem Mol Biol. 2017;171:209-17. https://doi.org/10.1016/j.jsbmb.2017.04.001.

25. Yoshida T, Eguchi H, Nakachi K, Tanimoto K, Higashi Y, Suemasu K, Iino Y, Morishita Y, Hayashi S. Distinct mechanisms of loss of estrogen receptor alpha gene expression in human breast cancer: methylation of the gene and alteration of trans-acting factors. Carcinogenesis. 2000;21(12):2193-201.

26. Tekmal RR, Liu YG, Nair HB, Jones J, Perla RP, Lubahn DB, Korach KS, Kirma N. Estrogen receptor alpha is required for mammary development and the induction of mammary hyperplasia and epigenetic alterations in the aromatase transgenic mice. J Steroid Biochem Mol Biol. 2005;95(1–5):9-15.

27. Watanabe J, Sasajima N, Aramaki A, Sonoyama K. Consumption of fructo-oligosaccharide reduces 2,4-dinitrofluorobenzene-induced contact hypersensitivity in mice. Brit J Nutr. 2008;100(2):339-46.

28. Russo J, Ao X, Grill C, Russo IH. Pattern of distribution of cells positive for estrogen receptor alpha and progesterone receptor in relation to proliferating cells in the mammary gland. Breast Cancer Res Treat. 1999;53(3):217-27.

29. Ewan KB, Oketch-Rabah HA, Ravani SA, Shyamala G, Moses HL, Barcellos-Hoff MH. Proliferation of estrogen receptor-alpha-positive mammary epithelial cells is restrained by transforming growth factor-beta1 in adult mice. Am J Pathol. 2005;167(2):409-17.

30. Band AM, Laiho M. Crosstalk of TGF-beta and estrogen receptor signaling in breast cancer. J Mammary Gland Biol Neoplasia. 2011;16(2):109-15.

31. Shepherd JA, Malkov S, Fan B, Laidevant A, Novotny R, Maskarinec G. Breast density assessment in adolescent girls using dual-energy X-ray absorptiometry: a feasibility study. Cancer Epidemiol Biomark Prev. 2008;17(7):1709-13.

32. Javed A, Lteif A. Development of the human breast. Semin Plast Surg. 2013;27(1):5-12.

33. Yaghjyan L, Colditz GA, Collins LC, Schnitt SJ, Rosner B, Vachon C, Tamimi RM. Mammographic breast density and subsequent risk of breast cancer in postmenopausal women according to tumor characteristics. J Natl Cancer Inst. 2011;103(15):1179-89.

34. Shepherd JA, Kerlikowske K, Ma L, Duewer F, Fan B, Wang J, Malkov S, Vittinghoff E, Cummings SR. Volume of mammographic density and risk of breast cancer. Cancer Epidemiol Biomark Prev. 2011;20(7):1473-82.

35. Harris HR, Tamimi RM, Willett WC, Hankinson SE, Michels KB. Body size across the life course, mammographic density, and risk of breast cancer. Am J Epidemiol. 2011;174(8):909-18.

36. Gaskins AJ, Pereira A, Quintiliano D, Shepherd JA, Uauy R, Corvalan C, Michels KB. Dairy intake in relation to breast and pubertal development in Chilean girls. Am J Clin Nutr. 2017;105(5):1166-75.

37. Boyd NF, Martin LJ, Bronskill M, Yaffe MJ, Duric N, Minkin S. Breast tissue composition and susceptibility to breast cancer. J Natl Cancer Inst. 2010;102(10):1224-37.

38. Swerdlow AJ, De Stavola BL, Floderus B, Holm NV, Kaprio J, Verkasalo PK, Mack T. Risk factors for breast cancer at young ages in twins: an international population-based study. J Natl Cancer Inst. 2002;94(16):1238-46.

39. MacMahon B, Cole P, Lin TM, Lowe CR, Mirra AP, Ravnihar B, Salber EJ, Valaoras VG, Yuasa S. Age at first birth and breast cancer risk. Bull World Health Organ. 1970;43(2):209-21.

40. Collaborative Group on Hormonal Factors in Breast C. Menarche, menopause, and breast cancer risk: individual participant meta-analysis, including 118 964 women with breast cancer from 117 epidemiological studies. Lancet Oncol. 2012;13(11):1141-51.

41. Mayer C, Acosta-Martinez M, Dubois SL, Wolfe A, Radovick S, Boehm U, Levine JE. Timing and completion of puberty in female mice depend on estrogen receptor alpha-signaling in kisspeptin neurons. Proc Natl Acad Sci U S A. 2010;107(52):22693-8.

42. Sano K, Nakata M, Musatov S, Morishita M, Sakamoto T, Tsukahara S, Ogawa S. Pubertal activation of estrogen receptor alpha in the medial amygdala is essential for the full expression of male social behavior in mice. Proc Natl Acad Sci U S A. 2016;113(27):7632-7.

43. Peper JS, Brouwer RM, van Leeuwen M, Schnack HG, Boomsma DI, Kahn RS, Hulshoff Pol HE. HPG-axis hormones during puberty: a study on the association with hypothalamic and pituitary volumes. Psychoneuroendocrinology. 2010;35(1):133-40.

44. Cho YH, Yazici H, Wu HC, Terry MB, Gonzalez K, Qu MX, Dalay N, Santella RM. Aberrant promoter hypermethylation and genomic hypomethylation in tumor, adjacent normal tissues and blood from breast cancer patients. Anticancer Res. 2010;30(7):2489-96.

45. Schwarzenbach H, Pantel K. Circulating DNA as biomarker in breast cancer. Breast Cancer Res. 2015;17(1):136.

46. Terry MB, McDonald JA, Wu HC, Eng S, Santella RM. Epigenetic biomarkers of breast cancer risk: across the breast cancer prevention continuum. Adv Exp Med Biol. 2016;882:33-68.

47. Galanter JM, Gignoux CR, Oh SS, Torgerson D, Pino-Yanes M, Thakur N, Eng C, Hu D, Huntsman S, Farber HJ, et al. Differential methylation between ethnic sub-groups reflects the effect of genetic ancestry and environmental exposures. elife. 2017;6. https://doi.org/10.7554/eLife.20532.

48. Biro FM, Greenspan LC, Galvez MP, Pinney SM, Teitelbaum S, Windham GC, Deardorff J, Herrick RL, Succop PA, Hiatt RA, et al. Onset of breast development in a longitudinal cohort. Pediatrics. 2013;132(6):1019-27.

49. Gonzalez L, Corvalan C, Pereira A, Kain J, Garmendia ML, Uauy R. Early adiposity rebound is associated with metabolic risk in 7-year-old children. Int J Obes. 2014;38(10):1299-304.

50. Tanner J. Growth at adolescence, 2nd ed. Oxford: Blackwell; 1962.

51. Pereira A, Garmendia ML, Gonzalez D, Kain J, Mericq V, Uauy R, Corvalan C. Breast bud detection: a validation study in the Chilean growth obesity cohort study. BMC Womens Health. 2014;14:96.

52. Shepherd JA, Herve L, Landau J, Fan B, Kerlikowske K, Cummings SR. Clinical comparison of a novel breast DXA technique to mammographic density. Med Phys. 2006;33(5):1490-8.

53. Maskarinec G, Morimoto Y, Daida Y, Laidevant A, Malkov S, Shepherd JA, Novotny R. Comparison of breast density measured by dual energy X-ray absorptiometry with mammographic density among adult women in Hawaii. Cancer Epidemiol. 2011;35(2):188-93.

54. Adiotomre E, Summers L, Allison A, Walters SJ, Digby M, Broadley P, Lang I, Morrison G, Bishop N, Arundel P, et al. Diagnostic accuracy of DXA compared to conventional spine radiographs for the detection of vertebral fractures in children. Eur Radiol. 2017;27(5):2188-99.

55. Ye X, Kuklenyik Z, Needham LL, Calafat AM. Automated on-line column-switching HPLC-MS/MS method with peak focusing for the determination of nine environmental phenols in urine. Anal Chem. 2005;77(16):5407-13.

56. Silva MJ, Samandar E, Preau JL Jr, Reidy JA, Needham LL, Calafat AM. Quantification of 22 phthalate metabolites in human urine. J Chromatogr B Analyt Technol Biomed Life Sci. 2007;860(1):106-12.

57. Boeniger MF, Lowry LK, Rosenberg J. Interpretation of urine results used to assess chemical-exposure with emphasis on creatinine adjustments - a review. Am Ind Hyg Assoc J. 1993;54(10):615-27.

58. Teass AW, Biagini RE, DeBord G, Hull RD. Application of Biological Monitoring Methods. NIOSH Man Anal Method. Cincinnati: National Institute for Occupational Safety and Health Division of Physical Sciences and Engineering; 1998.

59. Cediel G, Corvalan C, Aguirre C, de Romana DL, Uauy R. Serum 25-Hydroxyvitamin D associated with indicators of body fat and insulin resistance in prepubertal Chilean children. Int J Obes. 2016;40(1):147-52.

18

Loss of DNA methylation is related to increased expression of miR-21 and miR-146b in papillary thyroid carcinoma

Isabella Maria Dias Payão Ortiz[1†], Mateus Camargo Barros-Filho[1†], Mariana Bisarro dos Reis[1], Caroline Moraes Beltrami[1], Fabio Albuquerque Marchi[1], Hellen Kuasne[1], Luísa Matos do Canto[1,2], Julia Bette Homem de Mello[1], Cecilie Abildgaard[2], Clóvis Antônio Lopes Pinto[3], Luiz Paulo Kowalski[4] and Silvia Regina Rogatto[2*]

Abstract

Background: DNA methylation in miRNA genes has been reported as a mechanism that may cause dysregulation of mature miRNAs and consequently impact the gene expression. This mechanism is largely unstudied in papillary thyroid carcinomas (PTC).

Methods: To identify differentially methylated miRNA-encoding genes, we performed global methylation analysis (Illumina 450 K), integrative analysis (TCGA database), data confirmation (pyrosequencing and RT-qPCR), and functional assays.

Results: Methylation analysis revealed 27 differentially methylated miRNA genes. The integrative analyses pointed out miR-21 and miR-146b as potentially regulated by methylation (hypomethylation and increased expression). DNA methylation and expression patterns of miR-21 and miR-146b were confirmed as altered, as well as seven of 452 mRNAs targets were down-expressed. The combined methylation and expression levels of miR-21 and miR-146b showed potential to discriminate malignant from benign lesions (91–96% sensitivity and 96–97% specificity). An increased expression of miR-146b due to methylation loss was detected in the TPC1 cell line. The miRNA mimic transfection highlighted putative target mRNAs.

Conclusions: The increased expression of miR-21 and miR-146b due to loss of DNA methylation in PTC resulted in the disruption of the transcription machinery and biological pathways. These miRNAs are potential diagnostic biomarkers, and these findings provide support for future development of targeted therapies.

Keywords: DNA methylation, microRNA, miR-146b, miR-21, Papillary thyroid, Carcinoma

Background

Papillary thyroid carcinoma (PTC) is the most frequent thyroid malignant neoplasm and is responsible for the increased incidence of thyroid cancer worldwide [1, 2]. The main genetic alterations described in PTC are *BRAF* and *RAS* mutations and *RET* rearrangements [3]. Furthermore, *TERT* promoter mutations have been associated with more aggressive thyroid carcinomas [4, 5], especially in tumors harboring *BRAF* mutations [4].

DNA methylation and microRNA (miRNA) are events capable to regulate the expression of genes related to cancer development, as previously reported in PTC [6–9]. A recent study conducted by our group identified DNA methylation alterations related to prognosis in well differentiated thyroid lesions [10]. Using a robust methylation platform in 141 thyroid samples (non-neoplastic tissue, benign lesions, and carcinomas), we developed a prognostic classifier based on 21 CpGs. This classifier was able to distinguish well-differentiated thyroid carcinomas of patients showing worse prognosis (relapse

* Correspondence: silvia.regina.rogatto@rsyd.dk
†Isabella Maria Dias Payão Ortiz and Mateus Camargo Barros-Filho contributed equally to this work.
2Department of Clinical Genetics, Vejle Hospital, Institute of Regional Health Research, University of Southern Denmark, Beriderbakken 4, 7100 Vejle, Denmark
Full list of author information is available at the end of the article

during the follow-up) from those with good prognosis (without relapse in the follow-up) [10].

Similar to protein-encoding genes, miRNAs are transcribed and could be targets of epigenetic events that modulate their expression [11]. In the last few years, the number of miRNAs described as regulated by DNA methylation increased substantially [11–13]. However, the characterization of this epigenetic modification and its functional role in the control of miRNA expression are poorly explored in PTC. To our knowledge, only one study described miRNAs putatively regulated by methylation in thyroid cancer [7]. Nonetheless, neither confirmation nor functional experiments have been developed in this field. This knowledge can contribute to better understanding of PTC biology leading to the discovery of biomarkers and new therapeutic strategies.

Herein, a comprehensive DNA methylation data from PTC and matched NT (non-neoplastic tissue) samples, previously described by our group [8, 10], were re-evaluated focusing in the identification of miRNA genes potentially regulated by methylation. External molecular dataset from TCGA were assessed to perform integrative analysis using DNA methylation, miRNAs expression, and target mRNAs data. The miRNA-coding genes, *MIR21* and *MIR146B*, were further investigated in an independent sample set, and functional assays were carried out in PTC cell lines.

Results

MicroRNA genes differentially methylated in PTC

The main strategies to identify miRNAs potentially regulated by methylation are depicted in Fig. 1. DNA methylation analysis comparing paired PTC ($N = 50$) and NT ($N = 50$) samples revealed 50 CpG probes (34 miRNA genes) differentially methylated, of which 86% (42 probes mapped in 27 miRNA genes) was confirmed using the TCGA database (Table 1). A supervised hierarchical clustering analysis with all 42 probes revealed an enrichment of hypomethylation in both, our PTC cases and in the TCGA dataset (Additional file 1: Figure S1).

Impact of disrupted DNA methylation in miRNA expression

To identify alterations in the expression levels of miRNA genes in PTC, we assessed miRNA sequencing data from TCGA, revealing 58 miRNAs (27 up and 31 down expressed) (Additional file 2: Table S1). Only *MIR21* (hsa-miR-21-5p) and *MIR146B* (hsa-miR-146b-5p and hsa-miR-146b-3p) showed differential methylation and expression (hypomethylation with increased expression). The integrative analysis revealed highly significant negative correlation between methylation and miRNAs expression (Additional file 2: Table S2).

Alterations in mRNAs targeted by miRNAs potentially regulated by methylation

The mRNA data analysis from TCGA revealed 2432 differentially expressed coding transcripts in PTC (Additional file 2: Table S3), 452 of them were considered as targets of the miRNAs affected by DNA methylation. Among these, 250, 243, and 189 mRNAs are predicted to interact with hsa-miR-146b-3p, hsa-miR-146b-5p, or hsa-miR-21-5p, respectively (681 miRNA-mRNA predicted interactions with significant negative correlation) (Additional file 2: Table S4).

MicroRNAs and target genes associated with poor prognostic features

The DNA methylation levels of *MIR146B* and *MIR21*, expression of the miRNAs (*hsa-miR-146b-5p*, *hsa-miR-146b-3p*, and *hsa-miR-21*), and their target transcripts (452 mRNAs from the integrative analysis) were compared with the clinical-pathological findings (TCGA dataset). Hypomethylation and increased expression of *MIR146B*, as well as decreased target genes expression, were significantly associated with features related to poor prognosis (advanced clinical stage, lymph node metastasis, and extrathyroidal extension) and *BRAF* mutation (Additional file 2: Table S5).

Data confirmation by quantitative bisulfite pyrosequencing and RT-qPCR

Hypomethylation and overexpression of *MIR21* and *MIR146B* in PTC compared with NT and BTL were confirmed using quantitative bisulfite pyrosequencing and RT-qPCR, respectively (Fig. 2a, b). An additional analysis of PTC compared with NT samples from the same patients (18 matched samples for methylation and 17 for miRNA expression) also corroborated these findings (Additional file 1: Figure S2). A negative correlation between the methylation pattern and expression of *MIR21* ($r = -0.393$; $P < 0.001$) and *MIR146B* ($r = -0.649$; $P < 0.001$) was also observed (Fig. 2c).

Seven target genes selected for RT-qPCR evaluation (*DOK6*, *FHL1*, *FLRT1*, *MOB3B*, *MPPED2*, *MRO*, and *STXBP5L*) showed decreased expression in PTC compared to NT and BTL (Fig. 2d). The interactions among hsa-miR-146b-5p, hsa-miR-21-5p, and the seven targets, found in the integrative analysis using the TCGA dataset, supported the findings obtained in the RT-qPCR analysis (Fig. 2e).

The pyrosequencing and RT-qPCR results were also confronted with clinical-pathological features and *BRAF* mutation (observed in 59% of the PTC). A significant association was observed between lower methylation and higher expression levels of *MIR146B* and *MIR21* with *BRAF* mutation (Additional file 1: Figure S3).

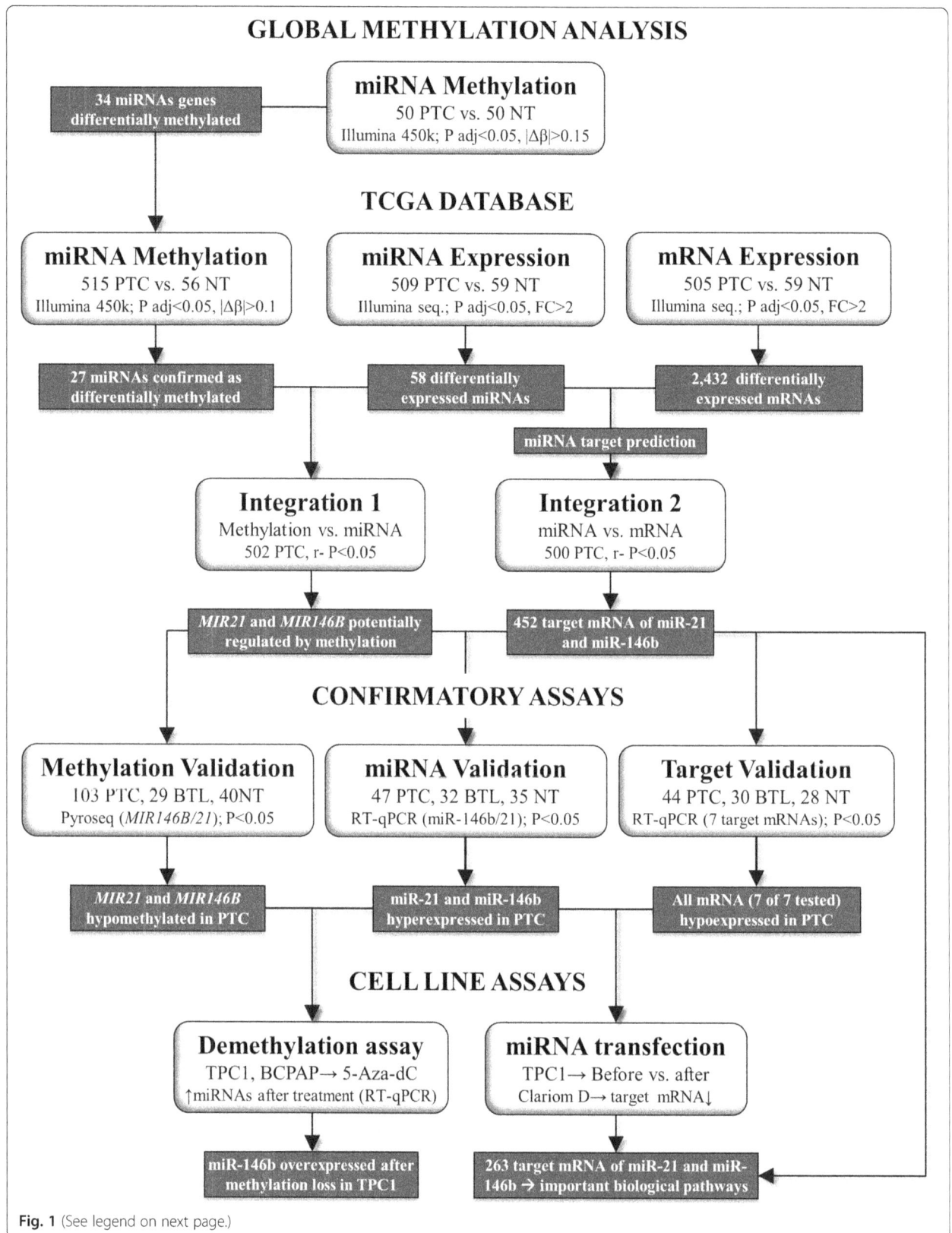

GLOBAL METHYLATION ANALYSIS

34 miRNAs genes differentially methylated

miRNA Methylation
50 PTC vs. 50 NT
Illumina 450k; P adj<0.05, |Δβ|>0.15

TCGA DATABASE

miRNA Methylation
515 PTC vs. 56 NT
Illumina 450k; P adj<0.05, |Δβ|>0.1

miRNA Expression
509 PTC vs. 59 NT
Illumina seq.; P adj<0.05, FC>2

mRNA Expression
505 PTC vs. 59 NT
Illumina seq.; P adj<0.05, FC>2

27 miRNAs confirmed as differentially methylated

58 differentially expressed miRNAs

2,432 differentially expressed mRNAs

miRNA target prediction

Integration 1
Methylation vs. miRNA
502 PTC, r- P<0.05

Integration 2
miRNA vs. mRNA
500 PTC, r- P<0.05

***MIR21* and *MIR146B* potentially regulated by methylation**

452 target mRNA of miR-21 and miR-146b

CONFIRMATORY ASSAYS

Methylation Validation
103 PTC, 29 BTL, 40NT
Pyroseq (*MIR146B/21*); P<0.05

miRNA Validation
47 PTC, 32 BTL, 35 NT
RT-qPCR (miR-146b/21); P<0.05

Target Validation
44 PTC, 30 BTL, 28 NT
RT-qPCR (7 target mRNAs); P<0.05

***MIR21* and *MIR146B* hypomethylated in PTC**

miR-21 and miR-146b hyperexpressed in PTC

All mRNA (7 of 7 tested) hypoexpressed in PTC

CELL LINE ASSAYS

Demethylation assay
TPC1, BCPAP→ 5-Aza-dC
↑miRNAs after treatment (RT-qPCR)

miRNA transfection
TPC1→ Before vs. after
Clariom D→ target mRNA↓

miR-146b overexpressed after methylation loss in TPC1

263 target mRNA of miR-21 and miR-146b → important biological pathways

Fig. 1 (See legend on next page.)

Development of a diagnostic tool in thyroid cancer

The DNA methylation (pyrosequencing) and expression (RT-qPCR) levels of *MIR21* and *MIR146B* were tested as a potential tool to discriminate malignant (PTC) from benign thyroid lesions (BTL). The combination of methylation values of both miRNAs allowed the discrimination of 87 out of 96 PTC and 25 out of 26 BTL (91% sensitivity and 96% specificity) (Fig. 2f). The hsa-miR-21-5p and hsa-miR-146b-5p relative expression was more efficient than methylation to classify correctly 45 of 47 PTC and 31 of 32 BTL (96% sensitivity and 97% specificity) (Fig. 2g). Curiously, the miRNA expression test correctly classified all NT samples as non-malignant (35 of 35), while the methylation test categorized 29 of 40 NT samples (73%) as malignant.

Global demethylation-induced *MIR146*B expression in TPC1 cell line

Firstly, we investigated the basal methylation of two PTC cell lines (TPC1 and BCPAP) to study hypomethylated CpGs. Whereas *MIR146B* showed high methylation levels in both cell lines (51–60% of methylated alleles), *MIR21* was completely unmethylated even at basal level (5–7% of methylated alleles), rendering no change in miR expression after 5-Aza-dC treatment (Fig. 3a). Loss of global methylation (*AlR1Sat* and *AluYB*8 repetitive regions) was confirmed after treatment with 5-Aza-dC. Specific loss of methylation in CpGs mapped in the *MIR146B* gene and an increased expression level of the hsa-miR-146b-5p in the TPC1 cell line was also observed (Fig. 3b).

No change in miR expression.

Decreased expression levels of target mRNAs after miRNA mimic transfection in the TPC1 cell line

A transfection assay using the TPC1 cell line for each miRNA mimic (hsa-miR-146b-3p, hsa-miR-146b-5p and hsa-miR-21-5p) was performed followed by global transcriptomic analysis. From the 452 mRNAs highlighted by the integrative analysis (681 miRNA-mRNA interactions), 168 also showed decreased expression levels after transfection (188 miRNA-mRNA interactions). This strategy gives additional evidence that 136, 112, and 134 mRNA targets are regulated by hsa-miR-146b-3p, hsa-miR-146b-5p, and hsa-miR-21-5p, respectively (Additional file 2: Table S6). The in silico pathway analysis (IPA and KOBAS 3.0) including the mRNA target candidates revealed the involvement of canonical pathways related to neuronal system, thyroid function (mainly for hsa-miR-146b-3p targets), and MAPK/ERK signaling (mainly for hsa-miR-146b-5p targets) (Additional file 2: Tables S7 and S8).

Discussion

Aberrant microRNA expression in thyroid neoplasia was previously reported [14, 15]; however, the mechanisms underlying the regulation of these miRNAs are poorly explored. As possible impact of DNA methylation was previously noticed [7]. In this study, we investigated the methylation profiles of PTC and NT in genes encoding miRNA using a high coverage platform (Illumina 450 k). Although the use of whole genome bisulfite sequencing would encompass more miRNA gene regions, an advantage of our strategy was the inclusion of 565 PTC and 106 NT evaluated by the same platform (internal and external samples from TCGA), which strengthened our findings.

MIR21 exhibited increased expression and decreased methylation levels in PTC compared to NT and BTL. *MIR21* overexpression was previously reported in thyroid cancer [16, 17]. The transcribed miRNA (hsa-miR-21) was one of the first oncomiR described and one of the most studied in several tumor types [18–20]. In prostate cancer cell lines, *MIR21* promoter hypermethylation resulted in its repressed expression [21]. Moreover, the 5-AZA-dC treatment stimulated the expression of this miRNA in prostate and ovary cancer cell lines [21, 22]. However, these studies were restricted to cell lines, and tumor samples were not evaluated to confirm the *MIR21* methylation pattern.

Similar to *MIR21*, *MIR146B* presented hypomethylation and increased expression levels in PTC. This miRNA was also previously described as overexpressed in PTC [7, 14, 15]. Contrarily, the hypermethylation and down-expression of *MIR146B* were reported in diffuse and anaplastic astrocytomas, gliomas, and breast cancer being the 5-AZA-dC treatment capable to induce the *MIR146B* expression [23, 24]. Taken together, these findings give evidences of the regulatory role of *MIR146B* in different tumor types, being able to act as tumor suppressor or oncomiR, depending on the context of altered regulatory pathways in each tumor type [25–28].

The identification of miRNAs target-genes is crucial to understand the regulatory mechanisms involved in thyroid cancer cells. In this context, 452 target transcripts were unveiled by the miRNA-mRNA integrative analysis (TCGA dataset). Interestingly, 168 of these 452 putative mRNA targets also exhibited decreased expression levels

Table 1 CpG probes mapped in miRNA-coding genes differentially methylated in PTC compared to NT

Probe (ID)	miRNA gene	Genomic functional distribution	CpG context	Internal data			TCGA data		
				Delta β	P	P adj.	Delta β	P	FDR
cg19019198	MIRLET7G	TSS200		− 0.36	< 1e-07	< 1e-07	− 0.49	< 1e-07	< 1e-07
cg07181702	MIR21	Body		− 0.19	< 1e-07	< 1e-07	− 0.20	< 1e-07	< 1e-07
cg04276626	MIR21	TSS200		− 0.18	< 1e-07	< 1e-07	− 0.16	< 1e-07	< 1e-07
cg02515217	MIR21	TSS200		− 0.17	< 1e-07	< 1e-07	− 0.16	< 1e-07	< 1e-07
cg15759721	MIR21	Body		− 0.17	< 1e-07	< 1e-07	− 0.14	< 1e-07	< 1e-07
cg04805065	MIR33B	TSS1500	Shore	− 0.25	< 1e-07	< 1e-07	− 0.29	< 1e-07	< 1e-07
cg09186408	MIR33B	TSS1500	Shore	− 0.20	< 1e-07	< 1e-07	− 0.23	< 1e-07	< 1e-07
cg19619576	MIR33B	TSS1500	Shelf	− 0.16	< 1e-07	1e-07	− 0.21	< 1e-07	< 1e-07
cg01243312	MIR128–1	Body		0.20	< 1e-07	< 1e-07	0.23	< 1e-07	< 1e-07
cg10734581	MIR134	TSS1500		− 0.19	< 1e-07	< 1e-07	NA	NA	NA
cg15857661	MIR146B	TSS200	Shelf	− 0.33	< 1e-07	< 1e-07	− 0.34	< 1e-07	< 1e-07
cg05858126	MIR146B	TSS200	Shelf	− 0.32	< 1e-07	< 1e-07	− 0.33	< 1e-07	< 1e-07
cg05251190	MIR146B	TSS200	Shelf	− 0.30	< 1e-07	< 1e-07	− 0.29	< 1e-07	< 1e-07
cg13442016	MIR146B	Body	Shelf	− 0.29	< 1e-07	< 1e-07	− 0.29	< 1e-07	< 1e-07
cg09701700	MIR146B	TSS1500	Shelf	− 0.20	< 1e-07	< 1e-07	− 0.19	< 1e-07	< 1e-07
cg13309012	MIR155	Body		− 0.30	< 1e-07	< 1e-07	− 0.30	< 1e-07	< 1e-07
cg13449535	MIR200B	TSS1500	Shore	− 0.25	< 1e-07	< 1e-07	− 0.37	< 1e-07	< 1e-07
cg14144728	MIR200B	TSS1500	Shore	− 0.23	< 1e-07	< 1e-07	− 0.21	< 1e-07	< 1e-07
cg08096702	MIR211	TSS1500		− 0.29	< 1e-07	< 1e-07	− 0.34	< 1e-07	< 1e-07
cg11721554	MIR377	TSS1500	Shelf	− 0.17	< 1e-07	< 1e-07	− 0.20	< 1e-07	< 1e-07
cg05138957	MIR377	TSS1500	Shelf	− 0.15	< 1e-07	< 1e-07	− 0.19	< 1e-07	< 1e-07
cg21513316	MIR410	Body	Island	− 0.16	< 1e-07	< 1e-07	− 0.14	< 1e-07	< 1e-07
cg20547131	MIR412	TSS1500	Shore	− 0.17	< 1e-07	< 1e-07	− 0.15	< 1e-07	< 1e-07
cg14910227	MIR495	Body		− 0.19	< 1e-07	< 1e-07	− 0.27	< 1e-07	< 1e-07
cg11978784	MIR512–1	TSS1500		− 0.17	< 1e-07	< 1e-07	NA	NA	NA
cg10583119	MIR518D	TSS1500		− 0.18	< 1e-07	< 1e-07	− 0.22	< 1e-07	< 1e-07
cg17670263	MIR520C	TSS1500		− 0.21	< 1e-07	1e-07	− 0.27	< 1e-07	< 1e-07
cg05865548	MIR543	TSS200		− 0.16	< 1e-07	< 1e-07	− 0.22	< 1e-07	< 1e-07
cg04522625	MIR548A2	Body		0.24	< 1e-07	< 1e-07	0.30	< 1e-07	< 1e-07
cg18697991	MIR548A2	Body		0.19	< 1e-07	< 1e-07	0.20	< 1e-07	< 1e-07
cg03221073	MIR548F1	Body		− 0.41	< 1e-07	< 1e-07	− 0.34	< 1e-07	< 1e-07
cg25874148	MIR548F5	Body		− 0.28	< 1e-07	< 1e-07	NA	NA	NA
cg01719718	MIR548F5	Body		− 0.17	< 1e-07	2e-07	− 0.18	< 1e-07	< 1e-07
cg05878887	MIR548G	Body		− 0.31	< 1e-07	< 1e-07	− 0.33	< 1e-07	< 1e-07
cg21175685	MIR548G	Body		− 0.31	< 1e-07	< 1e-07	− 0.24	< 1e-07	< 1e-07
cg02145866	MIR548G	Body		− 0.29	< 1e-07	< 1e-07	− 0.30	< 1e-07	< 1e-07
cg26664528	MIR548H4	Body	Shore	− 0.28	< 1e-07	< 1e-07	NA	NA	NA
cg11539052	MIR548N	Body	Shore	− 0.20	< 1e-07	< 1e-07	NA	NA	NA
cg05966699	MIR567	TSS1500		− 0.16	< 1e-07	< 1e-07	− 0.24	< 1e-07	< 1e-07
cg06277638	MIR570	TSS1500		− 0.17	< 1e-07	< 1e-07	NA	NA	NA
cg09031823	MIR575	TSS1500		− 0.17	< 1e-07	7e-04	− 0.25	< 1e-07	< 1e-07
cg18948646	MIR575	TSS200		− 0.16	< 1e-07	< 1e-07	− 0.13	< 1e-07	< 1e-07
cg26620021	MIR641	TSS1500	Shore	− 0.28	< 1e-07	< 1e-07	NA	NA	NA

Table 1 CpG probes mapped in miRNA-coding genes differentially methylated in PTC compared to NT *(Continued)*

Probe (ID)	miRNA gene	Genomic functional distribution	CpG context	Internal data			TCGA data		
				Delta β	P	P adj.	Delta β	P	FDR
cg11035122	MIR758	TSS1500		− 0.15	< 1e-07	2e-06	− 0.18	< 1e-07	< 1e-07
cg02558026	MIR762	TSS1500	Shore	− 0.20	< 1e-07	< 1e-07	− 0.24	< 1e-07	< 1e-07
cg13204193	MIR942	Body		0.19	< 1e-07	< 1e-07	NA	NA	NA
cg01940297	MIR1207	TSS1500		0.16	< 1e-07	3e-06	0.25	< 1e-07	< 1e-07
cg25037841	MIR1286	TSS1500		0.15	< 1e-07	< 1e-07	0.18	< 1e-07	< 1e-07
cg25591377	MIR1288	TSS1500		− 0.27	< 1e-07	< 1e-07	− 0.24	< 1e-07	< 1e-07
cg02746110	MIR1301	TSS1500		0.16	< 1e-07	4e-07	0.18	< 1e-07	< 1e-07

NA probes not available in the TCGA processed data (level 3); *P Adj* Bonferroni *P* value; *FDR* false discovery ratio; *TSS* transcription start sites; *Shelf*, 2–4 kb from CpG island; *Shore*, until 2 kb from CpG island

after the individualized mimic transfection assays using these three miRNAs (hsa-miR-146b-3p, hsa-miR-146b-5p, or hsa-miR-21-5p). Although the cell lines are very useful models, gene expression profiles are not identical with those found in primary tumor tissues. Differences based on epigenetic reprogramming have been reported as a causal effect of the in vitro conditions [29]. In addition, the induction of a single miRNA can influence the expression of many transcriptional factors, which enhances the complexity of the transcriptome regulation network and makes the outcome less predictable [30].

Seven selected transcripts were confirmed as having decreased expression levels in PTC compared to NT and BLT. Among the selected genes, *MPPED2*, *MRO*, *STXBP5L*, *FHL1*, and *FLRT1* were previously reported as down-regulated in PTC [31, 32]. In prostate [33], stomach [34], and breast cancer [35], *DOK6* and *MOB3B* were reported as putative tumor suppressor genes. In follicular tissues of the thyroid gland, these genes could have similar function of tumor suppressors.

We also investigated the association of miRNAs methylation and expression levels of the target-genes with clinical and pathological features of poor prognosis and *BRAF* mutation. Increased expression levels of *MIR146B* were related with advanced stage, tumor size, extrathyroidal extension, and *BRAF* mutation, as previously reported [36–39]. In our initial analysis using the TCGA cohort, *MIR21* and *MIR146B* hypomethylation and their increased expression levels, as well as decreased levels of several target-genes, were suggested as associated with poor prognosis features. Nevertheless, a clear distinction of the molecular profiles was confirmed using pyrosequencing and RT-qPCR analysis in our *BRAF*-mutated cases. The association between global DNA methylation and *BRAF* mutation in PTC has already been extensively explored, and a global hypomethylation in tumors harboring *BRAF* V600E was reported [8, 40, 41]. The mechanisms possibly involved in

the epigenetic control of genes by the *BRAF* mutation have been recently explored (42–44). In melanoma cells, the expression of 59 hypermethylated genes in the *BRAF* V600E knockdown were down-expressed suggesting that in mutated cells these genes were hypomethylated and over-expressed [42]. According to the authors, aberrant *EZH2* (histone methyltransferase) and *DNMT1* (DNA methyltransferase 1) expression were affected by the *BRAF* mutation [42]. A similar study performed by the same group was reported in two PTC cell lines (BCPAP and OCUT1), showing that *BRAF* mutation had an impact in the methylation and the expression of several genes, including *HMGB2* and *FDG1* [43]. A recent study demonstrated that the MAPK/ERK signaling pathway activated by the *BRAF* mutation was able to induce epigenetic aberrations by H3K27me3 and *MYC* [44]. Therefore, if *BRAF* mutation can trigger the epigenetic alterations in coding genes, the same effect is expected to occur in miRNAs.

MIR21 and *MIR146B* methylation and expression analysis revealed high sensitivity (91% and 96%, respectively) and specificity (96% and 97%, respectively) to distinguish PTC from benign lesions. Although the methylation classifier failed in distinguishing PTC from NT (73% of the NT samples were classified as malignant), the miRNA expression classifier categorized all NT as "non-malignant." These results suggest that our methylation markers could detect cells in the preliminary steps of malignant transformation (the non-neoplastic samples were obtained from the surrounding thyroid tissue from PTC patients). Epigenetic events are known to anticipate the phenotypic manifestation of malignancy [45, 46].

Considering the similarities observed in the classifiers for molecular diagnosis in thyroid nodules and the high complexity of the methylation assays, miRNAs expression analysis is more easily applicable in the clinical routine. Two recent studies [47, 48] reported the clinical validation of assays based on miRNA expression (Rosetta Genomics, Philadelphia, PA, USA). In these studies, a set of 24

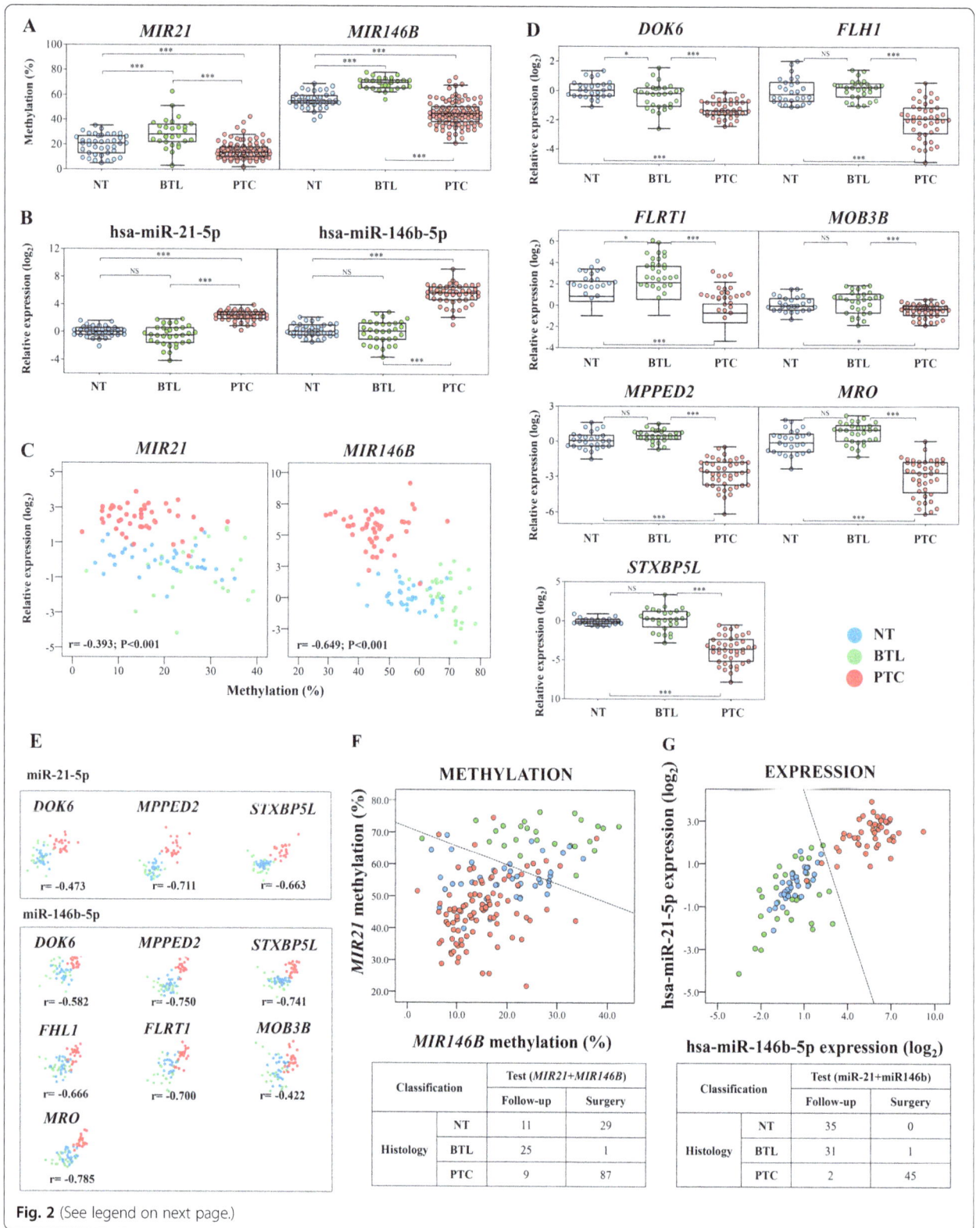

Fig. 2 (See legend on next page.)

(See figure on previous page.)
Fig. 2 Quantitative bisulfite pyrosequencing and RT-qPCR confirmed the data from the large-scale analysis. *MIR21* and *MIR146B* were significantly hypomethylated (**a**) and overexpressed (**b**) in PTC compared to non-neoplastic tissues (NT and BTL). **c** Significantly negative correlation between methylation and expression of *MIR21* and *MIR146B* was observed. **d** Five miRNA-target transcripts showed lower expression in PTC compared to NT and BTL. No significant differences were found between NT and BTL, in exception of *DOK6* and *FLRT1* genes. **e** All target transcripts demonstrated significant negative correlation with their miRNA regulators ($P < 0.001$ to all genes). Scatterplot representation of *MIR21* and *MIR146B* methylation (**f**) and expression (**g**) levels. A diagnostic classifier (dashed line) was designed to distinguish PTC from BTL using Fisher's linear discriminant analysis. The classification performance of the methylation and miRNA-based classifier is illustrated. Seven PTC and three BTL were excluded from the methylation diagnostic classifier (low pyrosequencing quality was observed for at least one of the miRNAs). NS, not significant; *$P < 0.05$; ***$P < 0.001$ (ANOVA followed by Tukey test). PTC, papillary thyroid carcinoma (red); NT, non-neoplastic thyroid tissue (blue); BTL, benign thyroid lesions (green); *r*, Pearson's correlation coefficient; *P*, *p* value obtained by Pearson's correlation test

miRNAs were evaluated (among them, hsa-miR-146b-5p) by RT-qPCR in thyroid nodules showing indeterminate cytology. First, an analytical validation was conducted to ensure the test robustness, proving the feasibility of the assay in fine-needle aspiration smears ($N = 576$ nodules) [47]. Subsequently, a classifier was developed to identify nodules as benign or suspect ($N = 189$ cases) showing 98% of sensitivity and 78% of specificity [48]. Despite our

malignant cohort was only represented by surgical specimens of PTC, we achieved a similar sensitivity and higher specificity.

Although most of studies focused in the discovery of tumor suppressor miRNAs repressed by epigenetic mechanisms [49, 50], only hypomethylated miRNA-encoding genes were detected in our study. Cell lines treated with demethylating agents, as 5-Aza-dC, is widely used to

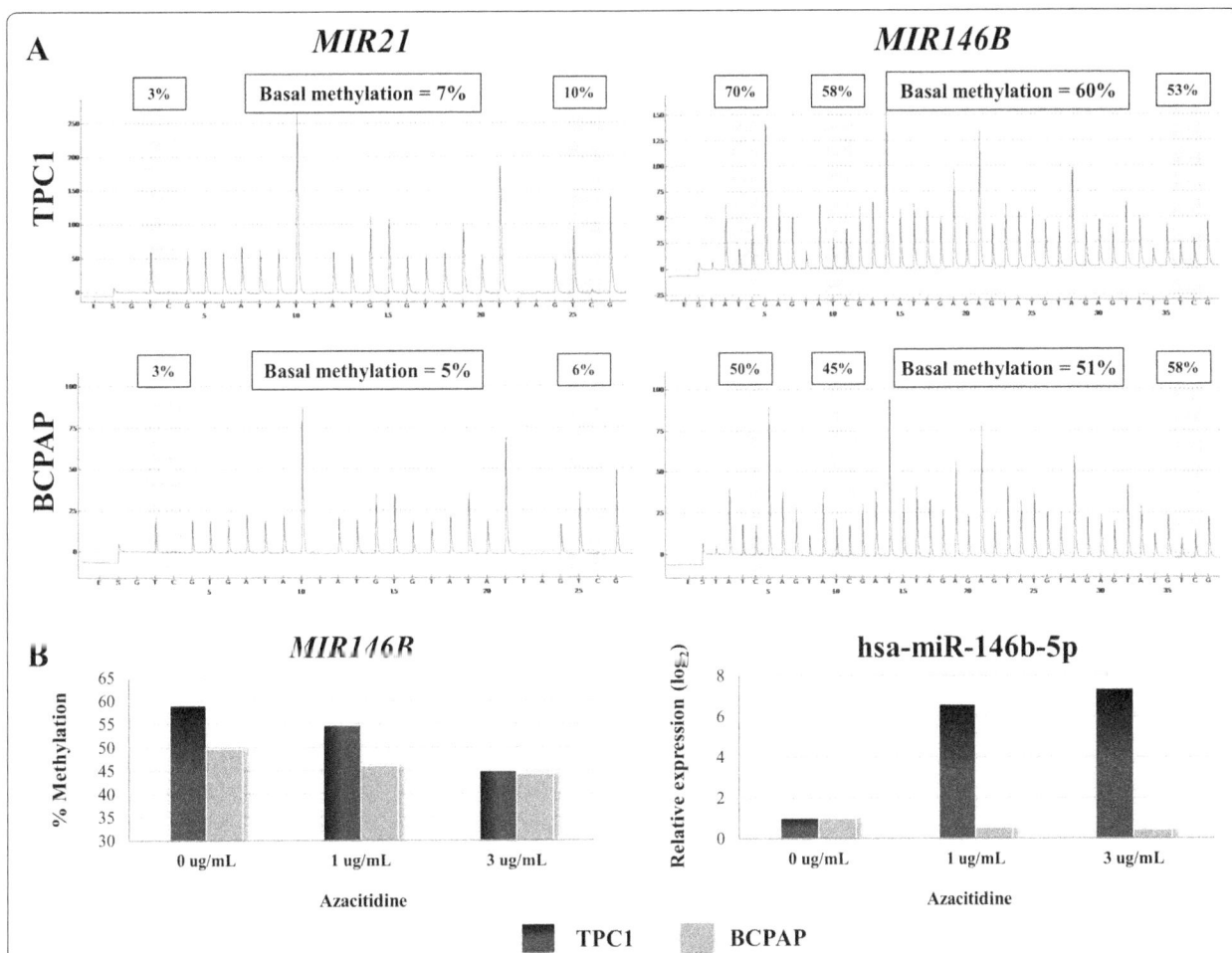

Fig. 3 Demethylation assays in thyroid cancer cell lines (TPC1 and BCPAP). **a** Pyrogram showing the percentage of basal methylation of *MIR21* (unmethylated in both cell lines) and *MIR146B* (> 50% methylation in both cell lines). **b** The demethylation in the mapped region of *MIR146B* was demonstrated after 5-Aza-dC treatment in TPC1 and BCPAP cell lines. BCPAP cell line had no changes in hsa-miR-146b-5p expression and TPC1 cell line presented seven-fold increased expression levels after the induced demethylation

demonstrate a direct regulation by methylation [51]. Even though *MIR21* and *MIR146B* were hypomethylated in PTC, the basal CpG methylation found in *MIR146B* was relatively high in two cell lines evaluated (TPC1 and BCPAP), allowing a functional assay using 5-Aza-dC. The increased expression of *MIR146B* after the treatment infers an association with the methylation loss in the miRNA gene promoter.

The role of hsa-mir-146b-5p in proliferation, migration, and invasiveness of thyroid cancer was previously investigated by others using mimics-miR transfection assays in thyroid cell lines [52, 53]. The functional role of hsa-mir-146b-5p in thyroid gland oncogenesis and its association with PTC aggressiveness was reported as involved with the down-regulation of *PTEN* and E-cadherin [53]. Likewise, it was previously described that inducing hsa-miR-21-5p in TPC1 cell line by plasmid transfection (pEZX-eGFP-miRNA-21) resulted in increased cell proliferation and invasion, and inhibited apoptosis, possibly mediated by *PDCD4* repression [16].

Conclusions

The mechanism underlying the overexpression of *MIR21* and *MIR146B* due to DNA methylation loss in PTC was explored in our study. We used, for the first time, small-scale (RT-qPCR and pyrosequencing) analysis and functional assays to corroborate the findings originated from large-scale screening in a large cohort of cases. The interconnections between these epigenetic events are potentially responsible for many deregulations in the thyroid transcriptome leading to cancer development. DNA methylation and expression levels of these miRNA-encoding genes were demonstrated as suitable PTC diagnostic markers. Moreover, the understanding of the mechanisms of upregulation of these oncomiRs in thyroid malignancies creates opportunities to develop miRNA-targeting therapies.

Methods
Sample population
Fifty matched PTC and NT samples from our previous DNA methylation profiling studies were re-evaluated as a discovery set. In addition, a confirmatory subset of 103 PTC, 40 NT, and 32 BTL (benign thyroid lesions: 14 follicular adenomas, 17 goiters, and 1 lymphocytic thyroiditis) snap-frozen tissues were obtained retrospectively from patients treated at A.C. Camargo Cancer Center, São Paulo, SP, Brazil. The Additional file 2: Table S9 summarizes the clinical features of PTC patients. Nucleic acid isolation and *BRAF* mutation genotyping are detailed in Additional file 3: Supplementary Methods.

Global DNA methylation analysis
DNA methylation profiling were obtained from the 50 paired PTC and NT samples using the Infinium® Human

Methylation450 BeadChip Platform (Illumina, San Diego, CA, USA). The data were retrieved from previously generated studies from our group [8, 10] and are available in the Gene Expression Omnibus database (GSE86961 and GSE97466). CpG probes differentially methylated in PTC compared to NT were detected using limma package [54] with adjusted P value (Bonferroni) < 0.05 and delta-beta ($\Delta\beta$) > 0.15 or < – 0.15. Quality controls and pre-processing data are detailed in Additional file 3: Supplementary Methods.

Integrative analysis using TCGA database
The available TCGA clinical and molecular data were retrieved using UCSC Xena (https://xenabrowser.net/datapages/—accessed in February 2018). DNA methylation data from 515 PTC and 56 NT (Infinium® Human Methylation450 BeadChip) from TCGA dataset were used to confirm the CpG probes differentially methylated identified in our study (t test adjusted $P < 0.05$, $\Delta\beta > 0.1$, or < – 0.1). Two strategies using integrative analysis were developed: (i) CpG probes differentially methylated in both cohorts were compared to miRNAs expression from TCGA (miRNASeq IlluminaHiSeq, 509 PTC and 59 NT), and (ii) miRNAs differentially expressed were contrasted with target-genes expression using the TCGA data (RNA-SeqV2 IlluminaHiSeq) in 505 PTC versus 59 NT (t test adjusted $P < 0.05$; fold change FC > 2 for both miRNA and mRNA). As different prediction methods are generally uncorrelated [55], miRNA target prediction was carried out with miRWalk 2.0 tool (http://zmf.umm.uni-heidelberg.de/apps/zmf/mirwalk2/), considering predicted interactions in at least two of four selected algorithms (miRWalk, miRanda, RNAhybrid, and Targetscan). Predictions were based on interactions between miRNA seed sequences (starting from the first position) and the 3′UTR region of the target mRNA. Pearson's correlation test was applied to investigate negatively correlated predicted interactions in PTC ($P < 0.05$).

DNA methylation analysis in miRNAs genes by pyrosequencing
To confirm the global DNA methylation results, 500 ng of genomic DNA samples were converted by sodium bisulfite using the EZ DNA Methylation Gold kit (Zymo, Irvine, CA, USA), according to the manufacturer's recommendations. Only independent samples (103 PTC, 29 BTL, and 40 NT) from the previous global methylation analysis [8, 10] were included. Forward and reverse biotinylated primers (Sigma, Darmstadt, Germany) were used to amplify the region of interest (Additional file 2: Table S10 and Additional file 1: Figure S4). Two probes representative of *MIR146B* and *MIR21* were selected, presenting the highest negative correlation with the corresponding miRNA expression. Primer design and PCR

conditions are detailed in Additional file 3: Supplementary Methods. Pyrosequencing (PyroMark Q24 system, Qiagen) was performed including methylated and unmethylated DNA controls according to the manufacturer's instructions (Zymo Research, Irvine, CA, USA).

MicroRNAs and target mRNAs expression analysis by RT-qPCR

Expression of miRNAs (hsa-miR-21-5p and hsa-miR-146b-5p) and mRNAs (*MPPED2*, *STXBP5L*, *MRO*, *FHL1*, *FLRT1*, *DOK6*, and *MOB3B*) were performed by RT-qPCR (detailed in Additional file 3: Supplementary Methods) using TaqMan® and SYBR® Green detection system, respectively (Applied Biosystems, CA, USA). The hsa-miR-146b-5p and hsa-miR-146b-3p showed redundant expression in the miRNA sequencing results using the TCGA dataset (PTC = 510, Pearson's r = 0.970, Pearson's P not computable). Based on these findings, we selected only hsa-miR-146b-5p to be evaluated by RT-qPCR (most prevalent mature form).

Seven of 452 target transcripts detected in the integrative analysis were selected according to the negative correlation coefficient values, expression levels in normal thyroid tissues (available at https://www.ncbi.nlm.nih.gov/gene), higher FC, and significant clinicopathological variables associated with poor prognosis (obtained from TCGA) (Additional file 2: Table S11). According to these parameters, all seven transcripts are targets of miR-146b-5p, and three of them (*DOK6*, *MPPED2*, and *STXBP5L*) are targets of miR-21-5p. The mRNA primer sequences are described in Additional file 2: Table S12.

For miRNA analysis, TaqMan® microRNA Reverse Transcription Kit (Applied Biosystems) and TaqMan® microRNA Assays (IDs: 000397 and 001097, Applied Biosystems) were used according to the manufacturer's instructions. miRNA normalization was performed using *RNU44* (ID 001094) and *RNU48* (ID 001006) [36, 56]. The highly stable references, *EIF2B1* and *PUM1*, were employed for mRNA normalization, as previously described [31]. The method proposed by Pfaffl (2001) [57] was used for normalization with a geometric mean of reference tests and efficiency equal to 100%.

Global demethylation assay in PTC cell lines

The human thyroid cancer cell lines TPC1 (*BRAF* wild type, received from Janete M Cerutti, Federal University of São Paulo, Brazil) and BCPAP (*BRAF* V600E, received from Edna T. Kimura, University of São Paulo, Brazil) were in vitro cultured in RPMI (Gibco, Grand Island, NY, USA) and DMEM/F-10 medium (Gibco), respectively, supplemented with 10% fetal bovine serum, 1% streptomycin (Gibco), and 1% penicillin (Gibco). Global demethylation assays were performed using 5-Aza-dC (Sigma, Darmstadt, Germany) at 1 μM and 3 μM

determined by cell viability assays (detailed in Additional file 3: Supplementary Methods). Loss of methylation after treatment was confirmed by pyrosequencing using AluYB8 and AlR1Sat primer pairs, as described by Choi et al. (2009) [58]. Basal methylation of *MIR21* and *MIR146B* regions and the corresponding mature miRNAs expression in the cell lines upon treatment were evaluated as described above. The samples treated with 5-Aza-dC were compared to vehicle using three replicates (independent assays) for each cell line.

MicroRNA mimics transfection in the TPC1 cell line

Due to the increased expression of *MIR146B* after azacitidine treatment in TPC1, this cell line was chosen to conduct the transfection experiments. The cells were seeded 24 h prior to the transfection in 6-well plates with 200,000 cells per well in the medium specific to the cell lines, without supplemented antibiotics. The transfection reagent Lipofectamine RNAiMAX (Invitrogen) was prepared in Opti-MEM medium (Invitrogen), as recommended by the manufacturer. The mirVana miRNA mimics (Invitrogen) hsa-miR-146b-3p, hsa-miR-146b-5p, and hsa-miR-21-5p were dissolved to the relevant concentrations in Opti-MEM medium. The diluted transfection reagent and mimics (final concentration of 30 nM) were then mixed and incubated at room temperature for 5 min. Afterwards, the complexes were added to each well containing cells and Opti-MEM medium. Negative control mimics (30 nM) and a mock control were included in the transfection experiments. The cells were incubated for 48 h before being harvested in trypsin followed by total RNA extraction. The mature miRNAs were reversely transcribed with targeted primers. Moreover, successful transfection was confirmed by RT-qPCR (> 100 increased expression levels for the three miRNAs).

Large-scale transcriptomic analysis after miRNA transfection

The RNA from mimics and control assays was amplified (200 ng), labeled, and hybridized using the Clariom D platform (Affymetrix, Santa Clara, CA, USA) following the manufacturer's instructions. Two biological replicates were included for each miRNA tested individually. The arrays hybridization was performed in a GeneChip® Hybridization Oven 645 (Affymetrix) and scanned using the GeneChip Scanner 3000 (Affymetrix). The data were analyzed using the Affymetrix Transcriptome Analysis Console software (v. 3.1.0.5) and normalized by the Robust Multiarray Average module. The analysis was focused in the target mRNAs found in the integrative analysis and specifically in transcripts down-expressed (in both duplicates) after the transfection with the mimics.

In silico canonical pathway analysis

Protein-encoding genes predicted as target of the miR-NAs potentially regulated by DNA methylation, found in the integrative analysis and down-expressed after the mimic transfection, were submitted to canonical pathway evaluation using the Ingenuity Pathway Analysis (IPA v2.1, Ingenuity Systems) and KOBAS 3.0 software (http://kobas.cbi.pku.edu.cn/).

Statistical analysis

The SPSS v. 21.0 (Statistics Packet for Social Sciences, Chicago, IL, USA) and BRB Array Tools v. 4.4.0 were used for statistical analysis. Graphical representations were implemented by GraphPad Prism v.5.0 (GraphPad Software Inc., La Jolla, CA, USA). The methylation, miR-NAs, and target gene expression from TCGA were compared with clinical and pathological data and $BRAF$ mutation using t test ($P < 0.001$; FDR $< 5\%$; $|\Delta\beta| > 0.10$ or FC > 1.5). Pyrosequencing (percentage of methylation in each CpG) and RT-qPCR data (miRNAs and mRNAs relative expression) were evaluated by parametric tests (paired and unpaired t test, ANOVA with Turkey's post hoc, and Pearson's correlation test). The null hypothesis was rejected when the two-tailed P value was < 0.05. Fisher discriminant analysis was used to construct diagnostic classifier algorithms.

Abbreviations

5-Aza-dC: 5-aza-deoxycytidine; BTL: Benign thyroid lesions; CpG: 5'-deoxycytosine-phosphate-deoxyguanosine-3; IPA: Ingenuity pathways analysis; KOBAS: KEEG orthology based annotation system; miRNA: MicroRNA; mRNA: Messenger RNA; NT: Non-neoplastic adjacent tissues; PTC: Papillary thyroid carcinoma; RT-qPCR: Reverse transcription quantitative polymerase chain reaction; TCGA: The Cancer Genome Atlas

Acknowledgements

The authors would like to thank the A.C. Camargo Cancer Center Biobank for providing the samples. Our gratitude to Dr. Mario Hiroyuki Hirata, Dra. Gisele Medeiros Bastos, and Ms. Jéssica Bassani Borges from the Molecular Biology Laboratory at the Dante Pazzanese Institute of Cardiology to assist with the pyrosequencing.

Funding

This study was supported by grants from the São Paulo Research Foundation (FAPESP 2015/20748-5 and 2015/17707-5).

Authors' contributions

SRR and LPK conceived and designed the experiments. IMDPO, MBR, CMB, HK, LMC, JBHM, CA, and MCBF conducted the experiments. MCBF and FAM analyzed the data. SRR contributed with reagents/materials. CALP performed the histopathological evaluation. IMDPO, MCBF, and SRR wrote and edited the manuscript. SRR and LPK supervised the study. All authors read and approved the final version of the manuscript.

Competing interests

The authors declare that they have no competing interests.

Author details

[1]International Research Center-CIPE, A.C. Camargo Cancer Center, Taguá Street 440, São Paulo 01508-010, Brazil. [2]Department of Clinical Genetics, Vejle Hospital, Institute of Regional Health Research, University of Southern Denmark, Beriderbakken 4, 7100 Vejle, Denmark. [3]Department of Pathology, A.C. Camargo Cancer Center, Professor Antonio Prudente Street 211, São Paulo 01509-900, Brazil. [4]Department of Head and Neck Surgery and Otorhinolaryngology, A.C. Camargo Cancer Center, Professor Antonio Prudente Street 211, São Paulo 01509-900, Brazil.

References

1. Ito Y, Nikiforov YE, Schlumberger M, Vigneri R. Increasing incidence of thyroid cancer: controversies explored. Nat Rev Endocrinol. 2013;9(3):178–84.
2. Lim H, Devesa SS, Sosa JA, Check D, Kitahara CM. Trends in thyroid cancer incidence and mortality in the United States, 1974-2013. JAMA. 2017; 317(13):1338–48.
3. Fagin JA, Wells SA. Biologic and clinical perspectives on thyroid cancer. N Engl J Med. 2016;375(11):1054–67.
4. Liu R, Zhang T, Zhu G, Xing M. Regulation of mutant TERT by BRAF V600E/ MAP kinase pathway through FOS/GABP in human cancer. Nat Commun. 2018;9(1):579.
5. Pozdeyev N, Gay LM, Sokol ES, Hartmaier R, Deaver KE, Davis S, et al. Genetic analysis of 779 advanced differentiated and anaplastic thyroid cancers. Clin Cancer Res. 2018;24(13):3059–68.
6. Rodríguez-Rodero S, Delgado-Álvarez E, Fernández AF, Fernández-Morera JL, Menéndez-Torre E, Fraga MF. Epigenetic alterations in endocrine-related cancer. Endocr Relat Cancer. 2014;21(4):R319–30.
7. Network CGAR. Integrated genomic characterization of papillary thyroid carcinoma. Cell. 2014;159(3):676–90.
8. Beltrami CM, Dos Reis MB, Barros-Filho MC, Marchi FA, Kuasne H, Pinto CAL, et al. Integrated data analysis reveals potential drivers and pathways disrupted by DNA methylation in papillary thyroid carcinomas. Clin Epigenetics. 2017;9:45.
9. Buj R, Mallona I, Díez-Villanueva A, Zafon C, Mate JL, Roca M, et al. Kallikreins stepwise scoring reveals three subtypes of papillary thyroid cancer with prognostic implications. Thyroid. 2018;28(5):601–12.
10. Bisarro Dos Reis M, Barros-Filho MC, Marchi FA, Beltrami CM, Kuasne H, Pinto CAL, et al. Prognostic classifier based on genome-wide DNA methylation profiling in well-differentiated thyroid tumors. J Clin Endocrinol Metab. 2017;102(11):4089–99.
11. Wang S, Wu W, Claret FX. Mutual regulation of microRNAs and DNA methylation in human cancers. Epigenetics. 2017;12(3):187–97.
12. Barros-Silva D, Costa-Pinheiro P, Duarte H, Sousa EJ, Evangelista AF, Graça I, et al. MicroRNA-27a-5p regulation by promoter methylation and MYC signaling in prostate carcinogenesis. Cell Death Dis. 2018;9(2):167.
13. Loginov VI, Pronina IV, Burdennyy AM, Filippova EA, Kazubskaya TP, Kushlinsky DN, et al. Novel miRNA genes deregulated by aberrant methylation in ovarian carcinoma are involved in metastasis. Gene. 2018; 662:28–36.
14. Wójcicka A, Kolanowska M, Jażdżewski K. Mechanisms in endocrinology: microRNA in diagnostics and therapy of thyroid cancer. Eur J Endocrinol. 2016;174(3):R89–98.
15. Wang T, Xu H, Qi M, Yan S, Tian X. miRNA dysregulation and the risk of metastasis and invasion in papillary thyroid cancer: a systematic review and meta-analysis. Oncotarget. 2018;9(4):5473–9.
16. Zhang J, Yang Y, Liu Y, Fan Y, Liu Z, Wang X, et al. MicroRNA-21 regulates biological behaviors in papillary thyroid carcinoma by targeting programmed cell death 4. J Surg Res. 2014;189(1):68–74.
17. Yoruker EE, Terzioglu D, Teksoz S, Uslu FE, Gezer U, Dalay N. MicroRNA expression profiles in papillary thyroid carcinoma, benign thyroid nodules and healthy controls. J Cancer. 2016;7(7):803–9.
18. Jiang J, Yang P, Guo Z, Yang R, Yang H, Yang F, et al. Overexpression of microRNA-21 strengthens stem cell-like characteristics in a hepatocellular carcinoma cell line. World J Surg Oncol. 2016;14(1):278.
19. Fang H, Xie J, Zhang M, Zhao Z, Wan Y, Yao Y. miRNA-21 promotes proliferation and invasion of triple-negative breast cancer cells through targeting PTEN. Am J Transl Res. 2017;9(3):953–61.
20. Koutsioumpa M, Chen HW, O'Brien N, Koinis F, Mahurkar-Joshi S, Vorvis C, et al. MKAD-21 suppresses the oncogenic activity of the miR-21/ PPP2R2A/ERK molecular network in bladder cancer. Mol Cancer Ther. 2018;17(7):1430–40

21. Hulf T, Sibbritt T, Wiklund ED, Bert S, Strbenac D, Statham AL, et al. Discovery pipeline for epigenetically deregulated miRNAs in cancer: integration of primary miRNA transcription. BMC Genomics. 2011;12:54.

22. Iorio MV, Visone R, Di Leva G, Donati V, Petrocca F, Casalini P, et al. MicroRNA signatures in human ovarian cancer. Cancer Res. 2007;67(18): 8699–707.

23. Xiang M, Birkbak NJ, Vafaizadeh V, Walker SR, Yeh JE, Liu S, et al. STAT3 induction of miR-146b forms a feedback loop to inhibit the NF-κB to IL-6 signaling axis and STAT3-driven cancer phenotypes. Sci Signal. 2014;7(310):ra11.

24. Wolter M, Werner T, Malzkorn B, Reifenberger G. Role of microRNAs located on chromosome arm 10q in malignant Gliomas. Brain Pathol. 2016;26(3): 344–58.

25. Haghpanah V, Fallah P, Tavakoli R, Naderi M, Samimi H, Soleimani M, et al. Antisense-miR-21 enhances differentiation/apoptosis and reduces cancer stemness state on anaplastic thyroid cancer. Tumour Biol. 2016;37(1): 1299–308.

26. Duan J, Zhang H, Qu Y, Deng T, Huang D, Liu R, et al. Onco-miR-130 promotes cell proliferation and migration by targeting TGFβR2 in gastric cancer. Oncotarget. 2016;7(28):44522–33.

27. Liu C, Zhang S, Wang Q, Zhang X. Tumor suppressor miR-1 inhibits tumor growth and metastasis by simultaneously targeting multiple genes. Oncotarget. 2017;8(26):42043–60.

28. Imamura T, Komatsu S, Ichikawa D, Miyamae M, Okajima W, Ohashi T, et al. Depleted tumor suppressor miR-107 in plasma relates to tumor progression and is a novel therapeutic target in pancreatic cancer. Sci Rep. 2017;7(1):5708.

29. Nestor CE, Ottaviano R, Reinhardt D, Cruickshanks HA, Mjoseng HK, McPherson RC, et al. Rapid reprogramming of epigenetic and transcriptional profiles in mammalian culture systems. Genome Biol. 2015;16:11.

30. Nazarov PV, Reinsbach SE, Muller A, Nicot N, Philippidou D, Vallar L, et al. Interplay of microRNAs, transcription factors and target genes: linking dynamic expression changes to function. Nucleic Acids Res. 2013;41(5):2817–31.

31. Barros-Filho MC, Marchi FA, Pinto CA, Rogatto SR, Kowalski LP. High diagnostic accuracy based on CLDN10, HMGA2, and LAMB3 transcripts in papillary thyroid carcinoma. J Clin Endocrinol Metabol. 2015;100(6):E890–E9.

32. Lan X, Zhang H, Wang Z, Dong W, Sun W, Shao L, et al. Genome-wide analysis of long noncoding RNA expression profile in papillary thyroid carcinoma. Gene. 2015;569(1):109–17.

33. Kim EA, Kim YH, Kang HW, Yoon HY, Kim WT, Kim YJ, et al. Lower levels of human MOB3B are associated with prostate cancer susceptibility and aggressive Clinicopathological characteristics. J Korean Med Sci. 2015;30(7): 937–42.

34. Leong SH, Lwin KM, Lee SS, Ng WH, Ng KM, Tan SY, et al. Chromosomal breaks at FRA18C: association with reduced. NPJ Precis Oncol. 2017;1(1):9.

35. Ghanem T, Bracken J, Kasem A, Jiang WG, Mokbel K. mRNA expression of DOK1-6 in human breast cancer. World J Clin Oncol. 2014;5(2):156–63.

36. Sheu SY, Grabellus F, Schwertheim S, Worm K, Broecker-Preuss M, Schmid KW. Differential miRNA expression profiles in variants of papillary thyroid carcinoma and encapsulated follicular thyroid tumours. Br J Cancer. 2010; 102(2):376–82.

37. Geraldo MV, Yamashita AS, Kimura ET. MicroRNA miR-146b-5p regulates signal transduction of TGF-β by repressing SMAD4 in thyroid cancer. Oncogene. 2012;31(15):1910–22.

38. Chou CK, Liu RT, Kang HY. MicroRNA-146b: A Novel Biomarker and Therapeutic Target for Human Papillary Thyroid Cancer. Int J Mol Sci. 2017; 18(3):e636.

39. Qiu Z, Li H, Wang J, Sun C. miR-146a and miR-146b in the diagnosis and prognosis of papillary thyroid carcinoma. Oncol Rep. 2017;38(5):2735–40.

40. White MG, Nagar S, Aschebrook-Kilfoy B, Jasmine F, Kibriya MG, Ahsan H, et al. Epigenetic Alterations and Canonical Pathway Disruption in Papillary Thyroid Cancer: A Genome-wide Methylation Analysis. Ann Surg Oncol. 2016;23(7):2302–9.

41. Mancikova V, Buj R, Castelblanco E, Inglada-Pérez L, Diez A, de Cubas AA, et al. DNA methylation profiling of well-differentiated thyroid cancer uncovers markers of recurrence free survival. Int J Cancer. 2014;135(3): 598–610.

42. Hou P, Liu D, Dong J, Xing M. The BRAF(V600E) causes widespread alterations in gene methylation in the genome of melanoma cells. Cell Cycle. 2012;11(2):286–95.

43. Hou P, Liu D, Xing M. Genome-wide alterations in gene methylation by the BRAF V600E mutation in papillary thyroid cancer cells. Endocr Relat Cancer. 2011;18(6):687–97.

44. Qu Y, Yang Q, Liu J, Shi B, Ji M, Li G, et al. C-Myc is required for BRAF(V600E)-induced epigenetic silencing by H3K27me3 in tumorigenesis. Theranostics. 2017;7(7):2092–107.

45. van Hoesel AQ, Sato Y, Elashoff DA, Turner RR, Giuliano AE, Shamonki JM, et al. Assessment of DNA methylation status in early stages of breast cancer development. Br J Cancer. 2013;108(10):2033–8.

46. Rodríguez-Paredes M, Bormann F, Raddatz G, Gutekunst J, Lucena-Porcel C, Köhler F, et al. Methylation profiling identifies two subclasses of squamous cell carcinoma related to distinct cells of origin. Nat Commun. 2018;9(1):577.

47. Benjamin H, Schnitzer-Perlman T, Shtabsky A, VandenBussche CJ, Ali SZ, Kolar Z, et al. Analytical validity of a microRNA-based assay for diagnosing indeterminate thyroid FNA smears from routinely prepared cytology slides. Cancer Cytopathol. 2016;124(10):711–21.

48. Lithwick-Yanai G, Dromi N, Shtabsky A, Morgenstern S, Strenov Y, Feinmesser M, et al. Multicentre validation of a microRNA-based assay for diagnosing indeterminate thyroid nodules utilising fine needle aspirate smears. J Clin Pathol. 2017;70(6):500–7.

49. Zhang L, Yan DL, Yang F, Wang DD, Chen X, Wu JZ, et al. DNA methylation mediated silencing of microRNA-874 is a promising diagnosis and prognostic marker in breast cancer. Oncotarget. 2017;8(28):45496–505.

50. Toll A, Salgado R, Espinet B, Díaz-Lagares A, Hernández-Ruiz E, Andrades E, et al. MiR-204 silencing in intraepithelial to invasive cutaneous squamous cell carcinoma progression. Mol Cancer. 2016;15(1):53.

51. Sato T, Issa JJ, Kropf P. DNA Hypomethylating Drugs in Cancer Therapy. Cold Spring Harb Perspect Med. 2017;7(5):a026948

52. Lima CR, Geraldo MV, Fuziwara CS, Kimura ET, Santos MF. MiRNA-146b-5p upregulates migration and invasion of different papillary thyroid carcinoma cells. BMC Cancer. 2016;16:108.

53. Ramírez-Moya J, Wert-Lamas L, Santisteban P. MicroRNA-146b promotes PI3K/AKT pathway hyperactivation and thyroid cancer progression by targeting PTEN. Oncogene. 2018;37(25):3369–83.

54. Ritchie ME, Phipson B, Wu D, Hu Y, Law CW, Shi W, et al. limma powers differential expression analyses for RNA-sequencing and microarray studies. Nucleic Acids Res. 2015;43(7):e47.

55. Gamazon ER, Im HK, Duan S, Lussier YA, Cox NJ, Dolan ME, et al. Exprtarget: an integrative approach to predicting human microRNA targets. PLoS One. 2010;5(10):e13534.

56. Dettmer M, Perren A, Moch H, Komminoth P, Nikiforov YE, Nikiforova MN. Comprehensive MicroRNA expression profiling identifies novel markers in follicular variant of papillary thyroid carcinoma. Thyroid. 2013;23(11):1383–9.

57. Pfaffl MW. A new mathematical model for relative quantification in real-time RT-PCR. Nucleic Acids Res. 2001;29(9):e45.

58. Choi SH, Worswick S, Byun HM, Shear T, Soussa JC, Wolff EM, et al. Changes in DNA methylation of tandem DNA repeats are different from interspersed repeats in cancer. Int J Cancer. 2009;125(3):723–9.

19

Comparing diagnostic and prognostic performance of two-gene promoter methylation panels in tissue biopsies and urines of prostate cancer patients

Catarina Moreira-Barbosa[1], Daniela Barros-Silva[1], Pedro Costa-Pinheiro[1], Jorge Torres-Ferreira[1,2], Vera Constâncio[1], Rui Freitas[3], Jorge Oliveira[3], Luís Antunes[4], Rui Henrique[1,2,5†] and Carmen Jerónimo[1,5,6*†] (iD)

Abstract

Background: Prostate cancer (PCa) is one of the most common cancers among men worldwide. Current screening methods for PCa display limited sensitivity and specificity, not stratifying for disease aggressiveness. Hence, development and validation of new molecular markers is needed. Aberrant gene promoter methylation is common in PCa and has shown promise as clinical biomarker. Herein, we assessed and compared the diagnostic and prognostic performance of two-gene panel promoter methylation in the same sample sets.

Methods: Promoter methylation of panel #1 (singleplex-*miR-34b/c* and *miR-193b*) and panel #2 (multiplex-*APC*, *GSTP1*, and *RARβ2*) was evaluated using MethyLight methodology in two different cohorts [prostate biopsy (#1) and urine sediment (#2)]. Biomarkers' diagnostic (validity estimates) and prognostic (disease-specific survival, disease-free survival, and progression-free survival) performance was assessed.

Results: Promoter methylation levels of both panels showed the highest levels in PCa samples in both cohorts. In tissue samples, methylation panel #1 and panel #2 detected PCa with AUC of 0.9775 and 1.0, respectively, whereas in urine samples, panel #2 demonstrated superior performance although a combination of *miR-34b/c*, *miR-193b*, *APC*, and *RARβ2* disclosed the best results (AUC = 0.9817). Furthermore, higher *mir-34b/c* and panel #2 methylation independently predicted for shorter DSS. Furthermore, time-dependent ROC curves showed that both *miR-34b/c* and *GSTP1* methylation levels identify with impressive performance patients that relapse up to 15 years after diagnosis (AUC = 0.751 and AUC = 0.765, respectively).

Conclusions: We concluded that quantitative gene panel promoter methylation might be a clinically useful tool for PCa non-invasive detection and risk stratification for disease aggressiveness in both tissue biopsies and urines.

Keywords: Prostate cancer, DNA methylation, Biomarkers, Methylation test, Detection, Prognosis

---

* Correspondence: carmenjeronimo@ipoporto.min-saude.pt;
cljeronimo@icbas.up.pt
†Rui Henrique and Carmen Jerónimo contributed equally to this work.
[1]Cancer Biology and Epigenetics Group, IPO Porto Research Center (CI-IPOP), Portuguese Oncology Institute of Porto (IPO Porto), Porto, Portugal
[5]Department of Pathology and Molecular Immunology, Institute of Biomedical Sciences Abel Salazar (ICBAS), University of Porto, Porto, Portugal
Full list of author information is available at the end of the article

Background

Prostate cancer (PCa) remains a major public health concern in male gender mainly due to increased life expectancy and population aging [1]. This neoplasm is usually clinically silent until extra-prostatic invasion or metastatic occurs, entailing the need for development and implementation of effective screening methods that allow for detection of PCa while still confined to the prostate, at a potentially curable stage. Moreover, PCa is a quite heterogeneous disease that ranges from clinical indolent to aggressive behavior and patients' risk stratification remains a clinical challenge [2, 3]. Notwithstanding recent advances in characterization of PCa biology, significant challenges concerning adequate PCa management remain, as new stratification methods and its clinical validation are still needed [4].

Aberrant DNA methylation, the most widely studied epigenetic mechanism in human cancers, is a very prevalent and specific feature of PCa [5]. Furthermore, altered DNA methylation patterns represent early events during prostate carcinogenesis and constitute the most frequent epigenetic phenomenon in both localized and metastatic PCa [6, 7]. Importantly, DNA methylation alterations are sufficiently stable and easily quantifiable in liquid biopsies [8, 9], which constitute a valuable and minimally invasive means of interrogating the presence of tumor cell DNA in bodily fluids.

Previous studies have identified several epigenetic-based biomarkers with great potential for detection of clinically relevant PCa [revised in [5]], including the ProCaM assay (which evaluates GSTP1, APC, and RARβ2 promoter methylation in urine samples), as a positive result correlates with increased likelihood of finding high-grade PCa in prostate biopsy [10]. More recently, we demonstrated that quantitative miR-193b and miR-34b/c promoter methylation might be useful for non-invasive detection/diagnosis and prognostication, both in tissue and urine samples [11]. Indeed, besides representing promising PCa detection/diagnostic biomarkers, several studies demonstrated that gene promoter hypermethylation might add relevant prognostic information, such as GSTP1 promoter methylation which independently predicted recurrence after radical prostatectomy [12] and higher APC promoter methylation levels which also showed independent prognostic value in addition to tumor stage [13]. Thus, DNA methylation-based biomarkers may add value in clinical practice as ancillary tests to assist in therapeutic decision-making.

Methods

Aim

Hence, the purpose of this study was to compare the diagnostic and prognostic value of two previously reported panels of methylated gene promoters, panel #1 (non-coding protein genes: miR-193b and miR-34b/c) [11] and panel #2 (protein coding genes: APC, GSTP1, and RARβ2) methylation levels [10] in the same series of samples, aiming at the establishment of an assay that may be further clinically validated.

Patients and sample collection

Two independent case control retrospective cohorts of PCa patients were included in this study. The first comprises 74 patients with elevated PSA levels submitted to prostate biopsy from 2001 to 2003 at Portuguese Oncology Institute of Porto (IPO Porto, cohort #1). For each case, in addition to the standard diagnostic biopsy cores, one tissue core sample was collected from the more suspicious area, frozen at − 80 °C and subsequently cut in a cryostat for DNA extraction. For each case, a 4-μm section was cut, stained, and examined by an experienced pathologist, to confirm the presence of malignant cells and grading. As control samples, 16 morphologically normal prostate tissues (MNPT) were collected from bladder cancer patients, without concomitant PCa, submitted to cystoprostatectomy. All specimens were immediately collected after surgical procedures and frozen at − 80 °C and histologically confirmed for the absence of any tumor foci. Additionally, a second cohort was composed of 87 PCa patients, primarily diagnosed from 1999 to 2002 at IPO Porto, which voluntarily provided early morning voided urine samples (20–30 mL) before radical prostatectomy without previous prostatic massage (cohort #2). For control purposes, urine samples were collected from 32 asymptomatic donors at IPO Porto (2009 to 2010). After collection, urine samples were centrifuged at 4000 rpm for 20 min at 4 °C, and the obtained pellets were washed in PBS 1× and frozen at − 80 °C.

Relevant clinical data was retrieved from clinical records and are shown in Tables 1 and 2. Concerning assessment of prognosis, disease-specific survival (DSS, i.e., time between diagnosis and death or last follow-up) and disease-free survival (DFS, i.e., time calculated using the interval between date of curative treatment and date of biochemical relapse or date of last follow-up or date of death, if relapse was not observed) were computed. Biochemical relapse was considered when patients presented two consecutive risings of serum PSA levels ≥ 0.2 ng/mL after surgery or 2 ng/mL above the PSA nadir after radiotherapy. Progression-free survival (PFS) was calculated from the date of androgen deprivation therapy to the date of biochemical progression, date of last follow-up, or death, if due to other causes but PCa.

DNA extraction and sodium bisulfite treatment

DNA was extracted from clinical samples using phenol-chloroform method as described elsewhere [13].

Table 1 Clinical and pathological data of morphologically normal prostatic tissue and prostate cancer patients submitted to a prostate biopsy (cohort #1) included in this study

Clinicopathological data	(Cohort #1)	
	MNPT	PCa (biopsies)
Patients, n	15	74
Median age, years (range)	64 (45–80)	69 (51–85)
Median PSA (ng/mL) (range)	n.a.	18.22 (4.52–542.00)
Clinical stage, n (%)		
II	n.a.	48 (64.86)
III	n.a.	12 (16.22)
IV	n.a.	14 (18.92)
Prognostic grade group, n (%)		
1	n.a.	30 (40.54)
2	n.a.	17 (22.97)
3	n.a.	16 (21.62)
4	n.a.	7 (9.46)
5	n.a.	4 (5.41)
CAPRA score, n (%)		
Low risk (0–2)	n.a.	7 (9.46)
Intermediate risk (3–5)	n.a.	26 (35.14)
High risk (6–10)	n.a.	41 (55.41)
D'Amico risk classification, n (%)		
Low risk		7 (9.46)
Intermediate risk		23 (31.08)
High risk		44 (59.46)
Treatment		
Radical prostatectomy/radiotherapy		39 (52.70)
Hormonotherapy		35 (47.30)
Follow-up		
Median (months, IQR)	n.a.	104.04 (67.03–145.48)
Patients without remission, n (%)	n.a.	3 (4.05)
Biochemical recurrence, n (%)	n.a.	13 (33.33)
Progression of disease, n (%)	n.a	16 (45.71)
Death due to PCa, n (%)	n.a.	13 (17.57)

MNTP morphologically normal prostate tissue, *PCa* prostate cancer, *IQR* interquartile range, *n.a* not applicable

Moreover, genomic DNA extracted from each clinical sample was submitted to bisulfite sodium conversion using EZ DNA Methylation-Gold™ Kit (Zymo Research, CA, USA) according to the manufacturer's recommendation.

Methylation analysis

The promoter methylation status of panel #1 (*miR-193b* and *miR-34b/c*) was determined as previously described in [11]. Briefly, methylation assessment of panel #1 was performed by quantitative methylation using KAPA SYBR FAST qPCR Kit (Kapa Biosystems, MA, USA).

Primer sequences (Additional file 1: Table S1) were designed using Methyl Primer Express 1.0 and purchased from Sigma-Aldrich (MO, USA).

Panel #2 (*APC*, *GSTP1*, and *RARβ2*) methylation levels were evaluated using multiplex MethyLight methodology. The multiplex MethyLight assay was carried out in a reaction volume of 10 μL in 96-well plates using a 7500 Sequence Detector. The scorpion primer-probe sequences were the previously published in [14, 15], except for *APC* (Additional file 1: Table S2). Briefly, per each well, 5 μL KiCqStart™ Probe qPCR ReadyMix™ (Low ROX) (Sigma-Aldrich, Germany), 300 nM of each

Table 2 Clinical and pathological features of urine samples from asymptomatic controls and prostate cancer patients enrolled in this study (cohort #2)

Clinicopathological data	Urine (cohort #2)	
	AC	PCa
Patients, n	32	87
Median age, years (range)	58 (50–64)	64 (47–75)
Median PSA (ng/mL) (range)	n.a.	8.80 (3.50–20.40)
Pathological stage, n (%)		
pT2	n.a.	43 (49.43)
pT3a	n.a.	35 (40.23)
pT3b	n.a.	9 (10.34)
Prognostic grade group, n (%)		
1	n.a.	34 (39.08)
2	n.a.	39 (44.83)
3	n.a.	7 (8.05)
4	n.a.	5 (5.75)
5	n.a.	2 (2.30)

AC asymptomatic controls, PCa prostate cancer, n.a not applicable

primer inner (Sigma-Aldrich, Germany); 100 nM of scorpion primer-probe for APC, RARβ2, and β-Actin, and 150 nM of scorpion primer-probe for GSTP1 (Sigma-Aldrich, Germany) and 3 μL of bisulfite modified DNA as a template were added. The PCR program consisted of 95 °C for 5 min and 40 cycles at 95 °C for 15 s, and 64 °C for 1 min and 72 °C for 10 s. All samples were run in triplicate, and β-Actin, a housekeeping gene, was used as reference gene to normalize the results obtained for each gene studied.

Statistical analysis

Differences in methylation levels and relationships between methylation and different clinical variables were assessed using the Kruskal-Wallis and Mann-Whitney non-parametric tests in multiple groups (more than two) and pairwise comparisons, respectively. P values were considered statistically significant if inferior to 0.05 for comparisons between two groups. In multiple comparisons and when statistically significant, Bonferroni's correction was applied for pairwise comparisons, dividing the original P value by the number of groups. Spearman non-parametric correlation test was performed to test for associations between methylation levels and patient's age and serum PSA.

For each gene promotor, receiver operator characteristics (ROC) curves were constructed by plotting the true positive (sensitivity) against the false-positive (1-specificity) rate, and area under the curve (AUC) was calculated. For the two panels, ROC curves were constructed using logistic regression model, to assess whether biomarker performance was increased using the panel.

Specificity, sensitivity, positive predictive value (PPV), negative predictive value (NPV), and accuracy were determined for the gene-panel considering positive for the test when at least one of the genes was plotted as positive in individual analysis. The positive (LR+) and negative (LR-) likelihood ratios were also determined, and as the quantitative value of a calculated likelihood ratio is further away from 1 in either direction (> 1 for LR+ and < 1 for LR−), there is increasing utility of a diagnostic test to point toward, or away from, a diagnosis which indicate the value of performing the respective diagnostic tests. For this, the empirical cutoff obtained by ROC curve analysis [sensitivity + (1-specificity)] was established for each gene. This cutoff value combines the maximum sensitivity and specificity, ensuring perfect categorization of the samples as positive and negative for methylation test. In addition, time-dependent ROC curves were constructed considering biochemical recurrence/progression of disease for all tested genes at three-time points (5, 10, and 15 years) as endpoint.

DSS, DFS, and PFS curves (Kaplan-Meier with log rank test) were constructed considering clinicopathological variables (PSA levels, histologic grade group according with Epstein classification [16], clinical stage, CAPRA score [17], D'Amico's risk group classification system [18]) and categorized promoter methylation status (using percentile 75 as cutoff). A Cox-regression model (multivariable model) was computed considering all significant clinical variables, to assess the relative contribution of each variable to the follow-up status. For multivariable testing, prognostic grade group (GG), clinical stage, PSA serum levels, CAPRA Score, and D'Amico's classification were coded into two groups each [GG1 vs. GG 2–5, T2 vs. T3–4, PSA < 10 ng/mL vs. PSA ≥ 10 < 20 ng/mL vs. PSA ≥20 ng/mL, CAPRA Score low and intermediate risk (0–5) vs. high risk (6–10) [19], D'Amico's classification low and intermediate risk vs. high risk].

Statistical analysis was carried out using SPSS Statistics, version 25 (IBM-SPSS, IL, USA), GraphPad Prism 7.01 (GraphPad Software, CA, USA) and R software version 3.2.5.

Results
Diagnostic performance of genes' promoter methylation in prostate biopsy (cohort #1) and urine sediments (cohort #2) using different panels
To determine the performance of the gene methylation panels as PCa detection tools, ROC curve analysis was carried out and an empirical cutoff value was defined for calculation of biomarker performance (Additional file 1: Tables S3 and S4).

In prostate biopsy (cohort #1), methylation levels of all gene promoters were significantly higher in PCa patients compared to controls (Additional file 2: Figure S1). Moreover, panel #1 (*miR-193b* and *miR-34b/c*) discriminated PCa from non-cancerous prostate tissue with 97.3% sensitivity and 80.0% specificity, whereas panel #2 (*APC*, *GSTP1*, and *RARβ2*) displayed maximal sensitivity and specificity (Table 3 and Fig. 1a).

In urine sediments (cohort #2), all tested genes, except for *GSTP1*, displayed significantly higher promoter methylation levels in samples from PCa patients comparing with controls (Additional file 3 Figure S2). Panel #1 disclosed the highest sensitivity (95.4%), providing 92.4% accuracy and an AUC of 0.8836 (Table 4 and Fig. 1b). Panel #2 also displayed high sensitivity and specificity, although with an inferior positive predictive value (84.4%) (Table 4 and Fig. 1b). Interestingly, when both panels were combined, PCa was detected in voided urine with 100% sensitivity and an AUC value of 0.9817 (Table 4 and Fig. 1b).

Association between promoter methylation levels and clinicopathological parameters

In cohort #1, higher methylation levels of panel #2 gene promoters significantly associated with higher prognostic grade group (GG2–5 vs. GG1; *APC* $P = 0.009$, *GSTP1* $P = 0.004$, *RARβ2* $P = 0.008$) (Fig. 2a), and the same was observed for *miR-34b/c* ($P = 0.006$) (Fig. 2b). Moreover, increased *APC* methylation levels significantly associated with higher CAPRA Score ($P = 0.005$) (Fig. 2c) and increased risk of recurrence, according with D'Amico's risk classification ($P = 0.038$) (Fig. 2d). Nevertheless, no association was depicted between promoter methylation levels and patient's age, diagnostic serum PSA levels, or clinical stage.

In cohort #2, no association between methylation levels and prognostic grade group, pathological stage, or diagnostic serum PSA levels was found. Nonetheless, *miR-34b/c* promoter methylation levels significantly associated (although modestly) with patients' age at diagnosis ($P = 0.018$, $r = 0.253$). Thus, ROC curves were normalized for this variable and diagnostic performance was calculated accordingly.

Table 3 Diagnostic performance of DNA methylation-based biomarkers in cohort #1

Parameters	Panel #1	Panel #2
Sensitivity %	97.3	100.0
Specificity %	80.0	100.0
Positive predictive value %	96.0	100.0
Negative predictive value %	85.7	100.0
Accuracy %	94.4	100.0
Positive likelihood ratio (LR+)	4.87	–
Negative likelihood ratio (LR–)	0.03	–

Prognostic value of panel #1 and panel #2 in cohort #1

Prognostic value was only tested in the cohort of PCa patients with longer follow-up (cohort #1), which displayed a median follow-up of 104.04 (range: 67.03–145.48) months. From the 74 patients, only 39 (52.70%) were treated curative intent. All patients were included in DSS analysis ($n = 74$), whereas for DFS, only patients with initial curative intention (RP/RT) but one (without remission) were included ($n = 38$). For PFS analysis, 3 patients were excluded from cohort #1 due to persistence of high serum PSA levels after treatment. During this period, 13/74 (17.57%) patients deceased from PCa, while disease progressed in 29/71 (40.85%). Moreover, 13/38 (34.21%) of patients with initial curative intention developed biochemical recurrence.

Regarding DSS, higher prognostic grade group ($P = 0.009$), advanced clinical stage ($P < 0.001$), high diagnostic serum PSA levels ($P = 0.010$), increased CAPRA score ($P = 0.004$), and D'Amico risk classification ($P = 0.001$) significantly associated with shorter survival. A similar result was found for higher *miR-34b/c* ($P = 0.035$) and panel #2 (*APC*, *GSTP1*, and *RARβ2*) ($P = 0.028$) promoter methylation levels (Fig. 3). Furthermore, in multivariable Cox-regression analysis, clinical stage (II vs. III/IV) and *miR-34b/c* or panel #2 methylation independently predicted DSS (Table 5). On the other hand, high prognostic grade group ($P = 0.004$), increased CAPRA score ($P = 0.001$) and higher panel #2 methylation levels ($P = 0.008$) significantly associated with biochemical relapse, but only in univariable analysis. Although panel #1 methylation levels did not associate with DFS, when *miR-34b/c* promoter methylation levels were added to panel #2, higher promoter methylation of this combination predicted shorter time to relapse ($P = 0.026$) (Fig. 4a). Indeed, the combination of *miR-34b/c* (panel #1) and panel #2 methylation levels also associated with shorter PFS in univariable analysis ($P = 0.011$), as well as clinical parameters [high prognostic grade group ($P = 0.017$) and increased CAPRA score ($P = 0.025$)] (Fig. 4b).

Furthermore, the prognostic performance of the methylation panels over time was analyzed by constructing time-dependent ROC curves (Fig. 5). Among panel #1 markers, *miR-34b/c* methylation levels showed the best performance at 15 years of follow-up (AUC = 0.751), whereas no significant information was provided by *miR-193b* methylation levels. Concerning panel #2, *APC* and *GSTP1* methylation levels displayed the best performance at 5 years (AUC = 0.681) and at 15 years (AUC = 0.765), respectively, whereas no significant information was provided by *RARβ2* methylation levels.

Discussion

Prostate cancer is the second most incident solid malignancy in men, being associated with significant morbidity

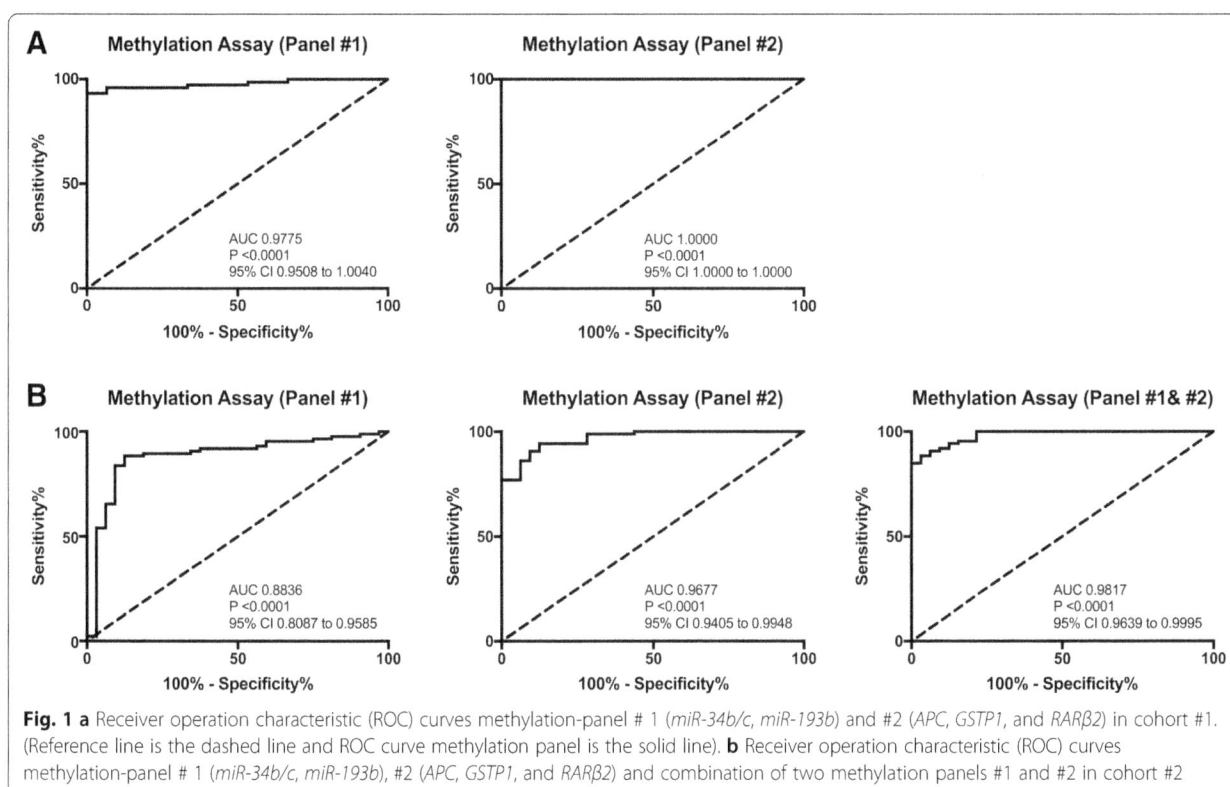

Fig. 1 a Receiver operation characteristic (ROC) curves methylation-panel # 1 (*miR-34b/c, miR-193b*) and #2 (*APC, GSTP1*, and *RARβ2*) in cohort #1. (Reference line is the dashed line and ROC curve methylation panel is the solid line). **b** Receiver operation characteristic (ROC) curves methylation-panel # 1 (*miR-34b/c, miR-193b*), #2 (*APC, GSTP1*, and *RARβ2*) and combination of two methylation panels #1 and #2 in cohort #2

and mortality (5th leading cause of cancer-related death) [20]. The implementation of serum PSA-based screening resulted in an increased number of men diagnosed with PCa at asymptomatic, early stage disease, but this was achieved at the cost of overdiagnosis and overtreatment of clinically insignificant disease. Indeed, serum PSA testing does not accurately discriminate between benign and malignant prostate disease, neither between indolent and clinically significant PCa [21]. Thus, the identification of robust and minimally invasive molecular biomarkers that may be used for screening, diagnosis, risk stratification, and prognostication is mandatory [22, 23]. Owing to the prevalence and cancer specificity of aberrant promoter methylation of both protein-coding and non-coding genes in PCa [24, 25], these constitute promising biomarkers for

Table 4 Diagnostic performance of DNA methylation-based biomarkers in cohort #2

Parameters	Panel #1	Panel #2	Panels #1 and #2
Sensitivity %	95.4	94.3	100.0
Specificity %	84.4	84.4	75.0
Positive predictive value %	94.3	94.3	91.6
Negative predictive value %	87.1	84.4	100.0
Accuracy %	92.4	91.6	93.3
Positive likelihood ratio (LR+)	6.12	6.04	4.00
Negative likelihood ratio (LR−)	0.05	0.07	-

clinical use [11]. Herein, we compared the biomarker performance of two methylation panels [panel #1 (*miR-193b/ miR-34b/c*) and panel #2 (*APC/GSTP1/RARβ2*)], for PCa diagnosis and prognostication, in the same series of prostate biopsies and urine sediments, from two independent cohorts.

In prostate biopsy samples, both panels demonstrated excellent performance for PCa detection, although panel #2 attained maximal performance, emphasizing the potential of these panels as ancillary tools for PCa detection in this setting. These results are in line with three previously reported multicenter studies, in which *APC/GSTP1/RASSF1A* multiplex quantitative methylation analysis in biopsy needle core tissue samples with histological negative result displayed 88–100% NPV, confirming methylation assays as helpful tools for assisting in decision of re-biopsy [26–28]. Indeed, besides the need to precisely identify PCa in biopsy, accurately deny of its presence is of paramount importance as this will allow for extending the time period until re-biopsy, significantly reducing costs and harmful side-effects of an invasive procedure. However, because only biopsy cores containing PCa were included and not negative cores, nor the respective prostatectomy specimens, this maximal sensitivity might not be confirmed definitively. Panel #1, however, displayed 97.3% sensitivity. This value obtained in the same sample set clearly indicates that although the vast

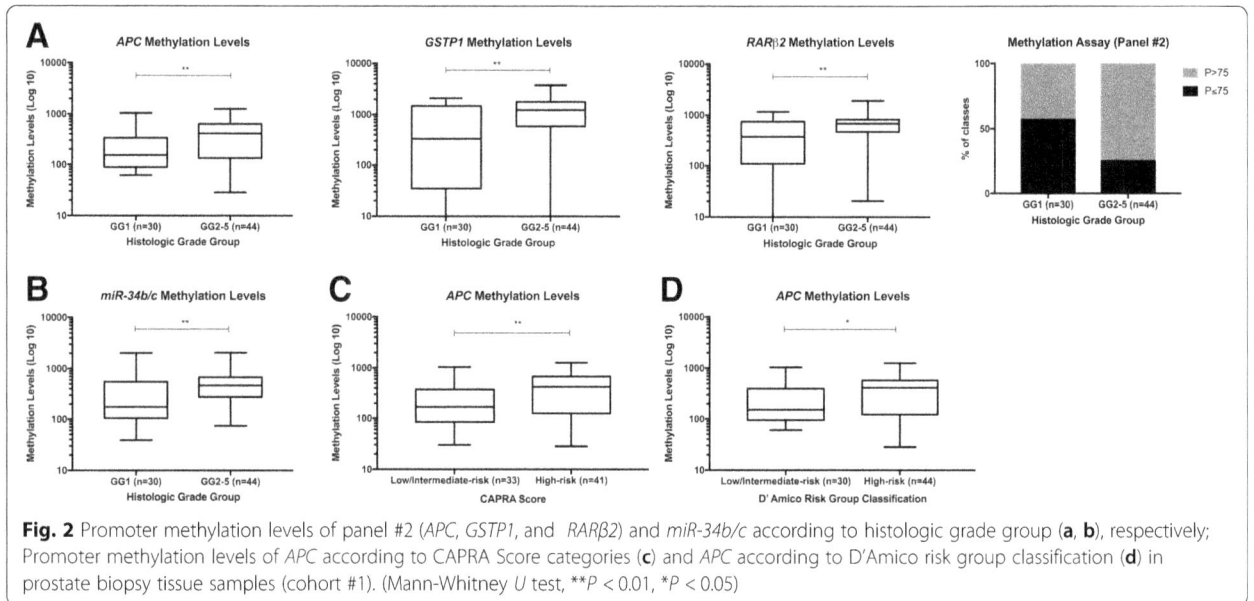

Fig. 2 Promoter methylation levels of panel #2 (*APC*, *GSTP1*, and *RARβ2*) and *miR-34b/c* according to histologic grade group (**a**, **b**), respectively; Promoter methylation levels of *APC* according to CAPRA Score categories (**c**) and *APC* according to D'Amico risk group classification (**d**) in prostate biopsy tissue samples (cohort #1). (Mann-Whitney *U* test, **$P < 0.01$, *$P < 0.05$)

majority of PCa cases display miR-34b/c and/or miR-193b promoter hypermethylation, 2.7% of cases do not, which might be due to tumor heterogeneity.

Notwithstanding the potential of methylation-based biomarkers in tissue samples, its use for early detection requires assessment in body fluids. In this setting, panel #1 identified PCa with higher sensitivity than panel #2, but with modest specificity, providing an AUC of 0.8836, in urine sediments. Unexpectedly, the panel #1 AUC was lower than previously reported by us [11] which

might be explained by differences in the control population. On the other hand, the methylation panel comprising *APC* and *RARβ2* identified PCa with only fair sensitivity and specificity, although with higher AUC compared to panel #1. The inclusion of only two genes (*APC* and *RARβ2*) was due to the lack of significant differences of *GSTP1* promoter methylation levels between PCa urine samples and controls. This was a rather unexpected finding considering previous reports from our group and others [14, 29–31], and it might be due to

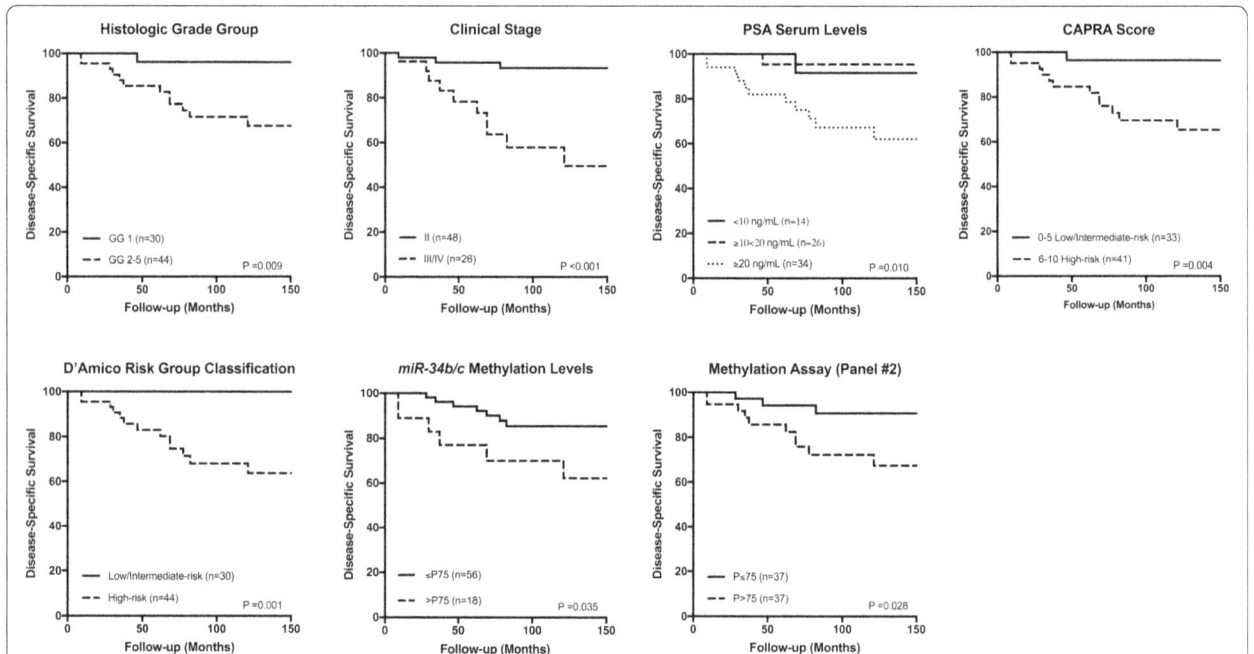

Fig. 3 Disease-specific survival curves according to standard clinicopathological parameters [histologic grade group, clinical stage, PSA serum levels, CAPRA Score, and D'Amico risk group classification] and epigenetic marks [*miR-34b/c* and panel #2] in prostate biopsy (cohort #1)

Table 5 Cox-regression models assessing the potential of clinical and epigenetics variables in the prediction of disease-specific survival in cohort #1

Disease-specific survival	Variable	Hazard ratio (HR)	95% CI for OR	P value
Multivariable	Clinical stage			
	III/IV	9.637	2.597–35.763	0.001
	Panel #1: *miR-34b/c*			
	Promoter methylation > P75	3.843	1.268–11.649	0.017
	Clinical stage			
	III/IV	8.334	2.274–30.548	0.001
	Panel #2			
	Promoter methylation > P75	3.786	1.038–13.810	0.044

HR hazard ratio

different procedures for urine collection. Indeed, the urine samples used in this study were not collected after DRE or prostatic massage, which increase shedding of prostate cells, thus improving sensitivity [32]. Nevertheless, the two-gene panel (*APC* and *RARβ2*), displayed better sensitivity and AUC than the ProCaM assay, which is a three-gene panel [10]. Moreover, in that study, promoter methylation analysis was performed in a two-step PCR, whereas we carried out a one-step PCR, allowing for faster and more cost-effective detection.

Remarkably, the combination of the two methylation panels depicted maximal sensitivity and NPV, improving accuracy (93.3%) and AUC (0.9817), thus augmenting PCa detection performance in urine. Also, the methylation test encompassing the two panels

present null LR–, indicating that there is no chance of disease when the test is negative, and a LR+ of 4. As previously mentioned, the accuracy of serum PSA testing to predict PCa is suboptimal [21] and regardless the efforts to improve its performance, namely through PSA-derived parameters, the added value is small [33]. On the contrary, our results show that a methylation assay combining panel #1 and panel #2 displays a diagnostic performance in urine sediments superior to serum PSA and urinary PCA3, which are currently used in clinical practice [34]. Nevertheless, future studies that include larger cohorts of PCa patients and healthy subjects are required to further validate these preliminary results and provide direct comparisons among the several tests.

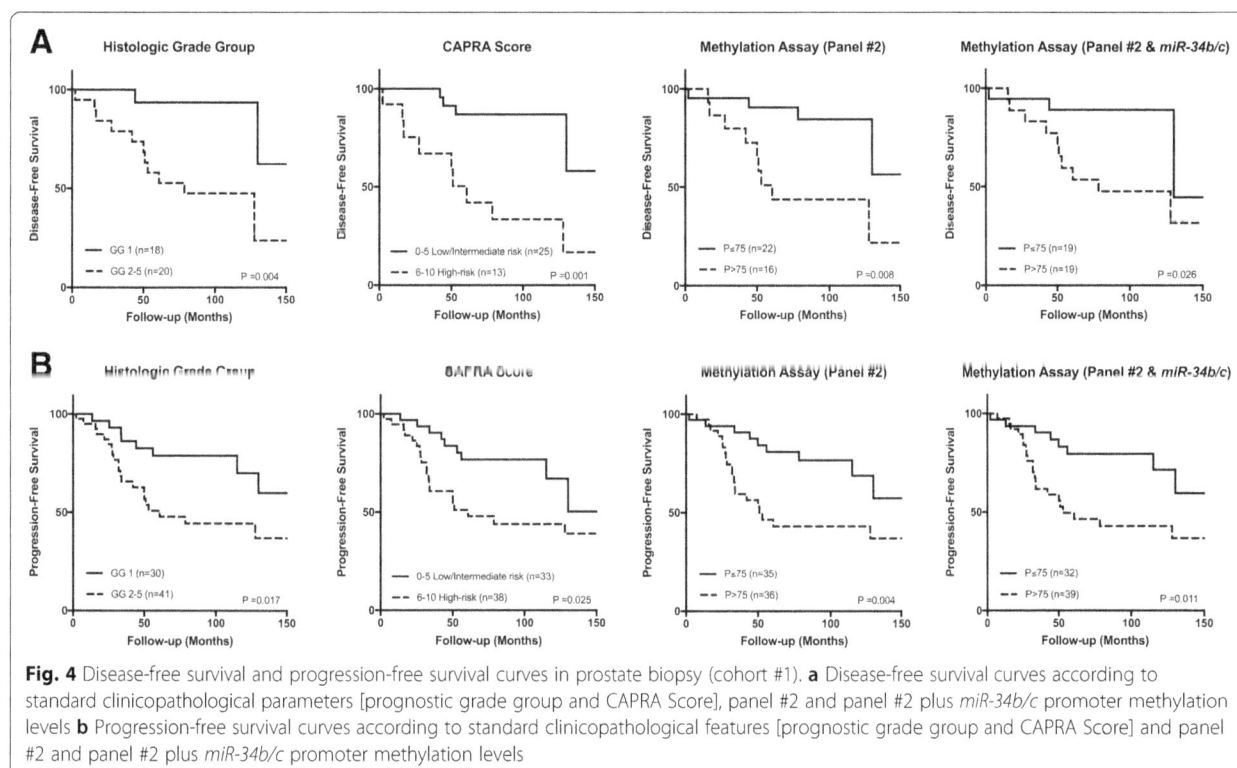

Fig. 4 Disease-free survival and progression-free survival curves in prostate biopsy (cohort #1). **a** Disease-free survival curves according to standard clinicopathological parameters [prognostic grade group and CAPRA Score], panel #2 and panel #2 plus *miR-34b/c* promoter methylation levels **b** Progression-free survival curves according to standard clinicopathological features [prognostic grade group and CAPRA Score] and panel #2 and panel #2 plus *miR-34b/c* promoter methylation levels

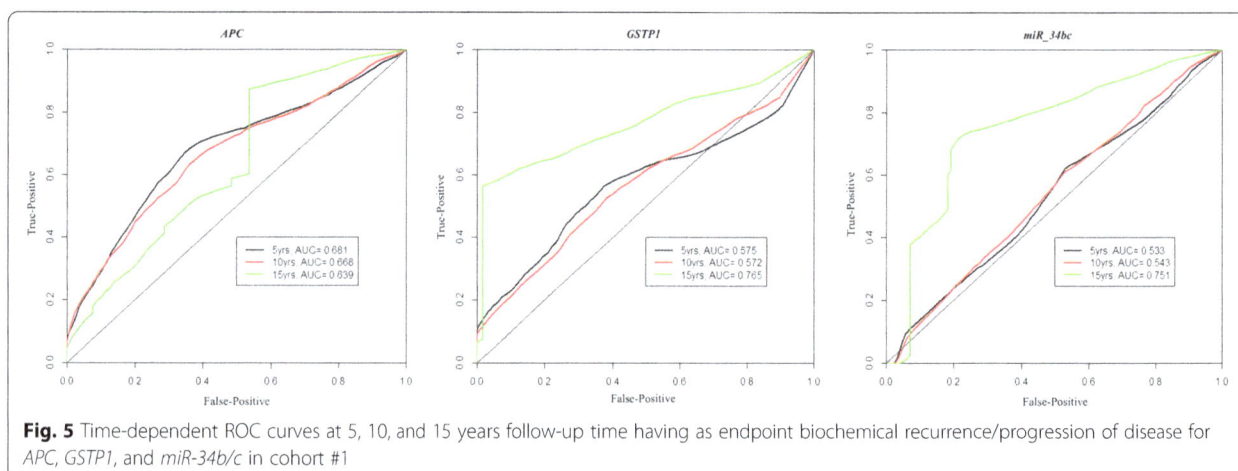

Fig. 5 Time-dependent ROC curves at 5, 10, and 15 years follow-up time having as endpoint biochemical recurrence/progression of disease for *APC, GSTP1,* and *miR-34b/c* in cohort #1

Because overdiagnosis and consequent overtreatment are a major concern, PCa detection should be accompanied by risk stratification for disease aggressiveness. Thus, the ability to convey relevant prognostic information is of chief importance. Interestingly, at the time of diagnosis, higher promoter methylation of *miR-34b/c* and panel #2 genes associated with clinicopathological features of disease aggressiveness (prognostic grade group, CAPRA score, D'Amico's risk classification), suggesting the ability to discriminate clinically significant from indolent PCa, in biopsy samples, probably due to the increased promoter methylation of several target genes along PCa initiation and progression. Notwithstanding these correlates, survival analysis is critical to assess the prognostic significance. Remarkably, *miR-34b/ c* from panel #1 and panel #2 promoter methylations disclosed independent prognostic significance, along with clinical stage, suggesting a role as stratification tool

for disease aggressiveness, and in line with a previous study from our group [11, 13]. Furthermore, we found that the prognostic ability of methylation biomarkers is time dependent. Indeed, both *miR-34b/c* and *GSTP1* promoter methylations increase its prediction accuracy over time, identifying patients that relapse up to 15 years after diagnosis and beyond. Thus, promoter methylation of these genes might allow for more personalized follow-up procedures, increasing the cost-effectiveness of PCa patients' management in the long term.

The main limitation of this study is the relatively small sample size, in both cohorts, that might preclude the identification of more significant differences between promoter methylation levels in tissue and urine samples and patient outcome. Furthermore, follow-up time of cohort #2 does not allow for the assessment of the prognostic value of methylation biomarkers in urine. Nevertheless, it should be emphasized that all samples

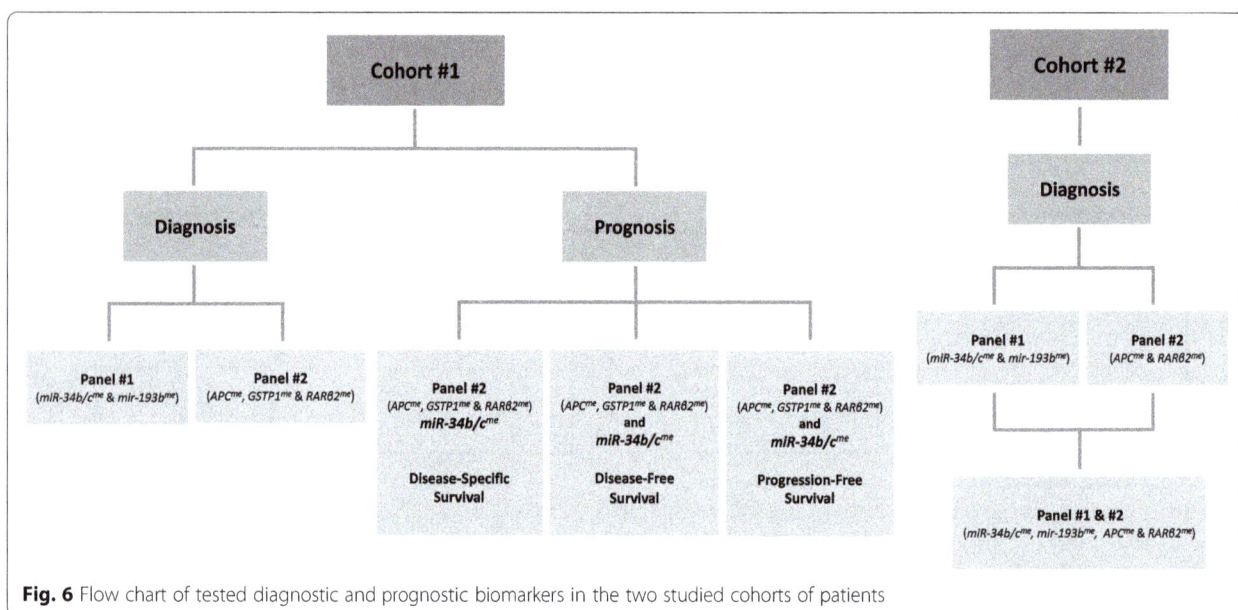

Fig. 6 Flow chart of tested diagnostic and prognostic biomarkers in the two studied cohorts of patients

were prospectively collected and that a multiplex assay was used, allowing for diagnostic and prognostic assessment of PCa suspects in a single analysis as a mean to improve the efficiency of the test, considering the limited amount of prostate cell-derived DNA present in urine. Importantly, although our results suggest a potential clinical usefulness, prospective validation (which we did not perform) in an independent cohort is mandatory.

Conclusions

In conclusion, this study highlights the potential of specific gene promoter methylation testing in biopsy and urine sediments for PCa detection and prognostication (Fig. 6). Furthermore, the multiplex methylation assay of panel #2 constitutes a powerful method for methylation analysis of samples with minimal DNA amounts. Nonetheless, the potential usefulness of these DNA methylation biomarkers requires further studies in larger series of PCa suspects, to develop a valid tool for accurate detection of clinically significant PCa.

Abbreviations

AC: Asymptomatic controls; APC: Adenomatosis polyposis coli; AUC: Area under curve; CAPRA score: Cancer of the prostate risk assessment score; DFS: Disease-free survival; DSS: Disease-specific survival; GSTP1: Glutathione S-transferase pi 1; IQR: Interquartile range; LR+/−: Positive/negative likelihood ratio; miR: MicroRNA; MNTP: Morphologically normal prostate tissue; NPV: Negative predictive value; PCa: Prostate cancer; PCR: Polymerase chain reaction; PFS: Progression-free survival; PPV: Positive predictive value; ProCAM: Prostate cancer methylation; PSA: Prostate-specific antigen; RARβ2: Retinoic acid receptor β 2

Acknowledgements
The authors are grateful to the Departments of Urology and of Laboratory Medicine of the Portuguese Oncology Institute of Porto for their collaboration in urine collection, in particularly to Ms. Berta Reis, Nursing D.

Funding
This work was funded by Research Center - Portuguese Oncology Institute of Porto (grant PI 74-CI-IPOP-19-2015). Catarina Moreira-Barbosa and Daniela Barros Silva were supported scholarships from Núcleo Regional da Madeira da Liga Portuguesa Contra o Cancro & Diário de Notícias and Research Center - Portuguese Oncology Institute of Porto (CI-IPOP-BI-GEBC2018/UID/DTP/00776/POCI-01-0145-FEDER-006868), respectively.

Authors' contributions
PCP, RH, and CJ conceived and designed the experiments. CM-B, DB-S, and JT-F performed the experiments. CM-B, DB-S, JT-F, VC, LA, RH, and CJ analyzed the data. RF and JO provided the clinical data from clinical charts. All authors read and approved the final manuscript.

Competing interests
The authors declare that they have no competing interests.

Author details
[1]Cancer Biology and Epigenetics Group, IPO Porto Research Center (CI-IPOP), Portuguese Oncology Institute of Porto (IPO Porto), Porto, Portugal. [2]Department of Pathology, Portuguese Oncology Institute of Porto (IPO Porto), Rua Dr. António Bernardino de Almeida, 4200-072 Porto, Portugal. [3]Department of Urology, Portuguese Oncology Institute of Porto (IPO Porto), Rua Dr. António Bernardino de Almeida, 4200-072 Porto, Portugal. [4]Department of Epidemiology, Portuguese Oncology Institute of Porto (IPO Porto), Rua Dr. António Bernardino de Almeida, 4200-072 Porto, Portugal. [5]Department of Pathology and Molecular Immunology, Institute of Biomedical Sciences Abel Salazar (ICBAS), University of Porto, Porto, Portugal. [6]Cancer Biology and Epigenetics Group - Research Center (LAB3), Portuguese Oncology Institute of Porto, Rua Dr. António Bernardino Almeida, 4200-072 Porto, Portugal.

References
1. Center MM, Jemal A, Lortet-Tieulent J, Ward E, Ferlay J, Brawley O, Bray F. International variation in prostate cancer incidence and mortality rates. Eur Urol. 2012;61(6):1079–92.
2. Shen MM, Abate-Shen C. Molecular genetics of prostate cancer: new prospects for old challenges. Genes Dev. 2010;24(18):1967–2000.
3. Roobol MJ, Carlsson SV. Risk stratification in prostate cancer screening. Nat Rev Urol. 2013;10(1):38–48.
4. Attard G, Parker C, Eeles RA, Schröder F, Tomlins SA, Tannock I, Drake CG, De Bono JS. Prostate cancer. Lancet. 2016;387(10013):70–82.
5. Jerónimo C, Henrique R. Epigenetic biomarkers in urological tumors: a systematic review. Cancer Lett. 2014;342(2):264–74.
6. Massie CE, Mills IG, Lynch AG. The importance of DNA methylation in prostate cancer development. J Steroid Biochem Mol Biol. 2017;166:1–15.
7. Gurioli G, Salvi S, Martignano F, Foca F, Gunelli R, Costantini M, Cicchetti G, Giorgi U, Sbarba PD, Calistri D. Methylation pattern analysis in prostate cancer tissue: identification of biomarkers using an MS-MLPA approach. J Transl Med. 2016;14(1):249.
8. Yegnasubramanian S. Prostate cancer epigenetics and its clinical implications. Asian J Androl. 2016;18:549.
9. Duffy M, Napieralski R, Martens J, Span P, Spyratos F, Sweep F, Brunner N, Foekens J, Schmitt M. Methylated genes as new cancer biomarkers. Eur J Cancer. 2009;45(3):335–46.
10. Baden J, Adams S, Astacio T, Jones J, Markiewicz J, Painter J, Trust C, Wang Y, Green G. Predicting prostate biopsy result in men with prostate specific antigen 2.0 to 10.0 ng/ml using an investigational prostate cancer methylation assay. J Urol. 2011;186(5):2101–6.
11. Torres-Ferreira J, Ramalho-Carvalho J, Gomez A, Menezes FD, Freitas R, Oliveira J, Antunes L, Bento MJ, Esteller M, Henrique R. MiR-193b promoter methylation accurately detects prostate cancer in urine sediments and miR-34b/c or miR-129-2 promoter methylation define subsets of clinically aggressive tumors. Mol Cancer. 2017;16(1):26.
12. Bastian PJ, Palapattu GS, Lin X, Yegnasubramanian S, Mangold LA, Trock B, Eisenberger MA, Partin AW, Nelson WG. Preoperative serum DNA GSTP1 CpG island hypermethylation and the risk of early prostate-specific antigen recurrence following radical prostatectomy. Clin Cancer Res. 2005;11(11):4037–43.
13. Henrique R, Ribeiro FR, Fonseca D, Hoque MO, Carvalho AL, Costa VL, Pinto M, Oliveira J, Teixeira MR, Sidransky D. High promoter methylation levels of APC predict poor prognosis in sextant biopsies from prostate cancer patients. Clin Cancer Res. 2007;13(20):6122–9.
14. Vener T, Derecho C, Baden J, Wang H, Rajpurohit Y, Skelton J, Mehrotra J, Varde S, Chowdary D, Stallings W. Development of a multiplexed urine assay for prostate cancer diagnosis. Clin Chem. 2008;54(5):874–82.
15. Baden J, Green G, Painter J, Curtin K, Markiewicz J, Jones J, Astacio T, Canning S, Quijano J, Guinto W. Multicenter evaluation of an investigational prostate cancer methylation assay. J Urol. 2009;182(3):1186–93.
16. Gordetsky J, Epstein J. Grading of prostatic adenocarcinoma: current state and prognostic implications. Diagn Pathol. 2016;11(1):1.
17. Cooperberg MR, Broering JM, Carroll PR. Risk assessment for prostate cancer metastasis and mortality at the time of diagnosis. J Natl Cancer Inst. 2009;101(12):878–87.
18. D'Amico AV, Whittington R, Malkowicz S, et al. Biochemical outcome after radical prostatectomy, external beam radiation therapy, or interstitial radiation therapy for clinically localized prostate cancer. JAMA. 1998;280(11):969–74.

19. Cooperberg MR, Freedland SJ, Pasta DJ, Elkin EP, Presti JC, Amling CL, Terris MK, Aronson WJ, Kane CJ, Carroll PR. Multiinstitutional validation of the UCSF cancer of the prostate risk assessment for prediction of recurrence after radical prostatectomy. Cancer. 2006;107(10):2384–91.

20. Ferlay J, Soerjomataram I, Dikshit R, Eser S, Mathers C, Rebelo M, Parkin DM, Forman D, Bray F. Cancer incidence and mortality worldwide: sources, methods and major patterns in GLOBOCAN 2012. Int J Cancer. 2015;136(5): E359–86.

21. Prensner JR, Rubin MA, Wei JT, Chinnaiyan AM. Beyond PSA: the next generation of prostate cancer biomarkers. Sci Transl Med. 2012;4(127): 127rv123.

22. Ramalho-Carvalho J, Henrique R, Jerónimo C. Chapter 14 - DNA methylation alterations as biomarkers for prostate cancer A2 - García-Giménez, José Luis. In: *Epigenetic Biomarkers and Diagnostics.* Edn. Boston: Academic Press; 2016. p. 275–96.

23. Ellinger J, Müller SC, Dietrich D. Epigenetic biomarkers in the blood of patients with urological malignancies. Expert Rev Mol Diagn. 2015;15(4): 505–16.

24. Ramalho-Carvalho J, Martins JB, Cekaite L, Sveen A, Torres-Ferreira J, Graca I, Costa-Pinheiro P, Eilertsen IA, Antunes L, Oliveira J, et al. Epigenetic disruption of miR-130a promotes prostate cancer by targeting SEC23B and DEPDC1. Cancer Lett. 2017;385:150–9.

25. Ramalho-Carvalho J, Graca I, Gomez A, Oliveira J, Henrique R, Esteller M, Jeronimo C. Downregulation of miR-130b~301b cluster is mediated by aberrant promoter methylation and impairs cellular senescence in prostate cancer. J Hematol Oncol. 2017;10(1):43.

26. Partin AW, Van Neste L, Klein EA, Marks LS, Gee JR, Troyer DA, Rieger-Christ K, Jones JS, Magi-Galluzzi C, Mangold LA, et al. Clinical validation of an epigenetic assay to predict negative histopathological results in repeat prostate biopsies. J Urol. 2014;192(4):1081–7.

27. Stewart GD, Van Neste L, Delvenne P, Delrée P, Delga A, McNeill SA, O'Donnell M, Clark J, Van Criekinge W, Bigley J. Clinical utility of an epigenetic assay to detect occult prostate cancer in histopathologically negative biopsies: results of the MATLOC study. J Urol. 2013;189(3):1110–6.

28. Van Neste L, Partin AW, Stewart GD, Epstein JI, Harrison DJ, Van Criekinge W. Risk score predicts high-grade prostate cancer in DNA-methylation positive, histopathologically negative biopsies. Prostate. 2016;76(12):1078–87.

29. Jernimo C, Usadel H, Henrique R, Silva C, Oliveira J, Lopes C, Sidransky D. Quantitative GSTP1 hypermethylation in bodily fluids of patients with prostate cancer. Urology. 2002;60(6):1131–5.

30. Hoque MO, Topaloglu O, Begum S, Henrique R, Rosenbaum E, Van Criekinge W, Westra WH, Sidransky D. Quantitative methylation-specific polymerase chain reaction gene patterns in urine sediment distinguish prostate cancer patients from control subjects. J Clin Oncol. 2005;23(27): 6569–75.

31. Roupret M, Hupertan V, Yates DR, Catto JW, Rehman I, Meuth M, Ricci S, Lacave R, Cancel-Tassin G, de la Taille A, et al. Molecular detection of localized prostate cancer using quantitative methylation-specific PCR on urinary cells obtained following prostate massage. Clin Cancer Res. 2007; 13(6):1720–5.

32. Ralla B, Stephan C, Meller S, Dietrich D, Kristiansen G, Jung K. Nucleic acid-based biomarkers in body fluids of patients with urologic malignancies. Crit Rev Clin Lab Sci. 2014;51(4):200–31.

33. Gaudreau P-O, Stagg J, Soulières D, Saad F. The present and future of biomarkers in prostate cancer: proteomics, genomics, and immunology advancements. Biomark Cancer. 2016;8(Suppl 2):15.

34. Sartori DA, Chan DW. Biomarkers in prostate cancer: what's new? Curr Opin Oncol. 2014;26(3):259.

20

Alterations of adiponectin gene expression and DNA methylation in adipose tissues and blood cells are associated with gestational diabetes and neonatal outcome

Raffael Ott[1], Jens H. Stupin[2], Kerstin Melchior[1], Karen Schellong[1], Thomas Ziska[1], Joachim W. Dudenhausen[2], Wolfgang Henrich[2], Rebecca C. Rancourt[1]*[†] (iD) and Andreas Plagemann[1†]

Abstract

Background: Adiponectin critically contributes to metabolic homeostasis, especially by insulin-sensitizing action. Gestational diabetes mellitus (GDM) is characterized by insulin resistance leading to materno-fetal hyperglycemia and detrimental birth outcomes. By investigating paired subcutaneous (SAT) and visceral adipose tissue (VAT) as well as blood (cell) samples of GDM-affected ($n = 25$) vs. matched control ($n = 30$) mother-child dyads of the prospective "*EaCH*" cohort study, we addressed whether alterations of adiponectin plasma, mRNA, and DNA methylation levels are associated with GDM and offspring characteristics.

Results: Hypoadiponectinemia was present in women with GDM, even after adjustment for body mass index (BMI). This was accompanied by significantly decreased mRNA levels in both SAT and VAT ($P < 0.05$), independent of BMI. Maternal plasma adiponectin showed inverse relations with glucose and homeostatic model assessment of insulin resistance (both $P < 0.01$). In parallel to reduced mRNA expression in GDM, significant ($P < 0.05$) yet small alterations in locus-specific DNA methylation were observed in maternal fat (~ 2%) and blood cells (~ 1%). While newborn adiponectin levels were similar between groups, DNA methylation in GDM offspring was variously altered (~ 1–4%; $P < 0.05$).

Conclusions: Reduced adiponectin seems to be a pathogenic co-factor in GDM, even independent of BMI, affecting materno-fetal metabolism. While altered maternal DNA methylation patterns appear rather marginally involved, functional, diagnostic, and/or predictive implications of cord blood DNA methylation should be further evaluated.

Keywords: Gestational diabetes mellitus, Epigenetics, DNA methylation, Adiponectin, Adipose tissue, Blood cells, Cord blood, Offspring

Background

Gestational diabetes mellitus (GDM) is one of the most frequent metabolic disorders in pregnancy affecting meanwhile > 10% of women in Western countries [1–3]. Both increased peripheral insulin resistance and failed compensation of insulin need are hallmarks of GDM [4]. While causes for these characteristics remain unclear, other endocrine factors are potentially contributing.

Adiponectin (*ADIPOQ*) is a key hormone in energy metabolism, critically involved in maintaining insulin sensitivity, glucose, and lipid homeostasis [5]. Accordingly, hypoadiponectinemia has been observed in insulin resistance, type 2 diabetes, GDM, and obesity [6, 7]. Interestingly, studies suggest that low adiponectin levels in early pregnancy represent a risk marker for GDM development [8], and the clinical relevance has been debated [9]. Furthermore, hypoadiponectinemia during

* Correspondence: rebecca.rancourt@charite.de
[†]Rebecca C. Rancourt and Andreas Plagemann contributed equally to this work.
[1]Division of 'Experimental Obstetrics,' Clinic of Obstetrics, Charité – Universitätsmedizin Berlin, Corporate Member of Freie Universität Berlin, Humboldt-Universität zu Berlin, and Berlin Institute of Health, Campus Virchow-Klinikum, Augustenburger Platz 1, 13353 Berlin, Germany
Full list of author information is available at the end of the article

gestation and/or post-partum is associated with poorer maternal insulin sensitivity after delivery and may predict future development of type 2 diabetes [10, 11]. In a normal pregnancy, maternal circulating adiponectin levels progressively decline particularly in the third trimester along with increasing insulin resistance [12]. Hence, a critical role of adiponectin in gestational metabolic adaptations has been proposed [13]. Adiponectin cannot cross the placenta but is able to influence materno-fetal nutrient transport directly by modulating insulin signaling in syncytiotrophoblast cells [14]. Collectively, adiponectin appears to be not only a specific factor for regulating materno-fetal metabolism but also an important candidate in GDM pathophysiology.

Adipose tissue represents the main source of adiponectin [5]. It has been proposed that production is higher in subcutaneous (SAT) than in visceral adipose tissue (VAT) [15–18]. In GDM, only two studies so far investigated *ADIPOQ* gene expression and found decreased mRNA levels in adipose tissues [19, 20]. However, both studies were rather limited in sample size, one had only access to SAT biopsies [19], or their group comparisons did not reach statistical significance in SAT and VAT, despite an even significant higher body mass index (BMI) in the GDM group [20]. Thus, it should be further evaluated if *ADIPOQ* gene expression is indeed altered in patients with GDM, in comparison to BMI-matched controls, as differential adiposity states impede the interpretation of a genuine GDM effect. Furthermore, if mRNA levels are affected, causal factors should be explored to gain more insights into the potential mechanisms of GDM.

Regulation of *ADIPOQ* mRNA expression is complex, and a variety of transcription factors has been identified [21]. Additionally, recent studies suggest a major role of epigenetic mechanisms, namely DNA methylation, in *ADIPOQ* transcription [22, 23]. DNA methylation occurs mainly on cytosine-guanine (CpG) dinucleotides. In general, increased methylation is commonly interpreted to be associated with repression of gene transcription; however, underlying mechanisms are more complex and certainly depend on the genomic/genetic location [24]. While patterns of DNA methylation can occur in a tissue-specific manner, they can be similar in other tissues, e.g., circulating blood cells, which would allow easy access for experimental and clinical purposes. Evaluation of potential functional relevance of DNA methylation signatures in the tissue of origin as well as cross-tissue reliability appears critical in this regard. Accordingly, DNA methylation represents a mechanism through which *ADIPOQ* transcription might be affected, but studies are lacking so far investigating this in adipose tissue from GDM patients.

Offspring of women with GDM are at increased risk for the development of glucose intolerance and associated disturbances later in life [4, 25]. The main (molecular) causes of this phenomenon remain unclear, but epigenetic mechanisms are increasingly suggested as a functional transmitter. Specifically, early in-life alterations of the DNA methylation pattern might lead to long-term dysregulation of gene expression, e.g., for *ADIPOQ*. Bouchard et al. [22] showed that maternal glucose levels at GDM screening are associated with placental DNA methylation of *ADIPOQ*. This may indicate that materno-fetal (hyper)-glycemia is involved in the programming of DNA methylation signatures. The placenta, however, does not appear to represent a key source tissue of adiponectin [9, 14, 20]. Therefore, further cross-tissue studies may provide additional information on whether and where *ADIPOQ* DNA methylation patterns are altered in the context of hyperglycemic materno-fetal conditions.

In the present study, we therefore analyzed adiponectin plasma levels and gene expression in SAT and VAT biopsies from women with GDM and matched normal glucose tolerant (NGT) controls. Furthermore, we investigated whether DNA methylation is associated with mRNA levels and shows consistency across maternal adipose tissues and blood (MB) cells. Finally, we determined DNA methylation of *ADIPOQ* in cord blood (CB) cells to evaluate the changes in offspring from GDM mothers and their potential implications.

Results

Study cohort

Table 1 shows general and specific characteristics of mothers and newborns. On average, both the GDM and NGT groups were overweight before pregnancy. Total gestational weight gain (GWG) was similar between the groups, while net GWG was significantly lower in diabetic subjects. At delivery, women of both groups showed comparable BMI. In GDM, maternal metabolic and hormonal state was still altered at the end of pregnancy as compared to controls. Fasting blood glucose, insulin, C-peptide, and homeostatic model assessment of insulin resistance (HOMA-IR) were higher in women with GDM. In contrast, plasma adiponectin was significantly lower in the GDM group (Table 1). This was independent of maternal BMI (adjusted for prepregnancy BMI, $P = 0.006$; adjusted for BMI at delivery, $P = 0.004$).

Across the whole cohort ($n = 55$), maternal plasma adiponectin correlated inversely with both BMI before and at the end of pregnancy, but not with total or net GWG, respectively (Table 1). Inverse relationships were observed between maternal adiponectin vs. glucose, C-peptide, insulin, and HOMA-IR. In addition, MB adiponectin was negatively related to CB glucose, C-peptide, and triglyceride levels.

Table 1 General and specific characteristics of study participants and relations with maternal blood adiponectin at delivery

	NGT	GDM	P value*	Spearman's r vs. MB adiponectin r (P value*)
n	30	25		
Maternal				
Age (years)	32.5 ± 1.0	32.4 ± 0.9	0.919	0.17 (0.210)
Ethnic origin—n (%)			1.000	n.a.
European	20 (66.7)	16 (64.0)		
Non-European	10 (33.3)	9 (36.0)		
Socio-economic status—n (%)†			0.215	n.a.
Lower SES category	21 (84.0)	20 (66.7)		
Higher SES category	4 (16.0)	10 (33.3)		
Smoking in pregnancy (any)—n (%)	7 (23.3)	3 (12.0)	0.318	n.a.
Nulliparous—n (%)	4 (13.3)	4 (16.0)	1.000	n.a.
Height (cm)	167.0 ± 1.2	164.6 ± 1.3	0.246	0.23 (0.100)
Prepregnancy weight (kg)	73.7 ± 3.9	77.7 ± 3.8	0.257	− 0.22 (0.114)
Prepregnancy BMI (kg/m^2)	26.4 ± 1.3	28.6 ± 1.3	0.105	− 0.31 (0.021)
Total GWG (kg)	17.2 ± 1.2	14.4 ± 1.4	0.127	0.03 (0.848)
Net GWG (kg)	13.9 ± 1.2	9.9 ± 1.4	0.028	0.14 (0.363)
BMI at delivery (kg/m^2)	32.5 ± 1.5	34.0 ± 1.2	0.124	− 0.31 (0.023)
Blood glucose at oGTT (mg/dL)				
Fasting	79.5 ± 1.7	99.0 ± 5.4	< 0.001	− 0.26 (0.086)
1 h	120.9 ± 6.3	207.0 ± 7.2	< 0.001	− 0.30 (0.041)
2 h	90.3 ± 4.2	161.4 ± 9.7	< 0.001	− 0.18 (0.243)
Area under the curve (mg/dL h)	205.8 ± 8.2	337.3 ± 13.5	< 0.001	− 0.28 (0.058)
Gestational age at delivery (weeks)	38.3 ± 0.1	37.8 ± 0.2	0.028	0.03 (0.841)
Mode of delivery—n (%)			1.000	n.a.
Primary cesarean section	9 (30.0)	7 (28.0)		
Repeat cesarean section	21 (70.0)	18 (72.0)		
Maternal fasting plasma levels at delivery				
Adiponectin (μg/mL)‡	9.9 ± 0.8	6.7 ± 0.5	0.002	n.a.
Glucose (mg/dL)	72.5 ± 2.0	85.0 ± 1.2	< 0.001	− 0.37 (0.007)
Insulin (μU/mL)	22.3 ± 2.7	40.1 ± 8.2	0.217	− 0.33 (0.014)
HOMA-IR	3.6 ± 0.3	8.3 ± 1.7	0.037	− 0.36 (0.009)
C-peptide (ng/mL)	2.0 ± 0.2	4.9 ± 0.7	< 0.001	− 0.53 (< 0.001)
Leptin (ng/mL)	28.9 ± 3.5	18.0 ± 2.6	0.017	0.04 (0.772)
Triglycerides (mmol/L)	2.4 ± 0.1	2.3 ± 0.1	0.554	0.11 (0.413)
Birth outcome/newborn				
Female sex—n (%)	18 (60.0)	11 (44.0)	0.285	n.a.
Placental weight (g)	658.7 ± 28.4	612.5 ± 37.8	0.337	− 0.15 (0.328)
Birth weight (g)	3368 ± 87	3578 ± 82	0.038	− 0.22 (0.113)
Birth length (cm)	51.1 ± 0.5	50.9 ± 0.3	0.890	− 0.03 (0.858)
Relative birth weight (g/cm)	65.8 ± 1.3	70.3 ± 1.5	0.022	− 0.23 (0.098)
Macrosomia—n (%)	3 (10.0)	4 (16.0)	0.689	n.a.
LGA—n (%)	3 (10.0)	9 (36.0)	0.026	n.a.
Hypoglycemia—n (%)	1 (3.6)	6 (24.0)	0.043	n.a.

Table 1 General and specific characteristics of study participants and relations with maternal blood adiponectin at delivery (*Continued*)

	NGT	GDM	P value*	Spearman's r vs. MB adiponectin r (P value*)
Cord blood plasma levels				
Adiponectin (µg/mL)	25.8 ± 1.6	28.5 ± 2.4	0.488	0.18 (0.182)
Glucose (mg/dL)	61.6 ± 2.0	72.0 ± 1.9	0.001	− 0.33 (0.015)
Insulin (µU/mL)	19.2 ± 2.0	26.9 ± 2.9	0.042	− 0.13 (0.366)
HOMA-IR	3.1 ± 0.4	5.0 ± 0.6	0.003	− 0.22 (0.117)
C-peptide (ng/mL)	1.0 ± 0.1	1.6 ± 0.1	< 0.001	− 0.31 (0.023)
Leptin (ng/mL)	10.8 ± 1.7	15.2 ± 2.6	0.247	− 0.21 (0.130)
Triglycerides (mmol/L)	1.1 ± 0.1	1.8 ± 0.1	< 0.001	−0.40 (0.003)

Data are means ± SEM or *n* (%)

NGT normal glucose tolerance, *GDM* gestational diabetes mellitus, *MB* maternal blood, *n.a.* not applicable, *SES* socio-economic status, *BMI* body mass index, *GWG* gestational weight gain, *oGTT* oral glucose tolerance test, *HOMA-IR* homeostatic model assessment of insulin resistance, *LGA* large-for-gestational age newborn

*Statistical significant (P value < 0.05)

[†]SES was categorized as previously described [36]

[‡]Continued to be significantly different between the groups after adjustment for prepregnancy BMI ($P = 0.006$) and BMI at delivery ($P = 0.004$)

Birth and newborn outcomes

Offspring of GDM women were significantly heavier at birth but similar in length compared to newborns of the NGT group (Table 1). CB plasma levels of glucose, insulin, C-peptide, and triglycerides were significantly increased in newborns of GDM mothers, accompanied by elevated HOMA-IR and leptin levels. There was no significant difference of CB adiponectin concentrations between the groups. Furthermore, female and male neonates showed equal amounts of CB adiponectin (female 27.8 ± 1.4 µg/mL vs. male 26.3 ± 2.5 µg/mL, $P = 0.299$). In the whole cohort, no correlations were present between CB adiponectin and newborns' anthropometry or CB metabolites/hormones. However, sex-specific subgroup analyses revealed positive associations between CB adiponectin vs. insulin and HOMA-IR in male neonates (insulin, $r = 0.41$, $P = 0.037$; HOMA-IR, $r = 0.41$, $P = 0.042$).

ADIPOQ gene expression in maternal adipose tissues

In both adipose tissue types, gene expression of *ADIPOQ* was significantly reduced in women with GDM (Fig. 1a, b). On average, diabetic subjects had 20–30% less mRNA levels compared to controls, with the difference higher in VAT than SAT. Again, these group differences were even independent of maternal BMI (adjusted for prepregnancy BMI—SAT: $P = 0.049$, VAT: $P = 0.008$, SAT+VAT: $P = 0.002$; adjusted for BMI at delivery—SAT: $P = 0.037$, VAT: $P = 0.006$, SAT+VAT: $P = 0.001$). Across the whole cohort, VAT, but not SAT, and *ADIPOQ* mRNA levels were inversely associated with maternal glucose concentrations at oral glucose tolerance test (oGTT) and at delivery (fasting glucose at oGTT: $r = -0.33$, $P = 0.029$; area under the curve of glucose (AUCG) at oGTT: $r = -0.43$, $P = 0.004$; fasting glucose at delivery: $r = -0.29$, $P = 0.040$). Gene expression in both fat depots was positively associated with maternal circulating adiponectin levels across the whole cohort (Fig. 1c–e), irrespective of the BMI (adjusted for prepregnancy BMI—SAT: $R = 0.44$, $P = 0.001$, VAT: $R = 0.34$, $P = 0.017$; SAT+VAT: $R = 0.51$, $P < 0.001$; and adjusted for BMI at delivery—SAT: $R = 0.45$, $P = 0.001$, VAT: $R = 0.35$, $P = 0.015$; SAT+VAT: $R = 0.52$, $P < 0.001$). SAT *plus* VAT mRNA levels showed the strongest correlations with plasma adiponectin.

DNA methylation at the ADIPOQ gene locus in maternal tissues

The overall DNA methylation pattern of the analyzed regions at the *ADIPOQ* gene locus was similar in SAT and VAT (Fig. 2b, c). All investigated CpG sites ($n = 10$) had moderate to high methylation levels (> 50%). Region R1 was hypermethylated as compared to R2 and R3. A generally higher variability of DNA methylation was observed in R2 and R3 in both fat depots.

In SAT, DNA methylation was consistent between both groups. Statistically, only the comparison at R2 CpG2 was close to significance ($P = 0.056$). Although similar to SAT regarding the overall pattern, methylation in VAT showed slightly less variability in R2 and R3. By groups, methylation of R3 in VAT appeared tighter in GDM subjects. Furthermore, DNA methylation of the two CpG sites was significantly altered in VAT of women with GDM vs. NGT. Compared to controls, R1 CpG4 was lower and R3 CpG1 higher methylated in VAT of the diabetic group (Fig. 2c). The mean methylation difference was around 2.1–2.4%. To evaluate the potential functional relevance of these two CpG sites, correlation analyses between DNA methylation at R1 CpG4 and R3 CpG1 and VAT gene expression were performed (Fig. 2f, g). Here, only the position R3 CpG1 showed a significant inverse relationship with mRNA levels. Further inverse correlations were found

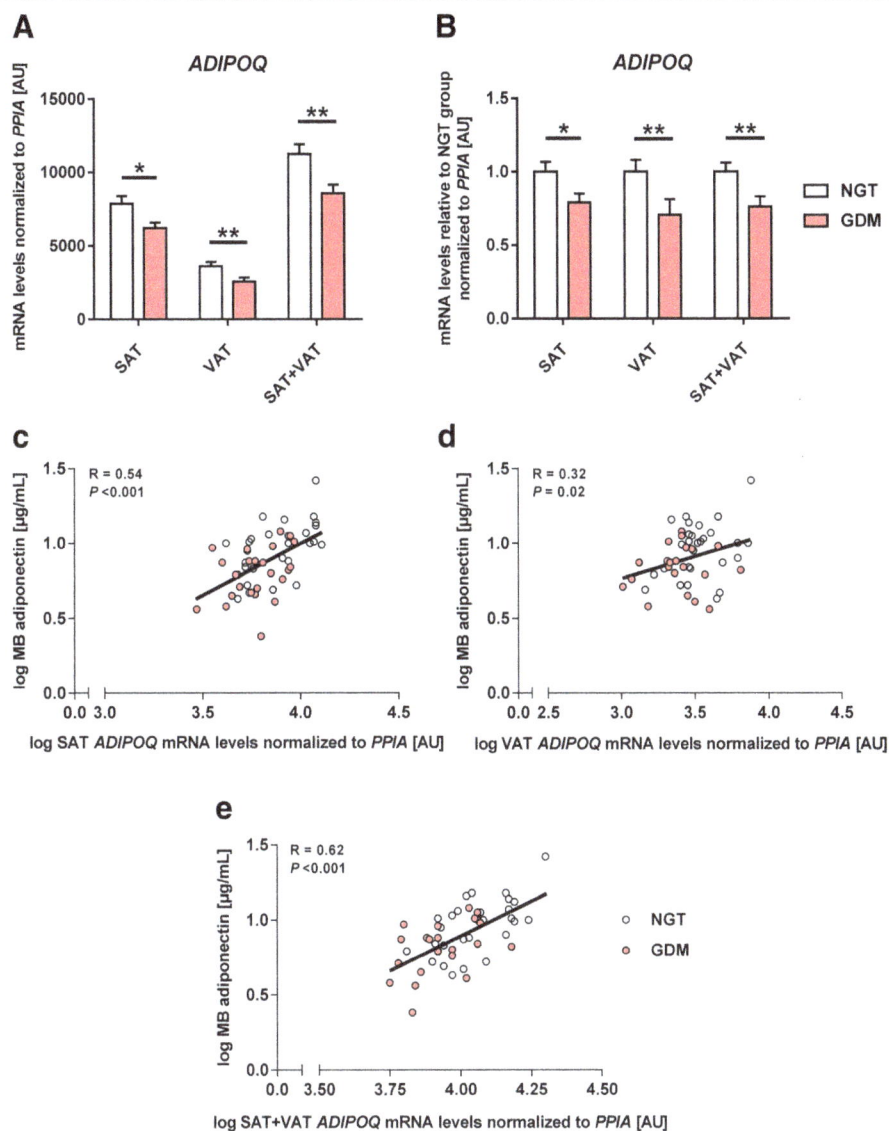

Fig. 1 Adiponectin mRNA levels in adipose tissues of women with NGT vs. GDM and their relations to plasma adiponectin. Gene expression of adiponectin (*ADIPOQ*) normalized to peptidylprolyl isomerase A (*PPIA*) analyzed in subcutaneous (SAT) and visceral adipose tissues (VAT), respectively, of normal glucose tolerance women (NGT; open bars; $n = 30$) vs. women with gestational diabetes mellitus (GDM; red bars; $n = 22–25$). Sum of expression of both fat depots (SAT+VAT) is plotted additionally (**a–b**). Data are means ± SEM, shown as raw data (**a**) or percentage of NGT levels (**b**). Pearson's correlation coefficients (*R*) calculating the relationship between maternal blood (MB) adiponectin levels and adipose tissue gene expression data (**c–e**). NGT, open circles; GDM, red circles. AU, arbitrary units. *$P < 0.05$, **$P < 0.01$

between gene expression and single CpG sites and/or mean methylation levels regarding R2 and R3, but not R1, across both fat depots. For example, the means of R2 and R3 were negatively associated with respective mRNA levels (SAT—R2 mean: $R = -0.31$, $P = 0.030$, R3 mean: $R = -0.40$, $P = 0.008$; VAT—R2 mean: $R = -0.33$, $P = 0.020$, R3 mean: $R = -0.45$, $P = 0.003$). Among all individual CpGs and the means of R1–R3, VAT CpG1 and CpG2 of R3 DNA methylation showed relations to maternal glucose levels, which were in a positive direction (CpG1—AUCG at oGTT:

$r = 0.37$, $P = 0.023$; fasting glucose at delivery: $r = 0.32$, $P = 0.034$; CpG2—AUCG at oGTT: $r = 0.34$, $P = 0.038$).

Despite the similarity of methylation pattern between SAT and VAT, cross-tissue correlations were rare and inconsistent. While R1 CpG1 and CpG2 patterns were inversely associated between both fat types (R1 CpG1: $r = -0.35$, $P = 0.014$; R1 CpG2: $r = -0.53$, $P < 0.001$), methylation at R2 CpG1 and R2 mean was related in a positive manner (R2 CpG1: $r = 0.32$, $P = 0.025$; R2 mean: $r = 0.30$, $P = 0.041$).

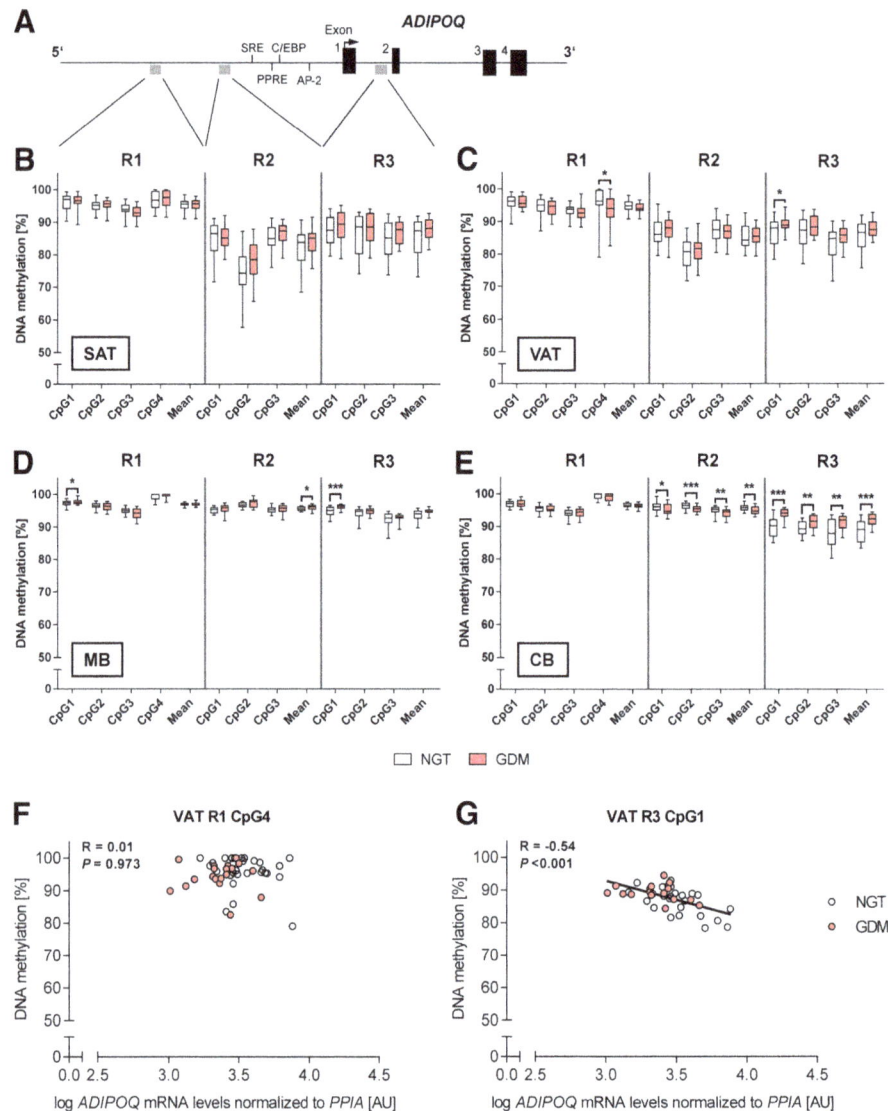

Fig. 2 CpG site-specific DNA methylation analyses at the adiponectin gene locus in adipose tissues and blood cells from mothers with NGT vs. GDM and their offspring. Schematic illustration of the adiponectin (*ADIPOQ*) gene locus, including characterized transcription factor binding sites (e.g., SRE, PPRE, C/EBP), and analyzed DNA methylation assays (R1-R3) (**a**). Percent DNA methylation is shown for each individual CpG site (numbering follows 5′ to 3′), analyzed per assay (R1–R3) for subcutaneous adipose tissue (SAT; **b**), visceral adipose tissue (VAT; **c**), maternal blood (MB; **d**), and cord blood (CB; **e**) in the normal glucose tolerant (NGT; open boxes; n = 30) vs. gestational diabetes mellitus group (GDM; red boxes; n = 22–25). Group comparisons in cord blood samples were adjusted for newborn sex. Box-whisker plots show the minimum and maximum values. Pearson's correlation coefficients (*R*) were calculated to determine the relationships between DNA methylation of significant CpG sites and respective *ADIPOQ* mRNA levels in VAT across the whole cohort (**f, g**). Gene expression of *ADIPOQ* was normalized to peptidylprolyl isomerase A (*PPIA*). NGT, open circles; GDM, red circles. AU, arbitrary units. *P < 0.05, **P < 0.01, ***P < 0.001

As compared to adipose tissues, MB was characterized by overall higher and rather tight methylation pattern (mostly > 90%; Fig. 2d). With regard to R3, the GDM group showed less variability compared to women with NGT, as observed in VAT. Group differences were detected at R1 CpG1, R2 mean, and R3 CpG1 (mean differences around 0.4–1.4%). Similar to VAT, R3 CpG1 in MB was hypermethylated in the GDM group. However, no correlation was found between methylation of VAT and MB.

Cord blood DNA methylation at the *ADIPOQ* gene locus
To evaluate a potential GDM effect on fetal DNA methylation, all regions were analyzed in CB cells, too. Across all investigated tissues, the CB methylation pattern was most similar to MB, showing the overall low variability (Fig. 2e). However, higher variation was observed at R3 in CB vs. MB, while methylation in CB from GDM-exposed newborns was more "compact." In comparison to controls, GDM offspring were characterized by significant

hypomethylation at all CpG sites and, accordingly, the mean of R2 (mean differences around 1%), while significant hypermethylation at all R3 CpG sites and the mean of R3 were observed (mean differences around 1.7–4.0%); even after adjustment for newborn sex (Fig. 2e). The most pronounced difference was observed at R3 CpG1, which followed the same pattern as in MB and VAT by showing higher methylation in the GDM group.

By analyzing the same CpG positions between maternal tissues and CB, the only positive correlations were found with the methylation levels of R3 of MB (CpG1: $r = 0.51$, $P = 0.001$; CpG2: $r = 0.43$, $P = 0.008$; CpG3: $r = 0.47$, $P = 0.003$). There were no relationships present between maternal age, prepregnancy BMI, total GWG, gestational age, or MB hormones and the CB methylation levels of these significant different regions. The mean CB DNA methylation levels of R2 correlated inversely with maternal BMI at delivery ($r = -0.31$, $P = 0.031$) and AUCG at oGTT ($r = -0.38$, $P = 0.013$). On the contrary, the mean DNA methylation levels of R3 were unrelated to maternal BMI but showed positive associations with AUCG at oGTT and fasting glucose at delivery (AUCG at oGTT: $r = 0.45$, $P = 0.004$; fasting glucose at delivery: $r = -0.44$, $P = 0.003$). Furthermore, Spearman's correlations revealed significant inverse relationships between R2 CpG1 and mean R2 methylation vs. (relative) birth weight (birth weight vs. R2 CpG1: $r = -0.32$, $P = 0.024$; relative birth weight vs. R2 CpG1: $r = -0.36$, $P = 0.012$; R2 mean: $r = -0.32$, $P = 0.024$). Furthermore, methylation of R3 CpG1, CpG3, and R3 mean was positively associated with CB adiponectin (R3 CpG1: $r = 0.34$, $P = 0.024$; R3 CpG3: $r = 0.38$, $P = 0.011$; R3 mean: $r = 0.34$, $P = 0.022$).

Discussion

This study demonstrates that plasma adiponectin and its gene expression in the two major adipose tissue types is consistently decreased in women with treated GDM as compared to matched healthy subjects, even independent of their BMI. Furthermore, our data indicate that DNA methylation of previously published regions (i.e., R2 and R3) indeed may be involved in respective gene regulation but are just slightly altered in patients with GDM. Overall, fat tissue DNA methylation patterns are not reliably reflected in MB cells. CB ADIPOQ DNA methylation profiles of R2 and R3, however, are significantly altered in affected offspring, irrespective of fetal sex, and associated with their phenotypic parameters.

The present study confirms that GDM is characterized by hypoadiponectinemia [7]. In addition, plasma adiponectin levels appear to be more related to the insulin-resistant state than to the maternal BMI/GWG, decisively specifying observations from other reports [6, 26]. Interestingly, GDM was associated here with significantly lower net GWG and circulating leptin levels at delivery. This may imply less

gestational adipose tissue accretion in these subjects, potentially due to GDM treatment. Thus, although adiposity became apparently reduced in the GDM group, adiponectin was still significantly decreased in comparison to controls. This argues in favor of a genuine GDM rather than a BMI (adiposity) effect. Considering its critical functions in enhancing insulin sensitivity and glucose/lipid disposal/oxidation, decreased adiponectin levels therefore probably affect materno-fetal metabolism and, consequently, nutrient supply to the fetus in GDM. Indeed, maternal adiponectinemia was inversely associated with blood glucose and HOMA-IR in both mothers and newborns. Potentially, this has adverse short- and long-term implications for the GDM offspring [4, 25].

CB adiponectin levels were similar between the groups and female/male offspring which support the findings from other studies [27, 28]. Interestingly, there was a positive link between CB adiponectin and insulin/insulin resistance in male offspring, which appears paradox compared with the adult situation, where adiponectin levels usually decline with increasing insulin resistance [6, 12]. However, CB adiponectin has been also suggested as a growth factor in early life [14, 27, 29], which may involve temporary synergistic effects with insulin. Fetal insulin is a potent anabolic factor contributing to higher in utero growth and has also been identified as a critical hormone for the early "programming" of later metabolic disease risk [30].

In adults, production of adiponectin is primarily located in white adipocytes [5]. Our data revealed reduced mRNA expression in SAT and VAT of women with GDM, even after adjustment for BMI. Reduced fat tissue expression, moreover, obviously affected the circulating plasma levels, as indicated by correlation analyses. Expression in both fat depots was associated with plasma adiponectin, while the relationship with the sum of SAT + VAT actually was the strongest. Interestingly, a large number of studies focused on circulating adiponectin [7], but only two investigated its expression in adipose tissues from women with GDM [19, 20]. In extension to these previous reports, the present study clearly shows altered ADIPOQ gene expression in SAT as well as VAT of GDM, even independent of their BMI. While the decrease in mRNA levels was relatively similar in both SAT and VAT in GDM subjects, the difference was more pronounced in VAT. In addition, maternal glucose levels were associated with VAT mRNA only indicating a particular regulatory role of VAT ADIPOQ gene expression on maternal glycemia. As the differential mRNA profiles are possibly a consequence of altered transcriptional mechanisms, analysis of regulatory factors appears critical to better understand the potential causes of this observation.

To the best of our knowledge, this is the first study determining DNA methylation of ADIPOQ in adipose tissues from women with GDM and NGT. Both fat depots were characterized by overall similar DNA methylation patterns irrespective of women's glucose tolerance. Furthermore, methylation of R2 and R3 was inversely associated with gene expression in SAT and VAT indicating the functional relevance of these two regions. While region R2 is able to serve as a transcription binding site for a variety of factors [23], a regulatory function of the intronic region R3 is unknown [22]. Interestingly, VAT R3 CpG1 was hypermethylated in GDM subjects as compared to controls. As DNA methylation at this site was correlated inversely with gene expression, this alteration might contribute to reduced transcription in VAT of women with GDM. However, the mean group difference was rather small, and therefore, it remains open if it plays, indeed, a relevant role. Thus, alterations of other regulatory mechanisms may be responsible for decreased mRNA levels. Moreover, there were obvious adipose tissue-specific DNA methylation patterns that were not associated with and reflected in DNA methylation of MB cells, even though only R3 CpG1 showed a consistent signature in MB and VAT across groups. Therefore, based on our findings, blood DNA methylation of investigated regions can hardly serve as a reliable indicator/ biomarker for adipose tissue methylation. Beyond the addressed study subject, this observation appears to deserve particular attention.

Exposure to a diabetic intrauterine environment may program the offspring for a higher susceptibility for "diabesity" development later in life [4, 25]. Alterations of DNA methylation are suggested to contribute to this phenomenon [25]. Pioneer work by Bouchard et al. [22] observed the relationships between maternal glucose levels at oGTT and placental DNA methylation of the two regions investigated here (R1 and R3). Intriguingly, we found indeed a significantly altered methylation pattern of R2 and R3, but not R1, in CB of GDM newborns. Moreover, maternal glucose at oGTT and/or at delivery was related to CB DNA methylation levels of R2 and, in particular, R3, which may suggest a potential influence of maternal hyperglycemia itself. Of note, R2 and R3 may be involved in gene regulation, as indicated by the adipose tissue data. In all cases, however, the mean methylation differences were rather small, as in other studies [31–33]. Paradoxically, the region R2 was consistently hypomethylated here, but R3 was hypermethylated at each analyzed CpG site in CB of GDM newborns. Considering the functional relevance of R2 as recently described [23], lower methylation could fit with the slightly higher circulating adiponectin levels observed in the GDM offspring. Since it is unclear whether ADIPOQ is expressed in CB cells, our ability to speculate about functional consequences of the observed alterations for ADIPOQ expression in the offspring is limited.

The associations found between methylation of R2 and (relative) birth weight seem to fit with the idea that lower methylation in R2 is related to increased ADIPOQ expression. Furthermore, it has been shown that CB adiponectin is positively associated with birth weight [27, 29]. However, the positive relation between methylation of R3 and CB adiponectin appears not in agreement with a functional role of R3, as higher methylation would result in lower expression. Notably, R3 CpG1 was hypermethylated in three tissues, i.e., VAT, MB, and CB, in the GDM group and might therefore have a diagnostic/ predictive potential for adiponectin dysregulation. Nevertheless, we cannot exclude that this finding has no decisive functional implications for the offspring, as CB adiponectin was not significantly altered in GDM offspring, and apparently, blood cells did not reflect maternal adipose tissue methylation. Interestingly and worth noting, however, a very recent study in adults born to mothers with GDM is showing significantly increased ADIPOQ DNA methylation, accompanied with lower gene expression in SAT [34].

A study limitation is that whole tissue biopsies were investigated, a common approach in the majority of such studies [19, 20, 22], and therefore, we cannot exclude that differences in cell-type heterogeneity between tissues, subjects, or GDM patients and controls influenced the molecular results. Furthermore, as adipose tissues are the major source of adiponectin, our expression analyses were solely in SAT and VAT and not in maternal and fetal blood cells, limiting our ability to evaluate the functional implications of blood DNA methylation on transcription. Still, as adipose tissues and other fetal tissues have been identified as tissues of origin for adiponectin in the newborn [35], the relative contribution of CB adiponectin expression, if there is any, to circulating levels might be comparably small. Larger human studies might be beneficial to evaluate the sex-specific effects of the role of fetal adiponectin and DNA methylation profiles in fetal tissues.

Conclusions

In conclusion, reduced adipose tissue ADIPOQ expression appears to be a genuine pathogenic co-factor in GDM, even irrespective of the maternal weight status. Accompanying, the DNA methylation of the two functional characterized regions (R2 and R3) is altered in CB cells of GDM-exposed newborns. Thus, future studies, especially in adiponectin-source tissues, should further evaluate the pathogenic, diagnostic, and/or therapeutic capability of adiponectin in GDM as well as the potential intrauterine-acquired DNA methylation patterns that affect gene transcription and, consequently, the phenotypic outcome and "diabesogenic" risk of GDM offspring.

Methods

This investigation is part of the prospective observational "Early CHARITÉ (*EaCH*)" cohort study [36]. Twenty-five women with GDM and 30 women with NGT were prospectively recruited before the scheduled delivery of singletons via cesarean section (CS) at the Clinic of Obstetrics of the Charité – Universitätsmedizin Berlin, Campus Virchow-Klinikum, Germany. Recruitment, exclusion criteria, standardized procedures, analytical methods, etc. are described in detail elsewhere [36]. The groups were matched for maternal age, ethnic origin, socio-economic status (SES), parity, and, in particular, prepregnancy BMI. Research design and methods were conducted in accordance with the Declaration of Helsinki, revised in 2004, and approved by the local Ethics Committee (EA2/026/04). Informed written consent was obtained from all subjects.

Subject data

Maternal data were collected as previously described [36]. Briefly, maternal height and weight before conception and the last measured weight within 1 week prior to delivery were abstracted from the "Mutterpass" (a standardized maternity record in Germany), and the BMI was calculated. Total gestational weight gain (GWG) was calculated as the difference between prepregnancy weight and nearest weight to delivery. Furthermore, to estimate the genuine maternal body habitus, net GWG was generated by subtracting birth weight and placental weight from women's total GWG. GDM screening was performed between the 24th and 28th week of gestation according to the national guidelines at the time of recruitment [37, 38]. Patients with GDM were treated either by dietary therapy alone or in combination with insulin therapy (*n* = 13) to achieve glucose targets according to the abovementioned guidelines [37, 38].

Newborn characteristics were abstracted from medical records. Anthropometric outcomes included birth weight, relative birth weight (g/cm), and macrosomia (defined as birth weight ≥ 4000 g). Further clinical parameters, including placental weight, were determined as described elsewhere [36].

Blood and adipose tissue sampling

Fasting maternal venous blood was collected prior to CS and venous umbilical CB was drawn immediately after birth and cord clamping. For further analyses, fractions of plasma and blood cells were stored separately at – 80 °C. Paired abdominal SAT and omental VAT biopsies were obtained during CS, snap frozen in liquid nitrogen, and stored at – 80 °C. For technical reasons, in one GDM subject, it was not possible to collect the VAT sample.

Blood hormone and metabolite analyses

Total plasma adiponectin was determined using a specific commercially available ELISA (Cat# RD191023100, BioVendor, Brno, Czech Republic). Plasma insulin, C-peptide, and leptin levels were measured using commercially available radioimmunoassays (insulin, Cat# RIA-1249; C-peptide, Cat# RIA-1252; leptin, Cat# RIA-1624; DRG Instruments, Marburg, Germany). The following are the inter-assay coefficients of variance: adiponectin 6.0%, insulin 3.4–6.0%, C-peptide 2.4–9.3%, and leptin 3.6–6.2%. Plasma glucose and triglyceride concentrations were quantified using the oxidase-peroxidase and the glyceride-3-phosphatoxidase-peroxidase method (both obtained from Dr. Lange, Berlin, Germany). As an indicator of insulin resistance, the homeostatic model assessment (HOMA-IR) was calculated [39].

Adipose tissue gene expression analyses

Total RNA was isolated from 100 mg adipose tissue using the RNeasy Lipid Tissue Mini Kit (Qiagen, Hilden, Germany) according to the manufacturer's protocol, including DNase treatment (Qiagen). Quantity and purity were assessed with a spectrophotometer (NanoDrop 1000, Thermo Scientific, Wilmington, DE, USA). Quality was evaluated using the Bioanalyzer 2100 (Agilent Technologies, Santa Clara, CA, USA). Overall, the samples showed high RNA integrity numbers (RIN; SAT: 7.8 ± 0.1, VAT: 7.7 ± 0.1); however, two VAT samples of the GDM group had to be excluded due to lower RNA quality (RIN < 6). For cDNA synthesis, 300 ng RNA was reverse transcribed using the iScript kit (Bio-Rad, Hercules, CA, USA) as recommended by the manufacturer. Quantitative real-time PCR was performed using TaqMan technology (Applied Biosystems, Waltham, MA, USA) in combination with a 7500 instrument (Applied Biosystems). All samples were run in triplicate, and all plates included respective controls to ensure run quality and confirm the absence of contamination. Protocol conditions were as follows: denaturation at 95 °C for 10 min, followed by 40 two-step cycles at 95 °C for 15 s and 60 °C for 1 min. A pre-designed exon-exon spanning TaqMan primer assay for *ADIPOQ* was obtained from Applied Biosystems (ID: Hs00605917_m1) and amplified in dualplex with the housekeeping gene peptidylprolyl isomerase A (*PPIA*; ID: Hs99999904_m1). *ADIPOQ* gene expression was normalized using the $2^{-\Delta Ct}$ method, including the correction for amplification efficiency calculated from standard curves of each primer set. Gene expression of *PPIA* was stable, as in a previous housekeeping gene study for adipose tissue [40], and was identical between the groups in both fat depots (SAT: 23.76 ± 0.09 vs. 23.72 ± 0.12; VAT: 23.39 ± 0.10 vs. 23.51 ± 0.08; NGT vs. GDM; arbitrary units). As both adipose tissue types contribute to circulating adiponectin, a sum of SAT and VAT mRNA levels was calculated and additionally analyzed.

DNA methylation analyses

Genomic DNA was extracted from 30 mg adipose tissue and 1 mL blood, respectively, using the Genomic DNA-Tissue kit or the Quick-gDNA Blood kit (both obtained from Zymo Research, Irvine, CA, USA), following the manufacturer's protocols. Quantity and purity of DNA were assessed with NanoDrop (Thermo Scientific). Sodium bisulfite treatment was performed on 400 ng DNA using the EZ DNA Methylation-Gold kit (Zymo Research) as recommended by the manufacturer. In silico analyses revealed that the *ADIPOQ* promoter has no classical CpG island and contains a low number of CpG sites (chromosomal location chr3:186,556,516-186,580,200, UCSC Genome browser on human Feb. 2009, GRCh37/hg19 assembly). Furthermore, characterized transcription factor binding sites, e.g., PPRE, SRE, include no CpG site [21, 41–44]. Thus, assays were selected based on recently published regions, obviously important for *ADIPOQ* gene regulation [22, 23]. The following regions were analyzed: R1 and R3 (similar to region "C" and "E" in Bouchard et al. [22]) and R2 (similar to "R2" in Kim et al. [23]). Methylation assays were designed using the PyroMark Assay Design Software v. 2.0 (Qiagen), and detailed information is given in Additional file 1: Table S1. Pyrosequencing was performed on amplified PCR products with the PyroMark Q24 pyrosequencer (Qiagen) as previously described [45]. Percent methylation was analyzed across individual CpG sites located within the following regions of interest: R1 (four CpGs), R2 (three CpGs), and R3 (three CpGs). Bisulfite treatment and pyrosequencing assays were tested and reproducibility validated using duplicate samples, various tissue types, and methylation scales (0–100%).

Statistical analyses

Data are presented as means ± SEM or number and percentage. Continuous variables were evaluated for normal distribution using Shapiro-Wilk tests. If necessary, skewed data were logarithmically transformed to achieve normal distribution. Group comparisons were analyzed by unpaired t test or Mann-Whitney U test or chi-squared/Fisher's exact test, as appropriate. ANCOVA was used to adjust for maternal BMI or newborn sex. To assess the associations between clinical and/or endocrine parameters and DNA methylation, Spearman's correlation coefficients (r) were calculated. Pearson's correlations coefficients (R) were used to test the relationships between molecular data, i.e., circulating adiponectin levels, gene expression, and DNA methylation. Potential confounding effects of maternal BMI were checked with partial Pearson's correlations. Statistical analyses were performed using SPSS v. 24.0 (IBM, Armonk, NY, USA). A P value < 0.05 was considered significant (two-tailed).

Abbreviations

ADIPOQ: Adiponectin gene; ANCOVA: Analysis of covariance; AUCG: Area under the curve of glucose; BMI: Body mass index; C/EBP: CCAAT/enhancer-binding protein; CB: Cord blood; CpG: Cytosine-guanine dinucleotide; CS: Cesarean section; EaCH: Early CHARITÉ study; ELISA: Enzyme-linked immunosorbent assay; GDM: Gestational diabetes mellitus; GWG: Gestational weight gain; HOMA-IR: Homeostatic model assessment of insulin resistance; LGA: Large-for-gestational age; MB: Maternal blood; n.a.: Not applicable; NGT: Normal glucose tolerant; oGTT: Oral glucose tolerance test; *PPIA*: Peptidylprolyl isomerase A; PPRE: Peroxisome proliferator-activated receptor response element; RIN: RNA integrity number; SAT: Subcutaneous adipose tissue; SES: Socio-economic status; SRE: Sterol regulatory element; VAT: Visceral adipose tissue

Acknowledgements

The authors acknowledge Thomas Harder, MD; Andrea Loui, MD; Elisabeth Eilers, MD; and Sandra Schulz, MSc, for the contributions to the initial study cohort design, subject recruitment, and sample/data collection. We are very grateful to all the participants of this study as well as the midwives and staff of the Clinic of Obstetrics at the Charité, Campus Virchow-Klinikum, Berlin, Germany, for their support in the subject recruitment and sample/data collection.

Funding

This study was supported in part by grants of the German Research Foundation (DFG: PL-241/5-1, GRK 1208) to Dr. Plagemann. The funder had no role in the study design, data collection and analysis, decision to publish, or preparation of the manuscript. We acknowledge support from the Open Access Publication Fund of Charité – Universitätsmedizin Berlin.

Authors' contributions

RO contributed to the design and conceptualization of the study, performed the experiments, analyzed and interpreted the data, and wrote the original draft. JHS contributed to the design and conceptualization of the study and data collection and reviewed the final draft. KM was involved in the data collection/management and laboratory measurements and reviewed the final draft. KS contributed to the data collection/management and interpretation and reviewed the final manuscript. TZ performed the laboratory measurements and revised the final manuscript. JWD contributed to the study design, provided the resources, and revised the final draft. WH provided the resources and reviewed the final draft. RCR contributed to the design and conceptualization of the study, performed the experiments, analyzed and interpreted the data, and wrote the original draft. AP contributed to the design and conceptualization of the study, analyzed and interpreted the data, and wrote the original draft. All authors critically read and approved the final manuscript.

Competing interests

The authors declare that they have no competing interests.

Author details

[1]Division of 'Experimental Obstetrics,' Clinic of Obstetrics, Charité – Universitätsmedizin Berlin, Corporate Member of Freie Universität Berlin, Humboldt-Universität zu Berlin, and Berlin Institute of Health, Campus Virchow-Klinikum, Augustenburger Platz 1, 13353 Berlin, Germany. [2]Clinic of Obstetrics, Charité – Universitätsmedizin Berlin, Corporate Member of Freie Universität Berlin, Humboldt-Universität zu Berlin, and Berlin Institute of Health, Campus Virchow-Klinikum, Berlin, Germany.

References

1. O'Sullivan EP, Avalos G, O'Reilly M, Dennedy MC, Gaffney G, Dunne F, on behalf of the Atlantic DIP collaborators. Atlantic Diabetes in Pregnancy (DIP): the prevalence and outcomes of gestational diabetes mellitus using new diagnostic criteria. Diabetologia. 2011;54:1670–5.

2. Sacks DA, Hadden DR, Maresh M, Deerochanawong C, Dyer AR, Metzger BE, Lowe LP, Coustan DR, Hod M, Oats JJN, Persson B, Trimble ER. Frequency of gestational diabetes mellitus at collaborating centers based on IADPSG Consensus Panel–recommended criteria the hyperglycemia and adverse pregnancy outcome (HAPO) study. Diabetes Care. 2012;35:526–8.

3. Melchior H, Kurch-Bek D, Mund M. The prevalence of gestational diabetes - a population-based analysis of a nationwide screening program. Dtsch Arztebl Int. 2017;114:412–8.

4. Metzger BE, Buchanan TA, Coustan DR, De Leiva A, Dunger DB, Hadden DR, Hod M, Kitzmiller JL, Kjos SL, Oats JN, Pettitt DJ, Sacks DA, Zoupas C. Summary and recommendations of the Fifth International Workshop-Conference on Gestational Diabetes Mellitus. Diabetes Care. 2007;30:S251–60.

5. Brochu-Gaudreau K, Rehfeldt C, Blouin R, Bordignon V, Murphy BD, Palin M-F. Adiponectin action from head to toe. Endocrine. 2010;37:11–32.

6. Weyer C, Funahashi T, Tanaka S, Hotta K, Matsuzawa Y, Pratley RE, Tataranni PA. Hypoadiponectinemia in obesity and type 2 diabetes: close association with insulin resistance and hyperinsulinemia. J Clin Endocrinol Metab. 2001;86:1930–5.

7. Fasshauer M, Blüher M, Stumvoll M. Adipokines in gestational diabetes. Lancet Diabetes Endocrinol. 2014;2:488–99.

8. Bao W, Baecker A, Song Y, Kiely M, Liu S, Zhang C. Adipokine levels during the first or early second trimester of pregnancy and subsequent risk of gestational diabetes mellitus: a systematic review. Metabolism. 2015;64:756–64.

9. Hauguel-De Mouzon S, Catalano P. Adiponectin: are measurements clinically useful in pregnancy? Diabetes Care. 2013;36:1434–6.

10. Winzer C, Wagner O, Festa A, Schneider B, Roden M, Bancher-Todesca D, Pacini G, Funahashi T, Kautzky-Willer A. Plasma adiponectin, insulin sensitivity, and subclinical inflammation in women with prior gestational diabetes mellitus. Diabetes Care. 2004;27:1721–7.

11. Retnakaran R, Qi Y, Connelly PW, Sermer M, Hanley AJ, Zinman B. Low adiponectin concentration during pregnancy predicts postpartum insulin resistance, beta cell dysfunction and fasting glycaemia. Diabetologia. 2010;53:268–76.

12. Catalano PM, Hoegh M, Minium J, Huston-Presley L, Bernard S, Kalhan S, Hauguel-De Mouzon S. Adiponectin in human pregnancy: implications for regulation of glucose and lipid metabolism. Diabetologia. 2006;49:1677–85.

13. Qiao L, Wattez J-S, Lee S, Nguyen A, Schaack J, Hay WW, Shao J. Adiponectin deficiency impairs maternal metabolic adaptation to pregnancy in mice. Diabetes. 2017;66:1126–35.

14. Aye ILMH, Powell TL, Jansson T. Review: adiponectin - the missing link between maternal adiposity, placental transport and fetal growth. Placenta. 2013;34:S40–5.

15. Motoshima H, Wu X, Sinha MK, Hardy VE, Rosato EL, Barbot DJ, Rosato FE, Goldstein BJ. Differential regulation of adiponectin secretion from cultured human omental and subcutaneous adipocytes: effects of insulin and rosiglitazone. J Clin Endocrinol Metab. 2002;87:5662–7.

16. Perrini S, Laviola L, Cignarelli A, Melchiorre M, De Stefano F, Caccioppoli C, Natalicchio A, Orlando MR, Garruti G, De Fazio M, Catalano G, Memeo V, Giorgino R, Giorgino F. Fat depot-related differences in gene expression, adiponectin secretion, and insulin action and signalling in human adipocytes differentiated in vitro from precursor stromal cells. Diabetologia. 2008;51:155–64.

17. Phillips SA, Ciaraldi TP, Oh DK, Savu MK, Henry RR. Adiponectin secretion and response to pioglitazone is depot dependent in cultured human adipose tissue. Am J Physiol Endocrinol Metab. 2008;295:E842–50.

18. Meyer LK, Ciaraldi TP, Henry RR, Wittgrove AC, Phillips SA. Adipose tissue depot and cell size dependency of adiponectin synthesis and secretion in human obesity. Adipocyte. 2013;2:217–26.

19. Ranheim T, Haugen F, Staff AC, Braekke K, Harsem NK, Drevon CA. Adiponectin is reduced in gestational diabetes mellitus in normal weight women. Acta Obstet Gynecol Scand. 2004;83:341–7.

20. Kleiblova P, Dostalova I, Bartlova M, Lacinova Z, Ticha I, Krejci V, Springer D, Kleibl Z, Haluzik M. Expression of adipokines and estrogen receptors in adipose tissue and placenta of patients with gestational diabetes mellitus. Mol Cell Endocrinol. 2010;314:150–6.

21. Liu M, Liu F. Transcriptional and post-translational regulation of adiponectin. Biochem J. 2010;425:41–52.

22. Bouchard L, Hivert MF, Guay SP, St-Pierre J, Perron P, Brisson D. Placental adiponectin gene DNA methylation levels are associated with mothers' blood glucose concentration. Diabetes. 2012;61:1272–80.

23. Kim AY, Park YJ, Pan X, Shin KC, Kwak S-H, Bassas AF, Sallam RM, Park KS, Alfadda A a, Xu A, Kim JB. Obesity-induced DNA hypermethylation of the adiponectin gene mediates insulin resistance. Nat Commun. 2015;6:7585.

24. Jones PA. Functions of DNA methylation: islands, start sites, gene bodies and beyond. Nat Rev Genet. 2012;13:484–92.

25. Plagemann A. Maternal diabetes and perinatal programming. Early Hum Dev. 2011;87:743–7.

26. Retnakaran R, Hanley AJG, Raif N, Connelly PW, Sermer M, Zinman B. Reduced adiponectin concentration in women with gestational diabetes: a potential factor in progression to type 2 diabetes. Diabetes Care. 2004;27:799–800.

27. Sivan E, Mazaki-Tovi S, Pariente C, Efraty Y, Schiff E, Hemi R, Kanety H. Adiponectin in human cord blood: relation to fetal birth weight and gender. J Clin Endocrinol Metab. 2003;88:5656–60.

28. Ballesteros M, Simon I, Ceperuelo-Mallafre V, Miralles RM, Albaiges G, Tinahones F, Megia A. Maternal and cord blood adiponectin multimeric forms in gestational diabetes mellitus: a prospective analysis. Diabetes Care. 2011;34:2418–23.

29. Mantzoros CS, Rifas-Shiman SL, Williams CJ, Fargnoli JL, Kelesidis T, Gillman MW. Cord blood leptin and adiponectin as predictors of adiposity in children at 3 years of age: a prospective cohort study. Pediatrics. 2009;123:682–9.

30. Dörner G, Plagemann A. Perinatal hyperinsulinism as possible predisposing factor for diabetes mellitus, obesity and enhanced cardiovascular risk in later life. Horm Metab Res. 1994;26:213–21.

31. El HN, Pliushch G, Schneider E, Dittrich M, Müller T, Korenkov M, Aretz M, Zechner U, Lehnen H, Haaf T. Metabolic programming of MEST DNA methylation by intrauterine exposure to gestational diabetes mellitus. Diabetes. 2013;62:1320–8.

32. Finer S, Mathews C, Lowe R, Smart M, Hillman S, Foo L, Sinha A, Williams D, Rakyan VK, Hitman GA. Maternal gestational diabetes is associated with genome-wide DNA methylation variation in placenta and cord blood of exposed offspring. Hum Mol Genet. 2015;24:3021–9.

33. Haertle L, El Hajj N, Dittrich M, Müller T, Nanda I, Lehnen H, Haaf T. Epigenetic signatures of gestational diabetes mellitus on cord blood methylation. Clin Epigenetics. 2017;9:28.

34. Houshmand-Oeregaard A, Hansen NS, Hjort L, Kelstrup L, Broholm C, Mathiesen ER, Clausen TD, Damm P, Vaag A. Differential adipokine DNA methylation and gene expression in subcutaneous adipose tissue from adult offspring of women with diabetes in pregnancy. Clin Epigenetics. 2017;9:37.

35. Corbetta S, Bulfamante G, Cortelazzi D, Barresi V, Cetin I, Mantovani G, Bondioni S, Beck-Peccoz P, Spada A. Adiponectin expression in human fetal tissues during mid- and late gestation. J Clin Endocrinol Metab. 2005;90:2397–402.

36. Ott R, Stupin JH, Loui A, Eilers E, Melchior K, Rancourt RC, Schellong K, Ziska T, Dudenhausen JW, Henrich W, Plagemann A. Maternal overweight is not an independent risk factor for increased birth weight, leptin and insulin in newborns of gestational diabetic women: observations from the prospective 'EaCH' cohort study. BMC Pregnancy Childbirth. 2018;18:250.

37. Deutsche Gesellschaft für Gynäkologie und Geburtshilfe. Diabetes und Schwangerschaft [Internet], 2008. Available from: https://www.dggg.de/fileadmin/documents/leitlinien/archiviert/beteiligt/057023_Diabetes_und_Schwangerschaft/057023_2008.pdf. Accessed 12 June 2018.

38. Kleinwechter H. Gestations diabetes mellitus (GDM). Dtsch Med Wochenschr. 2012;137:999–1002.

39. Matthews DR, Hosker JR, Rudenski AS, Naylor BA, Treacher DF, Turner RC. Homeostasis model assessment: insulin resistance and β-cell function from fasting plasma glucose and insulin concentrations in man. Diabetologia. 1985;28:412–9.

40. Neville MJ, Collins JM, Gloyn AL, McCarthy MI, Karpe F. Comprehensive human adipose tissue mRNA and microRNA endogenous control selection for quantitative real-time-PCR normalization. Obesity. 2011;19:888–92.

41. Iwaki M, Matsuda M, Maeda N, Funahashi T, Matsuzawa Y, Makishima M, Shimomura I. Induction of adiponectin, a fat-derived antidiabetic and antiatherogenic factor, by nuclear receptors. Diabetes. 2003;52:1655–63.

21

Idiopathic male infertility is strongly associated with aberrant DNA methylation of imprinted loci in sperm: a case-control study

Qiuqin Tang[1†], Feng Pan[2†], Jing Yang[3,4], Ziqiang Fu[3,4], Yiwen Lu[3,4], Xian Wu[5], Xiumei Han[3,4], Minjian Chen[3,4], Chuncheng Lu[3,4], Yankai Xia[3,4], Xinru Wang[3,4] and Wei Wu[3,4,6*]

Abstract

Background: Male infertility is a complex disease caused by a combination of genetic, environmental, and lifestyle factors. Abnormal epigenetic programming has been proposed as a possible mechanism compromising male fertility. Recent studies suggest that aberrant imprinting in spermatozoa in a subset of infertile men is a risk factor for congenital diseases in children conceived via assisted reproduction techniques. In this study, we examined the DNA methylation status of CpG sites within the differentially methylated regions (DMRs) of three imprinted genes, *H19*, *GNAS*, and *DIRAS3*, using combined bisulfite PCR restriction analysis and bisulfite sequencing in sperm obtained from 135 men with idiopathic male infertility, including normozoospermia ($n = 39$), moderate oligozoospermia ($n = 45$), and severe oligozoospermia ($n = 51$), and fertile controls ($n = 59$). The percentage of global methylation was compared between fertile controls and infertile patients displaying abnormal DNA methylation status of imprinted loci. Moreover, we also analyzed whether the DNA methyltransferases (DNMTs) polymorphisms impact upon the methylation patterns of imprinted genes in idiopathic infertile males.

Results: Aberrant methylation patterns of imprinted genes were more prevalent in idiopathic infertile males, especially in patients with oligozoospermia. Infertile males with aberrant methylation patterns of imprinted genes displayed a tendency of lower global methylation levels, although not reaching statistical significance ($P = 0.13$). In the genotype-epigenotype correlation analysis, no significant association was observed between aberrant methylation patterns of the three imprinted genes and genotypes of the four DNA methyltransferase (DNMT) genes.

Conclusion: We conclude that abnormalities of DMR within imprinted genes may be associated with idiopathic male infertility. Disruption in methylation pattern of the three imprinted genes does not occur in high-risk genotypes of DNMTs.

Keywords: DNA methylation, DNMT, Global methylation, Imprinted gene, Male infertility, Polymorphism, Sperm

Introduction

Male infertility is a multifactorial disorder which affects approximately 15% of couples at reproductive age globally with substantial clinical and social impact [1]. In spite of the magnitude of the problem and the considerable research efforts that have been made to understand its causes, a large proportion of male infertility cases remains idiopathic in nature [2]. In these patients, oligozoospermia is frequently observed, and most infertile men resort to some kinds of assisted reproductive technique (ART). Even though this method allows the infertile males to father their own children without knowing the cause of their infertility, it also carries the potential risk of transmitting genetic or epigenetic defects and impacting offspring [3, 4].

Genomic imprinting is an epigenetic phenomenon which mediates mono-allelic, parent-of-origin-specific expression

* Correspondence: wwu@njmu.edu.cn
†Qiuqin Tang and Feng Pan contributed equally to this work.
3State Key Laboratory of Reproductive Medicine, Institute of Toxicology, Nanjing Medical University, 101 Longmian Avenue, Nanjing 211166, China
4Key Laboratory of Modern Toxicology of Ministry of Education, School of Public Health, Nanjing Medical University, Nanjing, China
Full list of author information is available at the end of the article

of genes during embryonic development and after birth [5, 6]. Genomic imprints are erased in primordial germ cells and are newly established during later stages of germ cell development, which are stably inherited through somatic cell divisions during postzygotic development [7]. DNA methylation at differentially methylated regions (DMRs) is one of the regulatory mechanisms controlling the allele-specific expression of imprinted genes. DNA methylation of CpG dinucleotides at DMRs is the most studied epigenetic mark [7–10]. Genomic imprinting is vital for normal gene expression patterns in an individual, with errors sometimes resulted in inappropriate gene transcription or repression [6]. Aberrant regulation of imprinted genes is known to be responsible for various growth and behavioral syndromes [11]. Because imprinted genes escape epigenetic reprogramming after fertilization and maintain their parent-specific germline patterns, aberrant methylation imprints can be transmitted directly from the father's sperm into the developing embryo [12].

It has been suggested that intracytoplasmic sperm injection (ICSI), by canceling the natural selection of aberrant spermatozoa, may cause irregular embryo cell divisions due to the mechanical manipulation of the gametes and might transmit genetically related infertility [13, 14]. Although the overall rate of congenital anomalies in children conceived by ART is low (4–6%), this rate still represents a significant increase compared with the background rate of major malformations (3%) [15]. Several clinical studies reported an unexpected high incidence of imprinting disorders (e.g., Angelman syndrome (AS) and Beckwith-Wiedemann syndrome (BWS)) in children conceived with ART [16, 17]. Additionally, the demonstration of imprinting defects in cases of disrupted spermatogenesis raised the possibility that they could be associated with infertility itself [18]. Several studies have shown that infertile males with impaired spermatogenesis are prone to have a higher incidence of aberrant methylation in imprinted genes [18–26].

Although hints exist that spermatozoa from the infertile male can carry imprinting defects, relatively small sample size patient cohorts were investigated and few clinical details were given. In addition, most studies of the methylation status of imprinted genes usually select men diagnosed as infertile without the inclusion of any appropriate fertile controls [18–23]. These results can directly demonstrate the potential risk of imprinting defect on semen quality, but not male infertility. In this study, to test our hypothesis that imprinting defect is associated with idiopathic male infertility, we utilized carefully the selected fertile controls to evaluate the association between the imprinting defect of three imprinted genes and idiopathic male infertility. In addition, we analyzed the global methylation level of sperm DNA which represents epigenetic changes affecting multiple loci and explored the association between genotypes of four DNA methyltransferase (DNMT)

polymorphisms and risk of aberrant methylation of imprinted genes.

Methods

Subject recruitment and sample collection

Study subjects were volunteers form affiliated hospitals of Nanjing Medical University between July 2009 and September 2010. The study was approved by the Institutional Review Board of Nanjing Medical University, and subjects gave written informed consent. All activities involving human subjects were done under full compliance with the government policies and the Helsinki Declaration. Consecutive eligible men (without diagnosed infertile wives) were recruited to participate, 196 in total were asked. Of those approached, 87.2% consented (171 participants). A completed physical examination including height and weight was performed, and a questionnaire was used to collect information including personal background, lifestyle factors, environmental and occupational exposures, genetic risk factors, and medical history. Men with immune infertility, semen non-liquefaction, and medical history of risk factors for infertility (e.g., varicocele, orchidopexy, or postvasectomy), and receiving treatment for infertility (e.g., hormonal treatments) were excluded from the study (15 of 171 subjects). Men with other known causes related to male infertility, such as genetic disease, infection, and occupational exposure to the agents suspected to be associated with male reproduction, were also excluded (13 of 156 subjects). Furthermore, to avoid azoospermia or severe oligozoospermia caused by Y chromosome microdeletions, we excluded subjects with Y chromosome microdeletions of the azoospermia factor region (8 of 143 subjects). We selected 59 fertile men from the early pregnancy registry, from the same hospitals as the cases. All controls were healthy men with normal reproductive function and confirmed to have healthy babies 6–8 months later. All subjects were Han Chinese who came from Nanjing and neighborly suburban area.

Semen analysis

Semen samples were obtained in private by masturbation into a sterile wide-mouth and metal-free glass container after a recommended at least 3-day sexual abstinence. After liquefaction at 37 °C for 30 min, conventional semen analysis was conducted in accordance with the guidelines of the WHO Laboratory Manual for the Examination of Human Semen (World Health Organization, 1999), including semen volume, sperm number per ejaculum, sperm concentration, motility, progression, and motion parameters. Strict quality control measures were enforced throughout the study. Observation and counting in the semen analysis were automatic, and the backgrounds of the samples were blinded to avoid bias.

DNA extraction

Motile sperm cells were purified away from lymphocyte contamination, immature germ cells, and epithelial cells using a Percoll (GE Healthcare) gradient with two concentration layers (80% and 40%). A microscopic examination of the sperm fractions was performed to control the quality of cell preparations. The sperm pellets were resuspended twice in phosphate-buffered saline (PBS) and centrifuged at 400g for 10 min. Genomic sperm DNA isolation was performed as described [27]. DNA concentration was determined by spectrophotometry.

Bisulfite treatment and methylation analysis

Methylation assays were performed at the DMRs of three imprinted genes [*H19* (HGNC: 4713), *GNAS* (HGNC: 4392), and *DIRAS3* (HGNC: 687)] in humans using combined bisulfite PCR restriction analysis (COBRA) and bisulfite sequencing PCR (BSP). Genomic DNA (1 μg, or 500 ng when sperm DNA was not enough) was treated with sodium bisulfite using the EpiTect Bisulfite Kit (Qiagen) according to the protocol recommended by the manufacturer. Bisulfite converts unmethylated cytosine to uracil while 5-methylcytosine (5-MeC) remains unchanged. Three microliters of the final eluent was used for subsequent PCR amplification. PCR included an initial incubation at 94 °C for 5 min, followed by 40 cycles of 94 °C for 40 s; 60 °C (for *H19* and *GNAS*) and 54 °C (for *DIRAS3*) for 40 s; and 72 °C for 60 s, followed by one cycle of 72 °C for 10 min. The amplification products were separated on 2% agarose gels and stained with ethidium bromide. Most samples have been subject to two independent bisulfite treatments and were analyzed from two independent PCR products. The region analyzed for each of these genes was within the DMR of CpG islands. We examined 18 CpG sites in a 220-bp fragment of *H19* (chromosome 11: 1999796-2000015), 32 CpG sites in a 343-bp fragment of *GNAS* (chromosome 20: 58840057-58840399), and 13 CpG sites in a 207-bp fragment of *DIRAS3* (chromosome 1: 68050564-68050770) (Fig. 1).

To ensure that the sequencing results did not reflect a cloning bias, restriction analysis carried out on germ cell and somatic cell DNA, cutting the DNA with enzymes that could cleave only the methylated templates of the same bisulfite-treated PCR samples. After amplification, 20–50% of PCR products were digested with the restriction enzyme *TaqI* (New England Biolabs) for *H19* and *BstUI* (New England Biolabs) for *GNAS* and *DIRAS3*, both of which recognize sequences unique to the methylated (bisulfite-unconverted) templates but cannot recognize unmethylated (bisulfite-converted) templates. DNA was then electrophoresed on a 3% agarose gel. The intensity of methylated templates was calculated by densitometry using AlphaEaseFC software (Alpha Innotech), and the percentage of methylated restriction enzyme site in each genomic sample was calculated from the ratio between the enzyme-cleaved PCR products and the total amount of PCR products. In addition, the PCR products were purified and cloned into the pCR2.1 vector by TA Cloning kit (Invitrogen, Carlsbad, CA, USA). To determine the methylation status of DMR, an average of ten clones (each plate) were sequenced using M13 reverse primer and an automated ABI Prism 3730xl Genetic Analyzer (Applied Biosystems, Foster City, CA, USA).

Global methylation analyses

For each sample, methylation analysis was performed in triplicate and averaged (100 ng DNA each) using a Methylamp Global DNA Methylation Quantification Kit (Epigenetek, New York, NY) following the manufacturer's instructions. Briefly, the methylated fractions of DNA were recognized by an anti-5-methylcytosine antibody and quantified through an enzyme-linked immunosorbent assay-like reaction. The total amount of methylated DNA is proportional to the optical density (OD). Positive control and the negative control were provided with the kit and included in each experiment as an internal control. Global methylation percentage values were normalized to this internal control.

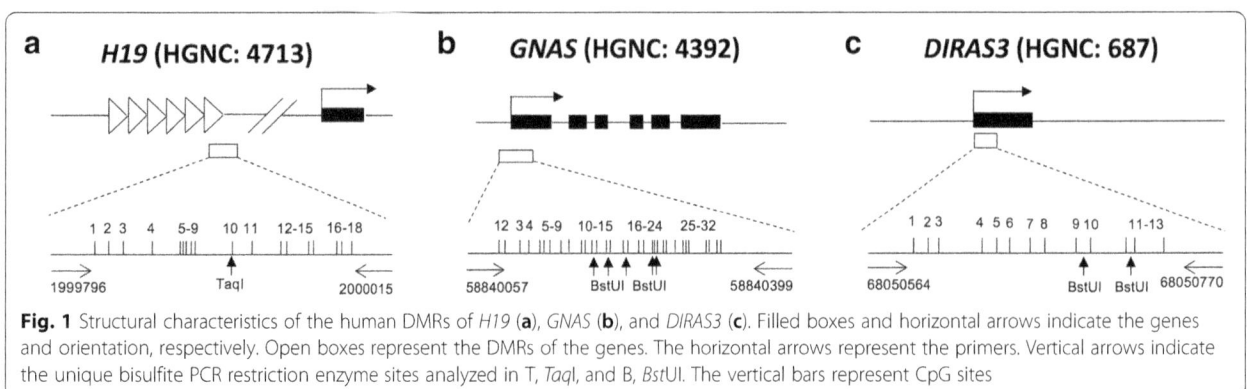

Fig. 1 Structural characteristics of the human DMRs of *H19* (**a**), *GNAS* (**b**), and *DIRAS3* (**c**). Filled boxes and horizontal arrows indicate the genes and orientation, respectively. Open boxes represent the DMRs of the genes. The horizontal arrows represent the primers. Vertical arrows indicate the unique bisulfite PCR restriction enzyme sites analyzed in T, *TaqI*, and B, *BstUI*. The vertical bars represent CpG sites

Variant genotyping

Genotype analyses of four polymorphisms in *DNMT1*, *DNMT3A*, *DNMT3B*, and *DNMT3L* were performed using the DNA obtained from the patient's blood. Genotypes were detected by allelic discrimination assay using TaqMan® MGB probes on a 7900HT Fast real-time PCR system (Applied Biosystems, CA). The gene variants studied were *DNMT1* (rs4804490), *DNMT3A* (rs1550117), *DNMT3B* (rs2424909), and *DNMT3L* (rs7354779) that have been described in our previous study [28]. Very rare variants are of limited value in association studies as they are only relevant to a small proportion of the population and their effects are difficult to detect in practice. Therefore, we selected only variants where the frequency of the minor allele was > 5%. For the quality control, the genotyping was done without the knowledge of case/control status of the subjects, a random 10% of cases and controls were genotyped twice by different individuals, and the reproducibility was 100%.

Statistical analysis

Analysis of variance was used to explore the relationships between fertility status and potentially important covariates, such as age, body mass index (BMI), ejaculate volume, sperm concentration, and motility. The χ^2 test was used to evaluate the differences in smoking status, alcohol drinking status, duration of sexual abstinence, and the frequency of aberrant methylation of imprinted genes between case and control groups. Logistic regression analysis was performed to obtain the odds ratios (ORs) for idiopathic male infertility and aberrant methylation and 95% confidence intervals (95% CI) with adjustment for age, BMI, smoking status, alcohol drinking, and duration of sexual abstinence, wherever it was appropriate. Results of global methylation are expressed as mean ± SD. All statistical analyses were carried out using Stata (Version 9.0, StataCorp, LP), and $P \leq 0.05$ was considered to be significant.

Results

We first analyzed the DNA methylation pattern of the three imprinted genes in sperm DNA samples from 135 idiopathic infertile males and 59 fertile male controls. Demographic categories by fertility and semen quality are described in Table 1. Briefly, each group of cases and controls were well matched for age, BMI, smoking status, and alcohol drinking (*P* > 0.05). As the analyzed genes were chosen as indicators of paternal and maternal imprinting, > 90% methylation was expected for the paternally imprinted *H19* and < 10% for the maternally imprinted *DIRAS3* and *GNAS* in sperm DNA [20].

In total, we identified the aberrant methylation of *H19*, *GNAS*, and *DIRAS3* in 19.3%, 21.5%, and 22.2% of the 135 infertile males, respectively (Additional file 1: Table S1).

The frequencies of aberrant methylation of the two maternal imprinted genes (*GNAS* and *DIRAS3*) were higher than those of the paternal imprinted gene (*H19*). However, cases with severe oligozoospermia were more prone to have aberrant methylation of the paternal imprinted gene than maternal imprinted genes (Additional file 1: Table S1). Notably, among 26 cases with aberrant methylation of *H19*, 29 cases with aberrant methylation of *GNAS*, and 30 cases with aberrant methylation of *DIRAS3*, 6 had all the three imprinted genes abnormally methylated, 9 had both *H19* and *GNAS* abnormally methylated, 8 had both *H19* and *DIRAS3* abnormally methylated, and 11 had both *GNAS* and *DIRAS3* abnormally methylated. Aberrant methylation of the three imprinted genes was also found in fertile controls (Table 2). Adjusted ORs and 95% CIs for associations between idiopathic male infertility and aberrant methylation status of imprinted genes are presented in Table 2. Compared with men of normal methylation status of imprinted genes, men with aberrant methylation status were more likely to have idiopathic infertility (for *H19*, OR = 7.61, 95% CI = 1.71–33.80; for *GNAS*, OR = 17.53, 95% CI = 2.29–134.19; for *DIRAS3*, OR = 9.02, 95% CI = 2.01–40.58; Table 2; Fig. 2), especially patients with severe oligozoospermia (for *H19*, OR = 28.52, 95% CI = 5.85–139.06; for *GNAS*, OR = 25.35, 95% CI = 3.10–207.00; for *DIRAS3*, OR = 19.79, 95% CI = 3.69–106.03; Table 2; Fig. 1). For a more detailed analysis, the subjects were categorized according to the concentration (< 5, 5–20, ≥ 20 million sperm/ml) of sperm. In all the three subgroups, there was a statistically significant increased frequency of aberrant methylation of *GNAS*. In contrast, the statistically significant increased frequency of aberrant methylation was observed only in case 3 subgroup for *H19* and in case 2 and case 3 subgroups for *DIRAS3* (Table 2). In addition, most patients with abnormalities in both imprint regions were severe oligozoospermia. These results suggested that aberrant methylation of imprinted genes was associated with increased idiopathic male infertility risks, while the idiopathic infertile subjects with oligozoospermia (especially severe oligozoospermia) might be at higher risk.

To further investigate whether sperm samples from patients with aberrant methylation of imprinted genes displayed global DNA methylation changes, we analyzed the global methylation of infertile men with aberrant methylation of imprinted genes (*n* = 20) and fertile controls (*n* = 20). Infertile men displayed a tendency of lower global methylation levels (4.25 ± 2.99% in infertile men versus 6.21 ± 4.83% in fertile controls), although not reaching statistical significance (*P* = 0.13; Fig. 3).

The previous study suggested that the epigenetic causal variation of male infertility should be considered together with genetic variations [29]. Therefore, we sought to analyze the correlation between the polymorphisms of DNMTs and aberrant methylation of imprinted genes in

Table 1 Characteristics of idiopathic infertile males and fertile controls

Characteristic	Controls $(n = 59)^a$	Cases			
		Case 1 $(n = 39)^b$	Case 2 $(n = 45)^c$	Case 3 $(n = 51)^d$	Case all $(n = 135)^e$
Age (years, mean ± SD)	29.08 ± 3.85	29.85 ± 4.84	28.71 ± 3.91	28.78 ± 4.07	29.07 ± 4.25
BMI (kg/m², mean ± SD)^f	23.93 ± 4.17	22.61 ± 3.54	22.99 ± 2.72	22.92 ± 3.36	22.86 ± 3.20
Smoking status [n (%)]					
No	27 (45.8)	21 (53.8)	26 (57.8)	23 (45.1)	70 (51.9)
Yes	32 (54.2)	18 (46.2)	19 (42.2)	28 (54.9)	65 (48.1)
Alcohol drinking [n (%)]					
No	46 (78.0)	33 (84.6)	37 (82.2)	41 (80.4)	111 (82.2)
Yes	13 (22.0)	6 (15.4)	8 (17.8)	10 (19.6)	24 (17.8)
Abstinence time [n (%)]					
< 4	15 (25.4)	7 (18.3)	10 (23.8)	4 (12.1)	21 (15.6)
4–7	38 (64.4)	41 (68.3)	24 (57.1)	23 (69.7)	88 (65.2)
≥ 7	6 (10.2)	12 (13.3)^g	8 (19.0)	6 (18.2)	26 (19.3)
Ejaculate volume (ml, mean ± SD)	4.29 ± 1.32	2.99 ± 1.21^g	3.30 ± 1.60^g	3.43 ± 1.47^g	3.26 ± 1.45^g
Sperm concentration (10⁶/ml, mean ± SD)	49.52 ± 33.85	76.92 ± 54.36^g	14.62 ± 2.91^g	4.35 ± 2.75^g	28.74 ± 42.58^g
Sperm motility (%, mean ± SD)	57.00 ± 16.05	53.81 ± 26.54	39.59 ± 20.12^g	31.48 ± 14.70^g	40.64 ± 22.27^g

^{a}Control: fertile men
^{b}Case 1: idiopathic infertile men with normozoospermia (sperm concentration ≥ 20 × 10⁶/ml)
^{c}Case 2: idiopathic infertile men with moderate oligozoospermia (sperm concentration 5–20 × 10⁶/ml)
^{d}Case 3: idiopathic infertile men with severe oligozoospermia (sperm concentration < 5 × 10⁶/ml)
^{e}Case all: the sum of case 1, case 2, and case 3
^{f}BMI body mass index
^{g}$P < 0.05$ when compared between case and control groups

the sperm of idiopathic infertile males. The genotypes of the four polymorphisms in DNMTs (rs4804490 in *DNMT1*, rs1550117 in *DNMT3A*, rs2424909 in *DNMT3B*, and rs7354779 in *DNMT3L*) were analyzed in the blood DNA of patients. Six patients showed aberrant methylation of all the three imprinted genes, four with wild-type homozygous of all four DNMTs, one with heterozygous of rs4804490, and one with variant homozygous of rs4804490. However, no statistically significant associations were observed between the distribution of any of the DNMT polymorphisms and aberrant methylation patterns of any of the imprinted genes as shown in Additional file 2: Table S2.

Discussion

This study adds to the growing literature that defects in spermatogenesis could be associated with the epigenetic regulation of imprinting in the male germ line [14, 30]. The DNA methylation of imprinted genes is established during spermatogenesis and maintained in mature spermatozoa. In fertile men with a normal ejaculate, paternal DMRs of the DNA should be methylated and the maternal DMRs should be unmethylated. Interestingly, even some fertile controls exhibited aberrant methylation of the three imprinted genes. As recently reported that environmental and lifestyle risk factors may affect DNA methylation of the imprinted gene in human sperm [10, 31], we speculated that the aberrant methylation of these fertile men might be

caused by environmental and lifestyle risk factors. Future studies are required to address this problem. In idiopathic infertile males, however, it showed variable aberrant methylation patterns that were proportional to the severity of the oligozoospermic phenotype. In this study, loss of methylation was detected in the paternally imprinted and methylated DMRs of *H19*, whereas the maternally imprinted and unmethylated DMR of *GNAS* and *DIRAS3* showed increased methylation in idiopathic infertile males, suggesting a simultaneous hypo- and hypermethylation of the haploid spermatozoa genome. Abnormal methylation was detected at the DMR of *H19* in 26 of 135 patients (19.3%), and one case of complete absence of methylation was observed. However, the patients with *H19* completely unmethylated did not acquire aberrant methylation of *GNAS* or *DIRAS3*.

In idiopathic infertile males, DNA methylation in sperm is frequently affected at one or multiple imprinting control regions. The studied loci represent only a small fraction of imprinted genes. However, methylation abnormalities in these imprinted genes may be considered as indicators for more profound epimutation at other loci. Therefore, we compared the global methylation levels of sperm DNA in idiopathic infertile males with aberrant methylation of imprinted genes and fertile controls. Alterations in tumor DNA methylation include locus-specific hypermethylation and generalized genome-wide hypomethylation [32, 33]. No significant difference in global methylation was

Table 2 Adjusted ORs (95% CIs) for idiopathic male infertility by methylation status of imprinted genes

Gene	Methylation	Control (n = 59)[a]	Case							
			Case 1 (n = 39)[b]		Case 2 (n = 45)[c]		Case 3 (n = 51)[d]		Case all (n = 135)[e]	
		n (%)	n (%)	OR (95% CI)[f]	n (%)	OR (95% CI)[e]	n (%)	OR (95% CI)[e]	n (%)	OR (95% CI)[e]
H19	Normal	57 (96.6)	37 (94.9)	1.00	44 (97.8)	1.00	28 (54.9)	1.00	109 (80.7)	1.00
	Aberrant	2 (3.4)	2 (5.1)	1.66 (0.20–13.48)	1 (2.2)	0.60 (0.05–7.43)	23 (45.1)	28.52 (5.85–139.06)	26 (19.3)	7.61 (1.71–33.80)
GNAS	Normal	58 (98.3)	33 (84.6)	1.00	36 (80.0)	1.00	37 (72.5)	1.00	106 (78.5)	1.00
	Aberrant	1 (1.7)	6 (15.4)	12.89 (1.35–122.79)	9 (20.0)	14.91 (1.76–126.58)	14 (27.5)	25.35 (3.10–207.00)	29 (21.5)	17.53 (2.29–134.19)
DIRAS3	Normal	57 (96.6)	35 (89.7)	1.00	35 (77.8)	1.00	35 (68.6)	1.00	105 (77.8)	1.00
	Aberrant	2 (3.4)	4 (10.3)	4.17 (0.61–28.58)	10 (22.2)	9.11 (1.76–47.16)	16 (31.4)	19.79 (3.69–106.03)	30 (22.2)	9.02 (2.01–40.58)

ORs adjusted for age, BMI, smoking status, alcohol drinking, and abstinence time

[a] Control: fertile men.

[b] Case 1: idiopathic infertile men with normozoospermia (sperm concentration $\geq 20 \times 10^6$/ml)

[c] Case 2: idiopathic infertile men with moderate oligozoospermia (sperm concentration 5–20×10^6/ml)

[d] Case 3: idiopathic infertile men with severe oligozoospermia (sperm concentration $< 5 \times 10^6$/ml)

[e] Case all: the sum of case 1, case 2, and case 3

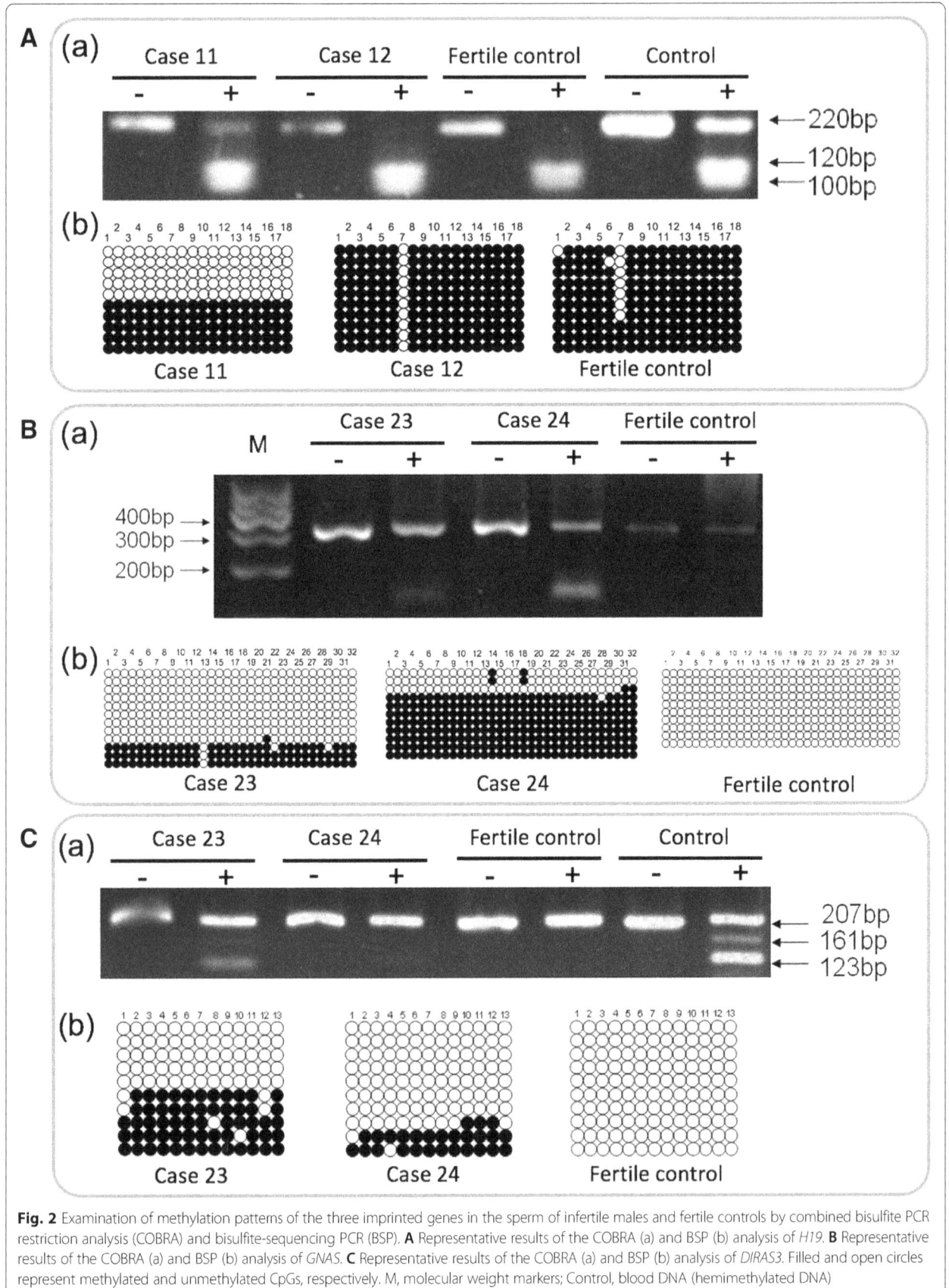

Fig. 2 Examination of methylation patterns of the three imprinted genes in the sperm of infertile males and fertile controls by combined bisulfite PCR restriction analysis (COBRA) and bisulfite-sequencing PCR (BSP). **A** Representative results of the COBRA (a) and BSP (b) analysis of *H19*. **B** Representative results of the COBRA (a) and BSP (b) analysis of *GNAS*. **C** Representative results of the COBRA (a) and BSP (b) analysis of *DIRAS3*. Filled and open circles represent methylated and unmethylated CpGs, respectively. M, molecular weight markers; Control, blood DNA (hemimethylated DNA)

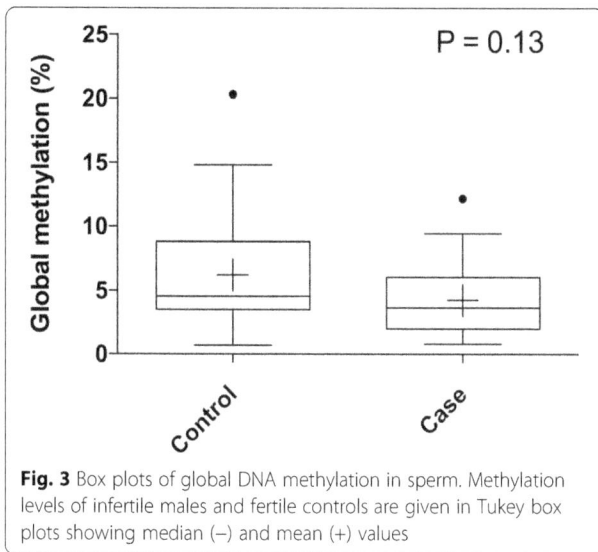

Fig. 3 Box plots of global DNA methylation in sperm. Methylation levels of infertile males and fertile controls are given in Tukey box plots showing median (−) and mean (+) values

observed between idiopathic infertile males and fertile controls but displayed a tendency of lower global methylation levels. Global hypomethylation is associated with genomic instability and an increased number of mutational events [34–37]. Furthermore, we found that the group with oligozoospermia had a higher frequent aberrant methylation of imprinted genes compared with the group with normozoospermia, suggesting a role of DNA methylation in regulating spermatogenesis in human males. We speculated that the altered methylation patterns of imprinted genes could be due to an improper erasure and establish of methylation imprints in the early germ cells since both gains, and loss of DNA methylation were observed and global methylation seemed unaffected.

Reduced sperm counts, low progressive motility, and abnormal morphology are indications for ART. We considered that low birth weight [38], congenital malformations [39, 40], and imprinting disorders [41] in some ART children can, at least partially, be attributed to epigenetic variations. The association between ART and both AS and BWS was studied and confirmed by research groups from the US, Europe, and Australia [16, 17, 42]. A previous study suggested that the increase in the incidence of imprinting disorders in individuals born by ART may be attributed to the use of sperm with imprinting defects [14]. The aberrant patterns of methylation at DMRs observed in sperm of oligozoospermic men could be transmitted to the zygote and might affect the expression of imprinted genes and phenotype in the developing embryo.

It has been noted that the developmental outcome of ART is generally poor when sperm showed to have an abnormal DNA methylation pattern [43]. Importantly, a previous study demonstrated that aberrant DNA methylation of DMRs in children of oligozoospermia males was inherited from the father [14]. Therefore, it is

necessary to add imprint methylation analysis to the routine sperm examination to identify preexisting imprint mutations when ART is applied in the fertility clinic to aid idiopathic infertile males to become fathers. Future studies are needed to determine whether infertility will be transmitted to offspring conceived by in vitro fertilization using the sperm of infertile men with aberrant methylation of imprinted genes. Additionally, we should pay special attention to the contamination of somatic cells in the purified sperm sample. Though we have done our very best to purify sperm and include a microscope to control the quality of cell preparations, contamination may remain a problem.

DNA methylation is performed by a group of proteins termed DNMTs. Embryogenesis is severely impaired in Dnmt1- or Dnmt3b-knockout mice, and spermatogenesis is impaired in Dnmt3a-knockout mice [44, 45]. DNMT3L, which is similar to DNMT3, is unique among DNMTs because it lacks enzymatic activity. The consequence of Dnmt3L deficiency in mice is the loss of imprints [46]. Our recent study has shown that DNA sequence variants were more prevalent in patients with oligozoospermia [28]. Therefore, we also analyzed the association between genetic variations of four DNMTs and the risk of aberrant methylation of imprinted genes. However, no significant association between the distribution of polymorphisms of DNMTs and risk of aberrant methylation of any of the imprinted genes was observed.

The findings obtained in the present study suggest that aberrant methylation patterns of imprinted genes were associated with the risk of spermatogenic failure in the Chinese population, although the global methylation levels do not seem to be associated with male infertility. Our results strengthen the premise that abnormal epigenetic reprogramming of the male germ line is a possible mechanism of compromised idiopathic male infertility. Our findings support the urgent need for research to better understand the potential mechanisms for aberrant methylation of imprinted genes in human spermatogenesis and the related pathology.

Abbreviations
5-MeC: 5-Methylcytosine; ART: Assisted reproductive technique; AS: Angelman syndrome; BMI: Body mass index; BSP: Bisulfite sequencing PCR; BWS: Beckwith-Wiedemann syndrome; COBRA: Combined bisulfite PCR restriction analysis; DMRs: Differentially methylated regions; DNMTs: DNA methyltransferases; ICSI: Intracytoplasmic sperm injection; OD: Optical density; PBS: Phosphate-buffered saline

Acknowledgements
We thank all the patients and donors who participated in our study.

Funding

This work was supported by the National Natural Science Foundation of China (81673217), Jiangsu Overseas Visiting Scholar Program for University Prominent Young & Middle-aged Teachers and Presidents, and the Priority Academic Program for the Development of Jiangsu Higher Education Institutions (Public Health and Preventive Medicine).

Authors' contributions

QT and WW conceived and designed the experiment. FP, JY, ZF, YL, XH, and WW performed the experiments. QT, MC, CL, and WW performed the statistical analysis. QT, WW, YX, and XW wrote and revised the manuscript. All authors read and approved the final manuscript.

Competing interests

The authors declare that they have no competing interests.

Author details

[1]Department of Obstetrics, The Affiliated Obstetrics and Gynecology Hospital of Nanjing Medical University, Nanjing Maternity and Child Health Care Hospital, Nanjing, China. [2]Department of Urology, The Affiliated Obstetrics and Gynecology Hospital of Nanjing Medical University, Nanjing Maternity and Child Health Care Hospital, Nanjing, China. [3]State Key Laboratory of Reproductive Medicine, Institute of Toxicology, Nanjing Medical University, 101 Longmian Avenue, Nanjing 211166, China. [4]Key Laboratory of Modern Toxicology of Ministry of Education, School of Public Health, Nanjing Medical University, Nanjing, China. [5]National Toxicology Program Laboratory, Division of the National Toxicology Program, National Institute of Environmental Health Sciences, Research Triangle Park, NC, USA. [6]Department of Health and Human Services, National Institute of Environmental Health Sciences, National Institutes of Health, Research Triangle Park, USA.

References

1. Jarow JP, Sharlip ID, Belker AM, et al. Best practice policies for male infertility. J Urol. 2002;167(5):2138–44 [published Online First: 2002/04/17].

2. Punab M, Poolamets O, Paju P, et al. Causes of male infertility: a 9-year prospective monocentre study on 1737 patients with reduced total sperm counts. Hum Reprod. 2017;32(1):18–31. https://doi.org/10.1093/humrep/dew284 [published Online First: 2016/11/20].

3. El Hajj N, Haertle L, Dittrich M, et al. DNA methylation signatures in cord blood of ICSI children. Hum Reprod. 2017;32(8):1761–9. https://doi.org/10.1093/humrep/dex209 [published Online First: 2017/06/03].

4. Stuppia L, Franzago M, Ballerini P, et al. Epigenetics and male reproduction: the consequences of paternal lifestyle on fertility, embryo development, and children lifetime health. Clin Epigenetics. 2015;7:120. https://doi.org/10.1186/s13148-015-0155-4 [published Online First: 2015/11/14].

5. Tilghman SM. The sins of the fathers and mothers: genomic imprinting in mammalian development. Cell. 1999;96(2):185–93 [published Online First: 1999/02/13].

6. Barlow DP, Bartolomei MS. Genomic imprinting in mammals. Cold Spring Harb Perspect Biol. 2014;6(2). https://doi.org/10.1101/cshperspect.a018382 [published Online First: 2014/02/05].

7. Reik W, Dean W, Walter J. Epigenetic reprogramming in mammalian development. Science. 2001;293(5532):1089–93. https://doi.org/10.1126/science.1063443 [published Online First: 2001/08/11].

8. Fagundes NS, Michalczechen-Lacerda VA, Caixeta ES, et al. Methylation status in the intragenic differentially methylated region of the IGF2 locus in Bos taurus indicus oocytes with different developmental competencies. Mol Hum Reprod. 2011;17(2):85–91. https://doi.org/10.1093/molehr/gaq075 [published Online First: 2010/09/14].

9. Peters FS, Peeters AMA, Mandaviya PR, et al. Differentially methylated regions in T cells identify kidney transplant patients at risk for de novo skin cancer. Clin Epigenetics. 2018;10:81. https://doi.org/10.1186/s13148-018-0519-7 [published Online First: 2018/06/28].

10. Soubry A, Guo L, Huang Z, et al. Obesity-related DNA methylation at imprinted genes in human sperm: Results from the TIEGER study. Clin Epigenetics. 2016;8:51. https://doi.org/10.1186/s13148-016-0217-2 [published Online First: 2016/05/10].

11. Ishida M, Moore GE. The role of imprinted genes in humans. Mol Aspects Med. 2013;34(4):826–40. https://doi.org/10.1016/j.mam.2012.06.009 [published Online First: 2012/07/10].

12. White CR, Denomme MM, Tekpetey FR, et al. High Frequency of Imprinted Methylation Errors in Human Preimplantation Embryos. Sci Rep. 2015;5:17311. https://doi.org/10.1038/srep17311 [published Online First: 2015/12/03].

13. Hewitson L, Dominko T, Takahashi D, et al. Unique checkpoints during the first cell cycle of fertilization after intracytoplasmic sperm injection in rhesus monkeys. Nat Med. 1999;5(4):431–3. https://doi.org/10.1038/7430 [published Online First: 1999/04/15].

14. Kobayashi H, Hiura H, John RM, et al. DNA methylation errors at imprinted loci after assisted conception originate in the parental sperm. Eur J Hum Genet. 2009;17(12):1582–91. https://doi.org/10.1038/ejhg.2009.68 [published Online First: 2009/05/28].

15. Katari S, Turan N, Bibikova M, et al. DNA methylation and gene expression differences in children conceived in vitro or in vivo. Hum Mol Genet. 2009; 18(20):3769–78. https://doi.org/10.1093/hmg/ddp319 [published Online First: 2009/07/17].

16. Mussa A, Molinatto C, Cerrato F, et al. Assisted Reproductive Techniques and Risk of Beckwith-Wiedemann Syndrome. Pediatrics. 2017;140(1). https://doi.org/10.1542/peds.2016-4311 [published Online First: 2017/06/22].

17. Lazaraviciute G, Kauser M, Bhattacharya S, et al. A systematic review and meta-analysis of DNA methylation levels and imprinting disorders in children conceived by IVF/ICSI compared with children conceived spontaneously. Hum Reprod Update. 2014;20(6):840–52. https://doi.org/10.1093/humupd/dmu033 [published Online First: 2014/06/26].

18. Marques CJ, Carvalho F, Sousa M, et al. Genomic imprinting in disruptive spermatogenesis. Lancet. 2004;363(9422):1700–2. https://doi.org/10.1016/S0140-6736(04)16256-9 [published Online First: 2004/05/26].

19. Marques CJ, Costa P, Vaz B, et al. Abnormal methylation of imprinted genes in human sperm is associated with oligozoospermia. Mol Hum Reprod. 2008;14(2):67–74. https://doi.org/10.1093/molehr/gam093 [published Online First: 2008/01/08].

20. Poplinski A, Tuttelmann F, Kanber D, et al. Idiopathic male infertility is strongly associated with aberrant methylation of MEST and IGF2/H19 ICR1. Int J Androl. 2010;33(4):642–9. https://doi.org/10.1111/j.1365-2605.2009.01000.x [published Online First: 2009/11/03].

21. Laurentino S, Beygo J, Nordhoff V, et al. Epigenetic germline mosaicism in infertile men. Hum Mol Genet. 2015;24(5):1295–304. https://doi.org/10.1093/hmg/ddu540 [published Online First: 2014/10/23].

22. Dong H, Wang Y, Zou Z, et al. Abnormal Methylation of Imprinted Genes and Cigarette Smoking: Assessment of Their Association With the Risk of Male Infertility. Reprod Sci. 2016. https://doi.org/10.1177/1933719116650755 [published Online First: 2016/06/02].

23. Xu J, Zhang A, Zhang Z, et al. DNA methylation levels of imprinted and nonimprinted genes DMRs associated with defective human spermatozoa. Andrologia. 2016;48(9):939–47. https://doi.org/10.1111/and.12535 [published Online First: 2016/01/26].

24. Montjean D, Zini A, Ravel C, et al. Sperm global DNA methylation level: association with semen parameters and genome integrity. Andrology. 2015; 3(2):235–40. https://doi.org/10.1111/andr.12001 [published Online First: 2015/03/11].

25. Li XP, Hao CL, Wang Q, et al. H19 gene methylation status is associated with male infertility. Exp Ther Med. 2016;12(1):451–6. https://doi.org/10.3892/etm.2016.3314 [published Online First: 2016/06/28].

26. Santi D, De Vincentis S, Magnani E, et al. Impairment of sperm DNA methylation in male infertility: a meta-analytic study. Andrology. 2017;5(4):695–703. https://doi.org/10.1111/andr.12379 [published Online First: 2017/07/19].

27. Wu W, Shen O, Qin Y, et al. Idiopathic male infertility is strongly associated with aberrant promoter methylation of methylenetetrahydrofolate reductase (MTHFR). PLoS One. 2010;5(11):e13884. https://doi.org/10.1371/journal.pone.0013884 [published Online First: 2010/11/19].

28. Tang Q, Chen Y, Wu W, et al. Idiopathic male infertility and polymorphisms in the DNA methyltransferase genes involved in epigenetic marking. Sci Rep. 2017;7(1):11219. https://doi.org/10.1038/s41598-017-11636-9 [published Online First: 2017/09/13].

29. Carrell DT, Aston KI. The search for SNPs, CNVs, and epigenetic variants associated with the complex disease of male infertility. Syst Biol Reprod Med. 2011;57(1–2):17–26. https://doi.org/10.3109/19396368.2010.521615 [published Online First: 2011/01/07].

30. El Hajj N, Zechner U, Schneider E, et al. Methylation status of imprinted genes and repetitive elements in sperm DNA from infertile males. Sex Dev. 2011;5(2):60–9. https://doi.org/10.1159/000323806 [published Online First: 2011/02/05].

31. Soubry A, Hoyo C, Butt CM, et al. Human exposure to flame-retardants is associated with aberrant DNA methylation at imprinted genes in sperm. Environ Epigenet. 2017;3(1):dvx003. https://doi.org/10.1093/eep/dvx003 [published Online First: 2018/03/02].

32. Esteller M. Cancer epigenomics: DNA methylomes and histone-modification maps. Nat Rev Genet. 2007;8(4):286–98. https://doi.org/10.1038/nrg2005 [published Online First: 2007/03/07].

33. Jones PA, Baylin SB. The epigenomics of cancer. Cell. 2007;128(4): 683–92. https://doi.org/10.1016/j.cell.2007.01.029 [published Online First: 2007/02/27].

34. Chen RZ, Pettersson U, Beard C, et al. DNA hypomethylation leads to elevated mutation rates. Nature. 1998;395(6697):89–93. https://doi.org/10.1038/25779 [published Online First: 1998/09/17].

35. Eden A, Gaudet F, Waghmare A, et al. Chromosomal instability and tumors promoted by DNA hypomethylation. Science. 2003;300(5618):455. https://doi.org/10.1126/science.1083557 [published Online First: 2003/04/19].

36. Gaudet F, Hodgson JG, Eden A, et al. Induction of tumors in mice by genomic hypomethylation. Science. 2003;300(5618):489–92. https://doi.org/10.1126/science.1083558 [published Online First: 2003/04/19].

37. Laird PW. Cancer epigenetics. Hum Mol Genet. 2005;1:R65–76. https://doi.org/10.1093/hmg/ddi113 [published Online First: 2005/04/06].

38. Schieve LA, Meikle SF, Ferre C, et al. Low and very low birth weight in infants conceived with use of assisted reproductive technology. N Engl J Med. 2002;346(10):731–7. https://doi.org/10.1056/NEJMoa010806 [published Online First: 2002/03/08].

39. Hansen M, Kurinczuk JJ, Bower C, et al. The risk of major birth defects after intracytoplasmic sperm injection and in vitro fertilization. N Engl J Med. 2002;346(10):725–30. https://doi.org/10.1056/NEJMoa010035346/10/725 [published Online First: 2002/03/08].

40. Katalinic A, Rosch C, Ludwig M. Pregnancy course and outcome after intracytoplasmic sperm injection: a controlled, prospective cohort study. Fertil Steril 2004;81(6):1604–1616. doi: https://doi.org/10.1016/j.fertnstert.2003.10.053 S0015028204004996 [pii] [published Online First: 2004/06/15].

41. Gosden R, Trasler J, Lucifero D, et al. Rare congenital disorders, imprinted genes, and assisted reproductive technology. Lancet. 2003;361(9373):1975–7. https://doi.org/10.1016/S0140-6736(03)13592-1 [published Online First: 2003/06/13].

42. Cortessis VK, Azadian M, Buxbaum J, et al. Comprehensive meta-analysis reveals association between multiple imprinting disorders and conception by assisted reproductive technology. J Assist Reprod Genet. 2018. https://doi.org/10.1007/s10815-018-1173-x [published Online First: 2018/04/27].

43. Kobayashi H, Sato A, Otsu E, et al. Aberrant DNA methylation of imprinted loci in sperm from oligospermic patients. Hum Mol Genet. 2007;16(21). 2542–51. https://doi.org/10.1093/hmg/ddm187 [published Online First: 2007/07/20].

44. Okano M, Bell DW, Haber DA, et al. DNA methyltransferases Dnmt3a and Dnmt3b are essential for de novo methylation and mammalian development. Cell. 1999;99(3):247–57 [published Online First: 1999/11/11].

45. Kaneda M, Okano M, Hata K, et al. Essential role for de novo DNA methyltransferase Dnmt3a in paternal and maternal imprinting. Nature. 2004;429(6994):900–3. https://doi.org/10.1038/nature02633 [published Online First: 2004/06/25].

46. Arima T, Hata K, Tanaka S, et al. Loss of the maternal imprint in Dnmt3Lmat −/− mice leads to a differentiation defect in the extraembryonic tissue. Dev Biol. 2006;297(2):361–73. https://doi.org/10.1016/j.ydbio.2006.05.003 [published Online First: 2006/08/22].

22

The DNMT1-associated lincRNA DACOR1 reprograms genome-wide DNA methylation in colon cancer

Saigopal Somasundaram[1], Megan E Forrest[1], Helen Moinova[1], Allison Cohen[1], Vinay Varadan[2], Thomas LaFramboise[1,2], Sanford Markowitz[1,2] and Ahmad M Khalil[1,2]*

Abstract

Background: DNA methylation is a key epigenetic mark in mammalian organisms that plays key roles in chromatin organization and gene expression. Although DNA methylation in gene promoters is generally associated with gene repression, recent studies demonstrate that DNA methylation in gene bodies and intergenic regions of the genome may result in distinct modes of gene regulation. Furthermore, the molecular mechanisms underlying the establishment and maintenance of DNA methylation in human health and disease remain to be fully elucidated. We recently demonstrated that a subset of long non-coding RNAs (lncRNAs) associates with the major DNA methyltransferase DNMT1 in human colon cancer cells, and the dysregulation of such lncRNAs contribute to aberrant DNA methylation patterns.

Results: In the current study, we assessed the impact of a key DNMT1-associated lncRNA, DACOR1, on genome-wide DNA methylation using reduced representation bisulfite sequencing (RRBS). Our findings demonstrated that induction of DACOR1 in colon cancer cells restores DNA methylation at thousands of CpG sites throughout the genome including promoters, gene bodies, and intergenic regions. Importantly, these sites overlap with regions of the genome that become hypomethylated in colon tumors. Furthermore, induction of DACOR1 results in repression of *FOS* and *JUN* and, consequently, reduced AP-1 transcription factor activity.

Conclusion: Collectively, our results demonstrate a key role of lncRNAs in regulating DNA methylation in human cells, and the dysregulation of such lncRNAs could emerge as a key mechanism by which DNA methylation patterns become altered in human tumors.

Keywords: Colon cancer, Epigenetics, lincRNAs, Tumorigenesis

Background

The epigenetic code is comprised of specific patterns of histone and DNA modifications [1–3], which cooperate to control gene expression without changing the underlying DNA sequence, typically through recruitment of various protein complexes to alter chromatin accessibility [4]. These epigenetic modifications are dynamic and critical for tissue-specific gene expression during development and cellular differentiation. Furthermore, many studies have now documented changes in the epigenetics landscape in human diseases, resulting in altered gene expression and, consequently, phenotype [4, 5]. In particular, there is global dysregulation of the epigenetic landscape in cancer cells, as compared to matched normal cells [4, 6–9]. These massive epigenetic alterations are thought to be critical events in the initiation and progression of tumorigenesis, and act in cooperation with somatic gene mutations to mediate tumor progression. Despite these extensive epigenetic changes in many tumor types, the underlying molecular mechanisms driving epigenetic changes are still emerging, as they are not always simply driven by mutations in key epigenetic modifiers [4–6, 9, 10].

One of the first epigenetic changes that were reported in cancer is DNA hypomethylation, which was first observed

* Correspondence: dr.ahmad.khalil@gmail.com
[1]Department of Genetics and Genome Sciences, Case Comprehensive Cancer Center, Case Western Reserve University School of Medicine, Cleveland, OH 44106, USA
[2]Case Comprehensive Cancer Center, Case Western Reserve University School of Medicine, Cleveland, OH 44106, USA

during colon tumorigenesis [11]. DNA methylation of cytosine residues within cytosine-phosphate-guanine site (CpG) dinucleotides to yield 5-methylcytosine is widespread throughout the mammalian genome and is catalyzed by DNA methyltransferases in response to various signals [12, 13]. DNA methyltransferase 1 (DNMT1) is the primary DNA methyltransferase responsible for maintaining DNA methylation patterns on newly synthesized DNA during cell division. Also, DNMT1, along with DNMT3a and DNMT3b, catalyzes de novo DNA methylation throughout development and cellular differentiation [12]. Aberrant DNA hypomethylation is an early epigenetic alteration in colon tumorigenesis that plays a key role in the transition from normal colon epithelium to hyperplastic epithelium by largely unknown mechanisms. During the course of tumorigenesis, DNA also becomes hypermethylated at specific gene promoters, often tumor suppressors, leading in some cases to gene repression. The mechanisms by which genome-wide changes in DNA methylation occur in colon cancer and other cancer types remain poorly understood.

In a recent publication from our laboratory, we demonstrated that many long non-coding RNAs are associated with DNMT1, suggesting that long non-coding RNAs (lncRNAs) have important functions in regulating genome-wide DNA methylation [14]. We further demonstrated that one such lncRNA, DNMT1-associated colon cancer repressed lncRNA 1 (DACOR1), is a positive regulator of DNA methylation in cell culture models of the disease. DACOR1 becomes repressed in colon tumors, and its re-expression in colon cancer cell lines resulted in re-methylation of specific CpG sites in gene promoters as assessed by the Illumina Infinium Human Methylation 450k beadchip microarray platform. However, these arrays have several limitations, including bias toward CpG methylation in promoter regions and potential false signals due to probe cross-reactivity and polymorphic CpGs. To identify the full impact of DACOR1 on DNA methylation on a genome-wide scale, we utilized reduced representation bisulfite sequencing (RRBS) [15], which led to the identification of thousands of CpG sites that are affected by DACOR1 induction. To determine if the CpG sites regulated by DACOR1 are relevant to colon cancer, we compared these sites to differentially methylated regions (DMRs) in two independent cohorts of colon tumors vs. normal colon tissues, and identified substantial overlap. Integration of these data sets with gene expression data sets, and functional studies of DACOR1 indicate a potential role of the ATF3 pathway in colon cancer (Additional file 1 and Additional file 2). Thus, these findings contribute to our understanding of how changes in DNA methylation in colon cancer affect gene expression, which is critical toward revealing the role of epigenetic changes in tumorigenesis and cancer progression [4, 9].

Results

Massive changes in genome-wide DNA methylation in colon tumors

To identify specific regions of the genome that undergo changes in DNA methylation in colon tumors versus normal colon tissue, we performed DNA methylation analysis on 40 normal colon and 83 colorectal tumor samples using reduced representation bisulfite sequencing (RBBS) assay. Over six million CpG sites per sample were analyzed for differential DNA methylation, including CpG sites in promoters, gene bodies, and intergenic regions (Fig. 1a, b, Additional file 3: Dataset 1). Using a stringent cutoff of greater than 30% change in average methylation in tumors vs. normal samples, we identified 204,313 differentially methylated CpG sites (Fig. 1c, Additional file 3: Dataset 1). Of these 204,313 CpG sites, 70,404 (34.5%) showed increased methylation (hypermethylation), whereas 133,909 (65.5%) showed decreased methylation (hypomethylation) in tumors. To determine where in the genome these changes in DNA methylation occur, we aligned the differentially methylated CpG sites to hg19 RefSeq gene track from the UCSC genome browser to categorize CpG sites in promoter regions, gene bodies, and intergenic regions of the genome. Promoter regions were defined as areas in the genome starting 2 kb upstream of the transcriptional start site (TSS), gene bodies were defined as the genomic areas between the transcriptional start and end sites, and intergenic regions were all those regions that were not in the promoter or gene bodies. Using these criteria, we found extensive changes in DNA methylation not only in gene promoters but also in gene bodies and intergenic regions of the genome, often observing both increases and decreases in methylation within a single gene region. (Figure 1c, Additional file 3: Dataset 1).

Changes in CpG methylation in colon tumors versus normal colon (Fig. 1c, Additional file 4: Dataset 7) are observed on all chromosomes (Fig. 2a, Additional file 3: Dataset 1). We also determined the number of CpG sites that are affected in gene promoters and gene bodies in our cohort, and identified genes that show increased and/or decreased methylation in gene promoters and gene bodies (Fig. 2b, Additional file 3: Dataset 1). Remarkably, we found some genes that show substantial changes in DNA methylation at over 100 CpG sites in tumors vs. normal samples (Fig. 2b). Collectively, these data demonstrate extensive changes in DNA methylation in colon tumors in gene promoters, gene bodies, and intergenic regions of the genome. To further confirm these observations in an independent cohort, we performed similar analysis using public datasets from The Cancer Genome Atlas (TCGA), see below.

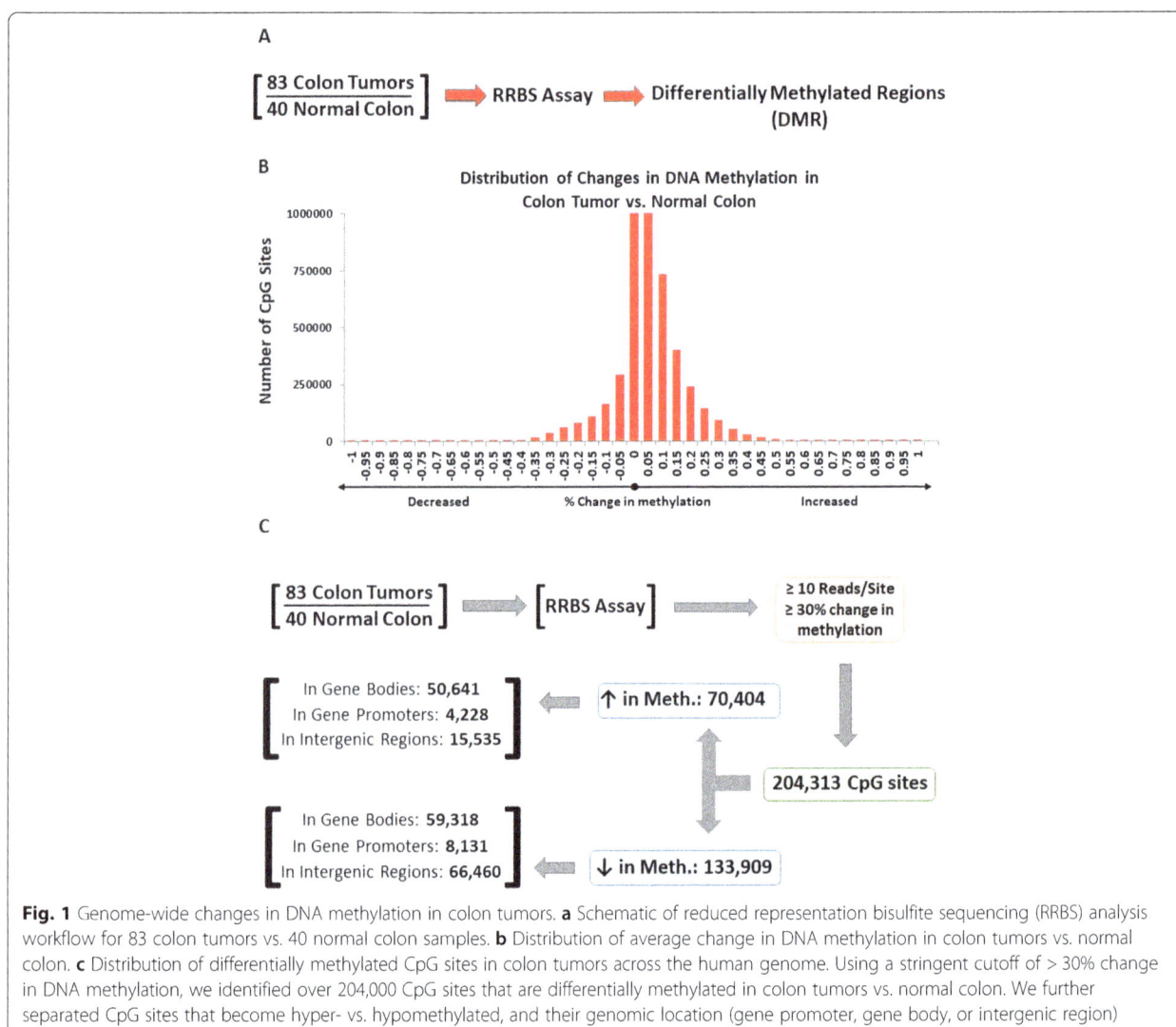

Fig. 1 Genome-wide changes in DNA methylation in colon tumors. **a** Schematic of reduced representation bisulfite sequencing (RRBS) analysis workflow for 83 colon tumors vs. 40 normal colon samples. **b** Distribution of average change in DNA methylation in colon tumors vs. normal colon. **c** Distribution of differentially methylated CpG sites in colon tumors across the human genome. Using a stringent cutoff of > 30% change in DNA methylation, we identified over 204,000 CpG sites that are differentially methylated in colon tumors vs. normal colon. We further separated CpG sites that become hyper- vs. hypomethylated, and their genomic location (gene promoter, gene body, or intergenic region)

DNA methylation is not a strong predictor of gene expression

To further test our observations in colon tumors vs. normal colon tissues, we downloaded DNA methylation data from TCGA from seven colon tumors that also had matched normal tissues. We restricted our analysis to tumor samples with matched normal tissues to account for differences that may result from human heterogeneity. TCGA DNA methylation studies were performed using HM450 arrays, which results in much less coverage than RRBS analysis. Nonetheless, these analyses supported our observations of both hypermethylation and hypomethylation occurring not only in promoters but also in gene bodies and intergenic regions (Fig. 3a–c, Additional file 5: Dataset 2). Also, we observed that the vast majority of changes in DNA methylation between tumors vs. normal samples show a difference of less than 50%, possibly due to tumor heterogeneity and/or aneuploidy (Fig. 3b, also see Fig. 1b). Furthermore, we did

not observe a chromosomal bias of differentially methylated CpGs (Fig. 4a, Additional file 5: Dataset 2). Lastly, we identified genes with changes in either promoters or gene bodies that show hyper- and/or hypomethylation (Fig. 4b, Additional file 5: Dataset 2, Additional file 6: Dataset 8) to assess how these changes affect gene expression, see below.

Next, we wanted to determine the relationship between DNA methylation at specific genomic regions (promoters, gene bodies) and gene expression. To that end, we analyzed the expression of mRNAs in 22 colon tumors vs. 22 matched normal tissues (TCGA RNA-seq). We identified 2442 mRNAs that are differentially expressed ($p < 0.05$, $\geq$ 2-fold change) (Fig. 5a, Additional file 5: Dataset 2, Additional file 7: Dataset 5). We intersected genes with changes in DNA methylation in either promoter regions or gene bodies with their expression in tumors vs. normal colon and did not observe a strong correlation between DNA methylation and gene

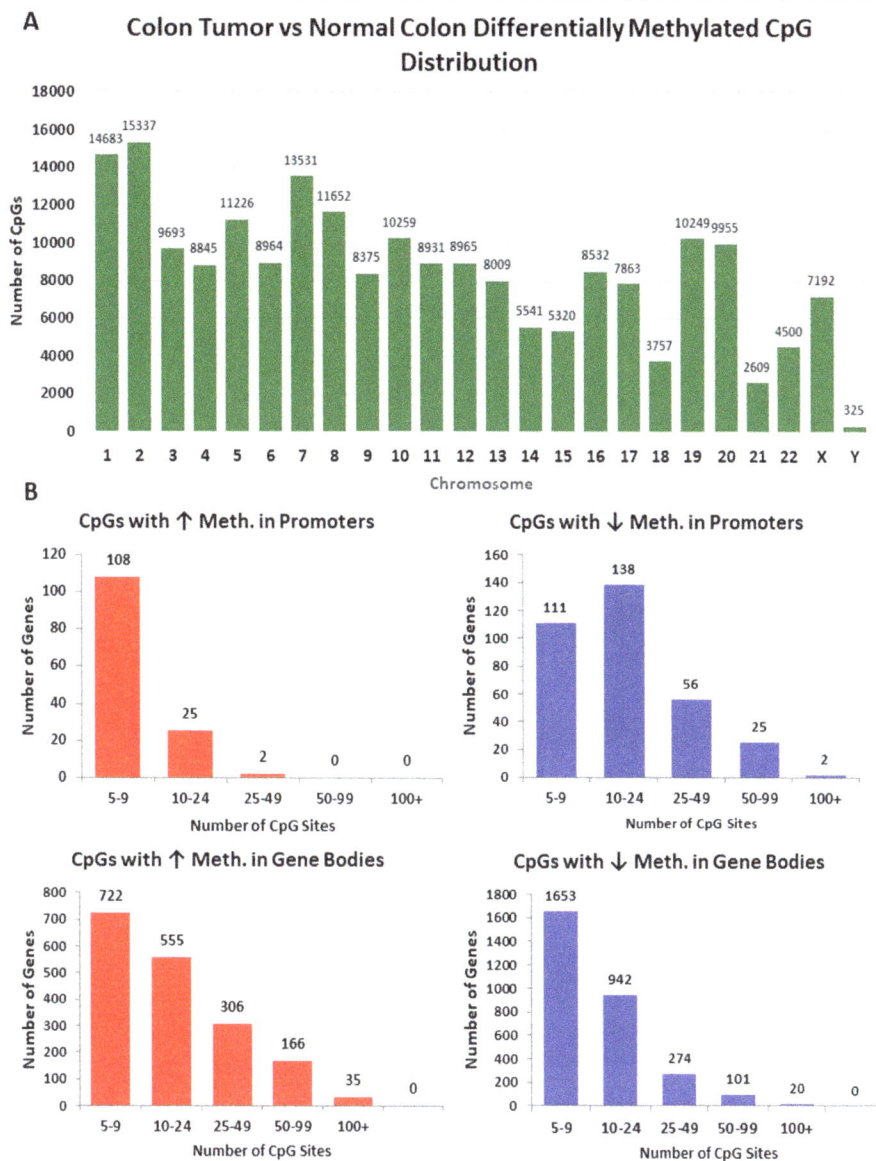

Fig. 2 Changes in DNA methylation in colon tumors occur on all human chromosomes. **a** Number of differentially methylated CpG sites per human chromosome as assayed by RRBS assay. **b** Number of genes with either increased or decreased DNA methylation in promoters or gene bodies with number of CpG sites affected listed on the x-axis

expression. For example, only ~ 52% of genes with increased DNA methylation in promoter regions showed decreased expression in tumors (Fig. 5b, Additional file 5: Dataset 2). These data demonstrate that DNA methylation is not sufficient to predict gene expression and that DNA methylation likely acts in conjunction with other changes in the epigenetic landscape to influence gene expression [9].

Induction of DACOR1 results in genome-wide changes in DNA methylation

We previously demonstrated that the expression of the DNMT1-associated lncRNA, DACOR1, results in increased CpG methylation as assessed by Illumina Infinium Human

Methylation 450k beadchip microarray platform. These findings suggest a novel mechanism of RNA-directed DNA methylation in human cells and could potentially shed light on global hypomethylation observed in colon tumors. To further explore this mechanism, we first assessed the role of DACOR1 in regulating genome-wide DNA methylation by performing reduced representation bisulfite sequencing (RRBS) assay in a patient-derived colon tumor cell line (V852), which has low endogenous expression of DACOR1. We had previously produced V852 cells with stable re-expression of DACOR1 using a lentivirus containing the full cDNA sequence of DACOR1. By assessing genome-wide DNA methylation in this line, as compared to V852 cells

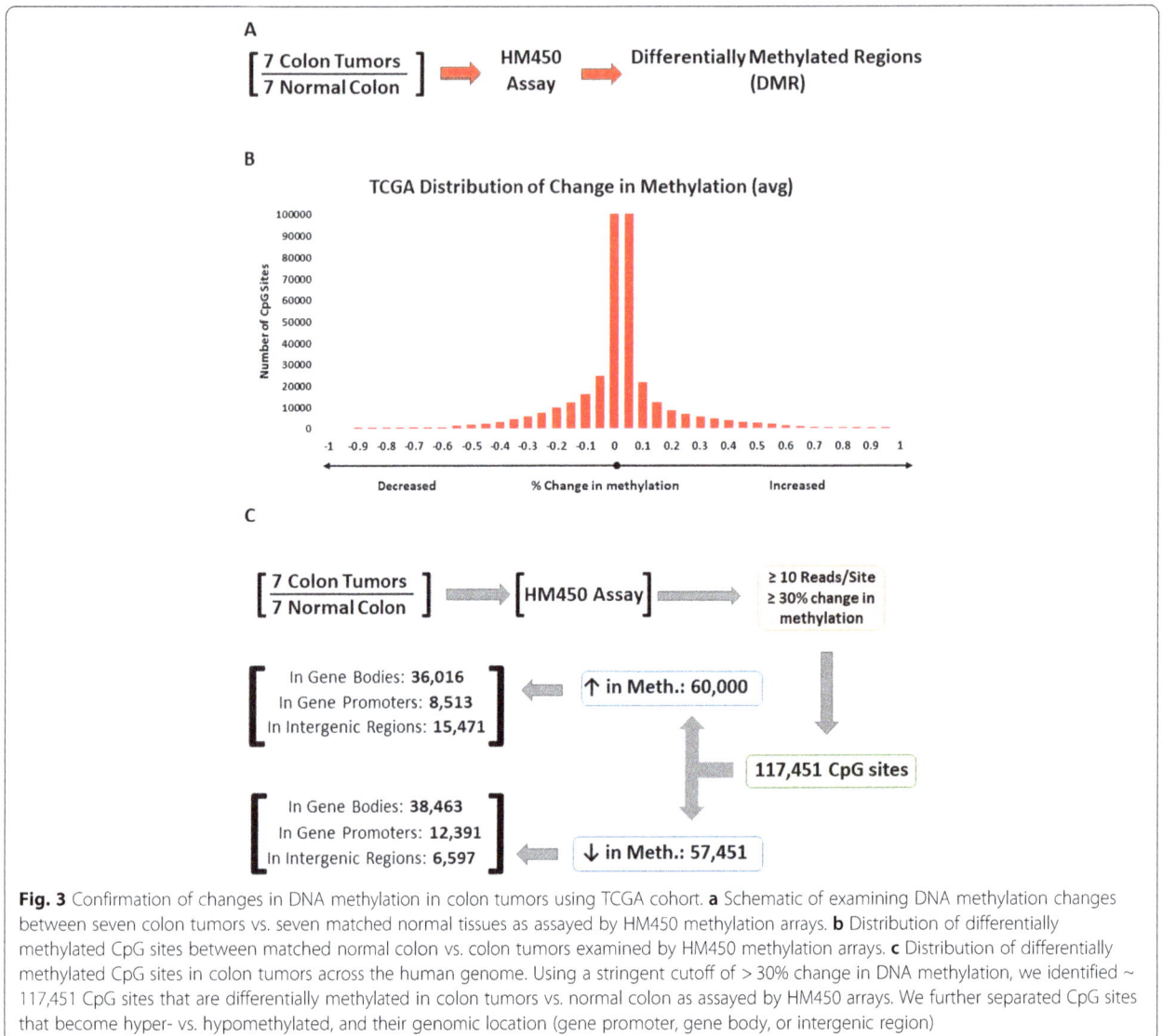

Fig. 3 Confirmation of changes in DNA methylation in colon tumors using TCGA cohort. **a** Schematic of examining DNA methylation changes between seven colon tumors vs. seven matched normal tissues as assayed by HM450 methylation arrays. **b** Distribution of differentially methylated CpG sites between matched normal colon vs. colon tumors examined by HM450 methylation arrays. **c** Distribution of differentially methylated CpG sites in colon tumors across the human genome. Using a stringent cutoff of > 30% change in DNA methylation, we identified ~ 117,451 CpG sites that are differentially methylated in colon tumors vs. normal colon as assayed by HM450 arrays. We further separated CpG sites that become hyper- vs. hypomethylated, and their genomic location (gene promoter, gene body, or intergenic region)

transduced with a control lentivirus, we identified CpG sites that become differentially methylated in response to DACOR1 re-expression (Fig. 6a, b, Additional file 8: Dataset 3). Strikingly, there was a strong bias toward increased DNA methylation upon DACOR1 induction as shown in Fig. 6b. Using a stringent cutoff of > 30% change in methylation between V852 control vs. DACOR1-expressing cells, we identified over 17,300 differentially methylated CpG sites. These differentially methylated CpG sites almost exclusively show an increase in DNA methylation; specifically, 17,280 (99.9%) of these CpG sites showed an increase in methylation in response to DACOR1 induction, while only 28 (0.01%) sites showed a decrease in methylation (Figs. 6c and 7a, Additional file 8: Dataset 3, Additional file 9: Dataset 6). These findings are in agreement with our previous findings that DACOR1 is a positive regulator DNA methylation in human cells.

To determine the genomic regions of DACOR1-mediated changes in DNA methylation, all affected CpG sites were mapped to individual human chromosomes; importantly, we did not observe any bias, with the exception of the Y chromosome showing only three affected CpG sites (Fig. 7b, Additional file 8: Dataset 3). We then aligned our list of differentially methylated CpG sites to the UCSC hg19 RefSeq gene track and identified specific genes that show increased DNA methylation in either gene promoters or gene bodies (Fig. 7c, Additional file 8: Dataset 3). By contrast, of the 28 CpG sites that showed a decrease in methylation in response to DACOR1 induction, two were mapped to promoter regions of two genes, while the remaining 26 CpG sites were within intergenic regions of the genome. Collectively, these findings demonstrate a key role for DACOR1 in positively mediating DNA methylation patterns genome-wide.

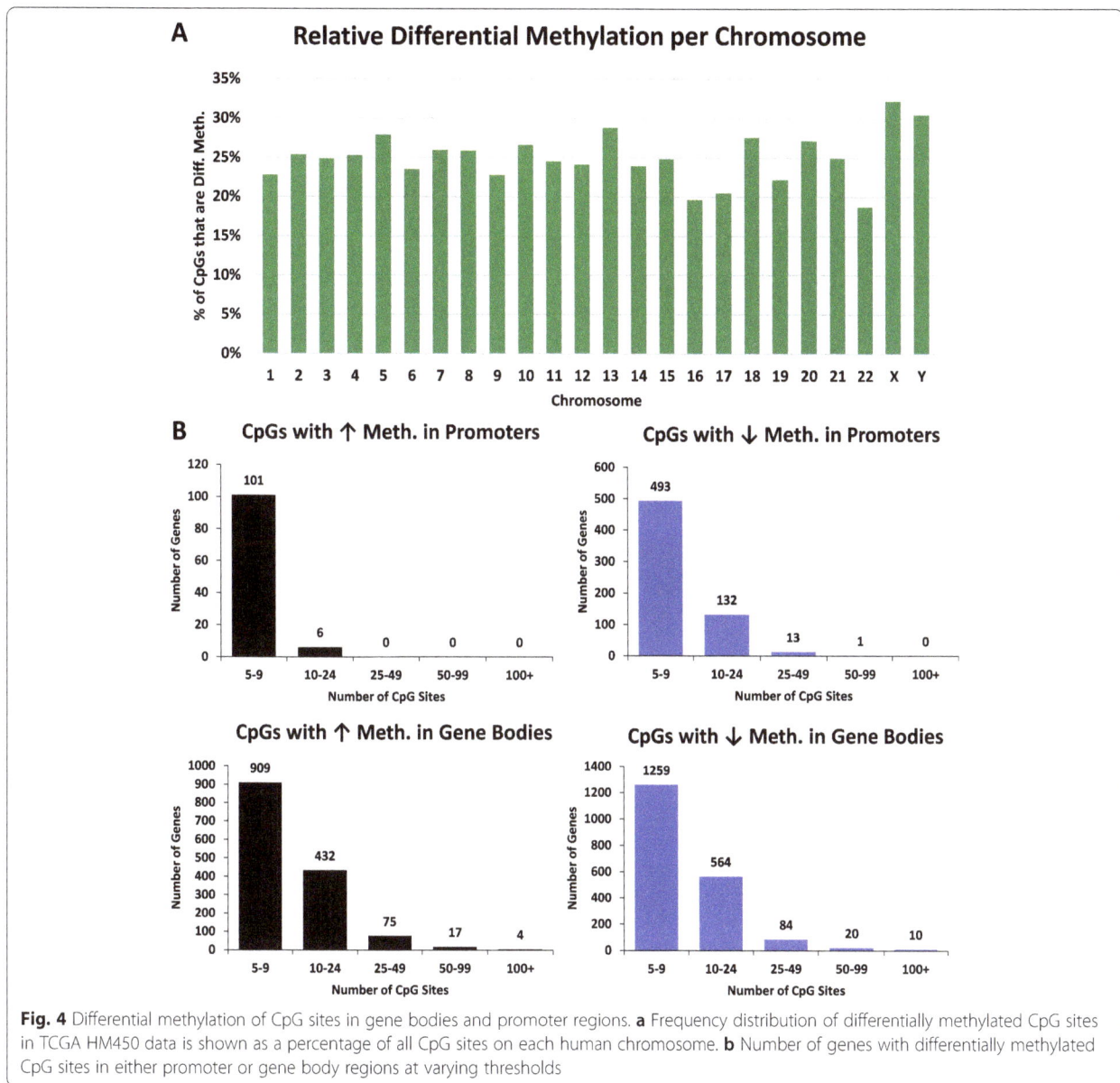

Fig. 4 Differential methylation of CpG sites in gene bodies and promoter regions. **a** Frequency distribution of differentially methylated CpG sites in TCGA HM450 data is shown as a percentage of all CpG sites on each human chromosome. **b** Number of genes with differentially methylated CpG sites in either promoter or gene body regions at varying thresholds

DACOR1 regulates clusters of CpG sites in gene promoters

We identified 86 genes that gain DNA methylation in promoter regions upon DACOR1 induction in V852 cells (Fig. 7c, Additional file 8: Dataset 3). Six genes with eight or more CpG sites that gained DNA methylation upon DACOR1 induction in promoters were assessed for the distribution of these CpG sites relative to all CpG sites within promoter regions (Fig. 8a, Additional file 8: Dataset 3). Notably, for all six genes examined, the differentially methylated CpG sites clustered together in regions smaller than 200 base pairs. To test if DACOR1 regulates clusters of CpG sites within CpG islands, we mapped the position and density of affected CpG sites as well as all

CpG sites for all six genes (Fig. 8b, Additional file 8: Dataset 3). Qualitatively, we observed that differentially methylated CpG sites are clustered together and are not dependent on the density or location of indexed CpG sites, suggesting that DACOR1 may target specific CpG clusters within gene promoters. To quantitatively assess if the clustering is not random, a MATLAB simulation (see "Methods" section) was performed to assess whether clustering, as measured by the number of adjacent differentially methylated CpG sites, was more than expected by chance. It was observed that for all 6 genes, such clustering in 100,000 simulations never surpassed what we observed in our RRBS data (p value 1×10^{-5}).

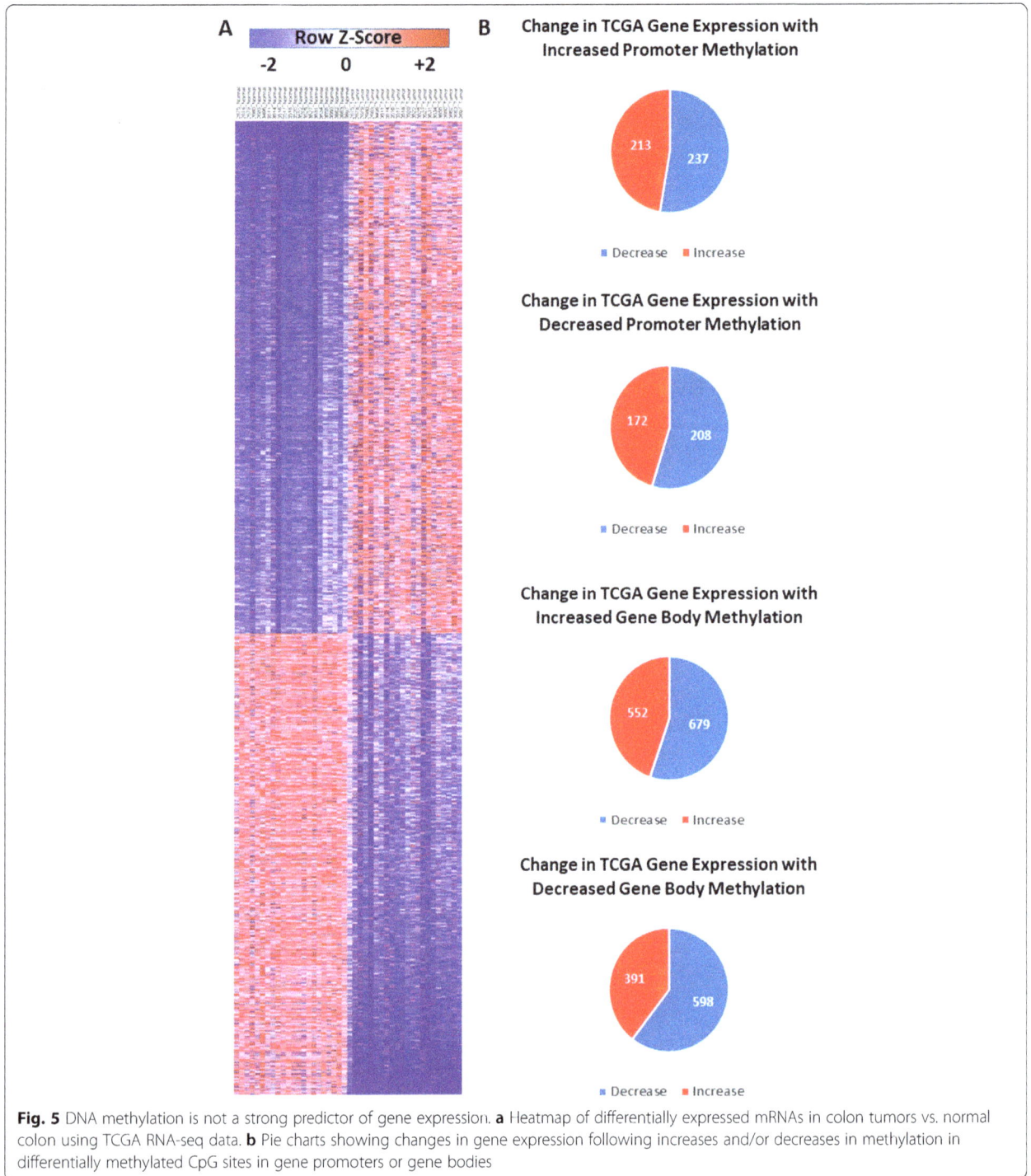

Fig. 5 DNA methylation is not a strong predictor of gene expression. **a** Heatmap of differentially expressed mRNAs in colon tumors vs. normal colon using TCGA RNA-seq data. **b** Pie charts showing changes in gene expression following increases and/or decreases in methylation in differentially methylated CpG sites in gene promoters or gene bodies

DACOR1-mediated DNA methylation in gene bodies is primarily in intronic regions

Given the numerous CpG sites that become hypermethylated in response to DACOR1 expression within gene bodies, we wanted to determine if these CpG sites are predominantly exonic, intronic, or equally distributed. The top ten genes with the highest differential methylation rate in gene bodies were identified (Additional file 1: Figure S1A-B, Additional file 10: Dataset 4), and CpG sites in gene bodies of these top ten genes with most CpG sites were sorted into either intronic or exonic regions. We found that 93.23% of DACOR1-regulated CpG sites in gene bodies are within intronic regions of protein-coding genes (Fig. 9, Additional file 10: Dataset 4).

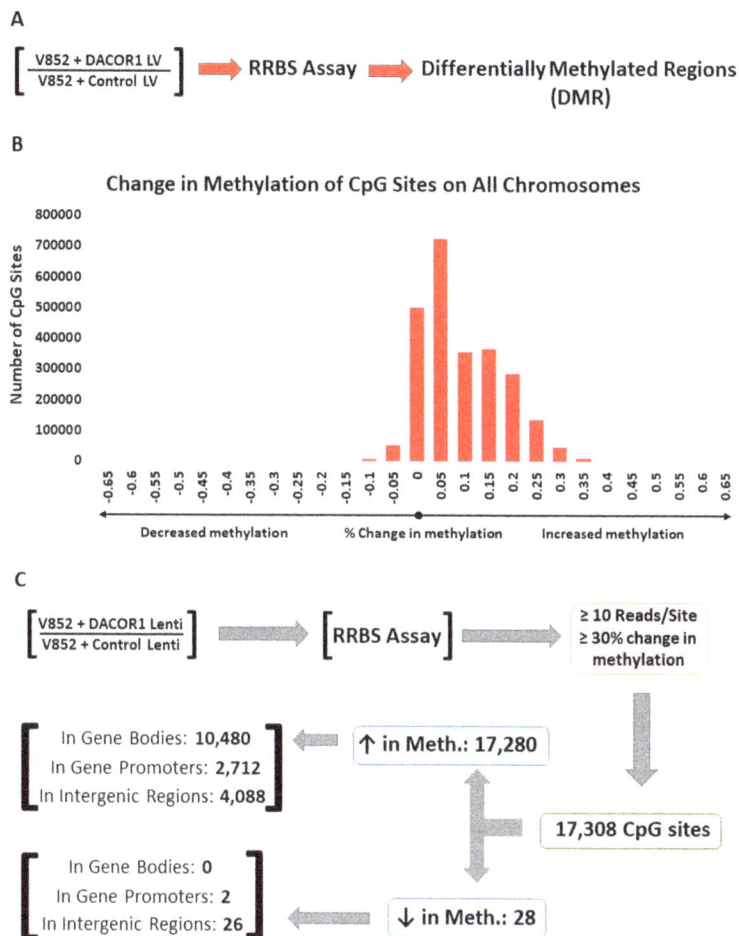

Fig. 6 Re-expression of DACOR1 in V852 colon cancer cells results in genome-wide changes in DNA methylation. **a** The patient-derived colon cancer cell line V852 was transduced with either an empty vector lentivirus or a lentivirus containing the full-length DACOR1, and DNA methylation was examined by RRBS assay under both conditions (*n* = 3 of each condition). **b** Distribution of changes in DNA methylation in V852 cells in response to DACOR1 induction. **c** Over 17,000 CpG sites are affected by DACOR1 induction with the vast majority of sites (99.9%) showing gain of methylation

DACOR1 regulates ATF pathway signaling in colon cancer

Given the extensive genome-wide changes in DNA methylation and the phenotypic effects of DACOR1 re-expression in colon cancer cells, we reasoned that DACOR1 expression is likely impacting key colon cancer-related pathways. First, we utilized The Broad Institute's gene set enrichment analysis (GSEA) tool to identify critical pathways that are deregulated in colon cancer based on differentially expressed genes in colon tumors vs. normal colon identified in our analysis of RNA sequencing (RNA-seq) from TCGA (see Fig. 5a, Additional file 7: Dataset 5). Using this approach, several key pathways emerged including well-established colon cancer-related pathways, such as the Wnt/β-catenin pathway and p53-related signaling (Additional file 2: Figure S2). This indicated that our analysis successfully identified relevant pathways to colon tumorigenesis. We also identified enrichment of genes in the activated transcription factor 2 (ATF2) signaling pathway ($p < 0.01$, FDR = 0.057). This pathway further stood out as DACOR1 regulates key genes in this pathway both at the expression level (RNA-seq studies) as well as promoter and gene body methylation. Although the ATF signaling pathway is an important pathway in colon cancer, it remains relatively understudied.

The ATF family is a group of basic leucine zipper (bZIP) transcription factors, including ATF1, ATF2, ATF3, and other cyclic AMP response element-binding (CREB) family members, which are closely related to activating protein-1 (AP-1) complexes. Canonical AP-1 complexes are typically composed of Jun-Jun homodimers or Jun-Fos heterodimers; ATF proteins, particularly ATF3, can also bind to c-Jun to form alternative AP-1 complexes. The AP-1 transcriptional regulation program is known to play a role in multiple cellular processes in

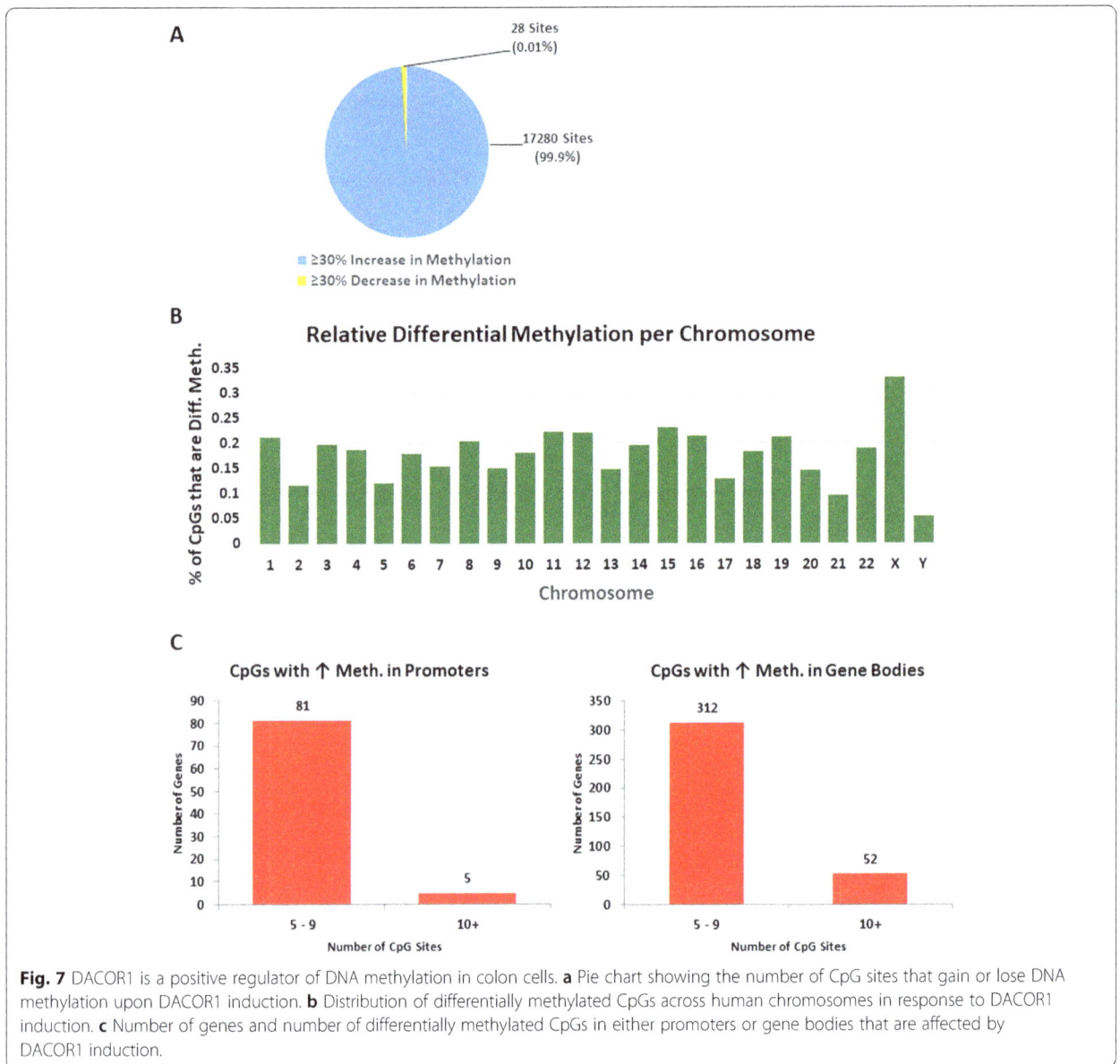

Fig. 7 DACOR1 is a positive regulator of DNA methylation in colon cells. **a** Pie chart showing the number of CpG sites that gain or lose DNA methylation upon DACOR1 induction. **b** Distribution of differentially methylated CpGs across human chromosomes in response to DACOR1 induction. **c** Number of genes and number of differentially methylated CpGs in either promoters or gene bodies that are affected by DACOR1 induction.

the context of cancer, including cell proliferation, differentiation, and regulation of both pro- and anti-apoptotic proteins. These complexes can either activate or repress transcription depending on the composition of the complex (e.g., Jun-Jun, Jun-Fos, Jun-ATF3), the promoter type, and the cell type, and can therefore act as either tumor suppressors or oncogenes in various cancer types.

DACOR1 induction affects DNA methylation of ATF3 in both the promoter and gene body regions; thus, we decided to test the effect of DACOR1 induction on the expression of ATF3 and several key genes involved in ATF3 signaling pathway. First, we examined the effect of DACOR1 expression on ATF3 in two distinct patient-derived colon cancer cell lines, V852 and V866. In both cell lines, the induction of DACOR1 resulted in

decreased expression of ATF3 (Fig. 10a). Next, we examined the effect of DACOR1 expression on FOS and JUN and observed significant decrease of both mRNAs upon DACOR1 induction (Fig. 10b). To test the functional consequences of the observed decrease in *ATF3*, *FOS*, and *JUN* gene expression, we performed an AP-1 luciferase reporter assay using a reporter plasmid containing tandem repeats of the AP-1 transcription factor consensus binding site coupled to firefly luciferase. AP-1 pathway activity was significantly decreased in DACOR1-expressing cells (Fig. 10c), consistent with the observed changes in gene expression. As discussed above, AP-1 transcription factor complexes are involved in the regulation of anti-apoptotic genes in the context of colon cancer. To test whether dysregulation of the AP-1

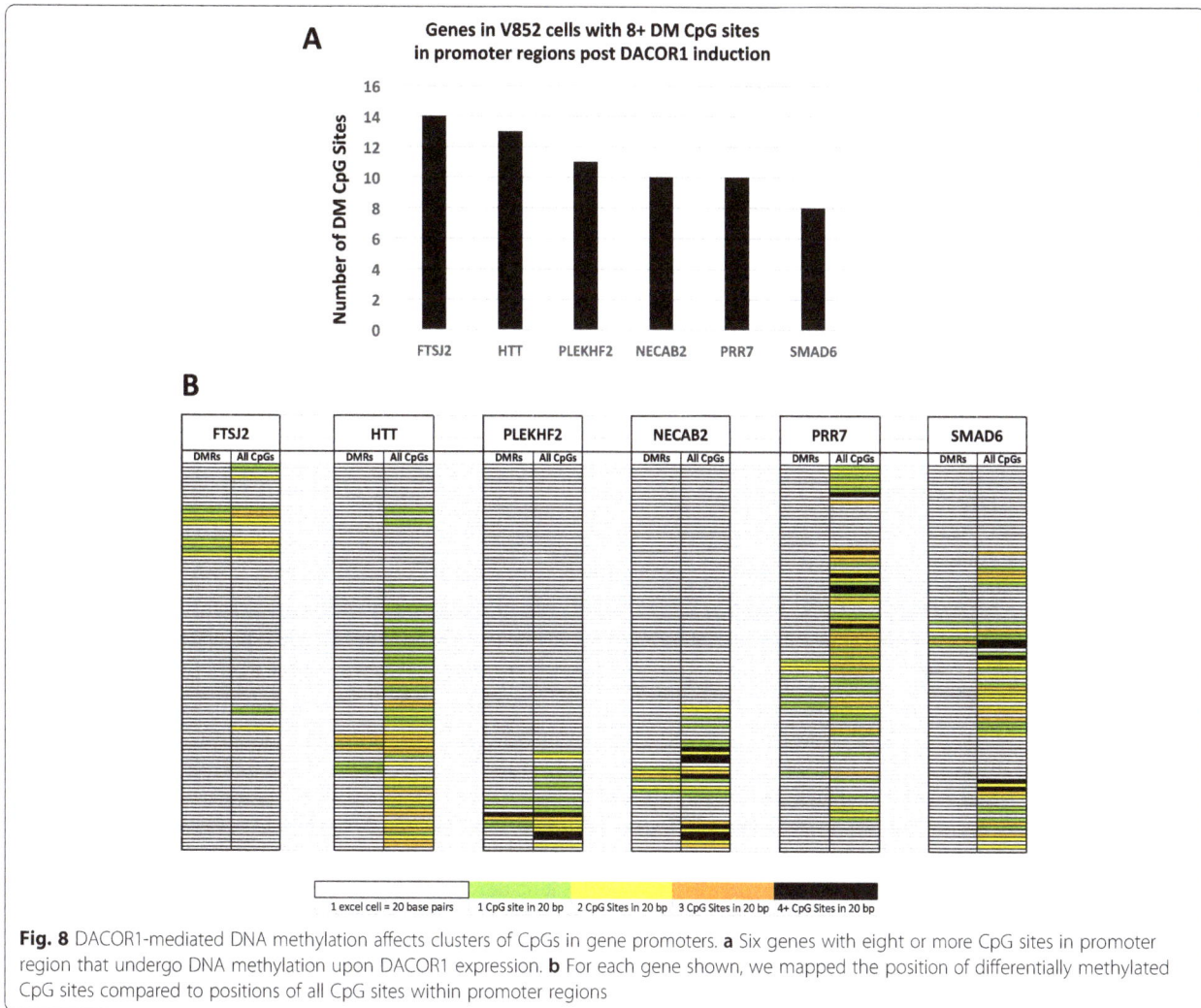

Fig. 8 DACOR1-mediated DNA methylation affects clusters of CpGs in gene promoters. **a** Six genes with eight or more CpG sites in promoter region that undergo DNA methylation upon DACOR1 expression. **b** For each gene shown, we mapped the position of differentially methylated CpG sites compared to positions of all CpG sites within promoter regions

pathway activity in DACOR1-expressing cells results in changes in apoptosis, we performed a caspase 3/7 cleavage assay. We observed a significant increase in apoptosis in DACOR1-expressing cells relative to control cells (Fig. 10d); this effect was also observed upon treatment with doxorubicin (Fig. 10e), a known pro-apoptotic agent in colon cancer. Taken together, these results suggest a possible role for DACOR1 in the regulation of the ATF pathway and downstream AP-1 complex formation. Thus, repression of DACOR1 during colon tumorigenesis may lead to resistance to apoptosis, further promoting cancer progression.

Discussion

In this study, we characterized differential DNA methylation patterns across colon tumors versus normal colon using RRBS technology, which led to the identification of over 204,000 differentially methylated CpGs in various regions of the genome (Additional file 11: Dataset 10). These data demonstrate extensive

genome-wide changes in the epigenome during colon tumorigenesis; however, the underlying mechanisms of these global changes are largely unknown. Our previous and current data provide evidence for a lncRNA-mediated regulation of DNA methylation. Specifically, we provide evidence that a DNMT1-associated lncRNA, DACOR1, regulates DNA methylation at thousands of CpG sites across the genome. Our current model proposes that when DACOR1 becomes repressed during colon tumorigenesis, this loss of expression leads to loss of DNMT1 targeting and/or loading to specific regions of the genome. This model is supported by our experimental data where the re-expression of DACOR1 leads to re-methylation of more than 17,300 CpG sites. These data clearly suggest that DACOR1 is a positive regulator of DNA methylation in human colon cells. It is possible that other DNMT1-associated lncRNAs also regulate DNA methylation either positively or negatively. However, experimental evidence is needed to demonstrate the

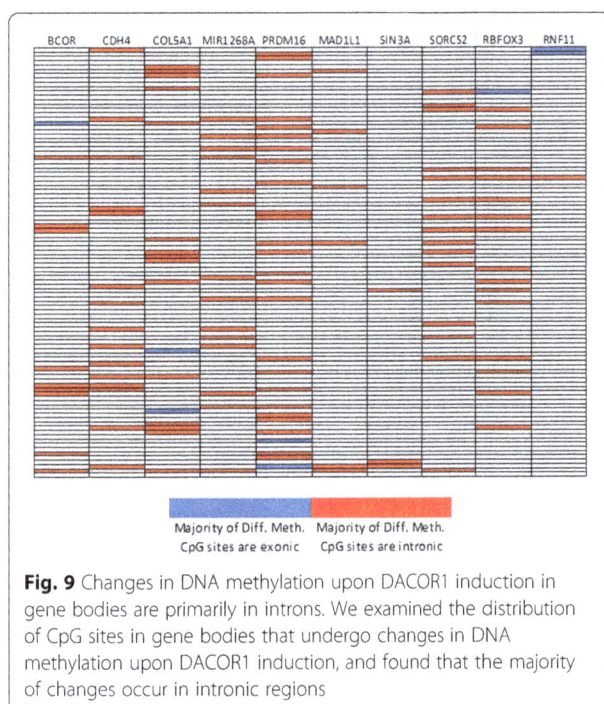

Fig. 9 Changes in DNA methylation upon DACOR1 induction in gene bodies are primarily in introns. We examined the distribution of CpG sites in gene bodies that undergo changes in DNA methylation upon DACOR1 induction, and found that the majority of changes occur in intronic regions

role of other DNMT1-associated lncRNAs in regulation of the epigenome.

The functional consequences of DNA methylation on gene expression are dependent upon the genomic location of DNA methylation (promoter, gene body, or intergenic) and cellular context. DNA methylation at CpG sites within promoters is frequently associated with gene silencing; however, recent studies suggest that there are additional consequences of promoter methylation. For example, DNA methylation in gene promoters has been shown to recruit activating transcription factors and chromatin-modifying complexes, demonstrating that the effects of DNA methylation on gene expression depend on additional epigenetic readers.

We also identified differentially methylated CpG sites that are outside of gene promoters, particularly within gene bodies. While some studies suggest that DNA methylation levels within gene bodies are positively correlated with gene expression, other studies suggest that gene body methylation exists as a mechanism for repression of spurious transcription contributing to transcriptional efficiency and genome stability. Thus, the consequences of aberrant gene body methylation, particularly in the context of cancer, remain to be elucidated. In addition, further studies are needed to determine the interplay between DNA methylation and other epigenetic marks to fully comprehend the functional consequences of changes in DNA methylation, both in normal cellular development and in disease states such as cancer.

A major challenge in the analysis of genome-wide DNA methylation in gene promoters and gene bodies in tumors is that hundreds of genes have both hyper- and hypomethylated CpGs; thus, it is challenging to classify these genes as hypo- or hyper-methylated without an arbitrary cutoff. This leads us to hypothesize that specific CpGs, based on their location in gene promoters or gene bodies, have stronger influence on gene expression than others. With the recent advent of genome editing technologies, it is now possible to perform experiments to test this hypothesis, and begin dissecting the effects of specific CpGs on gene expression.

Conclusion

Although DNA methylation has been studied for several decades in both health and disease, it remains unclear how this epigenetic mark contributes to gene regulation. With the advent of genome editing technologies, we now have the molecular tools to precisely alter specific CpG sites alone or in combinations to determine how they contribute to gene regulation. In summary, we have documented genome-wide changes in DNA methylation patterns in colon cancer and provided evidence that lncRNAs play a role in mediating DNA methylation. These studies should pave the way for a better understanding of how epigenetic alterations occur during tumorigenesis, and their contribution to disease state.

Methods

Cell culture

Patient-derived colon cancer cell lines were maintained in MEM 2+ media (2% FBS, 2 mM glutamine, 1 µg/mL hydrocortisone, 10 µg/mL insulin, 0.86 ng/mL selenium, 2 µg/mL transferrin, 50 µg/mL gentamicin) at standard conditions (37 °C, 5% CO_2) and passaged approximately every 3–5 days by trypsinization.

Reduced representation bisulfite sequencing assay and data analysis

Bisulfite treatment of DNA converts unmethylated cytosine residues into uracil, which enable the identification of methylated vs. unmethylated CpGs. Reduced representation bisulfite sequencing (RRBS) is an alternative to whole genome bisulfite sequencing that allows analysis of DNA methylation on a genome-wide scale, offering significantly increased CpG coverage versus array-based methods.

To identify DACOR1-regulated CpG sites, genomic DNA (gDNA) was isolated from three biological replicates of V852 cells stably transfected with a control lentiviral vector or a lentivirus expressing the full-length DACOR1 using the QIAGEN DNeasy Blood and Tissue Kit. Then, 100 ng of gDNA from each sample was digested with MspI restriction enzyme (New England Biosciences) at 37 °C overnight. Library preparation (consisting of end-repair, 3′-adenylation, and adapter

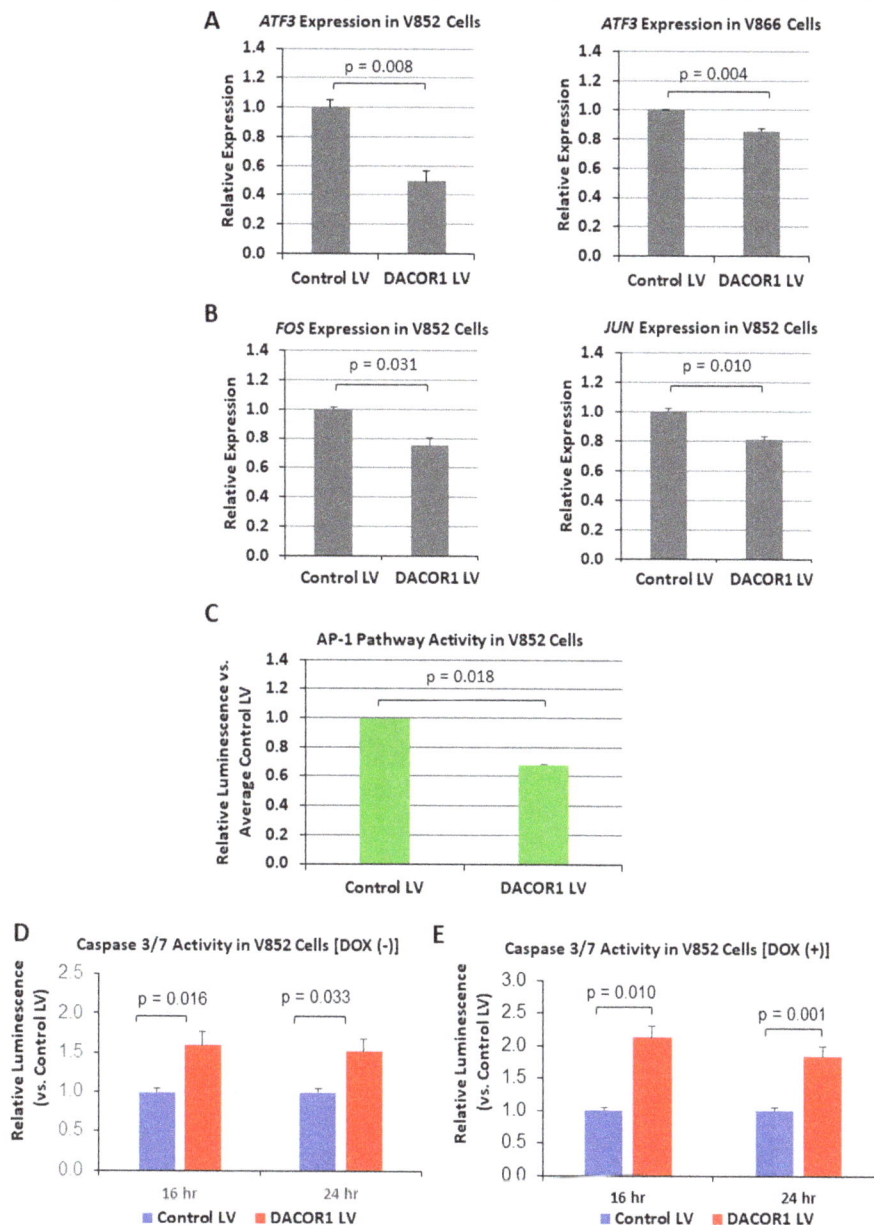

Fig. 10 The AP-1 transcription factor network is altered by DACOR1 re-expression. **a, b** Quantitative RT-PCR of selected AP-1 pathway genes in V852 and V866 cells with either a control lentivirus or a lentivirus expressing the full-length DACOR1. DACOR1 expression results in the repression of ATF3, FOS, and JUN. **c** AP-1 activity is measured in V852 cells upon DACOR1 expression using a luciferase reporter. We found that the induction of DACOR1 results in attenuation of AP-1 activity, consistent with the changes in gene expression of ATF3, FOS, and JUN. **d, e** DACOR1 induction results in increased susceptibility to apoptosis

ligation) was carried out using the NEXTflex Bisulfite Sequencing kit protocol (BIOO Scientific) with 6 NEXTflex Bisulfite-Seq barcodes. Resultant libraries were manually size-selected using gel electrophoresis and gel extraction (reagents included in NEXTflex Bisulfite Sequencing kit) to obtain fragments in the 200–400-bp range. Resultant fragments were bisulfite treated and purified using the QIAGEN EpiTect Bisulfite kit

protocol. Enrichment PCR was performed on bisulfite-treated sample using NEXTflex 0.5 µM primer mix, 0.4 mM dNTPs, 0.5 M betaine, and 0.2 µL Platinum Taq Polymerase with 1X PCR buffer and 2 mM $MgCl_2$ (Invitrogen). Enriched libraries were purified using Agencourt AMPure XP beads (Beckman Coulter) and analyzed for purity and proper size selection using the Agilent High Sensitivity DNA bioanalyzer chip. Final libraries were sequenced at McGill University and Génome Québec Innovation Center (Montreal, QC, Canada) on the Illumina HiSeq 2000 using paired-end 100-bp reads. Resultant reads were mapped to the genome (hg19), and differentially methylated CpGs were identified. Specifically, CpG sites that showed fewer than ten reads in any of the V852 Control-LV or V852 DACOR1-LV samples were trimmed from the dataset, and methylation averages for Control LV and DACOR1 LV samples were calculated. CpG sites that showed a change in average methylation of at least 30% between the two samples were designated as differentially methylated (Additional file 9: Dataset 6).

Similar RRBS preparation and data analysis was performed on gDNA obtained from normal vs. colon tumor samples presented in Fig. 1. Colon tumor and normal colon samples that showed fewer than ten reads for a specific CpG site were trimmed from the dataset for that CpG site. An average colon tumor and normal colon methylation value was calculated for each CpG site. CpG sites that presented a change in average methylation of at least 30% between colon tumors vs. normal colon samples were designated as differentially methylated (Additional file 4: Dataset 7). Differentially methylated CpG sites from Illumina HM450 (TCGA Samples) between primary tumors and normal samples are in Additional file 6: Dataset 8. Demographic and phenotypic data for the cohort in Fig. 1 is presented in Additional file 12: Dataset 9. Affected CpG sites according to their location in CpG islands, shores or shelves are in Additional file 11: Dataset 10.

RNA isolation and cDNA preparation

Trizol reagent (Life Technologies) was added directly to cell culture plate wells (1 mL per 1×10^7 cells) and incubated at room temperature for 5 min. Phenol/chloroform RNA isolation proceeded using the QIAGEN RNeasy Mini Kit protocol with DNase digestion. RNA was quantitated using the NanoDrop 1000 Spectrophotometer. cDNA was prepared using the RNA to cDNA EcoDry™ Premix kit protocol (Clontech). cDNA was diluted to 2 ng/μL for quantitative real-time PCR (qRT-PCR) analysis.

Quantitative real-time PCR

SYBR Green qRT-PCR was performed using 10 ng cDNA, 2× Maxima SYBR Green/ROX qPCR Master Mix (Thermo Scientific), and 0.3 μM forward primer and reverse primer. Samples were cycled using the standard SYBR Green protocol on an ABI StepOne qPCR instrument and analyzed using the comparative cycle threshold (C_T) method to obtain relative expression quantities.

Caspase 3/7 activity assay for apoptosis

Cells were plated in quadruplicate on two separate 96-well plates at a density of 5000–10,000 cells/well and allowed to incubate overnight (~ 16 h). Additional cells were plated in two sets of triplicates for DOX(+) and DOX(−) control to verify apoptosis induction. Then, 100 μM doxorubicin (DOX) stock solution (prepared from doxorubicin hydrochloride; Fisher Scientific, Cat #ICN15910101) was diluted to 1 μM in media and added to each test well and DOX(+) control wells; 100 μL fresh media was added to DOX (−) control wells. At 10 h and 24 h post DOX treatment, 100 μL of caspase 3/7 GLO reagent (Promega caspase 3/7 GLO Assay) was added to each test well, incubated at room temperature for 15 min, and read on the Wallac Victor2 1420 Multilabel Counter using the luminometer setting.

AP-1 luciferase reporter assay

3xAP1pGL3 (3xAP-1 in pGL3-basic) was a gift from Alexander Dent (Addgene plasmid # 40342). The 3x AP-1 reporter construct contains three tandem AP-1 binding sites (TGACTCA) upstream of a minimal promoter fragment in the firefly luciferase reporter plasmid pGL3-basic backbone (36). pcDNA 3.1 Hygro Renilla Luciferase vector was a gift from William Schiemann (Case Western Reserve University). 3xAP-1 firefly luciferase reporter and renilla luciferase control plasmids were co-transfected in a 3:1 ratio in V852 Control LV and V852 DACOR1 LV cells using the Lipofectamine 3000 transfection protocol (Invitrogen). Firefly and renilla luciferase signal was read 36 h post-transfection using the Dual-Glo® Luciferase Assay System (Promega). Results were expressed as relative firefly:renilla signal ratios.

Western blots

Protein was isolated from approximately one million cells using RIPA buffer and quantitated using the Pierce BCA Protein Assay kit protocol (Thermo Fisher Scientific). SDS-PAGE was performed using 4–20% Mini-PROTEAN® TGX™ Precast Protein Gels (BIO-RAD), and resultant proteins were transferred to nitrocellulose membrane (Thermo Fisher Scientific). Rabbit α-Histone H3 and Rabbit α-cleaved caspase 3 were obtained from Cell Signaling Technology, rabbit α-Phospo-c-Jun was obtained from Abgent, and goat α-rabbit-HRP conjugate secondary antibody was obtained from Abcam. Blots were blocked in appropriate blocking solution according to antibody product insert (5% milk in PBST for α-H3 and α-cleaved caspase 3; 3% BSA in PBST for α-Phospho-c-Jun). Following secondary antibody incubation, blots were developed using SuperSignal West Pico Chemiluminescent Substrate Solution and CL-X Exposure Film (both Thermo Fisher Scientific).

Differentially expressed genes in tumors vs. normal colon analysis

RNA-sequencing (RNA-seq) raw data for 22 colon tumors and 22 adjacent normal tissues were obtained from publicly available TCGA database. Fragments per kilobase of transcript per million mapped reads (FPKM) values for each gene in each samples was calculated and differentially expressed genes were identified based on a greater than a twofold change and $p < 0.05$ in a two-tailed T test. This analysis led to the identification of 2443 differentially expressed genes between tumor and normal samples (Additional file 10: Dataset 5).

Gene set enrichment analysis

The Broad Institute's gene set enrichment analysis tool was used for this analysis. A gene set enrichment analysis was performed using the MSigDB database C6: Oncogenic Signatures. A key pathway, the ATF2_UP.V1_UP family, which contained 33 of our ranked genes, was found to have an enrichment score of 0.33, with a nominal p value of < 0.01, a false discovery rate of 5.7%, and an FWER p value of 0.052.

Identification of CpG sites within gene promoters and bodies

Using the Table Browser function of the UCSC genome browser website, a database of 57,111 well-annotated coding and non-coding human genes was created from the RefSeq gene track and matched to genome build Hg19. The start and end positions of each gene were compared with the position of each differentially methylated CpG site using MATLAB scripts, allowing for the identification of CpG sites located within gene bodies, or in the promoter region of a gene (defined as the region 2 kb upstream of the transcription start site (TSS) of each gene) (Additional file 11).

Test for non-randomness in clustering of DACOR1-affected genes

Arrays were created in MATLAB to record the relative position of differentially methylated CpG sites in relation to all CpG sites indexed by the RRBS assay. Following this, a MATLAB script parsed through each array to identify the number of differentially methylated CpG sites that were adjacent to each other when indexed by the RRBS assay. The MATLAB script then proceeded to generate a pseudorandom distribution of differentially methylated CpG sites within an array of size corresponding to the number of CpG sites indexed by the RRBS assay for that gene, and then counted the number of adjacent differentially methylated CpG sites as before, i.e., if in gene A, 100 CpG sites were differentially methylated within a gene body region containing 5000 CpG sites indexed by RRBS assay, a pseudorandom distribution of these 100 sites was generated, followed by a count of adjacent sites. This count would then be compared

to the original count of adjacent sites (i.e., observed in data). This pseudorandom generation of sites followed by a count of adjacent differentially methylated sites was repeated 100,000 times for each gene or region of interest. P values were determined based on the number of trials where the count of adjacent sites from the pseudorandom distribution of differentially methylated sites exceeded or was equal to the count of adjacent sites from the observed data.

Additional files

Additional file 1: Figure S1. DACOR1-mediated DNA methylation affects CpGs in Gene Bodies. A) Ten genes with the highest proportions of differential methylation post DACOR1 induction are plotted, with the positions and count of differentially methylated CpG per 1/100th of Gene Body length (bp set) visualized. B) For each gene, we mapped the position and relative count of all CpG sites within gene body regions. (TIF 90 kb)

Additional file 2: Figure S2. Network map linking key genes within the ATF2 family. A) Links between ATF2 (yellow), ATF2 family genes identified from our GSEA analysis (green), and related intermediaries (orange) are shown in a network map leading to developmental cell activity or angiogenesis/metastasis. Both inhibitory (purple lines) and activating (black lines) interactions were identified through peer-reviewed literature. (TIF 160 kb)

Additional file 3: Dataset 1: RRBS methylation data from colon tumors vs. normal colon samples. Dataset contains methylated CpG sites for 83 colon tumors and 40 normal colon samples. Additionally, gene names with corresponding counts of differential methylation are provided for gene bodies and promoter regions. (XLSX 797 kb)

Additional file 4: Dataset 7: RRBS assay of 83 Colon Tumors and 40 Normal Colon Samples. Complete information on CpG sites analyzed from RRBS assay of Colon Tumors and Normal Colon samples, filtered to sites with at least a 30% change in methylation with all referenced samples having at least 10 reads per site. (XLSX 121505 kb)

Additional file 5: Dataset 2: Colon Tumor vs. Normal Colon from TCGA (COAD) – processed methylation and overlap with expression data. Dataset contains distribution of methylated CpG sites for seven matched colon tumor and normal colon samples from HM450 assay raw data. Additionally, gene names with corresponding counts of differentially methylated CpG sites are provided for gene bodies and promoter regions. A comparison of differentially expressed genes from TCGA samples is then intersected with genes that show differential methylation. (XLSX 659 kb)

Additional file 6: Dataset 8: Differentially Methylated CpG sites from HM450 assays of TCGA COAD. Data on individual CpG sites identified as differentially methylated between matched Colon Tumor and Normal Colon samples from TCGA COAD. (XLSX 18415 kb)

Additional file 7: Dataset 5; Gene expression in colon tumors vs. matched normal colon samples (TCGA RNA-seq). Calculated FPKM value for each gene in each sample is provided. Analysis of differentially expressed and statistically significant genes is provided. (XLSX 35769 kb)

Additional file 8: Dataset 3: DACOR1-mediated changes in DNA methylation from RRBS data. Dataset contains distribution of methylated CpG sites obtained from RRBS assay of V852 cells that were transduced with a control LV or a DACOR1-expressing LV vector. Differentially methylated CpG sites are also presented with gene names and corresponding counts of differentially methylated CpG sites for both gene bodies and gene promoter regions. (XLSX 950 kb)

Additional file 9: Dataset 6: RRBS assay of V852 Cells with DACOR 1 Re-expression vs. control cells. Complete information on differentially methylated CpG sites from RRBS assay output of read values and read depth. (XLSX 2964 kb)

Additional file 10: Dataset 4: DACOR1-mediated changes in Gene Body methylation. Dataset contains locations of all differentially methylated

CpG sites for top ten genes of interest, as well as identification if a specific site is located in an intron or an exon. (XLSX 34 kb)

Additional file 11: Dataset 10: Localization of modified CpGs. Modified CpGs according to their localization in CpG islands, CpG islands shores or shelves. (XLSX 774 kb)

Additional file 12: Dataset 9: RRBS Cohort demographic and Phenotypic data. Demographic and phenotypic information of the cohort analyzed in Fig. 1. (XLSX 14 kb)

Abbreviations

bZIP: Basic leucine zipper; COAD: Colon adenocarcinoma; CpG: Cytosine-phosphate-guanine site; CREB: Cyclic AMP response element-binding; DNMT1: DNA methyltransferase 1; FPKM: Fragments per kilobase of transcript per million mapped reads; gDNA: Genomic DNA; lncRNA: Long non-coding RNA; RNA-seq: RNA sequencing; RRBS: Reduced representation bisulfide sequencing; TCGA: The Cancer Genome Atlas; TSS: Transcriptional start site

Acknowledgements

We are grateful to Lydia Beard for guidance in the tissue culture of patient-derived colon tumor cell lines.

Funding

Funding for this work was supported by Institutional startup funds and NCI 1R01CA217992-01A1 to Dr. Ahmad Khalil, and U01CA152756 and 1P50CA150964 to Dr Sanford Marlowitz.

Authors' contributions

SS, TL, and AMK analyzed and interpreted DNA methylation and gene expression data. MEF and AC performed the experiments including RRBS assay and apoptosis studies. SS, MEF, and AMK wrote the manuscript with input from SM, HM, TL, VV, and AC. All authors read and approved the final manuscript.

References

1. Mohammad F, Mondal T, Kanduri C. Epigenetics of imprinted long noncoding RNAs. Epigenetics. 2009;4(5):277–86.
2. Bird A. Perceptions of epigenetics. Nature. 2007;447(7143):396–8.
3. Reik W, Dean W. DNA methylation and mammalian epigenetics. Electrophoresis. 2001;22(14):2838–43.
4. Dawson MA, Kouzarides T. Cancer epigenetics: from mechanism to therapy. Cell. 2012;150(1):12–27.
5. Egger G, Liang G, Aparicio A, Jones PA. Epigenetics in human disease and prospects for epigenetic therapy. Nature. 2004;429(6990):457–63.
6. Forrest ME, Khalil AM. Review: regulation of the cancer epigenome by long non-coding RNAs. Cancer Lett. 2017;407:106-112.
7. Wu H, Zhang Y. Reversing DNA methylation: mechanisms, genomics, and biological functions. Cell. 2014;156(1–2):45–68.
8. Stirzaker C, Taberlay PC, Statham AL, Clark SJ. Mining cancer methylomes: prospects and challenges. Trends Genet. 2014;30(2):75–84.
9. Suva ML, Riggi N, Bernstein BE. Epigenetic reprogramming in cancer. Science. 2013;339(6127):1567–70.
10. Sharma S, Kelly TK, Jones PA. Epigenetics in cancer. Carcinogenesis. 2010; 31(1):27–36.
11. Goelz SE, Vogelstein B, Hamilton SR, Feinberg AP. Hypomethylation of DNA from benign and malignant human colon neoplasms. Science. 1985; 228(4696):187–90.
12. Fatemi M, Hermann A, Gowher H, Jeltsch A. Dnmt3a and Dnmt1 functionally cooperate during de novo methylation of DNA. Eur J Biochem. 2002;269(20):4981–4.
13. Deplus R, Brenner C, Burgers WA, Putmans P, Kouzarides T, de Launoit Y, Fuks F. Dnmt3L is a transcriptional repressor that recruits histone deacetylase. Nucleic Acids Res. 2002;30(17):3831–8.
14. Merry CR, Forrest ME, Sabers JN, Beard L, Gao X-H, Hatzoglou M, Jackson MW, Wang Z, Markowitz SD, Khalil AM. DNMT1-associated long non-coding RNAs regulate global gene expression and DNA methylation in colon cancer. Hum Mol Genet. 2015;24(21):6240–53.
15. Gu H, Bock C, Mikkelsen TS, Jager N, Smith ZD, Tomazou E, Gnirke A, Lander ES, Meissner A. Genome-scale DNA methylation mapping of clinical samples at single-nucleotide resolution. Nat Methods. 2010;7(2):133–6.

23

Global DNA methylation changes spanning puberty are near predicted estrogen-responsive genes and enriched for genes involved in endocrine and immune processes

Emma E. Thompson[1]*[†], Jessie Nicodemus-Johnson[1,5†], Kyung Won Kim[1,6†], James E. Gern[2,3], Daniel J. Jackson[2,3], Robert F. Lemanske[2,3] and Carole Ober[1,4]

Abstract

Background: The changes that occur during puberty have been implicated in susceptibility to a wide range of diseases later in life, many of which are characterized by sex-specific differences in prevalence. Both genetic and environmental factors have been associated with the onset or delay of puberty, and recent evidence has suggested a role for epigenetic changes in the initiation of puberty as well.

Objective: To identify global DNA methylation changes that arise across the window of puberty in girls and boys.

Methods: Genome-wide DNA methylation levels were measured using the Infinium 450K array. We focused our studies on peripheral blood mononuclear cells (PBMCs) from 30 girls and 25 boys pre- and post-puberty (8 and 14 years, respectively), in whom puberty status was confirmed by Tanner staging.

Results: Our study revealed 347 differentially methylated probes (DMPs) in females and 50 DMPs in males between the ages of 8 and 14 years (FDR 5%). The female DMPs were in or near 312 unique genes, which were over-represented for having high affinity estrogen response elements (permutation $P < 2.0 \times 10^{-6}$), suggesting that some of the effects of estrogen signaling in puberty are modified through epigenetic mechanisms. Ingenuity Pathway Analysis (IPA) of the 312 genes near female puberty DMPs revealed significant networks enriched for immune and inflammatory responses as well as reproductive hormone signaling. Finally, analysis of gene expression in the female PBMCs collected at 14 years revealed modules of correlated transcripts that were enriched for immune and reproductive system functions, and include genes that are responsive to estrogen and androgen receptor signaling. The male DMPs were in or near 48 unique genes, which were enriched for adrenaline and noradrenaline biosynthesis (Enrichr $P = 0.021$), with no significant networks identified. Additionally, no modules were identified using post-puberty gene expression levels in males.

Conclusion: Epigenetic changes spanning the window of puberty in females may be responsive to or modify hormonal changes that occur during this time and potentially contribute to sex-specific differences in immune-mediated and endocrine diseases later in life.

Keywords: Epigenetics, Puberty, Differential methylation, Estrogen, Androgen, Immune response

* Correspondence: eethomps@uchicago.edu
†Equal contributors
[1]Department of Human Genetics, The University of Chicago, 920 E 58th St, CLSC Room 501, Chicago, IL 60637, USA
Full list of author information is available at the end of the article

Background

Many anatomical and physiological differences between boys and girls emerge around the time of puberty, a period marked by considerable metabolic and hormonal change as well as dynamic physiologic transitions. This period is characterized by shifts in male and female sex steroid hormone production [1], as well as sex disparities in the onset and remission of asthma [2, 3] and the development of autoimmune diseases and cardiometabolic risk factors, such as lipid profiles [4, 5], blood pressure [6, 7], and insulin resistance [8], among others.

In fact, the hormonal, immune and metabolic changes that occur during and following puberty have been implicated in susceptibility to a wide range of diseases later in life that differ in prevalence, age of onset, and/or severity between men and women [reviewed in ref. [9]]. It is possible, therefore, that puberty-associated hormonal changes result in profound effects on immune processes [3, 10] and could ultimately contribute to lifelong sex-specific risks for immune-mediated, cardiometabolic and endocrine diseases. Although the contribution of genetic factors to the onset of puberty is well established [11–13], only recently have epigenetic processes in the timing and control of puberty been reported. For example, an association was reported between LINE-1 methylation in peripheral blood cells from 9-year-old girls and decreased odds of experiencing menarche by age 12 [14]. Recently, a genome-wide methylation study in peripheral blood cells from 51 children (20 girls and 31 boys) sampled pre- and post-puberty identified 457 CpGs associated with pubertal age in the combined sexes [15]. Ninety-four of these CpGs predicted puberty status among all samples, and another set of 133 CpGs among boys (but not girls) were associated with circulating reproductive hormone levels. However, because boys and girls were analyzed together in this study, little is still known about epigenetic changes that arise during the window of puberty in males and females, which would differ if these changes are linked to the extreme dimorphism that arises during this period.

We undertook this study to identify global changes in an epigenetic mark, DNA methylation, that occur across the window of puberty in males and females separately and then characterize the genes and pathways associated with these epigenetic changes. We present here the results of a study of methylation patterns in DNA from peripheral blood mononuclear cells (PBMCs) collected pre- and post-puberty (8 and 14 years, respectively) from 30 girl and 25 boy participants in the Childhood Origins of ASThma (COAST) birth cohort study [16]. Our results show striking differences between boys and girls and suggest that epigenetic changes occurring between the ages of 8 and 14 in girls may contribute to estrogen, endocrine, and immune signaling pathways, and ultimately play a role in sex-specific differences in

susceptibility to immune-mediated and endocrine diseases later in life.

Methods

Sample composition

PBMCs were available for 100 children (50 boys, 50 girls) in the COAST study [16] at both ages 8 and 14 years. White blood cell differentials were performed at both ages, as previously described [17]; two individuals with missing differentials at either age were removed. Pubertal status was assessed by Tanner staging [18, 19]. Children who were not pre-puberty at age 8 (one boy, nine girls) or post-puberty at age 14 (18 boys, three girls) were removed, leaving 55 children for analysis of paired samples (25 boys, 30 girls).

The study was approved by the University of Wisconsin Human Subjects Committee and The University of Chicago Institutional Review Board.

Sample processing and analysis

PBMCs were stored at – 80 °C in cell culture freezing media (ThermoFisher Scientific, Waltham, MA) after collection. DNA for methylation studies was extracted from thawed PBMCs using the Qiagen AllPrep kit (QIAGEN, Valencia, CA). Genome-wide DNA methylation was assessed using the Illumina Infinium Human Methylation 450k BeadChip (Illumina, San Diego, CA) at the University of Chicago Functional Genomics Facility (UC-FGF). Data were processed using Minfi [20]; Infinium type I and type II probe bias were corrected using SWAN [21]. Raw probe values were corrected for color imbalance and background by control normalization. We removed probes that map to the sex chromosomes or to more than one location in a bisulfite-converted genome, had detection P values greater than 0.01 in 75% of samples, or overlapped with known single nucleotide polymorphisms (SNPs). Data quality was assessed using principal components analysis (PCA) [22], which identified chip and plate location as potential confounding variables. These effects were removed using ComBat [23]. Methylation levels are reported as β values at each CpG site, which is the fraction of signal obtained from the methylated beads over the sum of methylated and unmethylated bead signals. The Infinium HumanMethylation450 Manifest was used to generate chromosome coordinates based on hg19.

RNA for gene expression studies was isolated from PBMCs collected at the 14-year (post-puberty) time point and assessed using the Illumina Human HT-12 v4 array at the UC-FGF. RNA was not available at the 8-year (pre-puberty) time point. Probe level raw intensity values across arrays were normalized using quantile normalization, and background-corrected normalized expression values were obtained for each probe using the R package lumi [24]. Probes that were indistinguishable from background intensity ($P < 0.01$), contained more than one HapMap SNP, or mapped to multiple locations in the genome [25] were removed; 25,892 of the 47,265 transcripts present on the array remained after this step. The median probe intensity was used to represent the transcriptional abundance of each gene.

Extraction batch, chip, RNA concentration, and RNA quality were identified as potential confounders by PCA analysis of the gene expression data. The effects of batch and chip were removed using ComBat, and the effects of the quantitative variables (RNA concentration and quality) were regressed out using linear regression.

Network analysis
Weighted Gene Correlation Network Analysis (WGCNA) [26] was used to identify modules of correlated genes among the unique genes that were nearest to puberty-associated differentially methylated CpG sites. For this analysis, an FDR cutoff of 10% was used for differential methylation to increase the number of genes, and therefore power, yielding 893 female-specific DMPs, which mapped to 562 unique genes that were detected as expressed on the array, and 124 male-specific DMPs, which mapped to 81 unique genes that were detected as expressed on the array. The genes associated with each WGCNA module were used as input for gene enrichment analyses and IPA for the female samples, but the 81 genes in the males did not cluster into correlated modules of transcription.

Ingenuity pathway analysis
Using annotation provided by Illumina, the location of each CpG site was mapped to the closest transcription start site (TSS), according to ENSEMBL. Gene lists were interrogated using QIAGEN's Ingenuity Pathway Analysis (IPA; QIAGEN Redwood City, https://www.qiagenbioinformatics.com/products/ingenuity-pathway-analysis/), and network associations were constructed using the Ingenuity Knowledge Base. Network interactions were limited to those known to occur in primary cells or tissues; all other settings were left as the defaults. The score of each network is based on the network hypergeometric distribution and is calculated with the right-tailed Fisher's Exact Test to identify over-representation of the genes near DMPs relative to all genes present on the Illumina HT12 v4 array.

Statistical analyses
Data were analyzed with R software (version 3.3.0) using a 2×2 interaction test in limma [27]. A random effects model with individual ID coded as a random effect to account for the paired sample design was used to identify differentially methylated CpG sites in males and

females pre- and post-puberty. Race/ethnicity was not a significant covariate and was not included in the model; however, to exclude the possibility of confounding from these subjects, differential methylation analysis was repeated after excluding the five children of non-European ancestry (Table 1 and Additional file 1). Age-specific cell composition (% lymphocytes, % monocytes, and % eosinophils) was not included as a covariate; instead, we looked for effects of cell composition in downstream analyses. All enrichment analyses were conducted using Enrichr (http://amp.pharm.mssm.edu/Enrichr/) [28, 29]. Gene lists (genes nearest DMPs and genes comprising networks identified through WGCNA) were used as input and default settings were used for analysis. Permutations were performed by randomly selecting 312, 198, or 86 genes (for the data presented in Table 2 and Additional file 2, respectively) from the list of 3497 genes with high affinity estrogen receptor binding sites, then comparing the random sample with the observed gene list and recoding how many times (out of 500,000) the number of genes was equal to (or greater than) the observed value (63, 53, or 20, respectively). Correlations between differentially methylated CpGs and expression level of the nearest gene at age 14 were tested using Pearson coefficients as implemented in R.

Availability of data and materials
The datasets supporting the conclusions of this article will be made available at the time of publication.

Results
Identifying differentially methylated CpGs at 8 and 14 years of age
To assess global DNA methylation changes that occur between the ages of 8 and 14, we first identified differentially methylated probes (DMPs) (5% FDR) in the combined sample ($n = 55$ pairs), girls only ($n = 30$ pairs), and boys only ($n - 25$ pairs).

Overall, we detected a total of 445 DMPs: 48 in the combined sample (gray in Fig. 1), 347 unique to girls (shown in red in Fig. 1), and 50 unique to boys (shown in blue in Fig. 1; DMP lists are available in Additional files 3–5). Among the 347 female-specific DMPs, 155 (44.7%) became more methylated and 192 (55.3%) became less methylated between 8 and 14 years of age. Most of

Table 1 Size and ethnic composition of sample

	Males N (%)	Females N (%)
Sample size	25	30
Race/ethnicity		
European American	23 (92)	27 (90)
African American	2 (8)	1 (3)
Hispanic	0	2 (6)

Table 2 Predicted estrogen-responsive genes are over-represented near female puberty-associated DMPs. $P < 2.0 \times 10^{-6}$ by permutation testing

	No. of genes with high affinity estrogen-responsive elements (%)	No. of all other genes (%)	Total
Near a puberty DMP	63 (20.2)	249 (79.8)	312 (100)
Near a Non-DMP	3434 (14.7)	19,883 (85.3)	23,317 (100)
Total	3497 (14.5)	20,132 (85.5)	23,629 (100)

DMP, differentially methylated probe

these sites (263 of 347) are either in the body of a gene or within 1500 base pairs of a transcription start site (42.5 and 25.3%, respectively), slightly higher than the overall distribution of CpGs on the array (31 and 17%, respectively). In females, the median absolute change in methylation among DMPs was 2.6% (ranging from 1.6 to 10.5%); 9 CpGs (2.5%) had a change greater than 5%. The 347 female-specific DMPs are located in or near 312 unique genes.

Among the 50 male-specific DMPs, 29 (58%) became more methylated and 21 (42%) became less methylated between 8 and 14 years of age. As in the females, most of the sites (37 out of 50) are in the body of a gene or within 1500 base pairs of a transcription start site (40.0 and 34.0%, respectively). In males, the median absolute change in methylation was 3.2% (ranging from 2.6 to 6.

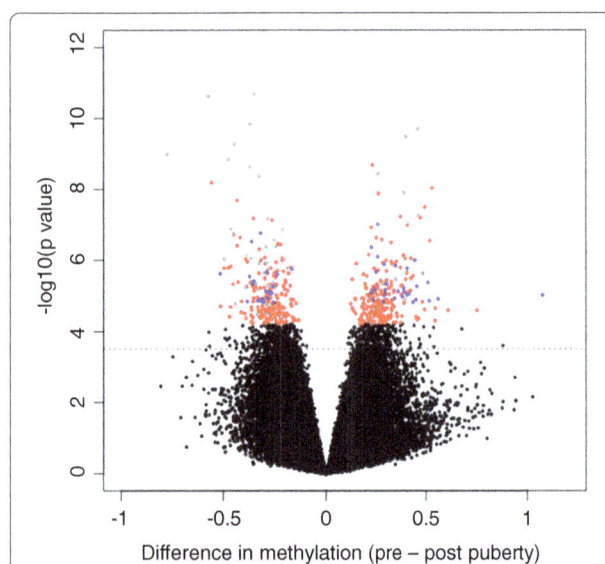

Fig. 1 Volcano plot showing differences in methylation between 8 and 14 years of age in males and females combined (DMPs in 55 paired samples). Significant (FDR = 5%) DMPs are shown as non-black circles. Female puberty-associated DMPs (347 in 30 paired female samples) are shown in red, male puberty-associated DMPs (50 DMPs in 25 paired samples) are shown in blue, and CpGs identified as being differentially methylated in the combined sample (48 in 55 paired samples) are shown in gray. The x axis shows –log10 P values and the y axis plots the mean difference in methylation β values. The horizontal line denotes significant CpGs at an FDR of 10%

9%); 5 CpGs (10%) had a change greater than 5%. The 50 male-specific DMPs are in or near 48 unique genes.

These results were not influenced by the inclusion of five children of non-European ancestry (Table 1). The beta values of the 347 DMPs ($N = 55$ vs 50 pairs) were significantly correlated between analyses with and without the five non-European individuals (Pearson correlation $r = 0.82$, Additional file 1). Therefore, all subsequent analyses include participants of all ancestries to maximize sample sizes.

Genes with high affinity estrogen response elements are over-represented among genes near female DMPs

Given the central role of estrogen in the developmental and reproductive changes that accompany puberty, we first asked whether genes near female puberty-associated DMPs were over-represented among potential estrogen-responsive genes. For this analysis, we used a list of genes from published studies revealing high-affinity genome-wide estrogen response elements [30] to represent predicted estrogen response genes (Additional file 6). A comparison of those genes to the genes nearest the 312 female puberty-associated DMPs revealed a significant excess of genes near female puberty-associated DMPs among predicted estrogen response genes ($n = 62$) compared to genes nearest to all CpGs on the array (Permutation $P < 2.0 \times 10^{-6}$; Table 2). These results suggest that at least some of the effects of estrogen signaling in puberty are modified through epigenetic mechanisms. As expected, there was no such pattern in the male-specific DMPs ($P = 0.57$; data not shown).

We next evaluated whether genes near female puberty-associated DMPs were functionally related to one another. To identify candidate pathways, we used Ingenuity Pathway Analysis (IPA) to construct protein-protein interaction networks using the list of 312 genes as input (Additional file 7). Remarkably, the genes nearest to each of the 347 female puberty-associated DMPs formed four significant networks that were enriched for genes implicated in pubertal timing and initiation, and endocrine system development using Enrichr (Table 3). For example, network 1 (score = 47) included 26 genes enriched for phosphatidylinositol signaling ($P = 0.0064$), which plays a key role in the integration of metabolic and neural signals regulating gonadotropin releasing hormone/luteinizing

Table 3 Enrichment categories of four significant protein-protein interaction networks in females constructed using Ingenuity Pathway Analysis (networks shown in Additional file 7)

Network (IPA Score)	Enrichr results		
	Enrichment category	Database	Adj. P value
1 (47)	Phosphatidylinositol signaling TGF-β receptor signaling	KEGG 2016	0.0064
		Panther 2016	0.043
2 (41)	FGF signaling pathway	Panther 2016	0.0073
3 (33)	Insulin-like growth factor-1 (IGF-1) signaling	NCI-Nature 2016	0.0098
4 (32)	Validated estrogen receptor alpha network	NCI-Nature 2016	0.0018

Adjusted P values were determined by performing the Fisher Exact Test for many random gene sets in order to compute a mean rank and SD from the expected rank for each term in the gene-set library

hormone release. Network 2 (score = 41) included 24 genes enriched for fibroblast growth factor (FGF) signaling ($P = 0.0073$). Network 3 (score = 33) included 21 genes enriched for insulin-like growth factor-1 (IGF-1) signaling ($P = 0.0098$), which has been implicated in growth and metabolism during female puberty (and IGF-1 levels are elevated among girls with precocious puberty [31]). Finally, network 4 (score = 32) included 20 genes enriched for estrogen receptor signaling ($P = 0.001845$). The 48 unique genes nearest to the 50 male puberty-associated DMPs were enriched for adrenaline and noradrenaline biosynthesis (Enrichr Adj $P = 0.021$; Panther 2016). Neither the genes nearest to 50 male puberty-associated DMP nor the genes nearest the 48 DMPs shared between males and females formed any significant networks using IPA, possibly due to the small number of genes use as input.

Genes near female puberty-associated DMPs are enriched for immune functions and sex hormone receptor signaling

To gain further insight into the processes and networks that are influenced by epigenetic changes during puberty, we measured transcript levels in post-puberty PMBCs collected at the same age 14 visit as those used for the methylation studies. We detected 18,756 transcripts as expressed in these samples, but for this analysis, we focused on the 562 genes near female puberty-associated DMPs and used a systems biology approach as implemented in Weighted Gene Correlation Network Analysis (WGCNA) to identify modules of correlated transcripts in the females. The motivation for this analysis is to identify

groups of functional molecules (based on transcript levels) near DMPs that are correlated with one another. WGCNA assigned 284 (50.5%) of these genes into two co-expression modules; the remaining 278 genes showed no correlation structure in the post-puberty samples. The 198 genes in the first module were significantly enriched for T cell receptor signaling ($P = 0.0038$) and activation ($P = 0.0021$) (Table 4) and were associated as a whole with inflammatory and respiratory diseases (IPA $P = 3.77 \times 10^{-4}$ for both). The second gene expression module consisted of 86 genes enriched for estrogen receptor beta signaling ($P = 0.0019$) and androgen receptor signaling ($P = 0.0067$). There was an over-representation of genes with high affinity estrogen response elements among genes in both modules compared to all other gene transcripts measured (Permutation $P < 2.0 \times 10^{-6}$ (module 1 and module 2); Additional file 2).

To investigate possible correlations between CpG methylation and gene expression, we further examined the 259 genes detected as expressed on the array (out of the 312 nearest genes). We observed correlations ($P < 0.05$) for 12/259 comparisons (5%), similar to rates reported in other studies [32, 33].

There were no modules of correlated gene expression using the genes nearest male puberty-associated DMPs, again potentially due to the small number of DMPs in the males ($N = 124$ DMPs and 81 unique genes at an FDR of 10%).

A subset of CpGs predicts pubertal status in COAST children

Almstrup et al. [15] identified a subset of 94 CpGs in peripheral blood cells that predicted pubertal status and

Table 4 Modules of correlated transcripts at genes near female puberty-associated DMPs are enriched for immune functions and hormone signaling

WGCNA Module (# of genes)	Pathway enrichment category (Adjusted P value)	Database
1 (198)	T cell receptor signaling ($P = 0.0038$) and activation ($P = 0.0021$)	KEGG 2016, BioCarta 2016
	Epidermal growth factor receptor (EGFR) signaling ($P = 0.029$)	Panther 2016
2 (86)	Estrogen receptor beta signaling ($P = 0.0019$)	KEGG 2016
	Androgen receptor signaling ($P = 0.0067$)	

133 CpGs that predicted circulating hormone levels in males in their study of 51 children (31 boys, 20 girls). Using 75 of the 94 puberty-predicting CpGs that were present in our dataset, we classified the COAST samples as pre- or post-puberty using unsupervised hierarchical clustering. Indeed, methylation changes at these 75 CpGs (Additional file 8) predicted pubertal status among the 55 COAST children, with a specificity of 92.7% and a sensitivity of 87.3% (Table 5). A subset of 104 of the 133 CpGs (Additional file 9) that predicted levels of six circulating sex hormones in males in the Almstrup study were present in our data set. Although hormone levels were not measured in the COAST children, the 104 CpGs separated the males on the basis of pubertal status with a specificity of 72.0% and a sensitivity of 96.0%. Curiously, in our study, we see the greatest overlap between the predictive CpGs reported by Almstrup et al. and the female-specific DMPs: 29% (22/75) of the CpGs used to predict puberty status and 27% (28/104) of the CpGs used to predict hormone levels in boys pre- and post-puberty are present among the 347 DMPs specific to females in our study (indicated in Additional files 8 and 9). In contrast, only 4% (3/75) and 2% (2/104) of the predictive CpGs were present among the male-specific DMPs reported here, and 24% (18/75) and 19% (20/104) were among the DMPs shared by girls and boys in this study.

Changes in cell proportions between 8 and 14 years of age are not associated with DMPs

Finally, we assessed whether changes in cell type proportions contributed to the observed puberty-associated DMPs. In fact, in both boys and girls, there were significant differences in lymphocyte (Wilcoxon Rank Test $P = 0.0036$ and $P = 0.00029$, respectively) and monocyte ($P = 3.05 \times 10^{-8}$ and $P = 2.67 \times 10^{-8}$, respectively), but not eosinophil ($P = 0.59$ and $P = 0.49$, respectively) proportions between pre- and post-puberty PBMCs. We next examined whether changes in cell proportions were correlated with changes in methylation levels between ages 8 and 14 years. Among females, changes in methylation levels were not correlated with changes in lymphocyte or eosinophil proportions ($P > 0.14$; Spearman correlation test). Among individual CpG sites, methylation level changes at three were correlated with changes in monocyte proportions at an FDR of 5%, but

none of the three CpG sites were puberty-associated DMPs in females. Among males, no significant correlations were observed between methylation changes and cell proportion changes pre- and post-puberty. Moreover, cell proportions were not associated with post-puberty transcript levels among the genes assigned to the two WGCNA modules, indicating that the correlations in gene expression post-puberty were not due to differences in cell proportions among subjects.

Discussion

Changes in DNA methylation can impact transcription of nearby genes and thereby modulate the effects of hormonal fluctuations in cells and tissues on gene expression. To our knowledge, this is the first report of sex-specific changes in methylation patterns across the window of puberty in humans, a period of dynamic change that can carry long-term implications for health and disease. The results of our unbiased, genome-wide study suggest that epigenetic modifications arise during early adolescence, particularly among females, and that many of these changes occur near genes implicated in traits that differ between males and females during or after sexual maturation. These findings may shed light on endocrine, metabolic, and immune disease susceptibility, among others, through either the identification of novel target genes near DMPs or the recognition of epigenetic mechanisms affecting these phenotypes.

Our study revealed an over-representation of genes near female DMPs, as well as among correlated modules of gene transcript levels measured post-puberty, that harbor high affinity estrogen response elements. These findings suggest the epigenetic changes that occur over the window of puberty are coordinated with estrogen signaling in females, potentially contributing to long-term health effects. Beyond the critical role estrogen is known to play in female puberty, it also modulates inflammation and immune responses [3, 34–36], influences the severity of a number of autoimmune diseases [37, 38], and is thought to play a role in protection against cardiovascular disease in women [39]. Our findings suggest that DMPs involved in estrogen signaling arise during puberty itself. As such, puberty may represent a unique window with regard to the influx of circulating hormones, and be a time during which girls are particularly sensitive to the effects of DNA

Table 5 Performance of predictive CpG sets reported by Almstrup et al. in this study

	Among COAST females (N = 30)		Among COAST males (N = 25)		Among COAST males and females combined (N = 55)	
	Specificity	Sensitivity	Specificity	Sensitivity	Specificity	Sensitivity
94 puberty classifiers (N = 75)	83.3%	96.7%	92.0%	92.0%	92.7%	87.3%
133 reproductive hormone[a] classifiers (N = 104)	86.7%	86.2%	72.0%	96.0%	90.9%	90.9%

[a]Follicle stimulating hormone (FSH), luteinizing hormone (LH), anti-Mullerian hormone (AMH), testosterone (T), estradiol (E2), inhibin B
Numbers in parentheses in first column refer to the number of CpGs in each subset reported by Almstrup that are present in this study

methylation changes. These changes and responses to hormones may ultimately influence a wide range of sex-specific traits. For example, *PRDM16*, identified as an estrogen-responsive gene in Network 1 (Fig. 2 and Additional files 6 and 7), controls brown adipose tissue (BAT) differentiation. BAT activity and volume increase during puberty [40], ultimately leading to gains in skeletal musculature consistent with pubertal development; significantly greater changes in BAT volume have been reported in males compared to females [41]. Metabolic and hormonal factors have been proposed to be responsible for this increase, although specific mechanisms have not been elucidated.

Moreover, the predicted estrogen-responsive genes were present as well-connected hubs in four networks. For example, PR/SET Domain 16 (*PRDM16*; network 1), discussed above, is also a regulator of TGF-β signaling; Runt-related transcription factor 2 (*RUNX2*; network 2) is a transcription factor involved in skeletal/bone development; FGF signaling, integrin subunit beta 3 (*ITGB3*; network 3) encodes a cell surface protein with a role in cell migration, adhesion and signaling; and cathepsin D (*CTSD*, network 4) is an A1 peptidase that plays a role in proteolytic activation of hormones and growth factors.

The identification of correlated modules of transcripts for genes involved in immune signaling and sex hormone receptor signaling is intriguing and points to the diverse array of puberty-associated developmental traits in which epigenetics likely plays a role. The enrichment of genes near female puberty-associated DMPs with correlated patterns of expression in protein networks that are centered on these phenotypes is indicative of both the sex-specific nature of many traits (particularly those that are endocrine or immune-related), and the expansive role of epigenetic modifications.

Further evidence for a critical role of DNA methylation during puberty comes from our demonstration that a subset of puberty-specific methylation changes in a combined sample of males and females in the Almstrup study [15] predicted puberty status in COAST children

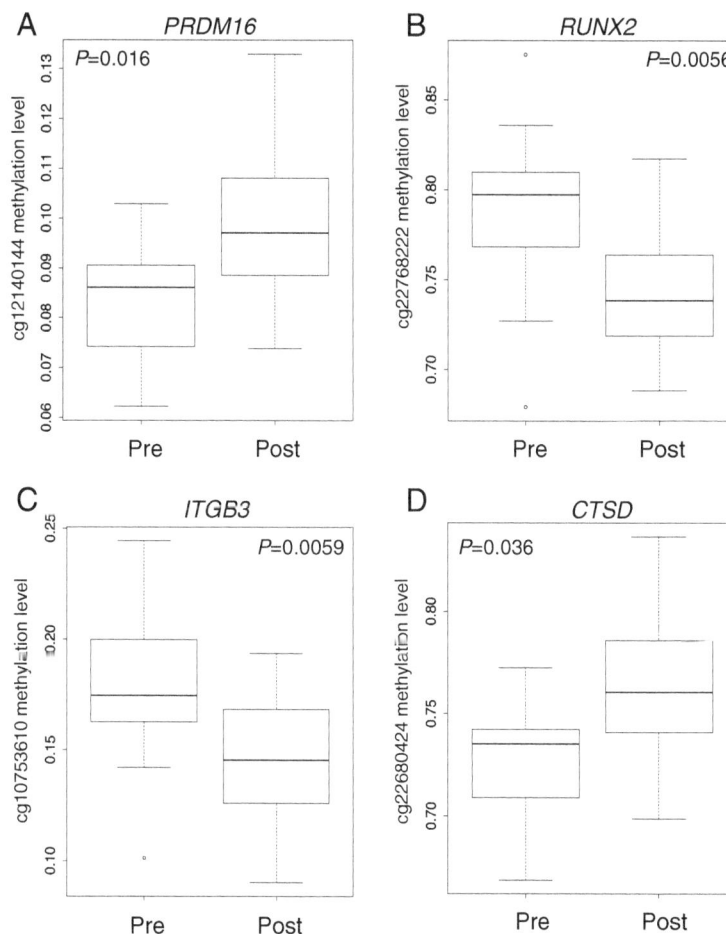

Fig. 2 Examples of changes in methylation levels (β values) in four estrogen-responsive genes present in the networks shown in Additional file 7. **a** Methylation levels of cg12140144 (*PRDM16*; network 1), **b** Methylation levels of cg22768222 (*RUNX2*; network 2), **c** Methylation levels of cg10753610 (*ITGB3*; network 3), and **d** Methylation levels of cg22680424 (*CTSD*; network 4)

with high sensitivity and specificity. Intriguingly, the greatest proportions of the puberty-predictive CpGs are within the sets of female-specific and shared DMPs in our study. This observation cannot be due simply to the smaller number of DMPs among males than females because the number of DMPs shared with those in the Almstrup study is similar to males and females (48 vs 50, respectively). Despite many parallels between our study and that of Almstrup et al., there are a number of important differences. Both studies evaluated genome-wide methylation patterns via the Illumina 450K array in blood cells collected pre-puberty (~ 8–9 year old) and post-puberty (~ 14–15 year old), and the combined sample sizes were similar (30 girls and 25 boys in our study compared to 20 girls and 31 boys in the Almstrup study). However, Almstrup et al. used peripheral blood leukocytes (PBLs) while we used peripheral blood mononuclear cells (PBMCs), and Almstrup et al. combined both sexes for analysis and used sex as a covariate to identify 457 DMPs in the combined sample, whereas we focused our studies on methylation changes that were unique to boys or to girls and identified sex-specific puberty DMPs (Fig. 1). Although Almstrup et al. did not specifically report sex-specific methylation changes, they state that only data from the boys resulted in significant CpGs when the two groups were analyzed separately, perhaps due to the relatively smaller number of girls in their study. Ultimately, the fact that two predictor sets of CpGs reported in the Almstrup study predict pubertal status in our study likely reflects common pathways involved in pubertal development in both sexes and the robustness and stability of the DNA methylation changes associated with puberty.

The small proportion of correlated DMP-transcript pairs in the post-puberty samples is not entirely unexpected. In fact, previous genome-wide studies have shown that overall few transcripts are correlated with nearby CpG methylation levels [42–44]. Our study was further limited because we did not have RNA for the pre-puberty time point. As a result, we could not test for correlations between changes in DNA methylation and changes in gene expression, a potentially more relevant comparison. In addition, we do not know the time or age at which puberty-associated methylation changes exert their effects on gene expression. It is possible, for example, that relevant changes in transcript abundance due to changes in methylation occur before 14 years of age. Longitudinal sampling over the window of puberty would be required to address these questions.

Our study has other limitations. First, despite discovering many significant DMPs, the size of our sample is relatively small and the observed effect sizes (absolute changes in methylation) were modest. Second, we cannot exclude the possibility that some of the changes in methylation we observe are simply due to age. For example, it is possible that the subset of DMPs that are common to both males and females represent age-specific methylation changes. Although only 1% of the puberty-associated CpG sites have been reported to undergo age-related methylation changes [45, 46] and methylation levels at the CpGs that are known to be associated with aging did not differ between males and females in our study ($P > 0.05$) [45, 46], it remains possible that some of the shared puberty DMPs are due to age-related changes that are unrelated to puberty itself. Third, our study is limited to data from PBMCs. It is possible, and even likely, that different patterns of epigenetic modifications would be present in other tissues.

In conclusion, our results provide evidence for significant female puberty effects on global DNA methylation patterns at CpGs whose nearby genes are enriched for estrogen responsiveness and form networks centered on immune processes and sex hormone signaling, findings that were validated in gene expression studies in the post-puberty period. In addition, two out of four significant protein interaction networks based on genes nearest the puberty DMPs include genes involved in puberty regulation and timing, supporting an important role for epigenetics in this process.

Conclusions

Genes near differentially methylated CpGs that arise during female puberty are over-represented for estrogen responsiveness and networks focused on endocrine system development as well as immune response. These results suggest that epigenetic changes across the window of puberty are, in part, responsive to the hormonal changes that occur during this time. Ultimately, this research may be useful in identifying genes that potentially contribute to sex-specific diseases later in life.

Abbreviations
DMP: Differentially methylated probe; IPA: Ingenuity Pathway Analysis; PBMC: Peripheral blood mononuclear cell; WGCNA: Weighted Gene Correlation Network Analysis

Acknowledgements
The authors thank Katherine Naughton at the University of Chicago and Christopher Tisler at the University of Wisconsin for the assistance with sample processing and the COAST participants and their families for making this study possible.

Funding
This work was supported by P01 HL070831, R01 HL129735, UL1 TR000427, 1UL1 TR002373, R01 HL113395, and U19 AI095230.

Authors' contributions
EET, JN-J, and KWK generated and analyzed the data and co-authored the manuscript. JEG, DJJ, RFL, and CO conceived, initiated, and designed the study. All authors read and approved the final manuscript.

Author details
[1]Department of Human Genetics, The University of Chicago, 920 E 58th St, CLSC Room 501, Chicago, IL 60637, USA. [2]School of Medicine and Public Health, University of Wisconsin-Madison, Madison, WI, USA. [3]Department of Pediatrics, Section of Allergy, Immunology and Rheumatology, University of Wisconsin School of Medicine and Public Health-Madison, Madison, WI, USA. [4]Department of Obstetrics and Gynecology, The University of Chicago, Chicago, IL, USA. [5]Present address: Research and Development, USANA Health Sciences Inc, Salt Lake City, Utah, USA. [6]Present address: Department of Pediatrics, Yonsei University College of Medicine, Seoul, South Korea.

References
1. Alonso LC, Rosenfield RL. Oestrogens and puberty. Best Pract Res Clin Endocrinol Metab. 2002;16:13–30.
2. Postma DS. Gender differences in asthma development and progression. Gend Med. 2007;4:S133–46.
3. Keselman A, Heller N. Estrogen signaling modulates allergic inflammation and contributes to sex differences in asthma. Front Immunol. 2015;6:568.
4. Altwaijri YA, Day RS, Harrist RB, Dwyer JT, Ausman LM, Labarthe DR. Sexual maturation affects diet-blood total cholesterol association in children: Project HeartBeat! Am J Prev Med. 2009;37:S65–70.
5. Morrison JA, Laskarzewski PM, Rauh JL, Brookman R, Mellies M, Frazer M, Khoury P, deGroot I, Kelly K, Glueck CJ. Lipids, lipoproteins, and sexual maturation during adolescence: the Princeton maturation study. Metabolism. 1979;28:641–9.
6. Shankar RR, Eckert GJ, Saha C, Tu W, Pratt JH. The change in blood pressure during pubertal growth. J Clin Endocrinol Metab. 2005;90:163–7.
7. Taittonen L, Uhari M, Turtinen J, Nuutinen M. Change in blood pressure during pubertal insulin resistance. Pediatr Res. 1997;41:272–5.
8. Kelsey MM, Zeitler PS. Insulin resistance of puberty. Curr Diab Rep. 2016;16:64.
9. Ober C, Loisel DA, Gilad Y. Sex-specific genetic architecture of human disease. Nat Rev Genet. 2008;9:911–22.
10. Straub RH. The complex role of estrogens in inflammation. Endocr Rev. 2007;28:521–74.
11. Elks CE, Perry JR, Sulem P, Chasman DI, Franceschini N, He C, Lunetta KL, Visser JA, Byrne EM, Cousminer DL, et al. Thirty new loci for age at menarche identified by a meta-analysis of genome-wide association studies. Nat Genet. 2010;42:1077–85.
12. Abreu AP, Kaiser UB. Pubertal development and regulation. Lancet Diabetes Endocrinol. 2016;4:254–64.
13. Perry JR, Day F, Elks CE, Sulem P, Thompson DJ, Ferreira T, He C, Chasman DI, Esko T, Thorleifsson G, et al. Parent-of-origin-specific allelic associations among 106 genomic loci for age at menarche. Nature. 2014;514:92–7.
14. Huen K, Harley K, Kogut K, Rauch S, Eskenazi B, Holland N. DNA methylation of LINE-1 and Alu repetitive elements in relation to sex hormones and pubertal timing in Mexican-American children. Pediatr Res. 2016;79:855–62.
15. Almstrup K, Lindhardt Johansen M, Busch AS, Hagen CP, Nielsen JE, Petersen JH, Juul A. Pubertal development in healthy children is mirrored by DNA methylation patterns in peripheral blood. Sci Rep. 2016;6:28657.
16. Lemanske RF Jr. The childhood origins of asthma (COAST) study. Pediatr Allergy Immunol. 2002;13(Suppl 15):38–43.
17. Neaville WA, Tisler C, Bhattacharya A, Anklam K, Gilbertson-White S, Hamilton R, Adler K, Dasilva DF, Roberg KA, Carlson-Dakes KT, et al. Developmental cytokine response profiles and the clinical and immunologic expression of atopy during the first year of life. J Allergy Clin Immunol. 2003;112:740–6.
18. Marshall WA, Tanner JM. Variations in pattern of pubertal changes in girls. Arch Dis Child. 1969;44:291–303.
19. Marshall WA, Tanner JM. Variations in the pattern of pubertal changes in boys. Arch Dis Child. 1970;45:13–23.
20. Aryee MJ, Jaffe AE, Corrada-Bravo H, Ladd-Acosta C, Feinberg AP, Hansen KD, Irizarry RA. Minfi: a flexible and comprehensive Bioconductor package for the analysis of Infinium DNA methylation microarrays. Bioinformatics. 2014;30:1363–9.
21. Maksimovic J, Gordon L, Oshlack A. SWAN: subset-quantile within array normalization for illumina infinium HumanMethylation450 BeadChips. Genome Biol. 2012;13:R44.
22. Leek JT, Scharpf RB, Bravo HC, Simcha D, Langmead B, Johnson WE, Geman D, Baggerly K, Irizarry RA. Tackling the widespread and critical impact of batch effects in high-throughput data. Nat Rev Genet. 2010;11:733–9.
23. Johnson WE, Li C, Rabinovic A. Adjusting batch effects in microarray expression data using empirical Bayes methods. Biostatistics. 2007;8:118–27.
24. Du P, Kibbe WA, Lin SM. lumi: a pipeline for processing Illumina microarray. Bioinformatics. 2008;24:1547–8.
25. Nicodemus-Johnson J, Naughton KA, Sudi J, Hogarth K, Naurekas ET, Nicolae DL, Sperling AI, Solway J, White SR, Ober C. Genome-wide methylation study identifies an IL-13-induced epigenetic signature in asthmatic airways. Am J Respir Crit Care Med. 2016;193:376–85.
26. Langfelder P, Horvath S. WGCNA: an R package for weighted correlation network analysis. BMC Bioinformatics. 2008;9:559.
27. Ritchie ME, Phipson B, Wu D, Hu Y, Law CW, Shi W, Smyth GK. limma powers differential expression analyses for RNA-sequencing and microarray studies. Nucleic Acids Res. 2015;43:e47.
28. Chen EY, Tan CM, Kou Y, Duan Q, Wang Z, Meirelles GV, Clark NR, Ma'ayan A. Enrichr: interactive and collaborative HTML5 gene list enrichment analysis tool. BMC Bioinformatics. 2013;14:128.
29. Kuleshov MV, Jones MR, Rouillard AD, Fernandez NF, Duan Q, Wang Z, Koplev S, Jenkins SL, Jagodnik KM, Lachmann A, et al. Enrichr: a comprehensive gene set enrichment analysis web server 2016 update. Nucleic Acids Res. 2016;44:W90–7.
30. Bourdeau V, Deschenes J, Metivier R, Nagai Y, Nguyen D, Bretschneider N, Gannon F, White JH, Mader S. Genome-wide identification of high-affinity estrogen response elements in human and mouse. Mol Endocrinol. 2004;18:1411–27.
31. Sorensen K, Aksglaede L, Petersen JH, Andersson AM, Juul A. Serum IGF1 and insulin levels in girls with normal and precocious puberty. Eur J Endocrinol. 2012;166:903–10.
32. Olsson AH, Volkov P, Bacos K, Dayeh T, Hall E, Nilsson EA, Ladenvall C, Ronn T, Ling C. Genome-wide associations between genetic and epigenetic variation influence mRNA expression and insulin secretion in human pancreatic islets. PLoS Genet. 2014;10:e1004735.
33. Medvedeva YA, Khamis AM, Kulakovskiy IV, Ba-Alawi W, Bhuyan MS, Kawaji H, Lassmann T, Harbers M, Forrest AR, Bajic VB, Consortium F. Effects of cytosine methylation on transcription factor binding sites. BMC Genomics. 2014;15:119.
34. Draijer C, Hylkema MN, Boorsma CE, Klok PA, Robbe P, Timens W, Postma DS, Greene CM, Melgert BN. Sexual maturation protects against development of lung inflammation through estrogen. Am J Physiol Lung Cell Mol Physiol. 2016;310:L166–74.
35. Klein SL, Flanagan KL. Sex differences in immune responses. Nat Rev Immunol. 2016;16:626–38.
36. Lamason R, Zhao P, Rawat R, Davis A, Hall JC, Chae JJ, Agarwal R, Cohen P, Rosen A, Hoffman EP, Nagaraju K. Sexual dimorphism in immune response genes as a function of puberty. BMC Immunol. 2006;7:2.
37. Liu HB, Loo KK, Palaszynski K, Ashouri J, Lubahn DB, Voskuhl RR. Estrogen receptor alpha mediates estrogen's immune protection in autoimmune disease. J Immunol. 2003;171:6936–40.
38. Khan D, Ansar AS. The immune system is a natural target for estrogen action: opposing effects of estrogen in two prototypical autoimmune diseases. Front Immunol. 2015;6:635.
39. Arnal JF, Fontaine C, Billon-Gales A, Favre J, Laurell H, Lenfant F, Gourdy P. Estrogen receptors and endothelium. Arterioscler Thromb Vasc Biol. 2010;30:1506–12.
40. Gilsanz V, Hu HH, Kajimura S. Relevance of brown adipose tissue in infancy and adolescence. Pediatr Res. 2013;73:3–9.
41. Gilsanz V, Smith ML, Goodarzian F, Kim M, Wren TA, Hu HH. Changes in brown adipose tissue in boys and girls during childhood and puberty. J Pediatr. 2012;160:604–9. e601
42. Long MD, Smiraglia DJ, Campbell MJ. The genomic impact of DNA CpG methylation on gene expression; relationships in prostate cancer. Biomol Ther. 2017;7:E15.
43. Schulz H, Ruppert AK, Herms S, Wolf C, Mirza-Schreiber N, Stegle O, Czamara D, Forstner AJ, Sivalingam S, Schoch S, et al. Genome-wide mapping of genetic determinants influencing DNA methylation and gene expression in human hippocampus. Nat Commun. 2017;8:1511.

Permissions

All chapters in this book were first published in CE, by BioMed Central; hereby published with permission under the Creative Commons Attribution License or equivalent. Every chapter published in this book has been scrutinized by our experts. Their significance has been extensively debated. The topics covered herein carry significant findings which will fuel the growth of the discipline. They may even be implemented as practical applications or may be referred to as a beginning point for another development.

The contributors of this book come from diverse backgrounds, making this book a truly international effort. This book will bring forth new frontiers with its revolutionizing research information and detailed analysis of the nascent developments around the world.

We would like to thank all the contributing authors for lending their expertise to make the book truly unique. They have played a crucial role in the development of this book. Without their invaluable contributions this book wouldn't have been possible. They have made vital efforts to compile up to date information on the varied aspects of this subject to make this book a valuable addition to the collection of many professionals and students.

This book was conceptualized with the vision of imparting up-to-date information and advanced data in this field. To ensure the same, a matchless editorial board was set up. Every individual on the board went through rigorous rounds of assessment to prove their worth. After which they invested a large part of their time researching and compiling the most relevant data for our readers.

The editorial board has been involved in producing this book since its inception. They have spent rigorous hours researching and exploring the diverse topics which have resulted in the successful publishing of this book. They have passed on their knowledge of decades through this book. To expedite this challenging task, the publisher supported the team at every step. A small team of assistant editors was also appointed to further simplify the editing procedure and attain best results for the readers.

Apart from the editorial board, the designing team has also invested a significant amount of their time in understanding the subject and creating the most relevant covers. They scrutinized every image to scout for the most suitable representation of the subject and create an appropriate cover for the book.

The publishing team has been an ardent support to the editorial, designing and production team. Their endless efforts to recruit the best for this project, has resulted in the accomplishment of this book. They are a veteran in the field of academics and their pool of knowledge is as vast as their experience in printing. Their expertise and guidance has proved useful at every step. Their uncompromising quality standards have made this book an exceptional effort. Their encouragement from time to time has been an inspiration for everyone.

The publisher and the editorial board hope that this book will prove to be a valuable piece of knowledge for researchers, students, practitioners and scholars across the globe.

List of Contributors

Gudrun Koppen, Sofie De Prins and Tijs Louwies
VITO- Sustainable Health, Boeretang 200, 2400 Mol, Belgium

Sabine A. S. Langie and Patrick De Boever
VITO- Sustainable Health, Boeretang 200, 2400 Mol, Belgium
Centre for Environmental Sciences, Hasselt University, Diepenbeek, Belgium

Matthieu Moisse and Diether Lambrechts
Laboratory for Translational Genetics, Center for Cancer Biology, VIB and KU Leuven, Campus Gasthuisberg, Leuven, Belgium

Wim Vanden Berghe
Proteinchemistry, Proteomics and Epigenetic Signaling (PPES), Department of Biomedical Sciences, University of Antwerp, Wilrijk, Belgium

Katarzyna Szarc vel Szic
VITO- Sustainable Health, Boeretang 200, 2400 Mol, Belgium
Proteinchemistry, Proteomics and Epigenetic Signaling (PPES), Department of Biomedical Sciences, University of Antwerp, Wilrijk, Belgium

Vera Nelen
Environment and Health unit, Provincial Institute of Hygiene, Antwerp, Belgium

Guy Van Camp
Center for Medical Genetics, University of Antwerp and Antwerp University hospital, Antwerp, Belgium

Ellen Van Der Plas
VITO- Sustainable Health, Boeretang 200, 2400 Mol, Belgium
Department of Biomedical Sciences, University of Antwerp, Wilrijk, Belgium

Greet Schoeters
VITO- Sustainable Health, Boeretang 200, 2400 Mol, Belgium
Department of Biomedical Sciences, University of Antwerp, Wilrijk, Belgium
Department of Environmental Medicine, Institute of Public Health, University of Southern Denmark, Odense, Denmark

Jiangxia Fan, Yan Zhang, Junhao Mu, Xiaoqian He, Bianfei Shao, Dishu Zhou, Weiyan Peng, Jun Tang, Yu Jiang, Guosheng Ren and Tingxiu Xiang
Chongqing Key Laboratory of Molecular Oncology and Epigenetics, the First Affiliated Hospital of Chongqing Medical University, Chongqing, China

Marija Klasić, Dora Markulin, Aleksandar Vojta, Ivana Samaržija, Ivan Biruš, Paula Dobrinić and Vlatka Zoldoš
Department of Biology, Division of Molecular Biology, Faculty of Science, University of Zagreb, Horvatovac 102a, 10000 Zagreb, Croatia

Nicholas T. Ventham
Gastrointestinal Unit, Centre for Genomics and Molecular Medicine, University of Edinburgh, Edinburgh EH4 6XU, UK

Irena Trbojević-Akmačić, Mirna Šimurina, Jerko Štambuk and Genadij Razdorov
Genos Glycoscience Research Laboratory, Borongajska cesta 83h, 10000 Zagreb, Croatia

Gordan Lauc and IBD consortium
Genos Glycoscience Research Laboratory, Borongajska cesta 83h, 10000 Zagreb, Croatia
Facult of Pharmacy and Biochemistry, University of Zagreb, Zagreb, Croatia

Nicholas A. Kennedy
Gastrointestinal Unit, Centre for Genomics and Molecular Medicine, University of Edinburgh, Edinburgh EH4 6XU, UK
IBD Pharmacogenetics, University of Exeter, Exeter, UK

Ana M. Dias and Salome Pinho
Institute of Molecular Pathology and Immunology of the University of Porto (IPATIMUP), Porto, Portugal

Vito Annese
Department of Medical and Surgical Sciences, Division of Gastroenterology, University Hospital Careggi, Florence, Italy

Anna Latiano
Department of Medical Sciences, Division of Gastroenterology, IRCCS-CSS Hospital, Viale Cappuccini, Rotondo, Italy

Renata D'Inca
Gastrointestinal Unit, University of Padua, Padua, Italy

Jack Satsangi
Gastrointestinal Unit, Centre for Genomics and Molecular Medicine, University of Edinburgh, Edinburgh EH4 6XU, UK
Translational Gastroenterology Unit, Nuffield Department of Medicine, University of Oxford, Oxford, UK

Alette Ortega Gómez and Oscar Arrieta
Thoracic Oncology Unit and Laboratory of Personalized Medicine, Instituto Nacional de Cancerología (INCan), San Fernando #22, Section XVI, Tlalpan, 14080 Mexico City, Mexico

Rubén Rodríguez Bautista
Thoracic Oncology Unit and Laboratory of Personalized Medicine, Instituto Nacional de Cancerología (INCan), San Fernando #22, Section XVI, Tlalpan, 14080 Mexico City, Mexico
Biomedical Science Doctorate Program, National Autonomous University of Mexico, Mexico City, Mexico

Alfredo Hidalgo Miranda
Cancer Genomics Laboratory, INMEGEN, Mexico City, Mexico

Alejandro Zentella Dehesa
Biochemistry Department, Instituto Nacional de Ciencias Médicas y Nutrición Salvador Zubirán, Mexico D.F, Mexico

Cynthia Villarreal-Garza
Breast Oncology Department, National Cancer Institute of Mexico, Mexico City, Mexico

Federico Ávila-Moreno
Lung Diseases And Cancer Epigenomics Laboratory, Biomedicine Research Unit (UBIMED), Facultad de Estudios Superiores (FES) Iztacala, National University Autonomous of México (UNAM), Mexico City, Mexico
Research Unit, National Institute of Respiratory Diseases (INER) "Ismael Cosío Villegas", Mexico City, Mexico

Igor Brikun and Diha Freije
Euclid Diagnostics LLC, 9800 Connecticut Dr., Crown Point, IN 46307, USA

Andrew Decatus and Lin Li
BioStat Solutions Inc., 5280 Corporate Dr., Suite C200, Frederick, MD 21703, USA

Eric Harvey
Health Decisions Inc., 2510 Meridian Parkway, Durham, NC 27713, USA

Deborah Nusskern
Euclid Diagnostics LLC, 9800 Connecticut Dr., Crown Point, IN 46307, USA
Luminex Corporation, 4088 Commercial Ave, Northbrook, IL 60062, USA

Eric S. Coker, Robert Gunier and Brenda Eskenazi
Center for Environmental Research and Children's Health (CERCH), School of Public Health, University of California, Berkeley, CA, USA
Berkeley, USA

Karen Huen and Nina Holland
Center for Environmental Research and Children's Health (CERCH), School of Public Health, University of California, Berkeley, CA, USA
Richmond, USA

Michael Borre
Department of Urology, Aarhus University Hospital, Aarhus, Denmark

Søren Høyer
Department of Pathology, Aarhus University Hospital, Aarhus, Denmark

Siri H. Strand, Torben F. Ørntoft and Karina D. Sørensen
Department of Molecular Medicine, Aarhus University Hospital, Aarhus, Denmark

Tine Maj Storebjerg and Anne-Sofie Lynnerup
Department of Urology, Aarhus University Hospital, Aarhus, Denmark
Department of Pathology, Aarhus University Hospital, Aarhus, Denmark
Department of Molecular Medicine, Aarhus University Hospital, Aarhus, Denmark

Fleur S. Peters, Annemiek M. A. Peeters, Jacqueline van de Wetering, Michiel G. H. Betjes, Carla C. Baan and Karin Boer
Neprology and Transplantation, Department of Internal Medicine, Rotterdam Transplant Group, Erasmus MC, Erasmus University Medical Center, Rotterdam, The Netherlands

Pooja R. Mandaviya and Joyce B. J. van Meurs
Department of Internal Medicine, Erasmus MC, Erasmus University Medical Center, Rotterdam, The Netherlands

Leo J. Hofland
Endocrinology, Department of Internal Medicine, Erasmus MC, Erasmus University Medical Center, Rotterdam, The Netherlands

Nora Knoblich, Annalena Wallisch, Katarzyna Glowacz, Julia Becker-Sadzio, Friederike Gundel, Christof Brückmann and Vanessa Nieratschker
Department of Psychiatry and Psychotherapy, University Hospital Tübingen, Calwerstr. 14, 72076 Tübingen, Germany

Mara Thomas
Department of Psychiatry and Psychotherapy, University Hospital Tübingen, Calwerstr. 14, 72076 Tübingen, Germany
Graduate Training Centre of Neuroscience, University of Tübingen, Tübingen, Germany

Iris Babion, Barbara C. Snoek, Annelieke Jaspers, Daniëlle A. M. Heideman, Chris J. L. M. Meijer, Peter J. F. Snijders and Renske D. M. Steenbergen
Cancer Center Amsterdam, Department of Pathology, VU University Medical Center, Amsterdam, The Netherlands

Putri W. Novianti
Cancer Center Amsterdam, Department of Pathology, VU University Medical Center, Amsterdam, The Netherlands
Department of Epidemiology and Biostatistics, VU University Medical Center, Amsterdam, The Netherlands

Nienke van Trommel
Center for Gynaecological Oncology, Antoni van Leeuwenhoek Hospital/ Netherlands Cancer Institute, Amsterdam, The Netherlands

Saskia M. Wilting
Department of Medical Oncology, Erasmus MC Cancer Institute, Erasmus University Medical Center, Rotterdam, The Netherlands

Daniel Castellano-Castillo
1Unidad de Gestión Clínica de Endocrinología y Nutrición del Hospital Virgen de la Victoria, Instituto de Investigación Biomédica de Málaga (IBIMA), Universidad de Málaga, Málaga, Spain

Sonsoles Morcillo
CIBER Fisiopatología de la Obesidad y Nutrición (CB06/03), Madrid, Spain

Mercedes Clemente-Postigo, Jose Carlos Fernandez-García, Francisco José Tinahones and Manuel Macias-Gonzalez
1Unidad de Gestión Clínica de Endocrinología y Nutrición del Hospital Virgen de la Victoria, Instituto de Investigación Biomédica de Málaga (IBIMA), Universidad de Málaga, Málaga, Spain
CIBER Fisiopatología de la Obesidad y Nutrición (CB06/03), Madrid, Spain

Ana Belén Crujeiras
Laboratory of Molecular and Cellular Endocrinology, Instituto de Investigación Sanitaria (IDIS), Complejo Hospitalario Universitario de Santiago (CHUS/ SERGAS), Santiago de Compostela University (USC), Santiago de Compostela, Spain
CIBER Fisiopatología de la Obesidad y la Nutrición (CIBERobn), Madrid, Spain

Esperanza Torres
Unidad de Gestión Clínica de Oncología Intercentros Hospital Universitario Virgen de la Victoria, Málaga, Spain

Vinod Dagar
Department of Paediatrics, University of Melbourne, Parkville 3052, Australia

Wendy Hutchison and Priscillia Siswara
Pathology, Monash Health, Clayton 3168, Australia

Andrea Muscat
School of Medicine, Deakin University, Geelong 3216, Australia

Anita Krishnan
Victorian Comprehensive Cancer Centre, Parkville 3052, Australia

David Hoke and Ashley Buckle
Department of Biochemistry and Molecular Biology, Monash University, Clayton 3800, Australia

George McGillivray and Susan White
Murdoch Children's Research Institute, Parkville 3052, Australia

David J. Amor
Department of Paediatrics, University of Melbourne, Parkville 3052, Australia
Murdoch Children's Research Institute, Parkville 3052, Australia

Jeffrey Mann
Department of Anatomy and Developmental Biology, Monash University, Clayton 3800, Australia

Jason Pinner
Department of Medical Genomics, Royal Prince Alfred Hospital, Camperdown 2050, Australia

Alison Colley
Clinical Genetics, Liverpool Hospital, Liverpool 2170, Australia

Meredith Wilson, Felicity Collins and Alan Ma
Clinical Genetics, Children's Hospital at Westmead, Westmead 2145, Australia

Rani Sachdev and Edwin Kirk
Centre for Clinical Genetics, Sydney Children's Hospital, Randwick 2031, Australia

Matthew Edwards
School of Medicine, University of Western Sydney, Penrith 2751, Australia

Kristi Jones
Clinical Genetics, Children's Hospital at Westmead, Westmead 2145, Australia
School of Medicine, University of Sydney, Camperdown 2006, Australia

Juliet Taylor and Ian Hayes
Auckland District Health Board, Auckland 1023, New Zealand

Christopher Barnett and Eric Haan
South Australian (SA) Clinical Genetics Service, SA Pathology, Women's and Children's Hospital, Adelaide 5000, Australia

Elizabeth Thompson
South Australian (SA) Clinical Genetics Service, SA Pathology, Women's and Children's Hospital, Adelaide 5000, Australia
School of Medicine, University of Adelaide, Adelaide 5000, Australia

Mary-Louise Freckmann
Department of Clinical Genetics, Royal North Shore Hospital, St Leonards 2065, Australia

Anne Turner
Centre for Clinical Genetics, Sydney Children's Hospital, Randwick 2031, Australia
School of Women's and Children's Health, University of NSW, Kensington 2052, Australia

Ben Kamien and Michael Field
Hunter Genetics, Hunter New England Local Health District, New Lambton 2305, Australia

Fiona Mackenzie, Gareth Baynam and Cathy Kiraly-Borri
Genetics Services of Western Australia, Crawley 6009, Australia

Tracey Dudding-Byth
Hunter Genetics, Hunter New England Local Health District, New Lambton 2305, Australia
University of Newcastle GrowUpWell Priority Research Centre, Callaghan 2308, Australia

Elizabeth M. Algar
Department of Paediatrics, University of Melbourne, Parkville 3052, Australia
Pathology, Monash Health, Clayton 3168, Australia
Hudson Institute of Medical Research, Clayton 3168, Australia
Department of Translational Medicine, Monash University, Clayton 3168, Australia

Varun Sasidharan Nair and Rowaida Z. Taha
Cancer Research Center, Qatar Biomedical Research Institute, College of Science and Engineering, Hamad Bin Khalifa University, Qatar Foundation, Doha, Qatar

Haytham El Salhat
Oncology Department, Al Noor Hospital, Abu Dhabi, United Arab Emirates
Oncology Department, Tawam Hospital, Al Ain, United Arab Emirates

Anne John
Department of Pathology, College of Medicine and Health Sciences, United Arab Emirates University, Al Ain, United Arab Emirates

Bassam R. Ali
Department of Pathology, College of Medicine and Health Sciences, United Arab Emirates University, Al Ain, United Arab Emirates
Zayed Center for Health Sciences, United Arab Emirates University, Al Ain, United Arab Emirates

Eyad Elkord
Cancer Research Center, Qatar Biomedical Research Institute, College of Science and Engineering, Hamad Bin Khalifa University, Qatar Foundation, Doha, Qatar
Institute of Cancer Sciences, University of Manchester, Manchester, UK

Yun Su
Department of Surgery, Jiangsu Province Hospital of Nanjing University of Chinese Medicine, 138 Xianlin Road, Nanjing 210023, China

Hong Bin Fang
Department of Biostatistics, Bioinformatics and Biomathematics, Georgetown University Medical Center, 4000 Reservoir Road, N.W, Washington D.C. 20057, USA

Feng Jiang
Department of Pathology, University of Maryland School of Medicine, Baltimore, MD, USA

Erin W. Hofstatter, Vikram B. Wali, Christos Hatzis, Gauri Patwardhan, Lianne Epstein and Lajos Pusztai
Department of Internal Medicine, Section of Medical Oncology, Yale School of Medicine, 300 George Street, Suite 120, New Haven, CT 06511, USA

Steve Horvath
Department of Human Genetics, David Geffen School of Medicine, University of California Los Angeles, Los Angeles, CA 90095, USA
Department of Biostatistics, Fielding School of Public Health, University of California Los Angeles, Los Angeles, CA 90095, USA

Disha Dalela, Meghan Butler, Karen Stavris, Tracy Sturrock and Stephanie Kwei
Department of Pharmacology, Yale School of Medicine, 333 Cedar Street, New Haven, CT 06511, USA

Piyush Gupta
Department of Surgery, Memorial Sloan Kettering Cancer Center, New York 10065, USA

Anees B. Chagpar
Department of Surgery, Yale School of Medicine, 330 Cedar Street, New Haven, CT 06511, USA

Veerle Bossuyt
Department of Pathology, Yale School of Medicine, 330 Cedar Street, New Haven, CT 06511, USA

Anna Maria Storniolo
Department of Internal Medicine, Indiana University Melvin and Bren Simon Cancer Center, Indianapolis, IN 46202, USA

Marie-Kristin Von Wahlde
Department of Internal Medicine, Section of Medical Oncology, Yale School of Medicine, 300 George Street, Suite 120, New Haven, CT 06511, USA
Department of Obstetrics and Gynecology, Münster University Hospital, Münster, Germany

Alexander Au
Department of Pharmacology, Yale School of Medicine, 333 Cedar Street, New Haven, CT 06511, USA

Department of Clinical Surgery, Perelman School of Medicine, University of Pennsylvania, Philadelphia, PA 19104, USA

Daniel Gackowski, Jolanta Guz, Kinga Linowiecka, Marta Starczak, Ewelina Zarakowska, Martyna Modrzejewska, Anna Szpila, Justyna Szpotan, Maciej Gawronski, Anna Labejszo and Marek Foksinski
Department of Clinical Biochemistry, Faculty of Pharmacy, Collegium Medicum in Bydgoszcz, Nicolaus Copernicus University in Torun, Torun, Poland

Andrzej Marszalek
Department of Clinical Pathomorphology, Faculty of Medicine, Collegium Medicum in Bydgoszcz, Nicolaus Copernicus University in Torun, Torun, Poland
Department of Oncologic Pathology and Prophylaxis, Poznan University of Medical Sciences and Greater Poland Cancer Center, Poznan, Poland

Zbigniew Banaszkiewicz
Department of Surgery, Faculty of Medicine, Collegium Medicum in Bydgoszcz, Nicolaus Copernicus University in Torun, Torun, Poland

Ariel Liebert and Maria Klopocka
Department of Vascular Diseases and Internal Medicine, Faculty of Health Sciences, Collegium Medicum in Bydgoszcz, Nicolaus Copernicus University in Torun, Torun, Poland

Magdalena Bodnar
Department of Clinical Pathomorphology, Faculty of Medicine, Collegium Medicum in Bydgoszcz, Nicolaus Copernicus University in Torun, Torun, Poland
Department of Otolaryngology and Laryngeal Oncology, K. Marcinkowski University of Medical Sciences, Poznan, Poland

Tomasz Dziaman and Ryszard Olinski
Department of Clinical Biochemistry, Faculty of Pharmacy, Collegium Medicum in Bydgoszcz, Nicolaus Copernicus University in Torun, Torun, Poland
Department of Clinical Biochemistry, Collegium Medicum in Bydgoszcz, Nicolaus Copernicus University, Karlowicza 24, 85-095 Bydgoszcz, Poland

Alexandra M Binder, Leah T Stiemsma and Karin B Michels
Department of Epidemiology, Fielding School of Public Health, University of California, Los Angeles 90095, USA

Kristen Keller
Department of Biostatistics, Fielding School of Public Health, University of California, Los Angeles 90095, USA

Sanne D van Otterdijk
Institute for Prevention and Cancer Epidemiology, Faculty of Medicine and Medical Center, University of Freiburg, Freiburg im Breisgau, Germany

Verónica Mericq and Ana Pereira
Institute of Nutrition and Food Technology, University of Chile, Santiago, Chile

José L Santos
Department of Nutrition, Diabetes and Metabolism, School of Medicine, Pontificia Universidad Católica de Chile, Santiago, Chile

John Shepherd
Population Sciences in the Pacific Program, University of Hawaii Cancer Center, Honolulu, HI 96813, USA

Isabella Maria Dias Payão Ortiz, Mateus Camargo Barros-Filho, Mariana Bisarro dos Reis, Caroline Moraes Beltrami, Fabio Albuquerque Marchi, Hellen Kuasne and Julia Bette Homem de Mello
International Research Center-CIPE, A.C. Camargo Cancer Center, Taguá Street 440, São Paulo 01508-010, Brazil

Cecilie Abildgaard and Silvia Regina Rogatto
Department of Clinical Genetics, Vejle Hospital, Institute of Regional Health Research, University of Southern Denmark, Beriderbakken 4, 7100 Vejle, Denmark

Luísa Matos do Canto
International Research Center-CIPE, A.C. Camargo Cancer Center, Taguá Street 440, São Paulo 01508-010, Brazil
Department of Clinical Genetics, Vejle Hospital, Institute of Regional Health Research, University of Southern Denmark, Beriderbakken 4, 7100 Vejle, Denmark

Clóvis Antônio Lopes Pinto
Department of Pathology, A.C. Camargo Cancer Center, Professor Antonio Prudente Street 211, São Paulo 01509-900, Brazil

Luiz Paulo Kowalski
Department of Head and Neck Surgery and Otorhinolaryngology, A.C. Camargo Cancer Center, Professor Antonio Prudente Street 211, São Paulo 01509-900, Brazil

Catarina Moreira-Barbosa, Daniela Barros-Silva, Pedro Costa-Pinheiro and Vera Constâncio
Cancer Biology and Epigenetics Group, IPO Porto Research Center (CI-IPOP), Portuguese Oncology Institute of Porto (IPO Porto), Porto, Portugal

Jorge Torres-Ferreira
Cancer Biology and Epigenetics Group, IPO Porto Research Center (CI-IPOP), Portuguese Oncology Institute of Porto (IPO Porto), Porto, Portugal
Department of Pathology, Portuguese Oncology Institute of Porto (IPO Porto), Rua Dr. António Bernardino de Almeida, 4200-072 Porto, Portugal

Rui Freitas and Jorge Oliveira
Department of Urology, Portuguese Oncology Institute of Porto (IPO Porto), Rua Dr. António Bernardino de Almeida, 4200-072 Porto, Portugal

Luís Antunes
Department of Epidemiology, Portuguese Oncology Institute of Porto (IPO Porto), Rua Dr. António Bernardino de Almeida, 4200-072 Porto, Portugal

Rui Henrique
Cancer Biology and Epigenetics Group, IPO Porto Research Center (CI-IPOP), Portuguese Oncology Institute of Porto (IPO Porto), Porto, Portugal
Department of Pathology, Portuguese Oncology Institute of Porto (IPO Porto), Rua Dr. António Bernardino de Almeida, 4200-072 Porto, Portugal
Department of Pathology and Molecular Immunology, Institute of Biomedical Sciences Abel Salazar (ICBAS), University of Porto, Porto, Portugal

Carmen Jerónimo
Cancer Biology and Epigenetics Group, IPO Porto Research Center (CI-IPOP), Portuguese Oncology Institute of Porto (IPO Porto), Porto, Portugal
Department of Pathology and Molecular Immunology, Institute of Biomedical Sciences Abel Salazar (ICBAS), University of Porto, Porto, Portugal
Cancer Biology and Epigenetics Group - Research Center (LAB3), Portuguese Oncology Institute of Porto, Rua Dr. António Bernardino Almeida, 4200-072 Porto, Portugal

Raffael Ott, Kerstin Melchior, Karen Schellong, Thomas Ziska, Rebecca C. Rancourt and Andreas Plagemann
Division of 'Experimental Obstetrics, ' Clinic of Obstetrics, Charité – Universitätsmedizin Berlin, Corporate Member of Freie Universität Berlin, Humboldt-Universität zu Berlin, and Berlin Institute of Health, Campus Virchow-Klinikum, Augustenburger Platz 1, 13353 Berlin, Germany

Jens H. Stupin, Joachim W. Dudenhausen and Wolfgang Henrich
Clinic of Obstetrics, Charité – Universitätsmedizin Berlin, Corporate Member of Freie Universität Berlin, Humboldt-Universität zu Berlin, and Berlin Institute of Health, Campus Virchow-Klinikum, Berlin, Germany

Qiuqin Tang
Department of Obstetrics, The Affiliated Obstetrics and Gynecology Hospital of Nanjing Medical University, Nanjing Maternity and Child Health Care Hospital, Nanjing, China

Feng Pan
Department of Urology, The Affiliated Obstetrics and Gynecology Hospital of Nanjing Medical University, Nanjing Maternity and Child Health Care Hospital, Nanjing, China

Jing Yang, Ziqiang Fu, Yiwen Lu, Xiumei Han, Minjian Chen, Chuncheng Lu, Yankai Xia and Xinru Wang
State Key Laboratory of Reproductive Medicine, Institute of Toxicology, Nanjing Medical University, 101 Longmian Avenue, Nanjing 211166, China
Key Laboratory of Modern Toxicology of Ministry of Education, School of Public Health, Nanjing Medical University, Nanjing, China

Xian Wu
National Toxicology Program Laboratory, Division of the National Toxicology Program, National Institute of Environmental Health Sciences, Research Triangle Park, NC, USA

Wei Wu
State Key Laboratory of Reproductive Medicine, Institute of Toxicology, Nanjing Medical University, 101 Longmian Avenue, Nanjing 211166, China
Key Laboratory of Modern Toxicology of Ministry of Education, School of Public Health, Nanjing Medical University, Nanjing, China
Department of Health and Human Services, National Institute of Environmental Health Sciences,
National Institutes of Health, Research Triangle Park, USA

Saigopal Somasundaram, Megan E Forrest, Helen Moinova and Allison Cohen
Department of Genetics and Genome Sciences, Case Comprehensive Cancer Center, Case Western Reserve University School of Medicine, Cleveland, OH 44106, USA

Vinay Varadan
Case Comprehensive Cancer Center, Case Western Reserve University School of Medicine, Cleveland, OH 44106, USA

Thomas LaFramboise, Sanford Markowitz and Ahmad M Khalil
Department of Genetics and Genome Sciences, Case Comprehensive Cancer Center, Case Western Reserve University School of Medicine, Cleveland, OH 44106, USA
Case Comprehensive Cancer Center, Case Western Reserve University School of Medicine, Cleveland, OH 44106, USA

Emma E. Thompson
Department of Human Genetics, The University of Chicago, 920 E 58th St, CLSC Room 501, Chicago, IL 60637, USA

James E. Gern, Daniel J. Jackson and Robert F. Lemanske
School of Medicine and Public Health, University of Wisconsin-Madison, Madison, WI, USA
Department of Pediatrics, Section of Allergy, Immunology and Rheumatology, University of Wisconsin School of Medicine and Public Health-Madison, Madison, WI, USA

Carole Ober
Department of Human Genetics, The University of Chicago, 920 E 58th St, CLSC Room 501, Chicago, IL 60637, USA
Department of Obstetrics and Gynecology, The University of Chicago, Chicago, IL, USA

Jessie Nicodemus-Johnson
Department of Human Genetics, The University of Chicago, 920 E 58th St, CLSC Room 501, Chicago, IL 60637, USA
Research and Development, USANA Health Sciences Inc, Salt Lake City, Utah, USA

Kyung Won Kim
Department of Human Genetics, The University of Chicago, 920 E 58th St, CLSC Room 501, Chicago, IL 60637, USA
Department of Pediatrics, Yonsei University College of Medicine, Seoul, South Korea

Index

www.ingramcontent.com/pod-product-compliance
Lightning Source LLC
Chambersburg PA
CBHW061330190326
41458CB00011B/3950